THE COMPLEMENT SYSTEM:
Novel Roles in Health and Disease

THE COMPLEMENT SYSTEM:
Novel Roles in Health and Disease

Edited by

Janos Szebeni
Walter Reed Army Institute of Research
Silver Spring, MD

KLUWER ACADEMIC PUBLISHERS
Boston / Dordrecht / New York / London

Distributors for North, Central and South America:
Kluwer Academic Publishers
101 Philip Drive
Assinippi Park
Norwell, Massachusetts 02061 USA
Telephone (781) 871-6600
Fax (781) 681-9045
E-Mail: kluwer@wkap.com

Distributors for all other countries:
Kluwer Academic Publishers Group
Post Office Box 322
3300 AH Dordrecht, THE NETHERLANDS
Telephone 31 786 576 000
Fax 31 786 576 254
E-Mail: services@wkap.nl

 Electronic Services <http://www.wkap.nl>

Library of Congress Cataloging-in-Publication Data

A C.I.P. Catalogue record for this book is available
from the Library of Congress.

The Complement System: Novel Roles in Health and Disease edited by Janos Szebeni.
ISBN 1-4020-8055-7
e-ISBN 1-2040-8056-5

Printed on acid-free paper.
Printed in the United States of America.

The Publisher offers discounts on this book for course use and bulk purchases.
For further information, send email to <joseph.burns@wkap.com>.

This book may provide relief for those

"hopelessly infected with the C bug"

Tibor Borsos, Chapter 1

CONTENTS

THE COMPLEMENT SYSTEM
NOVEL ROLES IN HEALTH AND DISEASE

CONTRIBUTORS

Ábel, György, M.D. Ph.D.
Medical Director, Department of
Laboratory Medicine, Lahey
Clinic Medical Center,
Burlington, MA, and Department
of Pathology, Harvard Medical
School, Boston, MA,
Gabel@hms.harvard.edu

Ambrus, Géza, Ph.D.
Postdoctoral Fellow
Institute of Enzymology
Biological Research Center
Hungarian Academy of Sciences
Budapest, Hungary
Geza@enzim.hu

Angello, Vincent, M.D.
Director, Immunology Research,
Department of Laboratory
Medicine, Lahey Clinic Medical
Center, Burlington, MA,
and Edith Nourse Rogers
Veterans Affairs Hospital
Bedford, MA,
Vincent.Agnello@Lahey.org

Bajtay, Zsuzsa, Ph.D.
Res. Assoc..Prof.
Department of Immunology,
Eötvös Loránd University,
Budapest, Hungary

Bánhegyi, Dénes , M.D.
Head, Department of
Immunology, St László Hospital
Budapest
immunol@mail.datanet.hu

Basta, Milan, M.D., Ph.D.
National Institute for
Neurological Disorders and
Stroke; National Institutes of
Health, Bethesda, Maryland, U.S.
BastaM@ninds.nih.gov

Bhole, Deepak
Postdoctoral fellow
Center for Experimental
Therapeutics and Reperfusion
Injury, Department of
Anesthesiology, Perioperative
and Pain Medicine
Brigham and Women's Hospital,
Harvard Medical School,
Boston, MA,

Borsos, Tibor, Sc.D.
Scientist Emeritus
4620 N Park Ave Apt. 608E
Chevy Chase, MD 20815,
Tborsos2@juno.com

Bourcier, Todd M.
Instructor, Center for
Experimental Therapeutics and
Reperfusion Injury,
Brigham and Women's Hospital,
Harvard Medical School,
Boston, MA,

Bradford, Roberta, B.Sc., DIBT
Head of Pharmacology and
Toxicology, Adprotech Ltd.
Cambridge, UK
R.bradford@adpro.co.uk

Bulla, Roberta, Ph.D.
Postdoctoral Fellow, Department
of Physiology and Pathology
University of Trieste, Italy

Csomor, Eszter
Department of Immunology,
Eötvös Loránd University,
Budapest, Hungary
Esztercsomor@yahoo.co.uk

Erdei, Anna, Ph.D., D.Sc.
Professor, Head of Department
and Research Group of the
Hungarian Academy of
Sciences, Eötvös Loránd
University, Budapest, Hungary
Anna.Erdei@freemail.hu

Esser, Dirk, Ph.D.
Senior Scientific Investigator
Adprotech Ltd., Cambridge, UK
D.esser@adpro.co.uk

Farkas, Henriette, M.D., PhD
Head, Angoedema and Allergy
Center, Semmelweis University,
Budapest, Hungary
Farkash@kut.sote.hu

Fischetti, Fabio, M.D.
Senior Scientific Investigator
Department of Medicine and
Neurology, University of Trieste
Trieste, Italy

Fishelson, Zvi, Ph.D.
Professor, Department of Cell and
Developmental Biology, Sackler
School of Medicine, Tel Aviv
University, Tel Aviv, Israel
lifish@post.tau.ac.il

Fleming, Sherry, D.
Research Ass. Professor, Dept. of
Cellular Injury, Walter Reed
Army Inst. of Research and Dept.
of Medicine, Uniformed Services
University of the Health Sciences,
Bethesda, MD,
Sherry.Fleming@na.amedd.army.
mil

Füst, George, M.D., Ph.D., D.Sc.
Professor, Chief, Research
Laboratory, Third Department of
Medicine, Faculty of Medicine
Semmelweis University, Budapest
Hungary
FustGe@kut.sote.hu

Gál, Péter, Ph.D.
Senior Scientist, Institute of
Enzymology, Biological Research
Center Hungarian Academy of
Sciences, Budapest, Hungary
Gal@enzim.hu

Girardi, Guillermina, Ph.D.
Department of Medicine
Hospital for Special Surgery
Weill Medical College of Cornell
University, New York, N.Y.
Girardig@hss.edu

Götze, Otto, M.D.
Emeritus Professor of
Immunology
Bodelschwingh Str. 20,
D 37075 Göttingen
Ogoetze@gwdg.de

Harris, Claire L., Ph.D.
Department of Medical
Biochemistry and Immunology,
University of Wales
College of Medicine, Cardiff, UK.
HarrisCL@cardiff.ac.uk

Hart, Melanie L.
Postdoctoral Fellow, Center for
Experimental Therapeutics and
Reperfusion Injury, Department
of Anesthesiology, Perioperative
and Pain Medicine, Brigham and
Women's Hospital, Harvard
Medical School, Boston, MA

Hawlisch, Heiko, Ph.D.
Senior Scientist, Division of
Mol.Immunology Cincinnati
Children's Hospital, Cincinnati,
OH,
Heiko.Hawlisch@chmcc.org

Huber-Lang, Markus S., M.D.
Resident, Department of
Traumatology, Hand- and
Reconstructive Surgery,
University of Ulm,
Ulm, Germany
Mshuberlang2000@aol.com

Karp, Christopher L., M.D.
Professor, Director
Division of Mol. Immunology,
Cincinnati Children's Hospital,
Cincinnati, OH,
Chris.Karp@chmcc.org

Kirschfink, Michael, M.D.
Professsor, Institute of
Immunology, University of
Heidelberg, Heidelberg, Germany
Michael.Kirschfink@urz.uni-
heidelberg.de

Köhl, Jörg, M.D.
Professor, Division of Molecular
Immunology, Cincinnati
Children's Hospital Cincinnati,
Ohio
Joerg.Koehl@chmcc.org

Kuttner-Kondo, Lisa, Ph.D.
Research Associate
Case Western Reserve University
Cleveland, Ohio
lak@pop.cwru.edu

Lőrincz, Zsolt, Ph.D.
Senior Scientist, Institute of
Enzymology
Biological Research Center
Hungarian Academy of Sciences
Hungary
Lorincz@enzim.hu

**Medof, Edward, M., M.D.,
Ph.D.**
Professor, Department of
Pathology, Case Western Reserve
University Cleveland, Ohio
mxm16@po.cwru.edu

Mollnes, Tom Eirik, M.D.
Professor, Institute of
Immunology, Rikshospitalet
University Hospital, Oslo,
Norway
T.e.mollnes@labmed.uio.no

Molnár, Eszter
Department of Immunology,
Eötvös Loránd University,
Budapest, Hungary
Eszterbembe@yahoo.co.uk

Morgan, B. Paul, Ph.D., FRC Path.
Professor, Department of Medical
Biochemistry and Immunology,
University of Wales, College of
Medicine, Cardiff, UK
MorganBP@cardiff.ac.uk

Prechl, József, MD, Ph.D.,
Research Group of the
Hungarian Academy of Sciences
Eötvös Loránd University,
Budapest, Hungary
Jprechl@yahoo.co.uk

Prohászka, Zoltán, M.D., Ph.D.
Vice-Head, Research Laboratory,
Third Department of Medicine,
Faculty of Medicine, Semmelweis
University, Budapest
Prohoz@kut.sote.hu

Ridley, Simon H., Ph.D.
Scientific Investigator
Adprotech Ltd., Cambridge, UK
S.ridley@adpro.co.uk

Salmon, Jane E., M.D.
Department of Medicine,
Hospital for Special Surgery-
Weill Medical College of Cornell
University, New York, NY
10021,

Sarma, J. Vidya, Ph.D.
Assistant Research Scientist,
Department of Pathology,
University of Michigan Medical
School, Ann Arbor, MI,

Stahl, Gregory L., Ph.D.
Associate Professor, Center for
Experimental Therapeutics and
Reperfusion Injury, Department
of Anesthesiology, Perioperative
and Pain Medicine, Brigham and
Women's Hospital, Harvard
Medical School, Boston, MA
Gstahl@zeus.bwh.harvard.edu

Smith, Richard A.G., D.Phil.
Chief Scientific Officer,
Adprotech Ltd., Cambridge, UK
R.a.smith@adpro.co.uk

Szebeni, Janos, M.D., Ph.D.
Senior Scientist, Walter Reed
Army Institute of Research, and
adjunct assistant professor of
Microbiology & Immunology,
Uniformed Services University of
the Health Sciences, Bethesda
MD
Jszebeni@aol.com

Takahashi, Minoru, Ph.D.
Researh Fellow, Center for
Experimental Therapeutics and
Reperfusion Injury,
Department of Anesthesiology,
Brigham and Women Hospital,
Harvard Medical School, Boston,
MA,

Tedesco, Francesco, M.D
Professor of Immunology,
Department of Physiology and
Pathology, University of Trieste,
Italy
Tedesco@univ.trieste.it

Tolnay, Mate, Ph.D.
Senior Scientist, Department of
Cellular Injury, Walter Reed
Army Institute of Research
Silver Spring, MD,
Mate.Tolnay@na.amedd.army.mil

**†Tóth, Ferenc D, M.D., Ph.D,
D.Sc.**
Professor, Institute of Medical
Microbiology,
Medical and Health Science
Center, University of Debrecen,
Debrecen, Hungary

Tsokos, George C., M.D.
Professor of Medicine and
Molecular Cell Biology,
Uniformed Services University of
the Health Sciences; and Chief,
Department of Cellular Injury,
Walter Reed Army Institute of
Research, Silver Spring, MD,
gtsokos@usa.net

Varga, Lillian, Ph.D.
Assistant professor,
Third Department of Medicine,
Faculty of Medicine, Semmelweis
University, Budapest
Lvarga@kut.sote.hu

Walsh, Mary C.
Postdoctoral fellow, Center for
Experimental Therapeutics and
Reperfusion Injury, Department
of Anesthesiology, Perioperative,
and Pain Medicine, Brigham and
Women's Hospital, Harvard
Medical School, Boston, MA

Ward, Peter A. M.D.
G.D. Stobbe Professor and
Chairman of Pathology,
Department of Pathology,
University of Michigan Medical
School, Ann Arbor, MI.
bschuman@med.umich.edu

Wills-Karp, Marsha, Ph.D.
Professor, Director
Division of Immunobiology,
Cincinnati Children's Hospital,
Cincinnati, OH
Marsha.Wills-Karp@chmcc.org

**Würzner, Reinhard, M.D.,
Ph.D.**
Professor, Institute for Hygiene
und Social Medicine, Medical
University of Innsbruck &
Ludwig-Boltzmann-Institute for
AIDS-Research,
Innsbruck, Austria
Reinhard.Wuerzner@uibk.ac.at

Závodszky, Péter
Professor, Institute of
Enzymology Biological Research
Center, Hungarian Academy of
Sciences Hungary
zxp@enzim.hu

Zetoune, Firas S., B.S.,
Research Associate II
Department of Trauma, Hand and
Reconstructive Surgery,
University of Ulm, Ulm,
Germany
Zipfel, Peter F., Ph.D.

Professor
Dept. Infection Biology,
Hans-Knöll-Institute for Natural
Products Research, Jena,
Germany
Peter.Zipfel@hki-jena.de

FOREWORD

As a phylogenetically old system complement is now regarded as a part of innate immunity. But it is much more than that. It bridges innate and adapted immunity, participates not only in host defense but also in many essential physiological processes, old and new diseases and adverse conditions. Indeed, complement became a term that almost defies categorization. What was for a long time a subject for a limited number of specialists has now moved into the mainstream of experimental and clinical immunology.

In 1973 I visited the Basel Institute of Immunology and met its director, the eminent scientist and Nobel laureate Nils Jerne. When I entered his office he greeted me with the following words: "Complement, does that really exist?" I was never certain whether he wanted only to tease me or whether he sincerely believed that the complement system was an unimportant biological curiosity, a misstep of evolution. But, of course, missteps do not survive the evolutionary process.

Little did I foresee the dramatic developments of recent years when Hans J. Müller-Eberhard and I started to unravel the specifics of the action of the cobra venom factor on the complement system in 1968 and defined a new pathway to its activation. An elucidation of the role of the system in diseases and its control for therapeutic reasons is now getting closer to actual realization in the clinic although many problems, in particular those of highly specific inhibition free of side effects, have still to be resolved.

This new and up-to-date book on the complement system presents and discusses the advances that have been made in recent years in the understanding of the roles of the system in the maintenance of health and its participation in pathology. The chapters from prominent experts cover the essentials as well as the hottest issues in complementology. The topics are ordered in increasing complexity from basic molecular to human clinical, building the case for the ultimate message: time has come to find new ways to modulate the system in-vivo in order to make better use of its protective powers and to prevent its adverse effects in disease. I am certain that this book will further these goals.

Otto Götze
Emeritus Professor of Immunology
University of Göttingen

PREFACE

The complement system, one of four proteolytic cascades in blood, is best known for its role in antimicrobial immunity. As the effector arm of non-specific humoral immunity, it provides first-line defense against all kinds of infectious agents including bacteria, viruses, fungi, yeasts and parasites. Complement research is only a year short of its 110th birthday. It was in 1895 that Jules Bordet, a young Belgian working in Metchnikoff's laboratory in Paris, observed that the destruction of V. cholerae required a heat-labile serum factor in addition to the specific antibodies. He called it "alexin". This name however, just as Metchnikoff's alternative term, "cytase", was soon replaced by Paul Ehrlich's functional term, "complement". The latter word captured the essence of the original observation, that a heat-labile plasma factor was "complementing" the bacteriolytic function of antibodies, and became widely accepted. Since then a century has passed, and the antibody-helping factor turned out to be a complex, multifaceted protein network whose function far exceeds the assistance of antibodies. For this reason, as explained below, complementologist colleagues with neologist vein might find substantial reason to consider updating this deeply rooted misnomer.

Considering its long history, today we are experiencing a renaissance of complement research, or rather a late "adolescence" with conspicuous growth day by day. To steal the words of Tom Eirik Mollnes from his chapter in this book, the question is no longer "In which conditions does complement activation contribute to the pathophysiology?" but rather "In which conditions is complement not involved?" Thousands of papers, dozens of reviews and numerous books have been published on complement to date, yet no topical workshop or general immunology conference passes without fundamental revelations or other surprises about the complement system.

Why write a book on a subject that's changing so rapidly, in our age of computers, when we can get updated information in matter of seconds? This question was my first reaction to an interest in books on the complement system by Mimi Thompson Breed, acquisitions editor at Kluwer Academic Publishers. Destiny sat us near one another at lunch at a Gordon Conference, and Ms. Breed somehow diagnosed my infection with the "C bug". She explained that for all the splendour of the computer age, the information explosion and mesmerizing advances in short-circuiting of library databases into our brain, professionals and students need, and many actually enjoy books that incisively cut to the fundamentals while providing a comprehensive account of the state of the field. She also said, however, that a precondition for successful selling of a book is that no similar volume had been published in the preceding couple of years. I could see the former argument, and, fortunately, the latter requirement with regard to the timeliness of a book was also met. Also fortunately, many prominent experts in the field agreed that the quantum of new information reached a critical level to warrant a qualitative update, motivating them to devote substantial time and effort and give their best to the present volume.

The chapters, sorted into six sections, cover almost all major themes in complement science today. The subjects addressed include the structure and function of soluble, membrane-regulator and terminal complex proteins, their roles in innate and adaptive immunity, immune evasion by infectious agents and tumor cells, and the role of complement in pregnancy. Other chapters focus on the various roles of complement in disease, such as autoimmune diseases, fetal loss, allergy and drug-induced hypersensitivity (pseudoallergic) reactions, myocardial infarction, acute respiratory disease syndrome and multiorgan failure. Of great pharmaco-therapeutical interest, the book contains the latest, most comprehensive information on complement inhibitors and their novel application areas. As an added curiosity, Tibor Borsos, a veteran of complement research, reminisces on life and science in the laboratory of Manfred M. Mayer, a highly esteemed pioneer of this field.

By way of disclaimer it should be mentioned that some basic facts and processes relating to complement activation, action and regulation are redundantly described in the various chapters. As editor I felt that all reviews are rounded and carry original information, and trimming repetitive elements would reduce their clarity. I comforted myself with the fact that repetitive structural elements, referred to as *short and long consensus repeats*, are abundant in complement proteins as well. They all contribute to the full function of the protein.

Mentioning a phrase unique to complement terminology brings us back to the initial note on the word "complement", which alludes to some kind of secondary role. A closer scrutiny of the relationship between antibodies and complement reveals, however, that the main player is complement and not the antibody. The "only" function of antibodies is to effectively and specifically direct the eliminatory immune mechanisms, such as the C cascade, against the invader. Thus, antibodies complement the opsonic-cytolytic-signaling function of complement proteins, and not the other way around. Having spent a decade in an army research institute I can best illustrate this point with an analogy to a combat scenario wherein the paratroopers reach strategically important targets by using landmarks, in order to set foot and launch a full-blown attack with a variety of weapon systems. Referring to the paratroopers' job as complementing the function of landmarks illustrates the oddness of current terminology, referring to a powerful protein armada with a variety of peacekeeping functions as "complement". Time may be ripe to start to think about possible linguistic innovations, although clearly, it will take a long time and new generations to rename a pillar of immunology, no matter how misleading and archaic its name is.

Finally, I would like to express sincere thanks to all contributors for their outstanding writings, their time and devotion to this project. Special thanks are also due to my family for various technical help, and to the publishers, for the commission that came along with enduring support and encouragement. The book is recommended for medical doctors and researchers interested in immune physiology and the immune basis of disease, as well as to medical and biology students to "complement" their immunology and microbiology textbooks.

Janos Szebeni
Bethesda

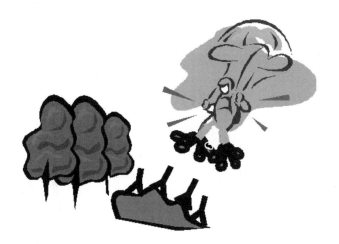

PART 1

A Piece of Complement History

1

The Development of the "One-Hit" or "Single Site" Theory of Complement Mediated Immune Hemolysis
A personal account

Tibor Borsos
Scientist Emeritus
National Cancer Institute, National Institutes of Health, Bethesda, MD, USA

Abstract: After a brief review of early experiments leading up to a multihit, or cumulative damage theory of immune hemolysis, the author describes the experiments by Mayer and associates that led to the development of the one hit theory. The author describes his personal experiences at and the workings of the Mayer laboratory at the Johns Hopkins School of Public Health and at the School of Medicine.   He discusses the development of the mathematical theory by Rapp for the interaction of C2 with the cell intermediate EAC142 and describes experimental confirmation for the one hit theory of immune hemolysis. The author places these events in historical context of the development of modern concepts of complement action.

Key words: Complement, hemolysis, single-site or one-hit mechanism, historical review

1.   INTRODUCTION

The term, complement, refers to a group or system of proteins in plasma that serves as the source of a large variety of biological activities. The first activity described that actually led to the discovery of the existence of this group of proteins was bacteriolysis. The nothing short of spectacular lysis of cholera bacilli by fresh serum of guinea pigs caused great deal of excitement and served as an explanation of why freshly drawn blood tended to remain sterile upon storage. Between 1880 and 1914 a firm foundation was laid for investigating the action of complement in the laboratories of two giants of immunology, Bordet and Ehrlich. The most important results from these studies were that 1. The cytolytic action of complement depended on the presence of an anti-cell antibody; 2. Complement was not a single substance but was comprised of several components; 3. Components had to act in a specific order; 4. Some component activity appeared to be bound in some manner to the target cell; 5. Physical-chemical properties of the components were different; 6. Complement activity was "consumed", inactivated, or "fixed" by antibody-antigen complexes, be they in solution or in an insoluble form. The last finding was used to invent the complement fixation test, a test that is even today is one of the most useful immunological tests for antibodies or antigens. Yet for the next 50 or 60 years most main-line immunologists (with very few exceptions) tended to ignore complement, or at best, to use the complement-fixation test without admitting that complement was an important constituent of plasma. Some went as far as declaring that the activity called complement was simply a physical state most likely generated as an artifact of obtaining plasma or serum and that these activities did not exist in vivo. The major problem of obtaining convincing evidence for the reality of complement was a lack of appropriate biological, chemical and physical tools to measure and quantitate its or its components' activity. The first real break occurred in Heidelberger's laboratory where it was shown that a defined and quantified antibody-antigen complex gained protein N upon mixing it with fresh serum. Controls indicated that the additional N was most likely some part of the complement system. Two of Heidelberger's young associates, Manfred M. Mayer and Abraham G. Osler became interested in complement and continued complement research after they became independent investigators. My story concerns contributions of Mayer's laboratory for it was there that the one-hit theory of immune hemolysis was developed and experimentally verified.

2.   THE BASIS FOR STUDIES OF IMMUNE HEMOLYSIS

It was Bordet (1) and his associates who discovered that complement was capable of lysing erythrocytes. It was, however, Ehrlich's laboratory that did the fundamental work in analyzing and partially elucidating the mechanism of red cell lysis by anti-red cell antibody and complement (2). For this purpose they used sheep erythrocytes (E), rabbit anti-sheep red cell antibody (amboceptor, A) and guinea pig serum as the source of complement (C). Few appreciate the important influence this research had on Ehrlich's ideas how antibodies functioned for he realized that antibodies have at least two functions (hence the term amboceptor), namely recognition of antigen and an effector function such as binding and/or activating C. From the results of ingenious experiments which involved manipulation of the physical-chemical environment of serum and the hemolytic reaction he and his colleagues deduced the following: lysis of amboceptor laden erythrocytes (EA) by C was a sequential process, where the results of each step could be isolated in form of an intact cell and where omission of any of the steps led to no cell lysis. Ehrlich and his associates also made extensive studies to define the effect of temperature, ionic environment, different sources of C and cells and finally to quantitate the activity of A and C (3,4). The next twenty or so years were spent in many laboratories in devising methods to quantitate C activity as a whole, and to quantitate the activity of each C component (4 by that time) and in attempting to formulate some theory that would help to explain the mechanism of lysis of E by C. Two fundamental observations were that the fraction of cells lysed was not a direct function of C concentration (a plot of fraction of cells lysed as a function of C concentration yielded an S shaped curve) and that the time course of lysis started with a lag (5). The primary explanation offered for the non-linearity of the dose-response curve and for the kinetic lag was that there was a variable resistance among the individual cells in addition to the fundamental reaction. This idea led to the notion that only after a critical number of lesions accumulated on a cell would that cell lyse. Curiously the theories advancing the multi-hit (cumulative damage) mechanism for the lytic action of C ignored the multi-component nature of C and the sequential action of its components. Attempts to develop reagents to quantitate the activity of each component were only partially successful because the reagents were generated by selectively depleting serum of the component being measured followed by reconstitution of the reagent by that component. Since neither depletion nor reconstitution was entirely specific for a given component the results were semi-quantitative at best and contradictory and confusing at worst. At the end of the 1930ies the word complement evoked in most mainstream immunologists a sense of hopeless confusion and complexity that defied analysis. It was left to Mayer and his associates to bring at least partial order to the confusion by developing methods that were in conformity with modern concepts of chemical kinetics and that permitted the analysis of the reaction of the individual components on a mathematical basis. Concurrently, new methods became available for the purification of proteins and these were applied to the isolation of C components in Mayer's and other investigators laboratories. Finally, the results of experiments in other laboratories laid the groundwork for the elucidation of the biochemical basis of C action. The formulation of the one-hit theory of immune hemolysis with the concomitant development of mathematical analysis of the hemolytic reaction, its application to the action of individual components and finally the explanation for the reason for the S-shaped dose-response curve were exclusively the product of the laboratory of Manfred Mayer and his associates. I was fortunate to be present in Mayer's laboratory 1955-1962 when many of these events occurred and I was instrumental in putting the mathematical models to experimental tests that ultimately furnished proof for their correctness. The ultimate triumph of the mathematical treatment of the one-hit theory was its ability of predicting experimental results that were intuitively not obvious.

3.   THE MAYER LABORATORY

The success of this major development in C research was due to Mayer's single-minded conviction that the hemolytic reaction could be put on a molecular basis and that it was possible to develop rational approaches to experiments that would permit this. To achieve this goal, Mayer believed that absolute control had to be gained over the seemingly capricious nature of C action. The first requirement in his laboratory was to follow rigid rules of quantitation to the extent that the junior members spent endless hours calibrating volumetric pipettes, performing Kjeldahl determinations, controlling the charge of car batteries that powered the DU spectrophotometers, washing glassware with utmost care, establishing rigid quality controls for buffers, solutions, and cell suspensions. He strove for almost absolute reproducibility of results and to achieve this he would go and drive others to go to almost any length. A fine example of this almost obsessive insistence on accuracy was the control of temperature of the water baths' used for incubating reagents and following the kinetics of a reaction. Each bath's temperature was controlled within 0.05 C! Another example of striving for accuracy was the use of a battery of electric clocks for timing kinetic reactions, where time of sampling, length of incubation and duration of reaction were timed in seconds even though the reactions may have lasted several hours. To ensure certainty of the results of an experiment each experiment was repeated almost endlessly under the same and under different conditions. Mayer was especially anxious to design variations of an experiment that were capable of disproving his theories or the results of a previous experiment. His credo was that if one could not disprove a result then maybe the theory supported by the result was correct... The consequence of this extreme preoccupation with precision and accuracy was that anything published from the Mayer laboratory was repeatable by anyone anywhere. One drawback was that to reduce pipetting errors, large volumes were used both in the reaction and in sampling. This was cumbersome and wasteful of valuable reagents. It took many years for Mayer to accept the necessity of miniaturizing experimental procedures.

When I arrived in Mayer's laboratory in the spring of 1955 as a student in his immunochemistry course, (I did not join his group full time until May

1958) Herb Rapp was the lab instructor (he received his Sc.D. in May 1955) and the only senior member of Mayer's lab. The pioneers of the early Hopkins days, Levine, Croft, Marucci, Cowan and others have already left, and only Rapp remained of that group after he got his doctorate.

The immunochemistry course as given by Mayer and Rapp was a revelation to me. I was a graduate student in a different department searching for an appropriate subject for my dissertation; my studies for the next three years concerned the pathogenesis of Rous sarcoma virus. Nevertheless, my summers and much of my spare time was spent with Rapp for I was hopelessly infected with the C bug, an infection from which I never recovered. And yet my training in Pathobiology and Tumor Virology came in good stead especially when I became deeply involved with the one-hit theory of immune hemolysis for I recognized that the problem of the distribution of viruses among the cells and the distribution of C components among red cells had certain similarities. The two-month course of Immunochemistry taught me to think quantitatively about complex reactions, to look for quantitative relations between molecules and their activities, to understand the exquisite specificity of antibodies, to understand cross reactions and their use in analysis of antibody-antigen complexes, to understand the vast difference in sensitivity of chemical reactions vs. biological activity; this latter insight became especially poignant when we compared the sensitivity of precipitin analysis with that of C fixation test for the same antibody-antigen complex. The text we used was the first edition of Kabat and Mayer's Immunochemistry, a unique and brilliant compendium of immunological, immunochemical, biochemical and analytical methods used in quantitative approaches to immunological problems. It was a book that for the first time summarized the theoretical and practical approaches of research into the molecular nature of the humoral immune system. It was replaced by the second edition in 1961 (6), which became the standard text for immunochemical theory and practice and continued to be so for the next decade or two.

4.   THE ROAD TO THE ONE-HIT THEORY

Mayer joined the faculty of the Johns Hopkins University School of Hygiene and Public Health in 1946. His goal was the elucidation of the action of C and thereby to contribute to our understanding of the physiologic significance of C. His approach was based on the conviction that the various activities of C were the property of molecules and as such they were subject to the rules of physical chemistry. Consequently, analysis of action of C or of its components had to be conducted under proper physical-chemical conditions. Since he realized that in the hemolytic reaction he was dealing with a tripartite system (cells, antibody and C) he initiated experiments where conditions were varied for each one at a time. At the same time he introduced time as a variable, which ultimately led to spectacular results. The first paper, followed by a long series of publications (reaching to his untimely death), was entitled "Kinetic Studies on Immune Hemolysis. I. A Method" (7) and set the tone of his laboratory for the next decade and a half. As Mayer put it "our work during this early period was concerned with the separation and definition of the individual steps that make up the complement system". The results of these experiments established certain fundamental facts that are as valid today as they were then. The first and perhaps most important concept introduced was the difference between excess antibody-limited C vs. limited antibody-excess C. It became obvious that both the kinetic behaviour and endpoint of reaction were strikingly different when the two conditions were studied. The most important observation was that with excess antibody-limited C the number of cells lysed by a given quantity of C became constant after a relatively short time while in the limited antibody-excess C system the number of cells lysed increased even after many hours of incubation. These experiments established the first cardinal condition for analyzing C action: anti-cell antibody must be used in true excess, i.e. changes in the concentration of anti-cell antibody must not affect the extent of lysis by a given amount of C. Put it in another way, the number of cells lysed must be solely the function of C concentration. Experiments performed under such conditions revealed that lysis of EA by limited C started with a lag of several minutes, that Ca^{++} and Mg^{++} were essential ions for the action of C, that the Ca^{++} dependent reaction preceded that depending on Mg^{++}, that the order of reaction was C1, C4, C2 and "C3", that the cell intermediate EAC14 was stable but EAC142 was not (EAC142 "decayed" i.e. lost reactivity with "C3"), that Ca^{++} was essential for the action of C1 and Mg^{++} for C2, and that the actual lytic process was independent of fluid phase components, i.e. a cell population washed free of fluid phase C could be isolated (E*) that had reacted with all the components necessary for lysis but that would lyse in a time dependent manner approaching first order kinetics (5). (As it turned out, Ueno (8) in 1938 in Japan, established the order of action of C components in the hemolytic reaction; it is not possible to tell if Mayer was aware of his results at the time his laboratory was analyzing the kinetics of the hemolytic reaction; it is only certain that in later publications Mayer acknowledged Ueno's contributions). A major advance was the introduction of EDTA treated serum (C-EDTA) as a converting agent of EAC142 to E* permitting the kinetic analysis of this conversion step the results of which became crucial in developing the one-hit theory. At this point Rapp began his mathematical analysis of the conversion of EAC142 to E* which ultimately resulted in the overthrow of the cumulative damage model of immune hemolysis and led to the present form of the one hit-theory. To summarize, three experiments formed the basis for the revolution in thinking about the nature of the hemolytic action of C: 1. the absolute number of EA lysed by C was independent of EA concentration; 2. competition between decay of EAC142 and its interaction with C3 could explain the sigmoid dose-response curve of C and 3. conversion of EAC142 to E* by "C3" started without a lag. (This last observation was shown by Rapp (9) to be incorrect who found that the exponential dose-response of "C3" was a consequence of "C3" not being a single substance). Thus the stage was set for the next step which was the transition from phenomenology to the description of the hemolytic reaction in molecular terms through the application of rigorous mathematical analyses to a single step in the reaction: the generation of EAC142 by action of purified C2 on EAC14. As a result of these analyses the cumulative damage hypothesis as an explanation for the sigmoid dose-response of C action was overthrown and the one-hit or single site theory for at least one step in the sequence was firmly established. It was my privilege to have participated in these developments.

5.   THE EXPERIMENTAL AND THEORETICAL BASIS OF THE ONE-HIT THEORY

The cumulative theory of Alberty and Baldwin (10) was a major advance in putting the action of C on a molecular basis. The theory had shown that the sigmoid dose-response of hemolytic action need not be the result of variable resistance of cells to lysis: it was sufficient to assume that a critical number of "hits" on cell had to accumulate for lysing that cell. From statistical considerations and the application of the binomial distribution equation it was deduced that about 10 critical "hits" per cell had to accumulate for lysis to occur. This explanation made eminent sense and was regarded as a useful hypothesis. Nevertheless, from the beginning there were obvious problems that Mayer thought were inconsistent with this interpretation of the action of C. First, the theory ignored the complex nature of C. Second, the number of critical hits varied when different number of cells was used or when the reaction volume changed. These latter problems may have been explainable as resulting from the complex nature of C. More serious doubts were raised by two different but related experiments. In studying the kinetics of hemolysis by excess A and limited C, it was found that the rate of lysis was the same for two different cell concentrations; furthermore, the absolute number of cells lysed was independent of the total number of cells in the system, i.e. the same number of cells was lysed regardless of the total number of cells (11). According to the cumulative theory, neither of these two observations was possible for an increase in cell concentration should have resulted in a large decrease in the number of cells lysable. To illustrate this point more simply if a cell required an average of 10 hits for lysis, doubling the cell concentration would have yielded an average of 5 hits per cell, a number insufficient to lead to significant lysis: if a quantity of C lysed 50% of a given cell population doubling the cell population would lead to 2% lysis under the Alberty-Balwin multihit theory; experimentally 25% lysis was found (i.e. the number of cells lysed did not change). On reflection these two results were consistent with a one-hit or single site mechanism of hemolysis, i.e. one critical lesion per cell was sufficient to lyse that cell. When Mayer first proposed this hypothesis at a meeting (11), it was received with little enthusiasm; it seemed unreasonable to accept that a single hit (of whatever nature) was sufficient to lead to the lysis of a cell. Furthermore, the sigmoid dose-response curve of hemolysis seemed an unassailable obstacle to the new hypothesis. At this point two events occurred that led to an explanation for the sigmoid dose-response curve: the Mayer laboratory discovered that EAC142 was not a stable intermediate, and Rapp began his brilliant mathematical analysis of the hemolytic reaction. (A detailed description of the mathematical analysis of C action can be found in reference 12) The instability of EAC142 (i.e. its loss of hemolytic activity with "C3" in generating E^*) and the exponential "C3" dose-response curve in lysing EAC142 could explain the sigmoid dose-response curve of C but they were not sufficient for proving the one-hit hypothesis.

Rapp's analysis of the reaction between EAC142 and "C3" yielded two important pieces of information. One was the recognition that mathematical analysis of the individual steps of the hemolytic reaction could not be properly carried out with cells as one of the terms. Instead, at the suggestion of Paul Meier the Poisson distribution was applied and hemolysis was analyzed in terms of sites on a cell. Second, by analyzing the data of the reaction between EAC142 and "C3" in terms of sites he formally showed that competition between the decaying SAC142 and the exponentially proceeding E^* generation led to a sigmoid dose-response curve virtually identical to the hemolytic dose-response curve of C (9). What was now needed was an analysis of one of the C reaction steps where, if the one-hit hypothesis was correct, the reaction had to start without a lag, the hemolytic dose-response curve for that step had to be concave to the abscissa and the fraction of cells lysed had to be independent of volume and concentration effects. Mayer and Rapp recognized that to achieve this at least one of the components had to be available in functionally pure form and the years between 1956 and 1958 were spent in devising procedures to achieve this. The tool that made this goal achievable was furnished by Petersen and Sober in form of cellulose derived ion exchange media. By using columns of (the anionic) DEAE-cellulose, we fractionated guinea pig serum and tested the effluents for activity of C1, C4, C2 and C3a and C3b. (By this time Rapp showed that "C3" was composed of at least two factors, (9)). Lou Hoffmann, who was working on his dissertation at that time, was helpful in testing for C1 and C4 activity and Rapp and I tested for C2 and C3a and C3b (12). The columns were set up in a cold room over a cantankerous fraction collector and as the fractions eluted we tested them immediately for activity. Since some of the runs lasted 48 hours (the columns ran excruciatingly slowly) we spent days and nights in the laboratory during a run. After establishing physical conditions for reasonable elution profile (i.e. pH, ionic strength, rate of flow) we were able to locate in the eluate C1, C4, C2, C3a and C3b. It became obvious that a single pass-through yielded overlapping patterns of activities and only very small quantities of useful materials. To solve these problems Rapp (with my help) came up with a method of rapid cellulose chromatographic separation of C components. This method was contrary to the then prevailing dogma of chromatography: slow and steady application and elution. One end of a large diameter glass tube (5-8 cm) was tapered to the form of a funnel. This end was plugged up with glass wool. On to of the glass wool we poured the slurry of the cellulose, packed it to its smallest volume and stabilized the top with glass wool and glass beads. Flow rates of 10ml/min were easily achieved with such columns. I applied this method for the purification of C2 and after a lot of trial and error I came up with a three step rapid method permitting the use of as much as 40 ml of serum. The final product was stable, highly active and was free of C1 and C4 activity, which was the first goal. Meanwhile, the preparation of EAC14 was proceeding well and we were able to generate and maintain cells in that state for many days. Thus for the first time it became possible to analyze an individual step in the hemolytic sequence. How to achieve this was a different matter. Up to this time the relative activity of EAC142 was assessed by determining the amount of "C3" in the form of CEDTA necessary to lyse a given amount of E. It was reasoned that the more C142 a cell carried that less CEDTA was needed for lysis. Unfortunately the "titers" still depended on cell concentration and reaction volume, mimicking the behavior of whole C. It was evident that this approach did not help in deciding if the process of hemolysis was due to single or to cumulative hits. Mayer, Rapp and I had numerous discussions about this problem without getting a solution. It was obvious that the less C2 activity was expressed on EAC142 the more concentration of "C3" was necessary for lysis to occur. Finally it dawned on me that since it was C2 that was titrated it had to be the variable component while all the others had to be in constant excess. On November 24 and 25, 1958 I performed the first molecular titration of guinea pig C2 by using as high a concentration of C in EDTA as was possible and by showing that EAC142 activity (for a given C2 concentration) approached a constant value with increasing CEDTA concentration. Because I was trained as a virologist, I plotted the results on a log dose of C2 vs. % of lysis and obtained a sigmoid curve that was essentially superimposable on a one-hit curve plotted the same way. When the fraction of cells lysed was plotted against relative C2 concentration we obtained a curve that was entirely concave to the abscissa. On November 26, 1958, I with the help of C. Cook performed the first Tmax experiment, i.e. the kinetics of EAC142 formation by the action of purified C2 on EAC14. The results showed that the reaction started without a lag, reached a maximal point (a point where generation of EAC142 and the decay of EAC142 exactly balanced) after which time the decay reaction predominated (13). Thus in three days, we were able to furnish evidence that fulfilled Mayer's conditions for a one-hit mechanism of immune hemolysis: a dose-response curve entirely concave to the abscissa and a reaction step starting without a lag. Since the reaction between EAC14 and C2 was a bimolecular event and the decay of EAC142 was a first order reaction, Rapp was able to begin the construction of a mathematical model for the reaction. One of the questions that had to be answered was what the products of the decay were. From Levine's data it was suspected that EAC142 decayed to EAC14 but formal experiments had not yet been performed to prove this (14). I designed a definitive experiment to find out if this suspicion was correct. EAC14 were exposed repeatedly to large excess of C2 followed at each cycle by decay and testing for EAC14 activity. It was found that there was no diminution of EAC14 activity in excess over the controls not exposed to C2 but otherwise treated the same way (15). (The slight diminution in EAC14 activity turned out to be due to dissociation of C1 occurring during repeated washing of the cells). The scheme that was analyzed was as follows:

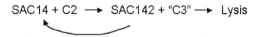

SAC14 + C2 ⟶ SAC142 + "C3" ⟶ Lysis

where S represent a reactive site on an E

The following constrains were applied to the reaction:

1) The number of SAC14 on an E was in large excess, i.e. only a small portion of SAC14 was occupied by C2 at any time during the reaction;
2) C2 was the sole limiting component, i.e. the extent of lysis was solely the function of C2;
3) The reaction between SAC14 and C2 was not measurably reversible and that the product of the decay of SAC142 was SAC14 plus a non-participating decay product of C2;
4) The decay was a first order process.

Rapp derived two equations: one describing the number of SAC142 at any time and the second the time of maximal SAC142 activity ("tmax"). The first equation was intuitively obvious: the reaction between SAC142 and C2 started without a lag, proceeded to maximal production of SAC142 followed by a decline in SAC142 activity due to the predominating decay reaction. The prediction of the second equation was intuitively not obvious: the time at which maximal amount of SAC142 was generated was independent of C2 concentration and was only dependent of SAC14 concentration. We performed two experiments to test these predictions. First we measured tmax as a function of C2 concentration and found that tmax was indeed constant for a given EAC14 preparation. To test the effect of SAC14 concentration on tmax we performed experiments under conditions where the number of EAC14 was varied while C2 was kept constant. The results were unequivocal: the fewer EAC14 were present the longer it took to reach tmax. We also prepared EAC14 with different amounts of SAC14 (something we could do at that time only with difficulty) and again the results were unequivocal: the fewer the SAC14/cell the later the tmax. The results of these and related experiments clearly explained the behavior of complement in lysing red cells under the usual experimental conditions. What became even more striking was that when the mathematical principles derived for the interaction of SAC14 with C2 were applied to the remaining C components (ultimately 9 "classical" components were isolated and shown to be necessary for the lysis of red cells by C) all except native C1 exhibited a one-hit curve as a function of concentration of any given component. The recognition that the dose response curve for native C1 was s-shaped led us to develop hemolytic tests for the idea (proposed earlier by Levine (16) and by Becker (17)) that C1 existed in plasma in a precursor form that was activated by the interaction of C1 with the antibody on the cell surface (18). C1 that was already activated either during the purification process or by certain enzymes showed an unequivocally one-hit dose-response curve. A spin-off of the analysis of the binding of activated C1 by cell surface antibodies led to the finding that while single cell-bound IgM molecules could bind (and activate) C1, at least two IgG molecules not more than 30 nm apart were necessary to bind and activate 1 C1 molecule (19).

6.   THE SIGNIFICANCE OF THE ONE-HIT THEORY

Many immunologists studying the nature of C and its components rapidly accepted the experimental methods that were so useful in proving the one-hit theory of immune hemolysis. Using the principles outlined above, it was possible to correlate the number of predicted sites/cell with the number of lesions visible by electron microscopy. Still there was little enthusiasm discernible for the idea that a single lesion in the cell membrane was sufficient to lead to the lysis of the cell. After all a given C concentration that was sufficient to lyse a given cell was not sufficient to lyse another type of cell. In addition, it was shown that because of the enzymic nature of activated C1 and of the complex SAC142 amplification reactions occurred i.e. one SAC142 complex could bind many C3 molecules to the cell surface raising the possibility that one SAC142 complex could generate many lesions on each cell. This raised the possibility that while the individual C components under limiting conditions indeed generated one-hit curves the final lytic process was multi-hit. Tschopp and I (in Henri Isliker's laboratory) using Tschopp's purified C9 showed that as few as 6 C9 molecules were sufficient to generate one lytic site/cell. Since it was known that one lesion could accommodate 6 C9 molecules (the size of the "hole" depending on the number of C9/site) it was clear that under the conditions developed in Mayer's laboratory a single lesion was sufficient to lyse the erythrocyte.

The ultimate significance of the principles developed by Mayer and his associates lay in the fact that C research became less chaotic and more standardized and that results obtained in different laboratories became more comparable. They emphasized that biological activities, no matter how complex are amenable to molecular analysis. That principle survives even to day albeit in a very different form.

7. REFERENCES

1. Bordet, J., Sur l'agglutination et la dissolution des globules rouges par le serum des animaux injcties de sang defibrine. Ann Inst Pasteur (Paris) 1898;12:688
2. Ehrlich, P., Morgenroth, J. Zur Theotie der Lysenwirkung. Berlin Klin Wochenschr. 1899; 36;6
3. Nathan, E. Ueber die Beziehungen der Komponenten des Komplements zu den ambozeptorbeladenen Blutkoerperchen. Z Immunitaetsforsch 1914; 21:259
4. Skwirsky, P. Ueber den Machnismus der Koplementbindungen. Z Immunitaestforsch 1910;5:538
5. Mayer, M. M., Complement and complement fixation In: Kabat and Mayer's Experimental Immunochemistry ed 2. Springfield Ill. Charles C Thomas, 1961
6. Kabat and Mayer's Experimental Immunochemistry ed 2 Springfield Ill Charles C Thomas 1961
7. Mayer, M.M., Croft, C. C. Gray, M. Kinetic studies on immune hemolysis. I. A method. J Exp Med 1948; 88:427
8. Ueno, S., Studien ueber die Komponenten des Komplements I and II 1938; 7:201,225
9. Rapp, H. J., Mechanism of immune hemolysis: Recognition of two steps in the conversion of EAC'142 to E* Science 1958; 127:234
10. Alberty, R. A., Baldwin, R. L., A mathematical theory of immune hemolysis J. Immunol 1951; 66:725
11. Mayer, M. M. Development of the one-hit theory of immune hemolysis In Immunochemical Approaches to Problems in Microbiology Rutgers University Press 1961
12. Rapp, H. J., Sims, M. R., Borsos, T. Separation of components of guinea pig complement by chromatography Pro Soc Exp Biol Med 1959; 100:730
13. Borsos,T., Rapp, H.J., Mayer, M. M .Studies on the second component of complement. I. The reaction between EAC'14 and C'2: evidence on the single site mechanism of immune hemolysis and determination of C'2 on a molecular basis J Immunol 1961; 87:310
14. Levine, L., Mayer, M. M., Kinetic studies on immune hemolysis. V. Formation of the complex EAC'x and its reaction with C'y J. Immunol 1953; 73:426
15. Borsos, T., Rapp, H.J., Mayer, M. M., Studies on the second component of complement. II. Nature of the decay of EAC"142 J Immunol 1961; 87:326
16. Levine, L., Inhibition of immune hemolysis by diisopropyl fluorophosphates Biochim Biophys Acta 1955; 18:283
17. Becker, Elmer., Concerning the mechanism of complement action. I. Inhibition of complement activity by diisopropyl fluorophosphates J. Immunol 1956; 77:462
18. Borsos, T., Rapp, H. J., Walz, U., Action of the first component complement: activation of C'1 to C'1a in the hemolytic system J Immunol 1964; 92:108
19. Borsos, T., Circolo, A., Effect of cell surface hapten density and immunoglobulin class on complement lysis and agglutination of cells In Recent Advances in Haematology, Immunology and Blood transfusion Akademiai Kiado Budapest 1983

PART 2

PATHWAYS, GENETICS AND GENE REGULATION OF COMPLEMENT

2

The Initiation Complexes of the Classical and Lectin Pathways

Péter Gál, Géza Ambrus, Zsolt Lőrincz and Péter Závodszky
Institute of Enzymology, Biological Research Center, Hungarian Academy of Sciences, Karolina 29-31, Budapest, Hungary

Abstract: Various antigen structures initiate the classical and the lectin pathways of complement activation. Multidomain modular proteases (C1r, C1s and MASPs) are involved in the initiation complexes of both pathways. Despite the identical domain organization of these serine proteases there are differences in their specificities and functions. A comparative analysis is given on the similarities and differences of the mechanism of action of these proteases, with emphasize on structural aspects. Recent structural and functional data underline the significance of molecular dynamics in the activation process of both C1 and MBL/MASPs. While the role of MASP-2 in the lectin pathway is supported by increasing number of evidence, the same can not be said about MASP-1 and MASP-3. The role of the initiation complexes in pathological processes such as inflammation and subsequent repair processes, apoptosis, susceptibility to infectious diseases etc. is also reviewed. C1 inhibitor is essential in regulating both pathways. This serpin interacts with several serine proteases including C1r, C1s and MASPs. C1 inhibitor deficiency related diseases, and C1 inhibitor as a therapeutic agent is also discussed.

Key words: classical pathway, lectin pathway, C1-inh, serine protease, complement deficiency

1.   INTRODUCTION

The classical pathway of complement activation is the initially discovered route for the initiation of the proteolytic cascade, which eventually leads to the destruction and elimination of invading pathogens and altered host structures. The multimolecular enzyme complex, which is responsible for the first step of the classical pathway of complement activation, is the C1 complex. The C1 complex consists of a recognition subunit, C1q, and associated serine proteases: C1r and C1s (Arlaud et al., 1987; Schumaker et al., 1987). The C1q molecule has a structure similar to a bunch of six tulips, with six globular head domains and six collagen-like arms. The globular domains bind to the activator structures, while the collagen-like arms convey the activation signal to the zymogen serine proteases, which are associated with them. The C1 complex has a well defined stoichiometry: a C1q molecule is associated with a C1s-C1r-C1r-C1s tetramer in a Ca^{2+}-dependent manner. The binding of C1q to the activator results in the autoactivation of the C1r zymogen. Activated C1r then cleaves and activates C1s, which in turn cleaves C2 and C4, the subsequent components of the complement system. Since C1q binds to the immune complexes, the classical pathway was first considered as an effector arm of the adaptive immunity. Later, a great number of so called "non-immune" activators of the classical pathway was discovered (e.g. CRP, nucleic acids, β-amiloid peptide aggregates, bacterial cell wall components, certain viruses, apoptotic cells, etc.), that linked this pathway to innate immunity, too.

Approximately one and a half decades ago another activation pathway, the lectin pathway was discovered (Ikeda et al., 1987; Kawasaki et al., 1989; Matsushita et al., 1992). The lectin pathway resembles the classical pathway in many respects. The initiation of the lectin pathway begins with the binding of mannose-binding lectin (MBL) to a carbohydrate array on the surface of the pathogen cell. The structure of MBL closely resembles that of C1q, having globular lectin domains and collagen-like arms. Since MBL binds directly to the foreign cell, this pathway is regarded as a component of innate immunity. Initially, it was believed that MBL triggers the complement system through C1r and C1s. Later it became gradually clear, that the picture is much more complex. First, it turned out that MBL has its own protease (MASP= MBL-associated serine protease), which is responsible for cleaving C2, C4, and probably C3. Later, MASP proved to be a mixture of two proteases: MASP-1 and MASP-2, with different substrate specificities. MASP-2 was shown to cleave C4 and C2, like C1s, while MASP-1 was suggested to cleave C3. Very recently a third MBL-associated protease, MASP-3, has been detected, but no corresponding natural substrate has been identified yet. Unlike C1, there is a small non-enzymatic protein also present in the MBL-MASPs complex, MAp19 or sMAP. The four MBL-associated proteins are the alternatively spliced products of two genes (Schwaeble et al., 2002). One gene encodes MASP-2 and MAp19, while another encodes MASP-1 and MASP-3. It is important to note at this point that the major components of the MBL-associated proteins are MASP-1 and MASP-2, associated to MBL in an approximately 3:1 ratio (Hajela et al., 2002), while MASP-3 and MAp19 are present only in trace amounts. The picture became even more complex, when it was shown that MASPs can bind to ficolins (Matsushita et al., 2000; Matsushita and Fujita, 2002). Ficolins also belong to the class of collectins, i.e. molecules with lectin domains and collagen-like arms.

The protease components of the C1 and MBL-MASPs complexes are composed of multiple, independently folded modules or domains. The domain organization of these proteases is identical, the C-terminal chymotrypsin-like serine protease (SP) domain is preceded by five non-catalytic modules (Figure 1).

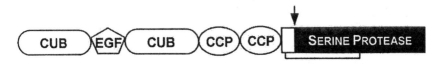

Figure 1. The schematic representation of domain organization of the serine proteases of the classical and lectin pathway initiator complexes C1r, C1s, MASP-1, MASP-2 and MASP-3. The Arg-Ile activation site is indicated by an arrow (↓) and the disulphide bridge connecting the split chains in the activated molecules is also shown (—). Potential glycolyzation sites are not indicated.

At the N-terminus an EGF-like domain is surrounded by two CUB domains. The CUB1-EGF-CUB2 triplet is followed by a tandem repeat of CCP modules. These non-catalytic domains modulate the substrate specificity of the SP domain and mediate important protein-protein interactions. Other common characteristics of these proteases are their highly restricted substrate specificities and low enzymatic activities. Due to the structural and functional similarities these proteases form a protease family, whose members are closely linked evolutionary. MASP-1 seems to be an ancient type of serine protease, since its SP domain, which is encoded by six exons, contains the so-called histidine loop, and its active site serine is encoded by a TCN codon. The SP domains of C1r, C1s, MASP-2 and MASP-3 are encoded by single exons, there is no histidine loop, and their active site serine is encoded by AGY (Endo et al., 1998; Krem and DiCera, 2002). As it will be outlined later, the functional properties of MASP-1 also underline the unique position of this enzyme within this protease family.The most important regulatory factor of the activity of C1r, C1s and MASP-2 proteases is the serpin C1-inhibitor. Lack of this important molecule leads to the uncontrolled activation of the classical and lectin pathways and depletion of numerous complement components. In this review we focus on the structure and function of the C1r, C1s, MASP-1 and MASP-2 proteases, as well as that of the C1-inhibitor, and their roles in certain disease conditions will also be discussed.

Either insufficient or uncontrolled activation of the complement system can lead to serious disorders. Deficiencies of C1r and C1s are rare but result in SLE-like symptomps and severe infections. There are also a few non-complement substrates of C1s which may have important role in pathogenic processes. Neurodegenerative diseases and ischemia-reperfusion are both associated with unwanted complement activation. In the case of the neurodegenerative diseases the uncontrolled activation of the classical pathway is responsible for the harmful effects, whereas in the case of ischemia-reperfusion the lectin pathway seems to be the key factor in the pathogenesis. In the literature there are abundant reports about disease associations of both MBL and C1 inhibitor. MBL deficiency can result in recurrent infection, especially in early childhood, when the adaptive immune system has not fully developed, yet, and there are numerous indications that MBL plays a modulatory role in adults with certain symptoms, as well. The most widely studied disease associated with low levels of functional C1 inhibitor is angioedema, where replacement therapy applications are already under way.

2.   THE CLASSICAL PATHWAY INITIATION COMPLEX

2.1   Overall Structure of the C1 Complex

Despite the rapid progress in the field of structure determination of the subcomponents of C1, we have only speculative models concerning the structure of the entire C1 complex (Schumaker et al., 1987; Arlaud et al., 1987; Tseng et al., 1997; Perkins and Nealis, 1989). Until recently the experimental data used for constructing the current C1 models came mainly from electron microscopy and neutron diffraction. These studies unambiguously indicate that the $C1r_2C1s_2$ tetramer binds to the collagen-like arms of C1q, however the details of this binding remain elusive. Recently the crystal structure of several fragments of the subcomponents of C1 has been determined. These fragments include the globular head of C1q (Gaboriaud et al., 2003), the CUB1-EGF (Gregory et al., 2003) and CCP2-SP (Gaboriaud et al., 2000) fragments of C1s, the CCP1-CCP2-SP fragment of zymogen C1r (Budayova-Spano et al, 2002a) and the CCP2-SP fragments of both the zymogen and activated C1r (Budayova-Spano et al., 2002b). C1q is composed of 18 polypeptide chains, which are made up from 6A, 6B and 6C chains with similar length (A chain 223, B chain 226, C chain 217 residues) and amino acid composition (Sellar et al, 1991). The three types of chains (A,B and C) trimerize to yield collagenous triple helices at the N-terminal part and globular heads at the C-terminal part of the molecule. The molecule is held together by strong non-covalent interactions, as well as by interchain disulfide bridges between the A and B chains and between pairs of C chains. The six collagen-like regions associate to form a stalk at the N-terminus from which the six arms diverge at a point where the Gly-Xaa-Yaa motif is interrupted. The C1s-C1r-C1r-C1s tetramer, which has a rather elongated structure, binds to the arms between the stalks and the heads. According to the most popular C1 models the $C1r_2C1s_2$ tetramer is folded around the collagen-like arms. The C1r subcomponents are inside the cone formed by the C1q arms, while the catalytic region of C1s can either be inside the cone, which enables its activation by C1r, or outside where it may engage substrates. The tetramer adopts a compact 8-shaped (Arlaud et al., 1987) or a more open S-shape (Schumaker et al., 1987; Tseng et al., 1997) conformation in the C1 complex. According to another model that is more consistent with neutron-scattering data, the $C1r_2C1s_2$ tetramer binds outside of the C1q cone adopting a W-like conformation (Perkins and Nealis, 1989). There are numerous arguments both in favor of and against these models, however due to lack of precise data all these models remain speculative.

2.2   Structure and Function of C1r and C1s

C1r and C1s are the serine protease subcomponents which are responsible for the enzymatic activity of the C1 complex. These proteases are of similar length (C1r has 688 amino acid residues, C1s has 673 amino acid residues), amino acid composition (38% sequence identity) and domain organization. C1r is a dimer in the presence or absence of Ca^{2+} ions. The dimerization occurs through the C-terminal catalytic region. Isolated C1s dimerizes through the N-terminal interacting regions in the presence of Ca^{2+}. If we mix equimolar amounts of C1r and C1s, they form Ca^{2+}-dependent tetramers. The core of a tetramer is formed by the C1r dimer whereas the C1s molecules are at the distal ends of it. The interaction between the C1r and C1s molecules takes place in the N-terminal region of both molecules. Electron microscopic studies visualized both the C1r and the C1s molecules as having a dumbbell-like shape, with two globular lobes and a short connecting segment (Weiss et al., 1986). Limited proteolysis experiments also yielded two major fragments: the N-terminal α-fragment, which consists of the entire CUB1 and EGF-like domains plus one third of the CUB2 domain, and the C-terminal γB-fragment, which encompasses the two CCP modules and the serine protease (SP) domain (Arlaud et al., 1987). The N-terminal α-fragments of C1r and C1s are responsible for the C1r-C1s interaction in the tetramer and for the interaction between C1q and the tetramer. Both interactions are Ca^{2+}-dependent. Recent structural studies on the CUB1-EGF fragment of C1s revealed the existence of two Ca^{2+} binding sites, one on the EGF module and another one on the distal end of the CUB1 module (Gregory et al., 2003). This is in agreement with the previous results of Rivas et al.(Rivas et al., 1992), who distinguished two Ca^{2+} binding sites on C1s with different affinities (Kd_1 = 30 μM, Kd_2 = 10 nM) using sedimentation equilibrium measurements. We can presume that the high affinity Ca^{2+} binding site is on the EGF module, which fulfills similar role in other proteins, whereas the low affinity binding site is on the CUB module. Both the C1s (Gregory et al., 2003) and the MASP-2 CUB1-EGF homodimers (Feinberg et al., 2003) show a head-to-tail structure involving interactions between the CUB1 module of one monomer and the EGF-like module of its counterpart. It is very likely that the C1rα-C1sα heterodimer has a similar structure. The C1sα fragment can bind to C1r dimer and the resulting C1sα-C1r-C1r-C1sα pseudo tetramer can bind to the C1q with an affinity similar to that of intact C1 (Busby and Ingham, 1990). This pseudo C1 complex also retained its ability to autoactivate (Tsai et al., 1997). It is very probably that the C1q binding sites of the $C1r_2C1s_2$ tetramer are in the C1sα-C1rα region, although we cannot exclude that other domains of C1r also participate in this interaction. It is important to note that the C1rα-C1sα dimer fails to bind to C1q. It could mean either that the divalent C1sα-C1r-C1r-C1sα ligand is necessary, or perhaps other regions of C1r than the CUB1-EGF motif play a role in this process. The status of the protease (γB) region also modulates the $C1q$-$C1r_2C1s_2$ interaction, indicating the flow of information between the C-and N-terminal parts of these protease molecules. The affinity of the $C1r_2C1s_2$ tetramer to C1q decreases significantly when C1r is activated (at 5°C K_d= 15 nM for zymogen and K_d=140 nM for the activated tetramer) (Siegel and Schumaker, 1983), and C1-inhibitor disrupts the C1 complex without disrupting the C1r-C1s interactions as it binds to the catalytic region of activated C1r and C1s forming C1-inh-C1r-C1s-C1-inh complexes, which dissociate from C1q.

The protease region of C1r and C1s consists of the two CCP modules and the SP domain. Structural studies indicate that the second CCP module is strongly associated with the SP domain (Gaboriaud et al., 2000). Although the SP domain alone can mediate important proteolytic functions (e.g.

autoactivation in the case of C1r) the contribution of the CCP domain to the proteolytic process is significant. The SP domain of C1s can be activated by C1r, and the active SP can cleave the C2 substrate as efficiently as the entire C1s (Rossi et al., 1998). The SP domain contains all the necessary contact sites for its efficient reaction with C1r and C2. C4 (M_r 201 kDa), the other substrate of C1s is much larger than C1r (M_r 87 kDa) and C2 (M_r 100 kDa), and for the efficient C4 cleavage both CCP modules are required. It is very probable that the CCP modules contain binding sites for the C4 substrate. We observed a similar phenomenon in the case of C1r, where the CCP2 domain significantly increases the efficiency of the cleavage of C1s (Kardos et al., 2001). Differential scanning calorimetry experiments demonstrated that the CCP2 module stabilizes the structure of the SP domain: the melting point of the isolated SP domain of C1r (47.3°C) is much less than that of the CCP2-SP fragment (55.4°C). The catalytic efficiency of the reactions with synthetic substrates and with C2, however, does not change with the stability changes. It is very likely therefore, that the increased catalytic efficiency on certain protein substrates is due to the additional substrate binding sites on the CCP modules. It has been shown, that the flexibility of the $C1r_2C1s_2$ tetramer and that of the entire C1 complex is a key element in the biological function of C1 (Lőrincz et al., 2000). The crystal structure of C1r (Budayova-Spano et al., 2002b) demonstrated some flexibility between the CCP2 and SP domains. It is also a general presumption that there is a considerable flexibility between the CCP1 and CCP2 modules (Arlaud et al., 2001) and that C1q itself is a flexible structure, as well. Although the X-ray structure of the C1 complex is not available, we can deduce from the set of indirect data that operation of this multimolecular complex is based on its flexibility.

2.3   Disease Associations of C1r and C1s

Deficiencies of C1r and C1s are rare but can cause severe disease conditions. The most common consequences of these deficiencies are *systemic lupus erythematosus* (SLE)-like syndromes and severe pyogenic infections. It has long been suggested that the SLE-like symptoms are the consequences of the inappropriate handling of immune complexes. Deficiency of C1r and C1s are almost exclusively coupled, probably due to the close physical proximity and the coordinated expression of the two genes (Morgan and Walport, 1991). However, recent studies revealed that selective and complete C1s deficiencies also exists (Inoue et al., 1998; Dragon et al., 2001). C1r and C1s have very restricted substrate specificities: C1r can autoactivate and cleave C1s while C1s can cleave C2 and C4. Several lines of evidence indicate that C1s has more relaxed substrate specificity than C1r and that C1s can participate in other physiological processes then complement activation. It has recently been demonstrated that cultured fibroblast and smooth muscle cells secrete C1r and C1s and that activated C1s cleaves insulin-like growth factor-binding protein-5 (IGFBP-5) (Busby et al., 2000; Moralez et al., 2003). IGFBP-5 regulates the action of insulin-like growth factor I (IGF-I) through tight binding. The cleavage of IGFBP-5 by C1s results in the release of IGF-I to receptors. This phenomenon could represent a linkage between inflammation and subsequent cellular repair processes. Human C1s has also been shown to cleave type I and type II collagens (Yamaguchi et al., 1990), as well as MHC class I antigens (Eriksson and Nissen, 1990). It was hypothesized therefore that C1s participates in the metabolism in cartilage matrix (Nakagawa et al., 1999) (and possibly in the pathogenesis of rheumatoid arthritis) and in the regulation of the immune response (Eriksson, 1996). Further studies are necessary to determine the physiological relevance of the proteolytic action of C1s on non-complement substrates.

Unwanted or uncontrolled activation of C1 can contribute to the pathogenesis of several diseases. The harmful effect of complement activation is suspected in the case of some neurodegenerative diseases in the CNS (Gasque et al., 2000) (e.g. Alzheimer disease (Jiang et al., 1994; Tachnet et al., 2001)) and in the inflammatory events occurring in ischemia and reperfusion (Weiser et al., 1996). The natural inhibitor of the C1r, C1s, and MASPs proteases is the serpin C1-inhibitor. In certain cases, however, endogenous C1-inhibitor might be insufficiently active (e.g. in the consequence of proteolysis by elastase) and uncontrolled C1 activation takes place. To prevent this type of complement activation small molecule inhibitors were synthesized, which block the action of C1s (Ueda et al., 2000; Buerke et al., 2001). *In vivo* administration of this C1s inhibitor, C1s-INH-248, attenuated myocardial injury following ischemia and reperfusion (Buerke et al., 2001). The potential disease associations of C1s are presented in Figure 2 (Figure 2).

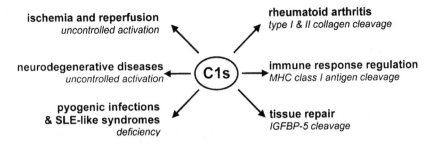

Figure 2. The possible disease associations of C1s. (Figure modified from Gál et al., 2002)

3. THE LECTIN PATHWAY INITIATION COMPLEX

The lectin pathway is an ancient constituent of the complement system predating the classical pathway of complement activation (Sekine et al., 2001). Its main function is the antibody independent activation of the complement cascade through the direct binding of mannose-binding lectin (MBL) to carbohydrate residues on the surface of invading pathogens and the subsequent activation of the MBL-associated serine proteases (MASPs) (Gál and Ambrus, 2001).

3.1 The Role and Structure of Mannose-Binding Lectin (MBL)

MBL is a multifunctional protein known to be exerting the following functions: i) initiation of the lectin pathway through the binding of carbohydrates; ii) opsonization of target structures; iii) modulation of inflammatory response; iv) promotion of apoptosis (Turner, 2003).

The initiation of the complement cascade is realized through the binding of the MBL lectin domains to sugar residues and the subsequent activation of the MASPs (Wong et al., 1999). Activated MASP-2 in turn activates C4 and C2, and from the cleavage products the classical pathway C3-convertase, the C4b2a protease complex is formed. MBL has been shown to bind to a variety of micro-organisms including bacteria, fungi, viruses and parasites (Neth et al., 2000; van Emmerik et al., 1994). Lectin pathway activation is especially important in early childhood in the window period when maternal antibodies are no longer found in the circulation and the self-antibody repertoire is not yet fully functional (Super et al., 1989). Nevertheless, the significance of lectin pathway activation in adults is gaining more ground which is in accordance of the ante-antibody property of MBL: its participation in the first line of defense before the generation of specific antibodies (Ezekowitz, 1991).

MBL has been suggested to opsonize through the binding of a number of receptors including cC1qR/calreticulin (Malhotra et al., 1990, Sim et al., 1998) C1qRp (Tenner et al, 1995) and CR1 (Ghiran et al., 2000; Klickstein et al., 1997). Nevertheless, the role of MBL as a direct opsonin or as an enhancer of opsonization is not yet clear (Turner, 2003).

The modulation of the inflammatory response by MBL is a relatively unexplored field. In a recent study MBL was shown to modulate the cytokine release by monocytes and the degree of TNF-α, IL-1β and IL-6 production was dependent on the MBL concentration of the sample (Jack et al., 2001). The apoptotic function of MBL is probably exerted through its interaction with cC1qR/calreticulin and it is suggested that CD91 is also involved in the process.

MBL is an oligomeric protein with an overall bouquet-like structure, resembling in this aspect C1q and lung surfactant protein-A (SP-A) (Lu et al., 1993). Three 32 kDa polypeptides trimerize through their N-terminal region to form one subunit of the oligomers. MBL is present in circulation as a mixture of variously sized proteins, the degree of oligomerization ranging from dimers to hexamers. Higher oligomerization structures have been reported to have an increased potential in activating complement, probably due to their higher avidity to bind sugar molecules. One polypeptide chain is composed of an N-terminal cysteine-rich region, a collagenous region which is followed by a hydrophobic neck region and the C-terminal lectin domain. The C-type lectin domains contain one binding site for calcium ions and thus one binding site for sugar residues. The affinity of the carbohydrate recognition domain (CRD) towards sugars is rather low and is in the milimolar range, but the hexameric MBL with 18 CRDs has a sufficiently high avidity to display strong binding towards arrays of such carbohydrates as N-acetyl glucoseamine, mannose, N-acetyl mannoseamine, fucose and glucose (Turner and Hamvas, 2000). Human MBL is encoded by the *mbl2* gene, which encompasses four exons and is located in the collectin gene cluster on chromosome 10 (the *mbl1* gene is a pseudogene) (Hansen and Holmskov, 1998).

3.2 The Role and Structure of MBL-Associated Serine Proteases (MASPs)

To date three serine proteases, namely MASP-1, MASP-2 and MASP-3 (Matsushita and Fujita, 1992; Thiel et al., 1997; Dahl et al, 2001) and a non-enzymatic component, MAp19 (Stover et al., 1999) were found to be associated with MBL. In a recent study it has been demonstrated that in serum, MASP-2 is entirely complexed with either MBL or ficolins (Møller-Kristensen et al., 2003), whereas MASP-1 circulates in both bound in unbound forms (Terai et al., 1997). Investigating MBL/MASPs complexes, in sucrose gradient experiments MASP-1 and MAp19 were found to be associated with smaller MBL oligomers, whereas MASP-2 and MASP-3 were in the same fraction with larger MBL oligomers (Dahl et al., 2001).

Previously, it has been suggested that MASP-1 is involved in the complement activation through the direct cleavage of C3 (Matsushita and Fujita, 1995; Matsushita et al., 2000), but independent *in vitro* experiments showed that this has a very low probability *in vivo* (Rossi et al., 2001, Ambrus et al., 2003). Although MASP-1 is a more efficient peptidase than MASP-2 (Ambrus et al., 2003) it does not display any efficient complement activating cleavages. Recently, a non-complement substrate of MASP-1 has been identified. It has been shown that MASP-1 cleaves fibrinogen at about 10-20% of the efficiency of thrombin, which might play a physiologically important role (Hajela et al., 2002). The MBL independent function of MASP-1 is in accordance with the observation that the major portion of MASP-1 is not bound to MBL (Terai et al., 1997).

MASP-2 is the key protease of the lectin pathway of complement activation. Its capacity to autoactivate, cleave C4 and C2 (Vorup-Jensen et al., 2000) incorporate all the functions conveyed by two proteases in the classical pathway of complement activation, C1r and C1s. Our knowledge about the substrate specificity of MASP-2 in terms of natural substrates has changed little from what was suggested in the seminal paper of Thiel and coworkers (Thiel et al., 1997). Nevertheless, recent works have provided an insight at the submolecular level how its function is actually accomplished. It is clear now, that MASP-1 and MASP-2, as well as MAp19 form homodimers and associate with MBL in a Ca^{2+} dependent manner through their CUB-EGF domains (Wallis and Dodd, 2000; Chen and Wallis, 2001; Thielens et al., 2001). It has been shown, that the autoactivation and the C2 cleaving property of MASP-2 is conveyed entirely through its serine protease (SP) domain, whereas in the efficient cleavage of C4 the second complement control protein (CCP2) module plays an important role (Ambrus et al., 2003). Recently, multidomain fragments of both the N-terminal and C-terminal parts have been crystallized and their structure determined (Feinberg et al., 2003; Harmat et al., unpublished).

An unclarified issue is the substrate specificity of MASP-3, as no natural substrate for this protease component has been identified, yet. It has been proposed that MASP-3 is a regulator of the lectin pathway activation through its competitive inhibition of MASP-2 binding to MBL (Dahl et al., 2001).

3.3   The Lectin Pathway in Health and Disease

The first study of linking recurrent infections to MBL deficiency was reported more than a decade ago (Super et al., 1989). Since then a large number of studies have been conducted on the association between MBL deficiency and the development or progression of various diseases, which have been extensively reviewed in recent years (Turner, 1998; Turner and Hamvas, 2000; Petersen et al, 2001; Turner, 2003). Three single nucleotide mutations in exon 1 of the *mbl2* gene have been identified as the major cause of decrease of functional MBL levels in sera. These single point mutations in codons 52, 54 and 57 (often referred to as alleles D, B, and C, respectively) have high incidence in many different populations. The B variant mutation appears in about 22-28% and the D variant in about 14% of the Eurasian population, whereas the C variant is prominent in the sub-Saharan population with occurrences reaching 50-60% (Turner, 2003). It has been proposed that these mutations interfere with the assembly of MBL into higher molecular weight oligomers. Sera from patients homozygous for the mutant alleles contain only low molecular weight non-functional MBL. A recent study on 1183 different sera identified another important factor contributing to apparent functional MBL levels. Garred and coworkers showed that in the sera of those individuals heterozygous for the variant alleles functional MBL levels were significantly dependent on the promoter type on the normal haplotype (Garred et al., 2003).

There is growing evidence that MBL deficiency is associated with increased susceptibility to many infectious diseases. In a study involving 228 patients with clinical symptoms such as recurrent lung infections, recurrent otitis media, diarrhoea and septicaemia were examined and their MBL genotype analyzed (Garred et al., 1995). The results showed a significantly higher incidence of patients with homozygous mutations in the *mbl2* gene

(8.3%) than in the control population (0.8%). It has been shown in a study involving 345 children that MBL deficiency increases the susceptibility towards extracellular pathogens (Summerfield et al., 1997) and another study demonstrated increased incidence of MBL deficiency among those with acute respiratory tract infections in early childhood (Koch et al., 2001). Moreover, a recent study on 90 Kawasaki disease patients revealed a higher frequency of MBL deficient subjects compared to the control group (Biezeveld et al., 2003).

Several reports have presented evidence about the contribution of MBL deficiency in autoimmune diseases. In a number of studies involving patients with systemic lupus erythematosus (SLE), a higher incidence of MBL deficient subjects was documented than in the control groups (Davies et al., 1995; Lau et al., 1996; Sullivan et al., 1996; Davies et al., 1997). The adverse effects of MBL mutations on the propagation of rheumatoid arthritis (RA) have also been recognized (Garred et al., 2000; Graudal et al., 1998; Graudal et al., 2000; Ip et al., 2000). In a study on 128 type I diabetes Japanese patients MBL deficiency has been suggested to be a minor risk factor for possessing the disease (Tsutsumi et al., 2003). In contrast to the above observations a study on Japanese patients failed to detect any significant correlation between mutant MBL alleles and the occurrence of SLE or RA (Horiuchi et al., 2000). Moreover, Garred and coworkers found that RA patients with normal MBL alleles are more likely to have persistent inflammation (Garred et al., 2000).

The effect of MBL deficiency on the susceptibility to HIV and the propagation of the disease has been a subject to a number of investigations. In studies involving a number of HIV patients it has been found that MBL deficiency slightly slowed down the progression from HIV to AIDS (Maas et al., 1998), and on the other hand it also decreased the median survival time of those patients who developed AIDS (Garred et al., 1997a). There is a controversy about the association of MBL deficiency and HIV infection. Quite a few cases have been reported where MBL deficiency had higher incidence among HIV infected individuals compared to the control group (Nielsen et al., 1995; Garred et al., 1997a; Garred et al., 1997b; Prohaszka et al., 1997), whereas in other cases no significant increase of MBL deficiency in HIV infected individuals has been detected (Senaldi et al., 1995).

Nevertheless, the high frequency of MBL mutations prompted investigators to search for beneficial effects of low MBL levels in circulation. It has been demonstrated that MBL binds to parasites such as

Leishmania major and *Leishmania mexicana* (Garred et al., 1994), *Trypanosoma cruzi* (Kahn et al., 1996), and *Schistosoma mansoni* (Klabunde et al., 2000). It has been suggested that the binding of MBL could promote the uptake of an intracellular parasite, either directly through MBL receptors or through subsequent complement component receptors. Indeed, a study involving Ethiopian subjects infected with *M. leprae* found significantly higher levels of MBL (Garred et al., 1994) and few other studies found significant correlation between MBL deficiency and protection against intracellular microorganisms (Bellamy et al., 1998; Hoal-Van Helden et al., 1999).

The involvement of MBL in other pathological processes has also been studied. Recently, it has been proposed that MBL (and possibly C1q) can be involved in allergen-induced activation of complement which may enhance pathological inflammatory response (Varga et al., 2003). In other studies it has been demonstrated that the lectin pathway of complement is activated after myocardial ischemia-reperfusion leading to tissue injury (Collard et al., 2000). In a rat animal model, blockade of the lectin pathway protected the heart from ischemia-reperfusion by reducing neutrophil infiltration and attenuating proinflammatory gene expression. (Jordan et al., 2001). Reperfusion injury appears in tissue temporarily deprived of oxygen as a result of heart attacks, angioplastic surgery, or pulmonary-cardiac by-pass surgery It is accompanied by a marked inflammatory reaction, which contributes to tissue injury. In addition to the role of oxygen free radicals and white blood cells, activation of the complement system represents one of the major contributors of the inflammatory reaction upon reperfusion. (Monsinjon et al., 2001)

Inhibition of the lectin pathway may represent a therapeutic strategy for ischemia-reperfusion injury (Collard et al., 2000; Petersen et al., 2000; Montalto et al., 2001; Lekowski et al., 2001) and other complement-mediated disease states, such as in chronic hepatitis C (Dumestre-Perard et al., 2002). An alternative approach to targeting MBL is to develop a specific inhibitor for MASP-2 and thereby block the activation of the lectin pathway.

4.   C1 INHIBITOR: A REGULATOR OF INITIATON COMPLEXES

4.1   The Structure and Function of C1 Inhibitor

The C1 and the MBL-MASPs complexes have a common serpin type specific regulator protein, C1 inhibitor. C1 inhibitor, forms covalent complexes with the activated C1r, C1s, MASP-1 and MASP-2 proteins, by freezing the proteolytic process in the acyl-enzyme intermediary state. C1 inhibitor prevents the autoactivation of C1, but does not prevent its appropriate activation by immune complexes. It also has physiologically relevant functions in other proteolytic systems, such as the coagulation and fibrinolysis and kinin systems, by inhibiting factor XIIa, kallikrein, and factor XIa (Davies et al., 1986).

The protein consists of 478 amino acids and contains two modules. A unique characteristic of C1 inhibitor, that it possesses a heavily glycosylated N-terminal domain with 113 amino acids that precedes the typical serpin domain (365 amino acids). The whole molecule contains 13 glycosylation sites, therefore the 76 kDa protein migrates on SDS-PAGE as a 104 kDa species. Two disulphide bridges connect the N-terminal and the C-terminal domains. Truncations conserving the disulphide bridges retain the inhibitory activity. The reduction by DTT causes a conformational change and the insertion of the Reactive Center Loop (RCL) into the central β-sheet (Simonovic et al., 2000). The function of the unique N-terminal domain is unclear, but deletion of the whole domain results in loss of inhibition. The N-terminal domain bears 10 of 13 glycosylation sites. The removal of sialic acid from C1 inhibitor decreases its half-life in a rabbit model (Minta, 1981), but it has no effect on the inhibition of C1s (Reboul et al., 1987). The role of the N-terminal region may be the maintenance of the metastable serpin conformation, as it happens in the case of heparin in antithrombin III (Bos et al., 2003). Another function of this domain might be the modification of endothelial-leukocyte interaction during inflammation (Cai et al., 2003). The serpin domain is essential for the inhibitory effect of the molecule. C1 inhibitor has a weak serpin activity, which can be enhanced by glycosaminoglicans (e.g. dextran sulphate, Chang et al., 1986).

C1 inhibitor has a flexible Reactive Center Loop (RCL) nearby its carboxy terminus. Due to the conformation of this loop it is presented as an ideal substrate for the target protease, with a cleavable bond between residues P1 (Arg444) and P1' (Thr445). The cleaved RCL moves to the opposite pole of the serpin, trapping the active protease. The reactive site loop is inserted into the central β-sheet, and a conformational change results in the formation of a covalent complex between inhibitor and protease. This tight association results in distortion and altered structure of the protease active center (Huntington et al., 2000).

C1 inhibitor has not been crystallized yet; however, based on four known 3D structures of serpins, a 3D homology model of C1 inhibitor has been constructed. Possible glycosaminoglycan binding sites and three heparin binding sites were identified in the model (Bos et al, 2002).

A great number of C1 inhibitor mutations have been described (Bos et al., 2002). Numerous active site mutations (Arg →His, Cys, Ser, Leu) inactivate the enzyme. Nevertheless, the Arg444His mutant has the ability to inhibit chymotrypsin. The Ala443Val mutation at the P2 position decreases the inhibition of C1s and C1r, but does not affect the inhibition of kallikrein or Factor XIIa. Mutations Val432Glu or Ala436Glu result in a loss of function by converting the inhibitor to a substrate, and some other mutations (e.g. Phe455Ser, Ala436Thr) lead to polymerization. Additional mutations of C1 inhibitor has been recently described among Hungarian patients with hereditary angioedema (HAE) (Kalmár et al., 2003).

4.2   C1 Inhibitor Related Diseases

C1 inhibitor has a broad spectrum of activity, inhibiting initial proteases of the classical (C1s, C1r) and lectin pathways of complement system (MASP-1, MASP-2), as well as, factor XIIa, kallikrein, and factor XIa of the coagulation contact system. Deficiency of C1 inhibitor leads to the defective regulation of these pathways.

Angioedema is a rare, but serious consequence of uncontrolled activation of complement, usually stemming from C1 inhibitor deficiency. Based on the relative levels of functional and antigenic C1 inhibitor, two types of hereditary angioedema have been described. In type I HAE, defective expression of one allele results in low antigenic and functional levels; whereas in type II HAE, the concentration of functional C1 inhibitor is low, while the C1 inhibitor antigen level is normal, due to the presence of a non-functional mutant protein. Individuals heterozygous for C1 inhibitor mutations typically express 5-30% active C1 inhibitor of normal levels. A third type of HAE with normal C1 inhibitor concentration, so far found only in women, has also been described (Bork et al., 2000). Acquired angioedema (AAE) is mostly antibody mediated (Jackson et al., 1986) or lymphoproliferative disease associated (Cicardi et al., 1996). In AAE the activity of C1 inhibitor is reduced unlike its antigenic level due to the slow clearance of degraded inhibitor from circulation. C1 inhibitor can be successfully used in replacement therapy in patients with hereditary or acquired angioedema. The effective and early inhibition of classical pathway activation with C1 inhibitor is an important issue in the case of ischemia/reperfusion injury, as well.

The regulation of complement and contact systems by C1 inhibitor may have therapeutic applications in the case of xenotransplantations (Davis et al., 1986, Kirschfink 2002). In a rat animal model, C1 inhibitor specifically prevented damage resulting from activation of these two systems (Casarsa et al. 2003) and also reduced complement mediated cytoxicity in other *in vitro* and *ex vivo* models of xenotransplantation (Bergamaschini et al., 2001).

Regulation of complement and contact systems is the most important action where C1 inhibitor has a therapeutic effect. Nevertheless, the appropriate dosing is essential, due to its side effects associated with the coagulation system (Bergamaschini et al., 2003). A low molecular weight specific inhibitor of C1 might be applied in the therapy of C1 inhibitor deficiency, but inhibitors of kallikrein or plasmin can have a similar effect, as well (Ritchie et al., 2003)

5. REFERENCES

Ambrus, G., Gál, P., Kojima, M., Szilágyi, K., Balczer, J., Antal, J., Gráf, L., Laich, A., Moffatt, B.E., Schwaeble, W., Sim, R.B., Závodszky, P. Natural Substrates and Inhibitors of Mannan-Binding Lectin-Associated Serine Protease-1 and -2: A Study on Recombinant Catalytic Fragments. J Immunol 2003; 170:1374-1382

Arlaud, G.J., Colomb, M.G., Gagnon, J. A functional model of the human C1 complex. Immun. Today 1987; 8:106-116.

Arlaud, G.J., Gaboriaud, C., Thielens, N.M., Rossi, V., Bersch, B., Hernandez, J-F., Fontecilla-Camps, J.C. Structural biology of C1: dissection of a complex molecular machinery. Immunological Reviews 2001; 180:136-145

Bellamy, R., Ruwende, C., McAdam, K.P., Thursz, M., Sumiya, M., Summerfield, J., Gilbert, S.C., Corrah, T., Kwiatkowski, D., Whittle, H.C., Hill, A.V. Mannose binding protein deficiency is not associated with malaria, hepatitis B carriage nor tuberculosis in Africans. QJM 1998; 91:13–18

Bergamaschini L., Gobbo G., Gatti S., Caccamo L., Prato P., Maggioni M., Braidotti P., Di Stefano R., Fassati L.R. Endothelial targeting with C1-inhibitor reduces complement activation in vitro and during ex vivo reperfusion of pig liver. Clin. Exp. Immunol. 2001; 126, 412–420

Bergamaschini L., Cicardi M. Recent advances in the use of C1 inhibitor as a therapeutic agent Mol. Immunol. 2003; 40. 155–158

Biezeveld, M.H., Kuipers, I.M., Geissler, J., Lam, J., Ottenkamp, J.J., Hack, C.E., Kuijpers, T.W. Association of mannose-binding lectin genotype with cardiovascular abnormalities in Kawasaki disease. Lancet 2003; 361:1268–70

Bork K, Barnstedt S.E, Koch P., Traupe H. Hereditary angioedema with normal C1-inhibitor activity in women Lancet 2000; 356, 213–217

Bos I.G., Hack C.E., Abrahams J.P. Structural and functional aspects of C1-Inhibitor Immunbiol. 2002; 205, 518-533

Bos I.G., Lubbers Y.T., Roem D., Abrahams J.P., Hack C.E., Eldering E.J. The functional integrity of the serpin domain of C1-inhibitor depends on the unique N-terminal domain, as revealed by a pathological mutant. Biol. Chem. 2003; 278; 29463-29470

Budayova-Spano, M., Lacroix, M., Thielens, N.M., Arlaud, G.J., Fontecilla-Camps, J.C., Gaboriaud,C. The crystal structure of the zymogen catalytic domain of complement protease C1r reveals that a disruptive mechanical stress is required to trigger activation of the C1 complex. EMBO J. 2002a; 21:231-239

Budayova-Spano, M., Grabarse, W., Thielens, N.M., Hillen, H., Lacroix, M., Schmidt, M., Fontecilla-Camps, J.C., Arlaud, G.J., Gaboriaud, C. Monomeric structures of the zymogen and active catalytic domain of complement protease C1r: further insights into the C1 activation mechanism. Structure, 2002b;10:1509-1519

Buerke, M., Schwetz, H., Seitzs, W., Meyer, J., Darius, H. Novel small molecule inhibitor of C1s exerts cardioprotective effects in ischemia-reperfusion injury in rabbits. J. Immunol. 2001; 167:5375-5380

Busby, T.F., Ingham, K.C. NH$_2$-terminal calcium-binding domain of human complement C1s mediates the interaction of C1r with C1q. Biochemistry 1990; 29:4613-4618

Busby, W. H., Nam, T-J., Moralez, A., Smith, C., Jennings, M., Clemmons, D.R. The complement component C1s is the protease that accounts for cleavage of insulin-like growth factor-binding protein-5 in fibroblast medium. J. Biol. Chem. 2000; 275:37638-37644

Cai S., Davis A.E.3rd. Complement regulatory protein C1 inhibitor binds to selectin and interferes with endothelial-leukocyte adhesion J. Immunol. 2003; 171, 4786-4791

Casarsa C., Luigi A.D., Pausa M., Simoni M.G., Tedesco F., Intracerebroventricular injection of the terminal complement complex causes inflammatory reaction in the rat brain. Eur. J. Immunol. 2003; 33, 1260–1270

Chang N.S, Boackle R J. Glycosaminoglycans enhance complement hemolytic efficiency: theoretical considerations for GAG-complement-saliva interactions. Mol. Immunol. 1986; 23: 887-893

Chen, C.B., Wallis, R. Stoichiometry of complexes between mannan-binding protein and its associated serine proteases. Defining functional units for complement activation. J Biol Chem 2001; 276:25894-902

Collard, C.D., Vakeva, A., Morrissey, M.A., Agah, A., Rollins, S.A., Reenstra, W.R., Buras, J.A., Meri, S., Stahl, G.L. Complement activation after oxidative stress: role of the lectin complement pathway. Am J Pathol 2000; 156:1549–1556

Cicardi M., Beretta A., Colombo M., Gioffre D., Cugno M., Agostoni A. Relevance of lymphoproliferative disorders and of anti-C1 inhibitor autoantibodies in acquired angiooedema Clin. Exp. Immunol 1996; 106, 475-480

Dahl, M.R., Thiel, S., Matsushita, M., Fujita, T., Willis, A.C., Christensen, T., Vorup-Jensen, T., Jensenius, J.C. A new mannan-binding lectin associated serine protease, MASP-3, and its association with distinct complexes of the MBL complement activation pathway. Immunity 2001; 15:1–10

Davies, E.J., Snowden, N., Hillarby, M.C., Carthy, D., Grennan, D.M., Thomson, W., Ollier, W.E. Mannose-binding protein gene polymorphism in systemic lupus erythematosus. Arthritis Rheum 1995; 38:110–114

Davies, E.J., Teh, L.S., Ordi-Ros, J., Snowden, N., Hillarby, M.C., Hajeer, A., Donn, R., Perez-Pemen, P., Vilardell-Tarres, M., Ollier, W.E. A dysfunctional allele of the mannose binding protein gene associates with systemic lupus erythematosus in a Spanish population. J Rheumatol 1997; 24:485–488

Davis A.E. III, Whitehead A.S., Harrison R.A., Dauphinais A., Bruns G.A.P., Cicardi M., Rosen F.S. Human inhibitor of the first component of complement, C1: characterization of cDNA clones and localization of the gene to chromosome 11. Proc. Nat. Acad. Sci. 1986; 83, 3161-3165

Dragon-Durey, M.A., Quartier, P., Fremeaux-Bacchi, V., Blouin, J., de Barace, C., Prieur, A.M., Weiss, L., Fridman, W.H. Molecular basis of a selective C1s deficiency associated with early onset multiple autoimmune diseases. J. Immunol. 2001; 166:7612-7616

Dumestre-Perard, C., Ponard, D., Drouet, C., Leroy, V., Zarski, J.P., Dutertre, N., Colomb, M.G. Complement C4 monitoring in the follow-up of chronic hepatitis C treatment. Clin Exp Immunol 2002; 127(1):131-6

Endo, Y., Takahashi, M., Nakao, M., Saiga, H., Sekine, H., Matsushita, M., Nonaka, M., Fujita, T. Two lineages of mannose-binding lectin-associated serine protease (MASP) in vertebrates. J. Immunol. 1998; 161:4924-4930.

Eriksson, H., Nissen, M.H. Proteolysis of the heavy chain of major histocompatibility complex class I antigens by complement component C1s. Biochim. Biophys. Acta 1990; 1037:209-215

Eriksson, H. Proteolytic cleavage of MHC class I by complement C1-esterases: an overlooked mechanism? Immunotechnology 1996; 2:163-168

Ezekowitz, R.A.B. Ante-antibody immunity. Curr Opin Immunol 1991; 1:60–62

Feinberg, H., Uitdehaag, J.C.M., Davies, J.M., Wallis, R., Drickamer, K., Weis,W.I. Crystal structure of the CUB1-EGF-CUB2 region of mannose-binding protein associated serine protease-2. EMBO J 2003; 22:2348-2359

Gaboriaud, C., Rossi, V., Bally, I., Arlaud, G.J, Fontecilla-Camps, J.C. Crystal structure of the catalytic domain of human complement C1s: a serine protease with a handle. EMBO J. 2000; 19:1755-1765

Gaboriaud, C., Juanhuix, J., Gruez, A., Lacroix, M., Darnault, C., Pignol, D., Verger, D., Fontecilla-Camps, J.C., Arlaud, G. J. The crystal structure of the globular head of complement protein C1q provides a basis for its versatile recognition properties. J. Biol. Chem. 2003; (Epub ahead of print)

Gál, P., Ambrus, G. Structure and Function of Complement Activating Enzyme Complexes: C1 and MBL-MASPs. Current Protein and Peptide Science 2001; 2:43-59

Gál, P., Ambrus, G., Závodszky, P. C1s, the Protease Messenger of C1. Structure, function and physiological significance. Immunobiol 2002; 205:383-394

Garred, P., Harboe, M., Oettinger, T., Koch, C., Svejgaard, A. Dual role of mannan-binding protein in infections: another case of heterosis? Eur J Immunogenet 1994; 21:125–131

Garred, P., Madsen, H.O., Hofmann, B., Svejgaard, A. Increased frequency of homozygosity of abnormal mannan-binding protein alleles in patients with suspected immunodeficiency. Lancet 1995; 346:941–943

Garred, P., Madsen, H.O., Balslev, U., Hofmann, B., Pedersen, C., Gerstoft, J., Svejgaard, A. Susceptibility to HIV infection and progression of AIDS in relation to variant alleles of mannosebinding lectin. Lancet 1997a; 349:236–240

Garred, P., Richter, C., Andersen, A.B., Madsen, H.O., Mtoni, I., Svejgaard, A., Shao, J. Mannan-binding lectin in the sub-Saharan HIV and tuberculosis epidemics. Scand J Immunol 1997b; 46:204–208

Garred, P., Madsen, H.O., Marquart, H., Hansen, T.M., Sorensen, S.F., Petersen, J., Volck, B., Svejgaard, A., Graudal, N.A., Rudd, P.M., Dwek, R.A., Sim, R.B., Andersen, V. Two edged role of mannose binding lectin in rheumatoid arthritis: a cross sectional study. J Rheumatol 2000; 27:26–34

Garred, P., Larsen, F., Madsen, H.O., Koch, C. Mannose-binding lectin deficiency—revisited. Mol Immunol 2003; 40:73–84

Gasque, P., Dean, Y.D., McGreal, E.P., Vanbeek, J., Morgan, B.P. Complement components of the innate immune system in health and disease in the CNS. Immunopharmacology 2000; 49:171-186

Ghiran, I., Barbashov, S.F., Klickstein, L.B., Tas, S.W., Jensenius, J.C., Nicholson-Weller, A. Complement receptor 1/CD35 is a receptor for mannan-binding lectin. J Exp Med 2000; 192:1797–1807

Graudal, N.A., Homann, C., Madsen, H.O., Svejgaard, A., Jurik, A.G., Graudal, H.K., Garred, P. Mannan binding lectin in rheumatoid arthritis. A longitudinal study. J Rheumatol 1998; 25:629–635

Graudal, N.A., Madsen, H.O., Tarp, U., Svejgaard, A., Jurik, G., Graudal, H.K., Garred, P. The association of variant mannose-binding lectin genotypes with radiographic outcome in rheumatoid arthritis. Arthritis Rheum 2000; 43:515–521

Gregory,L.A., Thielens,N.M., Arlaud,G.J., Fontecilla-Camps,J.C., Gaboriaud,C. X-ray structure of the Ca2+-binding interaction domain of C1s: insights into the assembly of the C1 complex of complement. J. Biol. Chem. 2003; 278:32157-32164

Hajela, K., Kojima, M., Ambrus, G., Wong, K.H.N., Moffatt, B.E., Ferluga, J., Hajela, S., Gál, P., Sim, R.B. The biological functions of MBL-associated serine proteases (MASPs). Immunobiology 2002; 205:467-476

Hansen, S., Holmskov, U., Structural aspects of collectins and receptors for collectins. Immunobiology 1998; 199:165–189

Harmat, V., Gál, P., Kardos, J., Szilágyi, K., Ambrus, G., Náray-Szabó, G., Závodszky, P. Crystal structure of the catalytic region of human mannose-binding lectin-associated serine protease-2. Manuscript in preparation

Hoal-Van Helden, E.G., Epstein, J., Victor, T.C., Hon, D., Lewis, L.A., Beyers, N., Zurakowski, D., Ezekowitz, A.B., Van Helden, P.D. Mannose-binding protein B allele confers protection against tuberculous meningitis. Pediatr Res 1999; 45:459–464

Horiuchi, T., Tsukamoto, H., Morita, C., Sawabe, T., Harashima, S., Nakashima, H., Miyahara, H., Hashimura, C., Kondo, M. Mannose binding lectin (MBL) gene mutation is not a risk factor for systemic lupus erythematosus (SLE) and rheumatoid arthritis (RA) in Japanese. Genes Immun 2000; 1:464–466

Huntington J.A., Read R.J., Carrell R.W. Structure of a serpin-protease complex shows inhibition by deformation. Nature 2000; 407, 923-926

Ikeda, K., Sannoh, T., Kawasaki, N., Kawasaki, T. Yamashina, I. Serum lectin with known structure activates complement through the classical pathway. J Biol Chem 1987; 262:7451-54

Inoue, N., Saito, T., Masuda, R., Suzuki, Y., Ohtomi, M., Sakiyama, H. Selective complement C1s deficiency caused by homozygous four-base deletion in the C1s gene. Hum. Genet. 1998; 103:415-418

Ip, W.K., Lau, Y.-L., Chan, S.Y., Mok, C.C., Chan, D., Tong, K.K., Lau, C.S. Mannose-binding lectin and rheumatoid arthritis in southern Chinese. Arthritis Rheum 2000; 43:1679–1687

Jack, D.L., Read, R.C., Tenner, A.J., Frosch, M., Turner, M.W., Klein, N.J., Mannose-binding lectin regulates the inflammatory response of human professional phagocytes to Neisseria meningitidis serogroup B J Infect Dis 2001; 184:1152–1162

Jackson J., Sim R.B., Whelan A., Feighery C. An IgG autoantibody which inactivates C1-inhibitor Nature 1986; 323, 722–724

Jiang, H., Burdick, D., Glabe, C.G., Cotman, C.W., Tenner, A.J. β-amyloid activates complement by binding to a specific region of the collagen-like domain of the C1q-A chain. J. Immunol. 1994; 152:5050-5058

Jordan, J.E., Montalto, M.C., Stahl, G. Inhibition of mannose-binding lectin reduces postischemic myocardial reperfusion injury. Circulation 2001; 104:1413–1418

Kahn, S.J., Wleklinski, M., Ezekowitz, R.A., Coder, D., Aruffo, A., Farr, A. The major surface glycoprotein of Trypanosoma cruzi amastigotes are ligands of the human serum mannose-binding protein. Infect Immun 1996; 64:2649–2656

Kalmár L., Bors A., Farkas H., Vas S., Fandl B., Varga L., Füst G., Tordai A. Mutation screening of the C1 inhibitor gene among Hungarian patients with hereditary angioedema. Hum Mutat 2003; 22(6):498

Kardos, J., Gál, P., Szilágyi, L., Thielens, N.M., Szilágyi, K., Lőrincz, Zs., Kulcsár, P., Gráf, L., Arlaud, G.J., Závodszky, P. The role of the individual domains in the structure and function of the catalytic region of a modular serine protease, C1r. J. Immunol. 2001; 167:5202-5208

Kawasaki, N., Kawasaki, T., Yamashina I. A serum lectin (mannan-binding protein) has complement-dependent bactericidal activity. 1989; J. Biochem. 106:483-489.

Kirschfink M. C1-inhibitor and transplantation Immunobiol. 2002; 205, 534–541

Klabunde, J., Berger, J., Jensenius, J.C., Klinkert, M.Q., Zelck, U.E., Kremsner, P.G., Kun, J.F. Schistosoma mansoni: adhesion of mannan-binding lectin to surface glycoproteins of cercariae and adult worms. Exp Parasitol 2000; 95:231–239

Klickstein, L.B., Barbashov, S.F., Liu, T., Jack, R.M., Nicholson-Weller, A. Complement receptor type 1 (CR1, CD35) is a receptor for C1q. Immunity 1997; 7:345–355

Koch, A., Melbye, M., Sørensen, P., Homøe, P., Madsen, H.O., Mølbak, K., Hansen, C.H., Andersen, L.H., Hahn, G.W., Garred, P. Acute respiratory tract infections and mannose-binding lectin insufficiency during early childhood. J Am Med Assoc 2001; 285:1316–1321

Krem, M.M., Di Cera, E. Evolution of enzyme cascades from embryonic development to blood coagulation. TIBS. 2002; 27:67-74.

Lau, Y.L., Lau, C.S., Chan, S.Y., Karlberg, J., Turner, M.W. Mannose-binding protein in Chinese patients with systemic lupus erythematosus. Arthritis Rheum 1996; 39:706–708

Lekowski, R., Collard, C.D., Reenstra, W.R., Stahl, G.L. Ulex europaeus agglutinin II (UEA-II) is a novel, potent inhibitor of complement activation. Protein Sci 2001; 10:277–284

Lőrincz, Zs., Gál, P., Dobó, J., Cseh, S., Szilágyi, K., Ambrus, G., ZávodszkyP. The cleavage of two C1s subunits by a single active C1r reveals substantial flexibility of the C1s-C1r-C1r-C1s tetramer in the C1 complex. J. Immunol. 2000;165:2048-2051.

Lu, J., Wiedemann, H., Timpl, R., Reid, K.B. Similarity in structure between C1q and the collectins as judged by electron microscopy. Behring Inst Mitt 1993; 93:6-16

Maas, J., Roda Husman, A.M., Brouwer, M., Krol, A., Coutinho, R., Keet, I., van Leeuwen, R., Schuitemaker, H. Presence of the variant mannose-binding lectin alleles associated with slower progression to AIDS. Amsterdam Cohort Study. AIDS 1998; 12:2275–2280

Malhotra, R., Thiel, S., Reid, K.B.M., Sim, R.B. Human leukocyte C1q receptor binds other soluble proteins with collagen domains. J Exp Med 1990; 172:955–959

Matsushita, M. Fujita, T. Activation of the classical complement pathway by mannose-binding protein in association with a novel C1s-like serine protease. J Exp Med 1992; 176:1497-1502

Matsushita, M., Fujita, T. Cleavage of the third component of complement (C3) by mannose-binding protein-associated serine protease (MASP) with subsequent complement activation. Immunobiology 1995; 194:443–448

Matsushita, M., Endo, Y., Fujita, T. Complement-Activating Complex of Ficolin and Mannose-Binding Lectin-Associated Serine Protease. J Immunol 2000; 164:2281-2284

Matsushita, M., Thiel, S., Jensenius, J.C., Terai, I., Fujita, T. Proteolytic activities of two types of mannose-binding lectin-associated serine protease. J Immunol 2000; 165:2637–2642

Matsushita, M., Fujita, T. The role of ficolins in innate immunity. Immunobiology 2002; 205:490-497

Minta J.O. The role of sialic acid in the functional activity and the hepatic clearance of C1-INH. J. Immunol. 1981; 126, 245-249.

Møller-Kristensen, M., Jensenius, J.C., Jensen, L., Thielens, N.M., Rossi, V., Arlaud, G., Thiel, S. Levels of mannan-binding lectin-associated serine protease-2 in healthy individuals J Immunol Meth 2003; 282:159– 167

Monsinjon T, Richard V, Fontaine M. Complement and its implications in cardiac ischemia/reperfusion: strategies to inhibit complement. Fundam Clin Pharmacol 2001; 15(5):293-306

Montalto, M.C., Collard, C.D., Buras, J.A., Reenstra, W.R., McClaine, R., Gies, D.R., Rother, R.P., Stahl, G.L. A keratin peptide inhibits mannose-binding lectin. J Immunol 2001; 166:4148–4153

Moralez, A., Busby, W.H., Clemmons, D. Control of insulin-like growth factor binding protein-5 protease synthesis and secretion by human fibroblast and porcine aortic smooth mucle cells. Endocrinology 2003; 144:2489-2495

Morgan, B.P., Walport, M.J.. Complement deficiency and disease. Immunol. Today 1991; 12: 301-306

Nakagawa, K., Sakiyama, H., Tsuchida, T., Yamaguchi, K., Toyoguchi, T., Masuda, R., Moriya, H. Complement C1s activation in degenerating articular cartilage of rheumatoid arthritis patients: immunohistochemical studies with an active form specific antibody. Ann. Rheum. Dis. 1999; 58:175-181

Neth, O., Jack, D.L., Dodds, A.W., Holzel, H., Klein, N.J., Turner, M.W. Mannose-binding lectin binds to a range of clinically relevant microorganisms and promotes complement deposition. Infect Immun 2000; 68:688–693

Nielsen, S.L., Andersen, P.L., Koch, C., Jensenius, J.C., Thiel, S. The level of the serum opsonin, mannan-binding protein in HIV-1 antibody-positive patients. Clin Exp Immunol 1995; 100:219– 222

Perkins, S. J., Nealis, A. S. The quaternary structure in solution of human complement subcomponent C1r2C1s2. Biochem, J. 1989; 263:463-469

Petersen, S.V., Thiel, S., Jensen, L., Vorup-Jensen, T., Koch, C., Jensenius, J.C. Control of the classical and the MBL pathway of complement activation. Mol Immunol 2000; 37:803–811

Petersen, S. V., Thiel, S. & Jensenius, J.C. The mannan-binding lectin pathway of complement activation: biology and disease association. Mol Immunol 2001; 38:133-149

Prohaszka, Z., Thiel, S., Ujhelyi, E., Szlavik, J., Banhegyi, D., Fust, G. Mannan-binding lectin serum concentrations in HIV-infected patients are influenced by the stage of disease. Immunol Lett 1997; 58:171–175

Reboul A., Prandini M.H., Colomb M.G. Proteolysis and deglycosylation of human C1 inhibitor. Effect on functional properties. Biochem J. 1987; 244, 117-121

Ritchie, B.C. Protease inhibitors in the treatment of hereditary angioedema Transf. and Aph. Sci. 2003; 29: 259-267

Rivas, G., Ingham, K.C., Minton, A.P. Calcium-linked self-association of human complement C1s. Biochemistry 1992; 31:11707-11712

Rossi, V., Bally, I. Thielens, N.M. Esser, A.F., Arlaud, G.J. Baculovirus mediated expression of truncated modular fragments from the catalytic region of human complement serine protease C1s. Evidence for the involvment of both complement control protein modules in the recognition of the C4 protein substrate. J. Biol. Chem. 1998; 273:1232-1239

Rossi, V., Cseh, S., Bally, I., Thielens, N.M., Jensenius, J.C., Arlaud, G.J. Substrate specificities of recombinant mannan-binding lectin-associated serine proteases-1 and –2. J Biol Chem 2001; 276:40880-7

Schumaker, V.N., Závodszky, P., Poon, P.H. Activation of the first component of complement. Ann. Rev. Immunol. 1987; **5:**21-42.

Schwaeble, W., Dahl, M.R., Thiel, S., Stover, C. Jensenius, J.C. The mannan-binding lectin-associated serine proteases (MASPs) and MAp19: four components of the lectin pathway activation complex encoded by two genes. Immunbiol., 2002; **205,** 455-466.

Sekine, H., Kenjo, A., Azumi, K., Ohi, G., Takahashi, M., Kasukawa, R., Ichikawa, N., Nakata, M., Mizuochi, T., Matsushita, M., Endo, Y., Fujita, T. An Ancient Lectin-Dependent Complement System in an Ascidian: Novel Lectin Isolated from the Plasma of the Solitary Ascidian, *Halocynthia roretzi*. J Immunol 2001; 167:4504-4510

Sellar, G.C., Blake, D.J., Reid, K.B.M. Characterization and organization of the genes encoding the A-, B- and C-chains of human complement component C1q: the complete derived amino acid sequence of human C1q. Biochem. J. 1991; 274:481-490

Siegel, R. C. and Schumaker, V. N. 1983. Measurement of the association constants of the complexes formed between intact C1q or pepsin-treated C1q stalks and the unactivated or activated C1r2C1s2 tetramers. Mol. Immunol. 20:53-66.

Sim, R.B., Moestrup, S.K., Stuart, G.R., Lynch, N.J., Lu, J., Schwaeble, W.J., Malhotra, R. Interaction of C1q and the collectins with the potential receptors calreticulin (cC1qR/collectin receptor) and megalin. Immunobiology 1998; 199(2):208-24

Simonovic I., Patston P.A. The native metastable fold of C1-inhibitor is stabilised by disulphide bonds Biochim. Biophys. Acta 2000; 1481, 97-102

Stover, C.M., Thiel, S., Thelen, M., Lynch, N.J., Vorup Jensen, T., Jensenius, J.C., Schwaeble, W.J. Two constituents of the initiation complex of the mannan-binding lectin activation pathway of complement are encoded by a single structural gene. J Immunol 1999; 162:3481–3490

Sullivan, K.E., Wooten, C., Goldman, D., Petri, M. Mannose-binding protein genetic polymorphisms in black patients with systemic lupus erythematosus. Arthritis Rheum 1996; 39:2046–2051

Summerfield, J.A., Sumiya, M., Levin, M., Turner, M.W. Association of mutations in mannose binding protein gene with childhood infection in consecutive hospital series. BMJ 1997; 314:1229–1232

Super, M., Thiel, S., Lu, J., Levinsky, R.J., Turner, M.W. Association of low levels of mannan-binding protein with a common defect of opsonisation. Lancet 1989; 2:1236–1239

Tacnet-Delorme, P., Chevallier, S., Arlaud, G.J. β-amyloid fibrils activate the C1 complex of complement under physiological conditions: evidence for a binding site for Aβ on the C1q globular regions. J. Immunol. 2001; 167:6374-6381

Tenner, A.J., Robinson, S.L., Ezekowitz, R.A.B. Mannose-binding protein (MBP) enhances mononuclear phagocyte function via a receptor that contains the 126,000 m(r) component of the C1q receptor. Immunity 1995; 3:485–493

Terai, I., Kobayashi, K., Matsushita, M., Fujita, T. Human serum mannose-binding lectin (MBL)-associated serine protease-1 (MASP-1): determination of levels in body fluids and identification of two forms in serum. Clin Exp Immunol 1997; 110:317–323

Thiel, S., Vorup Jensen, T., Stover, C.M., Schwaeble, W., Laursen, S.B., Poulsen, K., Willis, A.C., Eggleton, P., Hansen, S., Holmskov, U., Reid, K.B., Jensenius, J.C. A second serine protease associated with mannan-binding lectin that activates complement. Nature 1997; 386:506–510

Thielens, N.M., Cseh, S., Thiel, S., Vorup-Jensen, T., Rossi, V., Jensenius, J.C., Arlaud, G.J. Interaction properties of human mannan-binding lectin (MBL)-associated serine proteases-1 and -2, MBL-associated protein 19, and MBL. J Immunol 2001; 166:5068–5077

Tsai, S-W., Poon, P. K., Schumaker, V.N. Expression and characterization of a 159 amino acid, N-terminal fragment of human complement component C1s. Mol. Immunol. 1997; 34:1273-1280

Tseng, Y., Phillips, M.L., Schumaker, V.N. Probing the structure of C1 with an anti-C1s monoclonal antibody: the possible existence of two forms of C1 in solution. Mol. Immunol. 1997; 34: 671-679.

Tsutsumi, A., Ikegami, H., Takahashi, R., Murata, H., Goto, D., Matsumoto, I., Fujisawa, T., Sumida T. Mannose Binding Lectin Gene Polymorphism in Patients With Type I Diabetes. Human Immunol 2003; 64:621–624

Turner, M.W. Mannose-binding lectin (MBL) in health and disease. Immunobiology 1998; 199:327–339

Turner, M.W., Hamvas, R.M. Mannose-binding lectin: structure, function, genetics and disease associations. Rev Immunogenet 2000; 2:305–322

Turner M.W. The role of mannose-binding lectin in health and disease. Mol Immunol 2003; 40:423–429

Ueda, N., Midorikawa, A., Ino, Y., Oda, M., Nakamura, K., Suzuki, S., Kurunmi, M. Inhibitory effects of newly synthesized active center-directed trypsin-like serine protease inhibitors on the complement system. Inflamm. Res. 2000; 49:42-46

van Emmerik, L.C., Kuijper, E.J., Fijen, C.A.P., Dankert, J., Thiel, S. Binding of mannan-binding protein to various bacterial pathogens of meningitis. Clin Exp Immunol 1994; 97:411–416

Varga, L., Szilágyi, K., Lőrincz, Zs., Berrens, L., Thiel, S., Závodszky, P., Daha, M.R., Thielens, N.M., Arlaud, G.J., Nagy, K., Späth, P., Füst, G. Studies on the mechanisms of allergen-induced activation of the classical and lectin pathways of complement. Mol Immunol 2003; 39:839–846

Vorup-Jensen, T., Petersen, S.V., Hansen, A.G., Poulsen, K., Schwaeble, W., Sim, R.B., Reid, K.B., Davis, S.J., Thiel, S., Jensenius, J.C. Distinct pathways of mannan-binding lectin (MBL)- and C1-complex autoactivation revealed by reconstitution of MBL with recombinant MBL-associated serine protease-2. J Immunol 2000; 165:2093-2100

Wallis, R., Dodd, R.B. Interaction of mannose-binding protein with associated serine proteases: effects of naturally occurring mutations. J Biol Chem 2000; 275:30962–30969

Weiser, M.R., Williams, J.P., Moore, F.D., Kobzik, L., Ma, M., Hechtman, H.B., Carroll, M.C. Reperfusion injury of ischemic skeletal muscle is mediated by natural antibody and complement. J. Exp. Med. 1996; 183:2343-2348

Weiss, V., Fauser, C., Engel, J. Functional model of subcomponent C1 of human complement. J. Mol. Biol. 1986; 189:573-581

Wong, N.K.H., Kojima, M., Dobó, J., Ambrus, G., Sim, R.B. Activities of the MBL-associated serine proteases (MASPs) and their regulation by natural inhibitors. Mol Immun 1999; 36:853-861

Yamaguchi, K., Sakiyama, H., Matsumoto, M., Moriya, H., Sakiyama, S. Degradation of type I and II collagen by human C1s. FEBS Lett. 1990; 268:206-208

3

Complement Genetics

György Ábel[1,2] and Vincent Agnello[1,3]
[1]Department of Laboratory Medicine, Lahey Clinic, Burlington, Massachusetts, [2]Department of Pathology, Harvard Medical School, and [3]Edith Nourse Rogers Veterans Affairs Hospital, Bedford, Massachusetts, U.S.A.

Abstract: Clinical studies led to the discovery of complement deficient states several decades ago. With the advent of molecular biology the genetic basis of the deficient states has been revealed. In this chapter we review the current knowledge on the genetics of complement.

Key words: Complement deficiencies, MHC, HLA, haplotypes

1.   GENETICS OF COMPLEMENT COMPONENTS

The genes encoding the protein molecules of the complement system are located on at least six different chromosomes. The genes for C2, factor B, and two genes for C4, C4A, and C4B, are found on the short (p) arm of chromosome 6 within the major histocompatibility (HLA) complex (1-3) (Fig. 1). The genes in this chromosomal region control three different host-defense systems: self-recognition (HLA-A, B, C), immune response (HLA-Dr, Dp, Dq), and complement (C2, C4A, C4B, B). The genes of factor B and C2 are closely linked and separated from each other by 421 bases. They are approximately 30 kb apart from the locus of C4A, which is separated from the C4B locus by 10 kb. As with the HLA class I and class II genes, the complement genes within the HLA complex show considerable polymorphism both at the protein and DNA levels. These four genes are usually inherited as a single linkage group (haplotype) and their polymorphisms are characterized by complotypes.

Chromosome 6

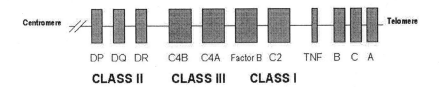

Figure 1. Simplified representation of the HLA gene complex on chromosome 6

1.1   C2

The structural gene for C2 is located within the major histocompatibility complex (MHC) between the gene for the HLA-B and that for complement factor B. In most patients with hereditary C2 deficiency, a single 28-bp mutation that results in a pseudogene incapable of producing C2 protein is present in essentially all Caucasian cases. This C2-deficiency gene is referred to as type I and is carried by the conserved extended MHC haplotype [HLA-B18, S042, DR2] or its complotype-containing fragments. The majority of patients have this mutation (4). In Swedish studies (5) the prevalence of type I complement C2 deficiency in SLE patients was investigated by DNA analysis. The characteristic 28 base pair deletion was determined by polymerase chain reaction analysis followed by gel electrophoresis. Five of the 86 patients (5.8%) were heterozygous for the C2Q0 gene compared with one heterozygote of 100 local blood donors (1%), the difference in prevalence not being significant. Among 26 other SLE patients, two patients who were siblings were C2Q0 homozygous. In Brazilian studies (6) the prevalence was 6.6% in SLE patients and 2.2% in blood donors. In a North American study (7) the prevalence of the 28-bp deletion gene was 2.46% in SLE patients and 0.7% in normal controls. The 28-bp deletion was not seen in any of the127 black SLE patients or 194 black controls.

A much less common heterogeneous group of genes determining C2 deficiency is associated with a variety of MHC haplotypes and is referred to as type II. Type II complement protein C2 deficiency is characterized by a selective block in C2 secretion. The Type II C2 null allele (C2Q0) is linked to two major histocompatibility haplotypes (MHC) that differ from the MHC of the more common Type I C2 deficiency. To determine the molecular basis of Type II deficiency the two Type II C2Q0 genes were isolated and transfected separately into L-cells. Subsequent molecular biology, biosynthetic, and immunofluorescence studies demonstrated that C2 secretion is impaired in Type II C2 deficiency because of different missense mutations at highly conserved residues in each of the C2Q0 alleles. One is in exon 5 (nucleotide C-->T; Ser-->Phe) of the C2Q0 gene linked to the MHC haplotype A11,B35,DRw1,BFS, C4A0B1. The other is in exon 11 (G-->A; Gly-->Arg) of the C2Q0 gene linked to the MHC haplotype A2,B5, DRw4,BFS,C4A3B1. Each mutant C2 gene product is retained early in the secretory pathway (8).

1.2   Factor B

The structural gene for factor B is located within the major histocompatibility complex (MHC) in the proximity of the gene for C2. Complement factor B (Bf) plays an important role in activating the alternative complement pathway Four allelic forms of factor B have been identified (S, F, F1, and S1) with gene frequencies of 0.71, 0.27, 0.01, and 0.01, respectively. Additional polymorphisms can also be demonstrated for factor B by restriction fragment length polymorphism (RFLP) (9). Complotypes missing the factor B gene have not yet been described (10). Factor B-deficient mice were particularly important to create because no complete factor B deficiency has been described in humans, leading to the interpretation that this state was likely to be lethal. Surprisingly, these mice were found to be viable and while their ability to activate the alternative pathway was missing and they displayed decreased activation of the classical pathway, no abnormalities of the immune system were noticed (11).

1.3   C4

There are two genes, C4A and C4B that encode C4 proteins and are highly homologous at both the protein and DNA sequence levels. The C4A gene is 22.5 kb long and positioned about 10 kb from the C4B gene (C4B long). A smaller, 16 kb C4B gene (C4B short), lacking a 6.5 kb intron near the 5′ end of the gene, occurs in about one-third of Caucasians and at a higher frequency of blacks (12, 13). This gene size variation is a result of an insertion of an endogenous retrovirus HERV-K (14,15). Polymorphism of C4 is very complex. C4 is comprised of two distinct but highly homologous (>99%) isotypes, C4A and C4B. Both are composed of 1,725 amino acids (12,16). There is an eight amino acid difference responsible for the electrophoretic, serologic (Chido and Rodgers blood group antigens), and hemolytic (C4B is more active than C4A) differences (17,18). There are additional polymorphisms producing 14 C4A and 17 C4B alleles (19). Sequencing revealed single amino acid differences in the thioester region

(C4d fragment) (20). Deletions and duplications of C4 and the nearby 21-hydroxylase genes are common (12-13, 20-27). The most studied deletion is on the DR3-B8 haplotype that results in loss of most of the C4A and all of the linked 21-hydroxylase pseudogene (CYP21A). Duplications in this region are thought to be a result of unequal crossing-over between C4A and C4B and associated genes. There are various combinations of one, two, or three C4A and C4B genes (21,22,28). C4A and C4B null alleles also seen from intact but noncoding C4A or C4B. This allele (HLA-B60 linked C4A null) is a result of a 2-bp insertion in exon 29 leading to a frame shift mutation and an early stop codon in exon 30 (29). Complete C4 deficiency is due to a null allele at all four loci (two C4A and two C4B null alleles). There have been only 50 individuals reported with this rare disorder, most of them having systemic lupus erythematosus. More common are homozygotes for null alleles in either the C4A or the C4B locus that results in abnormally low serum C4 levels.

1.4   C1

The C1 component consists of three subunits: C1q, C1r, and C1s. The C1q molecule consists of 6 units of polypeptide chains, A, B and C in triple helices that form a bouquet-like structure with 6 globular "flowers" at the carboxyl-terminus end and a stalk that has a collagen-like composition at the amino terminal end. The six globular structures each contain a combining site that are receptors for a specific sequence found on the Fc portion of IgG1, IgG2, IgG3, and IgM.

The C1 molecule is composed of one C1q, two C1r, and two C1s molecules. C1r and C1s are highly homologous proteins, each containing two short consensus repeats (SCRs). The molecules contain low-density lipoprotein (LDL) receptor type B sequences and serine protease portions. The genes for C1r and C1s are closely linked within 50 kb and found on chromosome 12. Three different genes within 24 kb on chromosome 1 encode the A, B, and C, and chains of C1q. In contrast to other complement component genes there is no polymorphism of the C1q genes. Single base mutations in one of the three genes are thought to be responsible for C1q deficiency phenotype. Two types of C1q deficiencies have been identified. In type I, no C1q protein is assembled, because premature chain termination takes place. In type II C1q deficiency, the quantity of C1 is normal but the molecule is nonfunctional. C1q molecules that cannot polymerize into the high-molecular-weight complex are formed and result in excess low-molecular-weight C1q in the plasma. Only individuals homozygous for the defective C1q genes have the C1q deficiency phenotype; heterozygous individuals have normal C1q and CH_{50} levels. Polymorphisms have not been identified at the protein level for C1r, C1s.

1.5 C3-C9

The genes for C6, C7, and the α and β chain genes of C8 are located on chromosome 1; C6 and C7 genes are very closely linked. An increased incidence of deficiencies of C6 and C8 has been described in blacks and deficiencies of C7 and C9 in Japanese. Two types of C8 deficiencies have been identified: type I, in which there are low levels of the β chain but normal levels of the α chain (which is functionally normal), and type II, in which there are dysfunctional α subunits and low levels of β chains in the plasma (30). The majority of C8 deficiencies are type I. Polymorphisms have also been demonstrated for the other complement proteins C3, C6, C7, and C8 (10) but these are much more limited than for the genes within the HLA complex. Polymorphisms have not been identified at the protein level for C5, or C9. The C6, C7, C8, and C9 proteins are all structurally similar to each other; C6 and C7 are single polypeptides, and C8 and C9 are dimers comprised of α and β chains.

There are two polymorphic forms of C3, and S and F. Studies comparing the S and F forms have demonstrated that the S form was slightly more efficient in hemolytic assays than was the F form (31). No differences were detected in the ability of the S and F forms to interact with factors H, 1, and CR1. The C3 protein has significant homology to both the C4 and C5 proteins. The C3 gene is located on chromosome 19. C3 deficiencies are very rare; in the single case analyzed at the DNA level, a stop codon was present within exon 18, leading to premature termination of the mRNA, and no C3 protein product was produced.

1.6 MBL

The mannan-binding lectin (MBL) gene encodes a peptide chain of 32 kDa. Three of these peptide chains associated together to form a basic subunit that has an N-terminal "neck" region, a collagenous triple helix "arm", and a C-terminal "flower" that is the lectin binding site. MBL can exist as dimers, trimers, tetramers, pentamers, and hexamers of this basic subunit bound together by disulfide bonds in the "neck" region. The three-dimensional structure of the MBL molecule is very analogous to the C1q structure. In the human plasma, the majority of MBL is dimer, trimer, or tetramer in structure.

The MBL gene contains four exons and is located on the long arm of chromosome 10 in a gene cluster that also contains the genes for SP-A and SP-D and a pseudogene SP-A. The DNA sequence has features typical for other acute phase proteins in the 5N region including a heat shock consensus element, three glucocorticoid responsive elements, and a sequence with similarity to that of serum amyloid A protein. The gene encodes protein with homology to a family of other proteins of the collectin family that includes pulmonary surfactant proteins SP-A and SP-D and conglutinin.

Three different point mutations in the MBL gene that cause immunodeficiency and significantly decreased MBL plasma levels have been identified (32,33). The mutations are in exon 1 at codons 52, 54, or 57 and cause amino acid substitutions that influence the protein function. The changes at 54 and 57 disrupt the structure of the collagen-like region and result in aberrant subunit structures that cannot form multimers. In addition, the codon 54 change results in the inability of the MASP (mannan-binding lectin (MBL)-associated serine proteases) protein to bind to the MBL protein and results in a lack of function of the complex (34). The codon 54 and 57 mutations show dominant inheritance and heterozygous individuals have MBL less than 10% of normal plasma levels. The change at position 52 introduces an additional cysteine residue and may result in extra disulfide bond formation. Patients heterozygous for the codon 52 mutation have MBL levels at 50% of normal plasma levels.

Patients homozygous for any of the three mutations have undetectable levels of serum MBL. MBL deficiency is common with the actual frequency of the mutation dependent on the racial makeup of the population (35). About 20% of the Caucasian population have at least one mutant allele, either the codon 52 or 54 alleles. Studies on British and Denmark Caucasian populations have shown gene frequencies of about 0.16 for codon 54 allele and 0.06 for the codon 52 allele. The frequency in Caucasian populations of individuals with homozygous codon 52 is about 0.2%, homozygous codon 54 individuals about 2.0%, and heterozygous codon 52/54 alleles about 0.6%. The codon 57 allele is found in high frequency in African populations. In a study done in the West Africa country of Gambia, the gene frequency in native Africans for codon 57 mutations were 0.29, for codon 52 were 0.02, and for codon 54 were 0.003. Gambians who were racially Caucasians (British) and Hong Kong Chinese had codon 54 gene frequencies of 0.17 and 0.11 but did not have any 57 mutations present.

Levels of MBL in the serum are also influenced by genetic elements in the promoter region of the MBL gene. Three haplotypes of protein expression, HY (high), LY (intermediate), and LX (low) phenotypes corresponding to the serum MBL levels have also been identified (36). These phenotypes are a result of two variants in the promoter region of the molecule that are in linkage disequilibrium located at codons 221 (X or Y) and 550 (H or L). The HY haplotype has a gene frequency of 0.38 in Caucasians and 0.11 in Africans, the LY haplotype is found at 0.38 in Caucasians and 0.65 in Africans, and the LX haplotype is found at 0.24 in Caucasians and 0.24 in Africans.

The MASP gene has been mapped to the long arm of chromosome 3 and contains six exons. The encoded protein has a molecular weight of 100 kDa and contains an epidermal growth factor-like domain, two SCR repeats, and a serine protease domain similar in structure to that of C1r and C1s. In addition, the MASP molecule has a histidine loop structure present in many serine proteases such as trypsin and chymotrypsin (37). It is this histidine structure that enables the molecule to have specificity for C3 cleavage.

2. GENETICS OF COMPLEMENT REGULATORY MOLECULES

2.1 C1-INH

C1-INH is a protein of the serpin family of protease inhibitors. There are two known allelic variants of C1-INH. Two types of deficiencies have been characterized: type I, in which normal molecules are produced but in levels only 5-30% of normal, and type II, in which the protein is present in normal levels but is nonfunctional. RFLP analysis of DNA from deficient patients has shown wide genetic variability at the DNA level.

2.2 Factor I

Factor I is a plasma glycoprotein of 88 kDa composed of two chains, a light chain (38 kDa) and a heavy chain (50 kDa) containing LDL receptor domains, a CD5 domain, and sequence unique to factor I, and a segment with sequence homology with C6 and C7 proteins. The gene for factor I is located on chromosome 4 and spans 63 kb with 13 exons. Polymorphism of factor I has been identified in Japanese individuals (38) and hereditary deficiency of factor I has been reported for 23 individuals from 19 families (39). Factor I DNA mutations have been studied for two families (40). In the first family a missense mutation led to the substitution of histidine by leucine in a semiconserved area near the enzyme active site. In the second, one allele had the same mutation as the patient in the first family (although there was no evidence that they were related) and the other allele had a splice site point mutation that led to the deletion of the fifth exon from the mRNA transcript. Both affected individuals had no detectable circulating factor I protein.

2.3   Transmembrane glycoproteins

The four transmembrane glycoproteins factor H, CR1, MCP, and DAF are highly homologous molecules with similar structures. The genes encoding these molecules are closely linked on chromosome 4 in the regulators of complement activation (RCA) gene cluster (41). Analysis of genes and amino acid sequences have identified common domain-like structures with SCRs of about 60-70 amino acids; factor H contains 20 SCRs; CR1, 33 SCRs; and DAF, 4 SCRs (42). Similar SCRs are also found in C4BP (56 SCRs); CR2, C2, and factor B (3 SCRs); and factor I (1 SCR). These highly homologous repeated sequences may be involved in the binding of C3. Because the transmembrane proteins have many SCRs, it is possible that a large number of C3 molecules interact with a single membrane protein. Factor H is transcribed into two messages, which are 4.3 and 1.8 kb. These are transcribed into a 155-kDa transmembrane protein with 20 SCR domains and a 45-kDa protein with 7 SCRs. All identified patients with factor H deficiency have been shown to have point mutations in either the SCR 9 or SCR 16 domains, which modify cysteine residues and are predicted to profoundly influence the three-dimensional structure of the 155-kDa protein (43). Two additional factor H-like proteins, FHL-1 and FHR-1-β have similar structures to the smaller factor H protein and each has seven repetitive SCR segments. The structure of the four NH-terminal SCRs are critical for the function of the FHL-1 and factor H molecules (44).

Decay-accelerating factor (DAF, CD55) is an intrinsic membrane glycoprotein present in red cells, granulocytes, platelets and lymphocytes, is widely distributed throughout the body and is also present in soluble form in body fluids. The functions of DAF are discussed in detail in Chapter 9. The length of the DAF gene is approximately 40 kb and it contains 11 exons (45). The DAF gene is located on chromosome 1q32 within the regulators of complement activation (RCA) gene cluster. Inherited forms of DAF deficiencies have been identified phenotypically. Deficiency of DAF can also be a result of defects in the gene of its regulatory molecules such as a defective PIG-A gene, which is located on the X chromosome that encodes a glycosyltransferase. The deficiency of the enzyme leads to the inability of the cells to link a number of glycoproteins to the membrane via their usual GPI (glycosylphosphatidyl- inositol)-linked anchors. The expression on the red cell and white cells of over 20 glycoproteins is deficient.

Four allelic forms of CR1 (CD35) have been identified: A, B, C, and D (46). The A (or F) allotype is found with a gene frequency of 0.87 in Caucasians, 0.74 in Blacks, and 0.98 in Asians. The B (or S) allotype is found with a gene frequency of 0.12 in Caucasians, 0.22 in Blacks, and 0.02 in Asians. The C allele is only found in Blacks at a frequency of 0.04 and the D allele in Caucasians at a frequency of 0.01. The CR1 molecules produced by the four different alleles are different sizes, the A protein is 190 kDa, the B protein is 220 kDa, the C protein is 160 kDa, and the D protein is 250 kDa. When the gene structure for the A, B, and C alleles was determined, significant differences in the genes for the alleles were found (47,48). The A gene contained 39 exons that encoded four long homologous repeats (LHRs) each of which encodes seven SCR repeated sequences. The B gene contained an additional eight exons and a fifth LHR. The C gene was truncated and only contained three LHR segments. Because each of the SCR repeated sequences binds to C3 and C4 molecules, the allelic forms could bind different quantities of complement fragments. The two most common alleles can be easily distinguished from each other at a DNA level by a Hind III restriction polymorphism detected by RFLP analysis with a CR1.1 probe (49). The A gene produces a 7.4-kb fragment whereas the B gene produces a 6.9-kb fragment.

The binding site for the CR1 molecule is located in the residues 727-768 on the C3 molecule. This area is also involved in the binding of C3 to factor H and factor B and involves at least two areas on the C3 molecule (50). The allelic forms of C3, C3S and C3F, bind with equal affinity to the CR1 receptor (51). The CR1 receptor also binds the C4 molecule. Studies with C4A and C4B show that erythrocyte bound CR1 as well as recombinant soluble CR1 (sCR1) bind with a significantly higher affinity to C4A than to C4B (52,53). A recent study also demonstrated that CRP bound to soluble ligands also can bind to the RBC CR1 (54). This suggests that CR1 may mediate a biological function of C-reactive protein (CRP).

2.4   C4 binding Protein

C4 binding protein (C4BP) is composed of multiple α chains (70 kDa) associated with a single β chain (45 kDa). C4BP is present in a variety of isoforms in plasma each of which has a different number of α chains present in the molecule. The relative level of each of the isoforms is determined by genetic factors that localize in the RCA gene cluster (55). Two genes, the

C4BPA and C4BPB genes, have been identified. The β chain contains three SCRs and contains a binding site for the anticoagulant protein S in the SCR-1 region (56). Enzyme assays have been developed to measure the serum levels of C4BP and protein S-C4BP complex. Levels of both of these proteins have been shown to be increased in patients with membranous nephropathy, decreased in liver cirrhosis patients, and unchanged in patients with IgA nephropathy (57). SLE patients have not yet been studied.

2.5   C3a and C5a Receptors

Receptors for the C3a and C5a molecules have been recently identified and cloned (58-60). The C5a (CD88) and C3a receptors have similar structures, both are within the G-protein superfamily of similar receptors that include receptors for IL-8, Mip-1/Rantes, thrombin, formyl peptide, and platelet-activating factor. Each of these receptors has seven hydrophobic domains that span the cell membrane and have a serpentine topology. The C5a receptor structure is complex and contains at least two separate C5a binding sites. Only one site needs to be activated to cause intracellular signaling (61). The C3a receptor has 37% homology to the C5a receptor but differs from it by the presence of a large extracellular loop with greater than 160 amino acids that is between transmembrane domains 4 and 5. Expression of mRNA for C3a and C5a has been found in tissues throughout the body and in the central nervous system (CNS). At least two monoclonal antibodies have been studied that react with the C5a receptor and inhibit the biological effects of C5a, which may in the future be useful to control anaphylactic responses in vivo (62,63).

2.6   C1q Receptor

The C1q receptor (collectin) has been identified as a single protein chain of 60 kDa. At an amino acid level it has homology to calreticulin, a component of the SS-A antigen, an *Onchocerca* antigen, and a murine melanoma antigen. The receptor is found on leukocytes, platelets, and endothelium where it binds to C1q, mannan-binding protein (MBP), lung surfactant protein A (SP-A), and conglutinin (64). The protein has three domains, the N, C, and central P domains, and recombinant studies have demonstrated that C1q binding site spans the N and P domains (65) and binds to the collagen stalk portion of the C1q molecule. The consequences of C1q binding to its receptor varies with the cell location, binding to monocytes enhances phagocytosis, while binding to granulocytes, eosinophils, endothelial cells, or smooth muscle cells generates toxic oxygen molecules. These consequences may aid in the destruction of foreign pathogens but also may damage host tissues (66). The C1qR also has been shown to prevent the association of C1q with C1r and C1s and functions to control complement activity (67). A second C1q binding protein receptor, gC1qR, has been identified that binds to the globular heads portion of C1q. The second protein receptor is present on vascular endothelium, platelets, neutrophils, and eosinophils and binds vitronectin in addition to C1q (68). A recent report has described that C1q may also bind to CR1 on leukocytes and RBCs (69).

3. SUMMARY

The genetics of all the known components of the complement system have been delineated, at least in part, except for the C1q, C3a, and C5a receptors. Genetic deficiencies of these three components have not been reported. Genetic deficiencies of all the other components have been reported and the genetic bases of deficiencies have also been delineated, at least in part.

4. REFERENCES

1. Fu, S.N., Kunkel, H.G,, Brusman, H.P., et al. Evidence for linkage between HL-A histocompatibility genes and those involved in the synthesis of the second component of complement. J Exp Med 1974; 140:1108-11
2. Allen F.H., Jr. Linkage of HL-A and GBG. Vox Sang 1974; 27:382-4
3. Hauptman, G., Grosshans, E., Heid, E. Lupus erythematosus syndrome and complete deficiency of the fourth component of complement. Ann Dermatol Syph 1974; 101:479-82.
4. Truedsson, L., Alper, C.A., Awdeh, Z.L., et al. Characterization of type I complement C2 deficiency MHC haplotypes. Strong conservation of the complotype/HLA-B-region and absence of disease association due to linked class II genes. J Immunol 1993; 151:5856-63
5. Truedsson, L., Sturfelt, G., Nived, O. Prevalence of the type I complement C2 deficiency gene in Swedish systemic lupus erythematosus patients. Lupus 1993; 2:325-7
6. Araujo, M.N., Silva, N.P., Andrade, L.E. et al. C2 deficiency in blood donors and lupus patients: Prevalence, clinical characteristics and HLA-associations in the Brazilian population. Lupus 1997; 6:462-6
7. Sullivan, K., Petri, M.A., Schmeckpeper, B.J., McLean, R.H., Winkelstein, J.A. Prevalence of a mutation causing C2 deficiency in systemic lupus erythematosus. J Rheumatol 1994; 21:1128-33.
8. Wetsel, R.A., Kulics, J., Lokki, M.L., Kiepiela, P., Akama, H., Johnson, C.A., Densen, P., Colten, H.R. Type II human complement C2 deficiency. Allele-specific amino acid substitutions (Ser189 --> Phe; Gly444 --> Arg) cause impaired C2 secretion. J Biol Chem. 1996; 271:5824-31

9.   Campbell, R.D. Molecular genetics of C2 and factor B. Br Med Bull 1987; 43:37-49
10. Raum, D., Donaldson, V.H., Rosen, F.S., et al. The complement system. 1980; Curr Top Hemat 1980; 3:111-74
11. Matsumoto, M., Fukuda, W., Circolo, A., Goellner, J., Strauss-Schoenberger, J., Wang X., Fujita, S., Hidvegi, T., Chaplin, D.D., Colten, H.R. Abrogation of the alternative complement pathway by targeted deletion of murine factor B. 1997; PNAS 94:8720-25
12. Campbell, R.D., Law, S.K.A., Reid, K.B.M., and Sim, R.B. Structure, organization and regulation of the complement genes. Annu Rev Immunol 1988; 6:161-95
13. Arnett, F.C., and Moulds, J.M. HLA class III molecules and autoimmune rheumatic diseases. Clin Exp Rheumatol 1991; 9:289-96
14. Dangel, A.W., Mendoza, A.R., Baker, B.J., Daniel, C.M., Carroll, M.C., Wu, L.C., Yu, C.Y. The dichotomous size variation of human complement C4 genes is mediated by a novel family of endogenous retroviruses, which also establishes species-specific patterns among old world primates. 1994; Immunogenetics 40:425-36
15. Chu, X., Rittner, C., Schneider, P.M. Length polymorphism of the human complement component C4 gene is due to an ancient retroviral integration. Exp Clin Immunogenet 1995; 12:74-81
16. Belt, K.T., Carroll, M.C., Porter, R.R. The structural basis of the multiple forms of human complement component C4. Cell 1984; 36:907-14
17. Yu, C.Y., Campbell, R.D., Porter, R.R. A structural model for the location of the Rodgers and the Chido antigenic determinants and their correlation with the human complement component C4A/C4B isotypes. 1988; Immunogenetics 27:399-405
18. Carroll, M.C., Fathallah, D.M., Bergamaschini, L., Alicot, E., Isenman, D.E. Substitution of a single amino acid (aspartic acid for histidine) converts the functional activity of human complement C4B to C4A. Proc Natl Acad Sci USA 1990; 87:6868-72
19. Mauff, G., Brenden, M., Braun-Stilwell, M. Relative electrophoretic migration distances for the classification of C4 allotypes. Complement Inflamm 1990; 7:277-281
20. Belt, K.T., Yu, C.Y., Carroll, M.C., Porter, R.R. Polymorphism of human complement component C4. Immunogenetics 1985; 21:173-180
21. Carroll, M.C., Palsdittir, A., Belt, K.T. Deletion of complement C4 and steroid 21-hydroxylase genes in the HLA class III region. 1985; EMBO J 4:2547-52
22. Schneider, P.M., Carroll, M.C., Alper, C.A. Polymorphism of the human complement C4 and steroid 21-hydroxylase genes. Restriction fragment length polymorphisms revealing structural deletions, homoduplications, and size variants. J Clin Invest 1986; 78:650-7
23. Yu, C.Y., Belt, K.T., Giles, C.M. Structural basis of the polymorphism of human complement component C4A and C4B: gene size, reactivity and antigenicity. EMBO J 1986; 5:2873-81
24. Tokunaga, K., Saueracker, G., Kay, P.H. Extensive deletions and insertions in different MHC supratypes detected by pulsed field gel electrophoresis. J Exp Med 1988; 168:933-40
25. Partanen, J., Campbell R.D. Restriction fragment analysis of non-deleted complement C4 null genes suggests point mutations in C4A null alleles but gene conversions in C4B null alleles. Immunogenetics 1989; 30:520-3
26. Steuer, M., Mauff, G., Adam, C. An estimate on the frequency of duplicated haplotypes and silent alleles of human C4 protein polymorphism. Investigations in healthy Caucasoid families. Tissue Antigens 1989;33:501-10

27. Braun, L., Schneider, P.M., Giles, C.G. Null alleles of human complement. Evidence for pseudogenes at the C4A locus and gene conversion at the C4B locus. J Exp Med 1990; 171:129-140.

28. Schneider, P.M. C4 DNA RFLP reference typing report. Complement Inflamm 1990; 7:21824

29. Barba, G., Rittner, C., Schneider, P.M. Genetic basis of human complement C4A deficiency. Detection of a point mutation leading to nonexpression. J Clin Invest 1993; 91:168186

30. Tedesco, F., Roncelli, L., Petersen, H., et al. Two distinct abnormalities in patients with C8 eficiency. J Clin Invest 1990; 86:884-8

31. Welch, T.R., Beischel, L., Kleesattel, A. Functional consequences of the genetic polymorphism of the third component of complement. J Pediatr 1990; 116:S92-7

32. Kurata, H., Cheng, H.M., Kozutsumi, Y., Yokata, Y., Kawasaki, T. Role of the collagen like domain of the human serum mannan-binding protein in the activation of complement and the secretion of this lectin. Biochem Biophys Res Commun 1993; 191:1204-10

33. Lipscombe, R.H.J., Sumiya, M., Summerfield, J.A., Turner, M.W. Distinct physiochemical characteristics of human mannose binding protein expressed by individuals of differing genotype. Immunology 1995; 85:660-7

34. Sato, T., Endo, Y., Matsushita, M., Fujita, T. Molecular characterization of a novel serine protease involved in activation of the complement system by mannose-binding protein. Int Immunol 1994; 6:665-9

35. Turner, M.W. Mannose-binding lectin: The pluripotent molecule of the innate immune system. Immunol Today 1995;17:532-40

36. Madsen, H.O., Garred, P., Thiel, S., et al. Interplay between promoter and structural gene variants control basal serum level of mannan-binding protein. J Immunol 1995; 155:3013-20

37. Sato, T., Endo, Y., Matsushita, M., Fujita, T. Molecular characterization of a novel serine protease involved in activation of the complement system by mannose-binding protein. Int Immunol 1994; 6:665-9

38. Rasmussen, J.M., Teisner, B., Brandslund, J., et al. A family with complement factor I deficiency. Scand J Immunol 1986; 23:711-5

39. Vyse, T.J., Spath, P.J., Davies, K.A., et al. Hereditary complement factor I deficiency. Q J Med 1994; 87:385-405

40. Vyse, T.J., Morley, B.J., Bartok,I., et al. The molecular basis of hereditary complement factor I deficiency. J Clin Invest 1996; 97:925-33

41. Hourcade, D., Holers, V.M., Atkinson, J.P. The regulators of complement activation (RCA) gene cluster. Adv Immunol 1989; 45:381-401

42. Ahern J.M, Fearon D.T. Structure and function of the complement receptors CRI (CD35) and CR2 (CD21). Adv Immunol 1989; 46:183-219

43. Ault, B.H., Schmidt, B.Z., Fowler, N.L., et al. Human factor H deficiency. Mutations in framework cysteine residues and block in H protein secretion and intracellular catabolism. J Biol Chem 1989; 272:25168-75

44. Kuhn, S., Skerka, C., Zipfel, P.F. Mapping of the complement regulatory domains in the human factor H-like protein 1 and in factor H1. 1995; J Immunol 155:5663-70

45. Post, T.W., Arce, M.A., Liszewski, M.K., Thompson, E.S., Atkinson, J.P., Lublin, D.M. (1990) Structure of the gene for human complement protein decay accelerating factor. J Immunol 1990; 144, 740-744

46. Van Dyne, S., Holers, V.M., Lubin, D.M., Atkinson, J.P. The polymorphism of the
     C3b/C4b receptor in the normal population and in patients with systemic lupus
     erythematosus. Clin Exp Immunol 1987; 68:570-9
47. Vik, D.P., Wong, W.W. Structure of the gene for the F allele of complement receptor
     type 1 and sequence of the coding region unique to the S allele. J Immunol 1993;
     151:6214-24
48. Wong, W.W., Cahill, J.M., Rosen, M.D., et al. Structure of the human CR1 gene.
     Molecular basis of the structural and quantitative polymorphisms and identification of a
     new CR1-like allele. J Exp Med 1989; 169:847-63
49. Wilson, J.G., Wong, W.W., Murphy, E.E., Schur, P.H., Fearon, D.T. Deficiency of the
     C3b/C4b receptor (CR1) of erythrocytes in systemic lupus erythematosus: Analysis of
     the stability of the defect and of a restriction fragment length polymorphism of the CR1
     gene. J Immunol 1987; 138:2708-10
50. Lambris, J.D., Lao, Z., Oglesby, T.J., et al. Dissection of CR1, factor H, membrane
     cofactor protein, and factor B binding and functional sites in the third complement
     component. J Immunol 1996; 156:4821-32
51. Bartok, I., Walport, M.J. Comparison of the binding of C3S and C3F to complement
     receptors type 1, 2, and 3. J Immunol 1995; 154:5367-75
52. Gibb, A.L., Freeman, A.M., Smith, R.A., Edmonds, S., Sim, E. The interaction of
     soluble human complement receptor type 1 (sCR1, BRL55730) with human
     complement component C4. Biochim Biophys Acta 1993; 1180:313-20
53. Reilly, B.D., Mold, C. Quantitative analysis of C4Ab and C4Bb binding to the C3b/C4b
     receptor (CR1, CD35). 1997; Clin Exp Immunol 110:310-20
54. Mold, C., Gurule, C., Otero, D., Du Clos, T.W. Complement-dependent binding of
     C-reactive protein complexes to human erythrocyte CR1. Clin Immunol Immunopathol
     1996; 81:153-60
55. Sanchez-Corral, P., Criado Garcia, O., Rodriguez de Cordoba, S. Isoforms of human
     C4b-binding protein. I. Molecular basis for the C4BP isoform pattern and its variations
     in human plasma. J Immunol 1995; 155:4030-6
56. Hardig, Y., Dahlback, B. The amino-terminal module of the C4b-binding protein
     beta-chain contains the protein S-binding site. J Biol Chem 1996; 271:20861-7
57. Tamei, H., Hoshino, T., Yoshida., S. et al. One-step sandwich enzyme immunoassays
     for human C4b-binding protein (C4BP) and protein S-C4BP complex using monoclonal
     antibodies. Clin Chim Acta 1995; 234:115,
58. Ames, R.S., Li, Y., Sarau, H.M., et al. Molecular cloning and characterization of the
     human anaphylatoxin C3a receptor. 1996; J Biol Chem 271:20231-4
59. Gerard, C., Gerard, N.P. C5A anaphylatoxin and its seven transmembrane-segment
     receptor. Annu Rev Immunol 1994; 12:775,
60. Wetsel RA: Structure, function and cellular expression of complement anaphylatoxin
     receptors. Curr Opin Immunol 1995; 7:48-53
61. Siciliano, S.J., Rollins, T.E., DeMartino, J., Konteanis, Z., Malkowitz, L., Van Riper,
     G., Bondy, S., Rosen, H., Springer M.S. Two-site binding of C5a by its receptor: An
     alternative binding paradigm for G protein-coupled receptors. Proc Natl Acad Sci USA
     1994; 91:1214-8
62. Elsner, J., Oppermann, M., Kapp, A. Detection of C5a receptors on human eosinophils
     and inhibition of eosinophil effector functions by anti-C5a receptor (CD88) antibodies.
     Eur J Immunol 1996; 26:1560-4
63. Morgan, E.L., Ember, J.A., Sanderson, S.D., Scholz, W., Buchner, R., Ye, R.D., Hugli
     T.E. Anti-C5a receptor antibodies. Characterization of neutralizing antibodies specific

for a peptide, C5aR-(9-29), derived from the predicted amino-terminal sequence of the human C5a receptor. J Immunol 1993; 151:377-88

64. Malhotra, R. Collectin receptor (C1q receptor): Structure and function. Behring Inst Mitt 1993;93:254-8

65. Stuart, G.R., Lynch, N.J., Lu, J., et al. Localisation of the C1q binding site within C1q receptor/calreticulin. FEBS Lett 1996; 397:245-9

66. Tenner, A.J. Functional aspects of the C1q receptors. Behring Inst Mitt 93:241, 1993

67. van den Berg, R.H., Faber-Krol, M., van Es, L.A., Daha, M.R. Regulation of the function of the first component of complement by human C1q receptor. Eur J Immunol 1995; 25:2206-10

68. Lim, B.L., Reid, K.B., Ghebrehiwet, B., et al. The binding protein for globular heads of complement C1q, gC1qR. Functional expression and characterization as a novel vitronectin binding factor. 1996; J Biol Chem 271:26739-44

69. Klickstein, L.B., Barbashov, S.F., Liu, T., Jack, R.M., Nicholson-Weller, A. Complement receptor type 1 (CR1, CD35) is a receptor for C1q. Immunity 1997; 7:345-55

4

Regulation of Complement Receptor Gene Expression
Regulators and Inhibitors

Mate Tolnay and George C. Tsokos
Department of Cellular Injury, Walter Reed Army Institute of Research, Silver Spring, MD 20910, USA

Abstract: Complement receptors form a critical interface between extracellular complement activation and intracellular signaling. The proper cellular response to complement fragments depends on cell-specific expression of complement receptors at precise cell surface densities. An array of transcription factors binding to promoter elements of the complement receptor genes regulate complement receptor mRNA and, ultimately, protein levels. In addition, specific extracellular stimuli modify complement receptor expression levels that, in turn, alter the capacity of the cell to respond to complement fragments.

Key words: CR1, CR2, CR3, CR4, C3aR, C5aR, gene expression, transcription, transcription factors

1.   INTRODUCTION

Many of the biological activities of the complement system are mediated by complement receptors (CR) expressed on various immune and non-immune cell types (Table 1). Importantly, only activation products generated during complement activation, but not native complement components, bind to these receptors. In addition, a number of ligands unrelated to complement are known.

Transcriptional control of complement receptor gene expression is an important regulatory step that ensures the specificity and efficiency of CR-mediated responses. Mechanisms that control the expression of the various CR genes evolved so that each receptor is expressed in a cell-specific manner. Importantly, and perhaps this is less appreciated, the expression of CRs at the appropriate amount is required for a balanced cellular response to complement fragments. Furthermore, external stimuli can modulate the expression levels of all CRs, providing additional regulatory opportunities. Our aim here is to discuss (a) the regulation of the expression of CR genes, (b) the stimuli and mechanisms that alter basal levels of expression, and (c) the functional repercussions of altered CR expression.

2.   TRANSCRIPTIONAL REGULATION OF COMPLEMENT RECEPTOR GENE EXPRESSION

The number of CR1 per erythrocyte varies between approximately 100 and 1000, and is genetically regulated by two alleles [1]. In comparison, leukocytes express between 10,000 and 50,000 CR1 on the surface membrane. Although the number of CR1 per erythrocyte is low, as compared to other cell types, the abundance of erythrocytes in the circulation means that erythrocytes are the major carriers of CR1. Surprisingly little is known about the transcriptional regulation of CR1 (Fig. 1). The only study that we are aware of found that a 38-nucleotide proximal segment of the

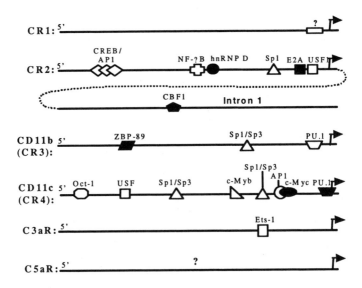

Figure 1. Transcriptional regulation of complement receptor expression. The promoter regions of human complement receptors are depicted with interacting transcription factors. External Empty objects represent activators, whereas filled objects represent repressors

promoter is active in erythroleukemia cells, in addition to unidentified more distal elements [2].

Expression of CR2 is restricted to mature B cells and follicular dendritic cells. In addition, a subpopulation of T cells express 10-times less CR2 than B cells [3]. A number of cell types were found to express low levels of CR2 (Table 1).

Table 1. Complement Receptors

Receptor	Ligands	Distribution
Complement receptor 1 (CR1, CD35)	C3b>C4b>iC3b	All PB cells (except platelets), FDC, peripheral nerve fibers, endothelial cells.
Complement receptor 2 (CR2, CD21)	C3dg>iC3b EBV, CD23, IFNα	Mature B cells, FDC, activated T cells, epithelial cells, platelets.
Complement receptor 3 (CR3, CD11b/CD18)	iC3b, ICAM-1, factor X, fibrinogen, LPS	Monocytes, macrophages, neutrophils, NK cells, dendritic cells, T cells, mast cells.
Complement receptor 4 (CR4, CD11c/CD18)	iC3b, fibrinogen	Monocytes, macrophages, neutrophils, NK cells, dendritic cells, T cells, mast cells, activated B cells.
C3a receptor (C3aR)	C3a	Mast cells, neutrophils, monocytes, eosinophils, basophils, activated lymphocytes, dendritic cells, smooth muscle cells, nervous tissue.
C5a receptor (C5aR)	C5a	Mast cells, neutrophils, monocytes, eosinophils, basophils, T cells, dendritic cells, smooth muscle cells, endothelial cells.

Several studies addressed transcriptional regulation of CR2, and a very complex network of transcription factors has emerged (Fig. 1). An approximately 1.2 kb segment of the 5'-promoter region of the human CR2 gene is essential for CR2 expression [4,5]. Moreover, a silencing element located in the first intron regulates cell-specific expression of CR2 in humans [6] and mice [7]. A nucleotide sequence in the first intron that interacts with the transcriptional repressor CBF1 and other unidentified proteins was shown to be critical to silencing of the human gene [8]. On the other hand, binding of the transcriptional activator NFAT-4 to murine intronic elements has been suggested to release inhibition of CR2 expression in mature B cells [9]. Subsequently, another cell type-specific repressor element that interact with E2A proteins was identified in the proximal promoter of the human gene [10]. The functional interactions between transcription factors binding to intronic and promoter elements are yet to be defined. Several recent studies shed light on transcriptional mechanisms that are involved in the regulation of CR2 expression on mature B cells. TATA-proximal promoter elements that bind the transcription factors USF1 and Sp1 and regulate basal activity have been identified [11]. Our studies have demonstrated that expression of the CR2 gene can be induced by a cell-permeable cAMP analogue, and a protein kinase A and C-responsive heterogeneous nuclear ribonucleoprotein (hnRNP D) binds to a novel element in the promoter region of the CR2 gene [12,13]. Transcription of the murine CR2 gene is positively regulated by histone acetylation, suggesting an important role for the acetylation-dependent accessibility of DNA by transcription factors [14;15]. A role for AP1 and CREB proteins have been proposed [16]. NF-κB has recently been implicated in regulating the expression of the CR2 gene in peripheral blood B cells [17]. NF-κB proteins bind to two CR2 promoter elements, resulting in enhanced promoter activity and enhanced expression of the CR2 gene. Stimuli that activate NF-κB enhance the activity of the CR2 promoter, and known NF-κB-inducers, such as LPS, rapidly increase the number of CR2 proteins on the surface of B cells.

CR3, CR4, as well as LFA-1, consist of a distinct alpha subunit non-covalently attached to an identical beta subunit. The tissue distributions of CR3 and CR4 are similar, it is thus not surprising that the transcriptional regulation of the two genes is related. The CD11b and CD11c genes, which encode the C3 fragment-binding alpha subunit of CR3 and CR4, respectively, are both controlled by the transcription factor Sp1 in a cell-specific manner [18,19]. Because Sp1 is a ubiquitous protein, it is likely that the binding of Sp1 to the CD11b and CD11c promoters is influenced by other factors. Indeed, Sp1 was found to cooperate with c-Jun and c-Fos to activate the CD11c promoter [18]. However, neither c-Jun nor c-Fos are cell-specific, thus their functional interplay with Sp1 can not explain the limited expression profile of CR3 and CR4. The answer may be that several additional transcription factors bind to the promoters, and the pattern of interacting factors, including recruited transcriptional coactivators, imparts cell-specific expression. Alternatively, cell-specific secondary modifications of transcription factors may be involved. Indeed, the following list of additional factors regulating the activity of the CD11b and CD11c promoters suggests the existence of a very complex controlling mechanism. The Sp1-related factor Sp3 also enhances the activity of the endogenous CD11b and CD11c promoters, in cooperation with c-Jun [20]. Another transcription factor, c-Myc, functions as a transcriptional repressor of CD11c through an AP-1 site [21]. The zinc finger transcription factor ZBP-89 is a repressor of the CD11b gene [22]. Interestingly, the transcription factor PU.1 decreases the activity of the CD11c promoter while enhances the activity of the CD11b and CD18 promoters [23;24]. Transcription factors Oct-1 [25], Ets [26], c-Myb [27] and Pur-α [28] have also been implicated in the transcriptional regulation of CD11c gene (see [29] for a review).

Among human leukocytes neutrophils and monocytes express the most C5aR, and 5-20-times less C3aR [30]. On the other hand, eosinophils and basophils express C3aR and C5aR in comparable numbers. During the last couple of years a number of additional cells were shown to express C3aR and C5aR. Although unstimulated T and B lymphocytes were initially reported not to express C3aR or C5aR [31], more recently a subpopulation of T lymphocytes was shown to carry C5aR [32], and also C3aR following IFN-α treatment [33]. B lymphocytes have been shown to express C3aR [34]. Skin-derived dendritic cells express both C3aR and C5aR [35]. Importantly, hematopoetic stem cells and progenitor cells express functional C3aR [36]. However, the transcriptional regulation of the C3aR and C5aR genes have not been explored. A preliminary report has indicated that the transcription factor Ets-1 enhances the activity of the C3aR promoter [37].

3.   REGULATION OF COMPLEMENT RECEPTOR EXPRESSION

Any stimulus or condition that alters the expression level of a CR has the potential to impact on the cellular response to complement fragments. A number of stimuli were shown to affect CR expression. The relative changes in the amount of CR range from 0.5 to 10-fold, and indicate a generally modest alteration of expression levels. Some stimuli produce very rapid changes that peak within minutes, and are the result of the release of stored proteins, whereas in other cases the response can take days. Below we discuss known examples of stimuli affecting CR expression. Nevertheless, many more cases are likely to await discovery.

Human vascular endothelial cells express functional CR1, and exposure of the cells to hypoxia, or treatment with LPS or TNF-α enhances CR1 protein expression [38] (Table 2). Endothelial cells that expressed more CR1, as a result of exposure to hypoxia, bind more immune complexes [38]. The control of endothelial CR1 expression may have important therapeutic implications in diseases in which complement contributes to vascular endothelial cell injury. CR1 expression in erythrocytes is a special case, because erythrocytes have lost their nucleus during maturation, and thus can not produce more CR1 mRNA. As a result of the inability of erythrocytes to produce more CR1, the protein is lost progressively from the cell surface during in vivo aging, so that old cells are almost devoid of CR1 [39].

Morphine has been shown to downregulate CR1 and CR3 levels in neutrophils, and the decreased receptor expression may contribute to morphine-induced inhibition of neutrophil phagocytic and oxidative activity [40]. In addition, endogenous morphine-like substances could play a role in downregulating the immune response following stimulation.

Table 2. Stimuli that result in altered CR levels

Receptor	Cell type*	Stimulus	Change (Time)	Ref.
CR1	Endothelial cell	Hypoxia	3.7-fold (48 hr)	[38]
CR1	Endothelial cell	LPS	2.6-fold (18 hr)	[38]
CR1	Endothelial cell	TNF-α	3.5-fold (18 hr)	[38]
CR1	T lymphocyte	PHA	- (6 hr)	[52]
CR1	Neutrophil	Morphine	0.6-fold (2.5 hr)	[40]
CR2	B lymphocyte	LPS	1.5-fold (2.5 hr)	[17]
CR3/ CD11b	Granulocyte	GM-CSF	2-3-fold (5 min - 12 hr)	[44;45]
CR3/ CD11b	Neutrophil	fMLP	- (30 min)	[53]
CR3/ CD11b	Neutrophil	Morphine	0.5-fold (2.5 hr)	[40]
CR3/ CD11b	Neutrophil	PACAP	10-fold (20 min)	[46]
CR3/ CD11b	T lymphocyte	Anti-CD3/IL-2	- (4-6 days)	[47]
CR3/ CD11b	Myeloid line	G-CSF	-	[24]
CR4/ CD11c	Granulocyte	GM-CSF	2-fold (15 min)	[44]
C3aR	Monocytic line	IFN-γ	5-fold (48 hr)	[54]
C3aR	T lymphocyte	IFN-α	1.6-fold (48 hr)	[33]
C5aR	Monocytic line	IFN-γ	5-fold (72 hr)	[54]
C5aR	T lymphocyte	PHA	- (1 - 60 hr)	[32]

*All cells are human.

Bacterial LPS, through NF-κB, has been shown to enhance the number of CR2 proteins on the surface of primary B cells 2-3 hours after stimulation [17]. There are indications that the modest, 1.5-fold, increase in CR2 expression by LPS could significantly affect B cell antigen receptor signaling and activation [41-43]. The extremely rapid and transient increase in CR2 protein levels by LPS indicates tight regulation that would only allow enhanced B cell antigen receptor signaling within a narrow time window, ensuring a localized response. Thus, at the onset of an infection, the NF-κB pathway could sensitize the B cell to antigen by increasing the number of CR2 co-stimulatory molecules available to interact with antigen-C3d complexes.

Granulocytes as well as monocytes have been shown to possess intracellular pools of CD11b that can be rapidly mobilized to the cell surface upon cell activation. Brief, 5-15 minutes, exposure of granulocytes to GM-CSF in vitro increases 2-3-fold the surface expression of both CD11b and CD11c, and enhances granulocyte adhesiveness [44]. In vivo administration of GM-CSF in humans increased the surface expression of CD11b in granulocytes as early as 30 minutes, with maximal response after 1 hour [45]. Although the surface expression level of CD11c did not change in vivo, the percentage of CD11c-positive granulocytes increased from 9% to 50% after 1 hour. CD11b expression was also enhanced by G-CSF in a myeloid cell line [24]. The neuropeptide pituitary adenylate cyclase-activating peptide (PACAP) markedly increased the expression of CD11b in neutrophils [46]. A subpopulation of T lymphocytes expresses CR3, and this population could be expanded by antigen receptor stimulation (anti-CD3) and IL-2 [47].

Increased C3aR and C5aR expression have been reported in a number of cells and organs upon injury and inflammation. C5aR expression is strikingly increased, in an IL-6-dependent manner, in several organs of mice during experimental sepsis [48;49]. C5aR expression is induced, mainly on neurons, following closed head injury in mice [50]. Murine bronchial epithelial and smooth muscle cells express C3aR and C5aR, and the density of both receptors are enhanced by endotoxin (LPS) or experimental asthma [51]. C5aR is expressed at a low basal level on a subset of human T lymphocytes, and is induced as early as 1 hour upon mitogen (PHA) stimulation [32]. Accordingly, T lymphocytes are chemoattracted to C5a, and PHA-stimulation enhances their ability to migrate toward C5a.

4.   FUNCTIONAL CONSEQUENCES OF ALTERED CR EXPRESSION

It is obvious that stimuli that induce CR expression on previously CR-negative cells will enable the cell to respond to complement fragments. This can happen during embryonic development as part of the development program, or later as a result of an extracellular stimulus. One example is C3aR on T lymphocytes. C3aR is not present on unstimulated T lymphocytes, but is induced upon IFN-α treatment, making the cells responsive to C3a [33].

In addition, conditions or stimuli that quantitatively modulate CR protein levels can reasonably be expected to affect CR-modulated cellular functions. The impact of altered protein expression on cellular function will depend on how rate-limiting is the amount of CR on that particular function, and whether the amount of CR linearly or exponentially correlates to function. For example, the amount of CR1 on erythrocytes, and the efficiency of immune complex clearance, is expected to display linear correlation (until saturation is reached), because immune complexes are essentially carried on the erythrocyte attached to CR1. Accordingly, a hypothetical 1.5-fold increased CR1 expression on erythrocytes is expected to result in 1.5-times more effective clearance of circulating IC. On the other hand, the amount of CR2 on B lymphocytes could affect cell activation exponentially, because CR2 on B cells functions as a co-receptor of the antigen receptor, and was shown to amplify the B cell response to antigen up to 10,000-fold [55]. In this case, a 1.5-fold increase in B cell CR2 expression levels might be predicted to result in higher than 1.5-fold enhanced B cell response.

Establishing experimentally a direct quantitative link between altered CR expression and the functional capacity of the cell to respond to complement fragments can be challenging. Even more complex task is to demonstrate the physiological significance of altered CR expression. One source of uncertainty is that the stimulus that result in altered CR level may have multiple effects on the cell. For example, a stimulus that alters the level of CR3 might as well change the level of another CR or Fc-receptor, making a direct conclusion on phagocytic capacity difficult. Nevertheless, there are examples of external stimuli quantitatively modulating cell surface CR densities that result in a corresponding shift in the ability of the cells to respond to complement fragments. As an example, CR1 surface expression in endothelial cells is induced 3.7-fold upon exposure of the cells to hypoxia, and this change is accompanied by a same-degree enhancement in the ability of the cells to bind immune complexes [38].

It is important to note that we have just begun to explore the physiological significance of altered expressions of the different CR and the correlations with various functions. Nevertheless, it is already clear that mechanisms that govern basal and induced expression levels of CR are important regulators of CR-associated cellular functions, and their disturbances may contribute to various diseases. On the other hand, these mechanisms, once understood, could be exploited therapeutically.

5. CONCLUDING REMARKS

CRs on the surface membrane of cells function as molecular sensors. It is clear that the expression levels of CRs are regulated by external stimuli, and as a result the ability of cells to respond to complement fragments is altered. It is thus surprising that so little is known about the transcriptional regulation of several CRs. But how functional dissection of promoters can contribute to deciphering physiologically relevant questions regarding regulation of complement protein synthesis? As exemplified by the regulation of CR2 expression by the NF-κB signaling pathway, investigation of the molecular details of promoter-protein interactions can point to unexpected mechanisms that alter the ability of the cell to respond to complement fragments under physiological conditions. In addition, pharmacological targets for intervention in pathological conditions may be obtained. The understanding of the dynamics of CR expression in a quantitative manner will provide us with a better picture of how cells respond to complement fragments, and with tools to intervene.

Disclaimer. The opinions and assertions contained herein are the private views of the authors and are not to be construed as official or as reflecting the views of the Department of the Army or the Department of Defense.

6. REFERENCES

1. Wilson,J.G., Wong,W.W., Schur,P.H., and Fearon,D.T., Mode of inheritance of decreased C3b receptors on erythrocytes of patients with systemic lupus erythematosus. N.Engl.J Med. 1982. 307: 981-986.
2. Funkhouser,T. and Vik,D.P., Promoter activity of the 5' flanking region of the complement receptor type 1 (CR1) gene: basal and induced transcription. Biochim.Biophys.Acta 2000. 1490: 99-105.
3. Fischer,E., Delibrias,C., and Kazatchkine,M.D., Expression of CR2 (the C3dg/EBV receptor, CD21) on normal human peripheral blood T lymphocytes. J Immunol 1991. 146: 865-869.
4. Rayhel,E.J., Dehoff,M.H., and Holers,V.M., Characterization of the human complement receptor 2 (CR2, CD21) promoter reveals sequences shared with regulatory regions of other developmentally restricted B cell proteins. J.Immunol. 1991. 146: 2021-2026.
5. Yang,L.M., Behrens,M., and Weis,J.J., Identification of 5'-regions affecting the expression of the human CR2 gene. J.Immunol. 1991. 147: 2404-2410.
6. Makar,K.W., Pham,C.T., Dehoff,M.H., O'Connor,S.M., Jacobi,S.M., and Holers,V.M., An intronic silencer regulates B lymphocyte cell- and stage-specific expression of the

human complement receptor type 2 (CR2, CD21) gene. J.Immunol. 1998. 160: 1268-1278.

7. Hu,H., Martin,B.K., Weis,J.J., and Weis,J.H., Expression of the murine CD21 gene is regulated by promoter and intronic sequences. J.Immunol. 1997. 158: 4758-4768.

8. Makar,K.W., Ulgiati,D., Hagman,J., and Holers,V.M., A site in the complement receptor 2 (CR2/CD21) silencer is necessary for lineage specific transcriptional regulation. Int.Immunol. 2001. 13: 657-664.

9. Zabel,M.D., Wheeler,W., Weis,J.J., and Weis,J.H., Yin Yang 1, Oct1, and NFAT-4 form repeating, cyclosporin-sensitive regulatory modules within the murine CD21 intronic control region. J Immunol 2002. 168: 3341-3350.

10. Ulgiati,D. and Holers,V.M., CR2/CD21 proximal promoter activity is critically dependent on a cell type-specific repressor. J Immunol. 2001. 167: 6912-6919.

11. Ulgiati,D., Pham,C., and Holers,V.M., Functional analysis of the human complement receptor 2 (CR2/CD21) promoter: characterization of basal transcriptional mechanisms. J Immunol 2002. 168: 6279-6285.

12. Tolnay,M., Lambris,J.D., and Tsokos,G.C., Transcriptional regulation of the complement receptor 2 gene: role of a heterogeneous nucler ribonucleoprotein. J.Immunol. 1997. 159: 5492-5501.

13. Tolnay,M., Vereshchagina,L.A., and Tsokos,G.C., Heterogeneous nuclear ribonucleoprotein D0B is a sequence-specific DNA- binding protein. Biochem.J 1999. 338: 417-425.

14. Zabel,M.D., Byrne,B.L., Weis,J.J., and Weis,J.H., Cell-specific expression of the murine CD21 gene depends on accessibility of promoter and intronic elements. J Immunol. 2000. 165: 4437-4445.

15. Zabel,M.D., Weis,J.J., and Weis,J.H., Lymphoid transcription of the murine CD21 gene is positively regulated by histone acetylation. J Immunol. 1999. 163: 2697-2703.

16. Vereshchagina,L.A., Tolnay,M., and Tsokos,G.C., Multiple transcription factors regulate the inducible expression of the human complement receptor 2 promoter. J Immunol. 2001. 166: 6156-6163.

17. Tolnay,M., Vereshchagina,L.A., and Tsokos,G.C., NF-kappaB regulates the expression of the human complement receptor 2 gene. J Immunol 2002. 169: 6236-6243.

18. Noti,J.D., Reinemann,B.C., and Petrus,M.N., Sp1 binds two sites in the CD11c promoter in vivo specifically in myeloid cells and cooperates with AP1 to activate transcription. Mol.Cell Biol 1996. 16: 2940-2950.

19. Chen,H.M., Pahl,H.L., Scheibe,R.J., Zhang,D.E., and Tenen,D.G., The Sp1 transcription factor binds the CD11b promoter specifically in myeloid cells in vivo and is essential for myeloid-specific promoter activity. J Biol Chem 1993. 268: 8230-8239.

20. Noti,J.D., Sp3 mediates transcriptional activation of the leukocyte integrin genes CD11C and CD11B and cooperates with c-Jun to activate CD11C. J Biol Chem 1997. 272: 24038-24045.

21. Lopez-Rodriguez,C., Delgado,M.D., Puig-Kroger,A., Nueda,A., Munoz,E., Leon,J., Bernabeu,C., and Corbi,A.L., c-Myc inhibits CD11a and CD11c leukocyte integrin promoters. Eur.J Immunol 2000. 30: 2465-2471.

22. Park,H., Shelley,C.S., and Arnaout,M.A., The zinc finger transcription factor ZBP-89 is a repressor of the human beta 2-integrin CD11b gene. Blood 2003. 101: 894-902.

23. Lopez-Rodriguez,C. and Corbi,A.L., PU.1 negatively regulates the CD11c integrin gene promoter through recognition of the major transcriptional start site. Eur.J Immunol 1997. 27: 1843-1847.

24. Panopoulos,A.D., Bartos,D., Zhang,L., and Watowich,S.S., Control of myeloid-specific integrin alpha Mbeta 2 (CD11b/CD18) expression by cytokines is regulated by Stat3-dependent activation of PU.1. J Biol Chem 2002. 277 : 19001-19007.
25. Lopez-Rodriguez,C., Zubiaur,M., Sancho,J., Concha,A., and Corbi,A.L., An octamer element functions as a regulatory element in the differentiation-responsive CD11c integrin gene promoter: OCT-2 inducibility during myelomonocytic differentiation. J Immunol 1997. 158: 5833-5840.
26. Noti,J.D., Reinemann,C., and Petrus,M.N., Regulation of the leukocyte integrin gene CD11c is mediated by AP1 and Ets transcription factors. Mol.Immunol 1996. 33: 115-127.
27. Rubio,M.A., Lopez-Rodriguez,C., Nueda,A., Aller,P., Armesilla,A.L., Vega,M.A., and Corbi,A.L., Granulocyte-macrophage colony-stimulating factor, phorbol ester, and sodium butyrate induce the CD11c integrin gene promoter activity during myeloid cell differentiation. Blood 1995. 86: 3715-3724.
28. Shelley,C.S., Teodoridis,J.M., Park,H., Farokhzad,O.C., Bottinger,E.P., and Arnaout,M.A., During differentiation of the monocytic cell line U937, Pur alpha mediates induction of the CD11c beta 2 integrin gene promoter. J Immunol 2002. 168: 3887-3893.
29. Corbi,A.L. and Lopez-Rodriguez,C., CD11c integrin gene promoter activity during myeloid differentiation. Leuk.Lymphoma 1997. 25: 415-425.
30. Zwirner,J., Gotze,O., Begemann,G., Kapp,A., Kirchhoff,K., and Werfel,T., Evaluation of C3a receptor expression on human leucocytes by the use of novel monoclonal antibodies. Immunology 1999. 97: 166-172.
31. Martin,U., Bock,D., Arseniev,L., Tornetta,M.A., Ames,R.S., Bautsch,W., Kohl,J., Ganser,A., and Klos,A., The human C3a receptor is expressed on neutrophils and monocytes, but not on B or T lymphocytes. J Exp.Med. 1997. 186: 199-207.
32. Nataf,S., Davoust,N., Ames,R.S., and Barnum,S.R., Human T cells express the C5a receptor and are chemoattracted to C5a. J Immunol 1999. 162: 4018-4023.
33. Werfel,T., Kirchhoff,K., Wittmann,M., Begemann,G., Kapp,A., Heidenreich,F., Gotze,O., and Zwirner,J., Activated human T lymphocytes express a functional C3a receptor. J Immunol 2000. 165: 6599-6605.
34. Fischer,W.H. and Hugli,T.E., Regulation of B cell functions by C3a and C3a(desArg): suppression of TNF-alpha, IL-6, and the polyclonal immune response. J Immunol 1997. 159: 4279-4286.
35. Kirchhoff,K., Weinmann,O., Zwirner,J., Begemann,G., Gotze,O., Kapp,A., and Werfel,T., Detection of anaphylatoxin receptors on CD83+ dendritic cells derived from human skin. Immunology 2001. 103: 210-217.
36. Reca,R., Mastellos,D., Majka,M., Marquez,L., Ratajczak,J., Franchini,S., Glodek,A., Honczarenko,M., Spruce,L.A., Janowska-Wieczorek,A., Lambris,J.D., and Ratajczak,M.Z., Functional receptor for C3a anaphylatoxin is expressed by normal hematopoietic stem/progenitor cells, and C3a enhances their homing- related responses to SDF-1. Blood 2003.
37. Schaefer,M., Konrad,S., Sohns,B., Hetfeld,B., Rheinheimer,C., Bautsch,W., and Klos,A., Transcriptional regulation of the human C3a-receptor: Ets-1 as one important factor. Abtracts of the 19th International Complement Workshop; 2002 Sept. 22-26, Palermo, Italy: Int.Immunopharmacol. 2002; 2: 1305-1305.
38. Collard,C.D., Bukusoglu,C., Agah,A., Colgan,S.P., Reenstra,W.R., Morgan,B.P., and Stahl,G.L., Hypoxia-induced expression of complement receptor type 1 (CR1, CD35) in human vascular endothelial cells. Am.J.Physiol. 1999. 276: C450-C458.

39. Lach-Trifilieff,E., Marfurt,J., Schwarz,S., Sadallah,S., and Schifferli,J.A., Complement receptor 1 (CD35) on human reticulocytes: normal expression in systemic lupus erythematosus and HIV-infected patients. J Immunol 1999. 162: 7549-7554.

40. Welters,I.D., Menzebach,A., Goumon,Y., Langefeld,T.W., Teschemacher,H., Hempelmann,G., and Stefano,G.B., Morphine suppresses complement receptor expression, phagocytosis, and respiratory burst in neutrophils by a nitric oxide and mu(3) opiate receptor-dependent mechanism. J Neuroimmunol. 2000. 111 : 139-145.

41. Boyd,A.W., Anderson,K.C., Freedman,A.S., Fisher,D.C., Slaughenhoupt,B., Schlossman,S.F., and Nadler,L.M., Studies of in vitro activation and differentiation of human B lymphocytes. I. Phenotypic and functional characterization of the B cell population responding to anti-Ig antibody. J.Immunol. 1985. 134: 1516-1523.

42. Takahashi,K., Kozono,Y., Waldschmidt,T.J., Berthiaume,D., Quigg,R.J., Baron,A., and Holers,V.M., Mouse complement receptor type 1 (CR1; CD35) and type 2 (CR2; CD21) expression on normal B cell subpopulations and decreased levels during the development of autoimmunity in MRL/lpr mice. J.Immunol. 1997. 159: 1557-1569.

43. Zhou,L.J., Smith,H.M., Waldschmidt,T.J., Schwarting,R., Daley,J., and Tedder,T.F., Tissue-specific expression of the human CD19 gene in transgenic mice inhibits antigen-independent B-lymphocyte development. Mol.Cell Biol 1994. 14: 3884-3894.

44. Arnaout,M.A., Wang,E.A., Clark,S.C., and Sieff,C.A., Human recombinant granulocyte-macrophage colony-stimulating factor increases cell-to-cell adhesion and surface expression of adhesion- promoting surface glycoproteins on mature granulocytes. J. Clin. Invest. 1986. 78:597-601.

45. Socinski,M.A., Cannistra,S.A., Sullivan,R., Elias,A., Antman,K., Schnipper,L., and Griffin,J.D., Granulocyte-macrophage colony-stimulating factor induces the expression of the CD11b surface adhesion molecule on human granulocytes in vivo. Blood 1988. 72: 691-697.

46. Kinhult,J., Egesten,A., Uddman,R., and Cardell,L.O., PACAP enhances the expression of CD11b, CD66b and CD63 in human neutrophils. Peptides 2002. 23: 1735-1739.

47. Wagner,C., Hansch,G.M., Stegmaier,S., Denefleh,B., Hug,F., and Schoels,M., The complement receptor 3, CR3 (CD11b/CD18), on T lymphocytes: activation-dependent up-regulation and regulatory function. Eur.J Immunol 2001. 31: 1173-1180.

48. Riedemann,N.C., Neff,T.A., Guo,R.F., Bernacki,K.D., Laudes,I.J., Sarma,J.V., Lambris,J.D., and Ward,P.A., Protective effects of IL-6 blockade in sepsis are linked to reduced C5a receptor expression. J Immunol 2003. 170 : 503-507.

49. Riedemann,N.C., Guo,R.F., Neff,T.A., Laudes,I.J., Keller,K.A., Sarma,V.J., Markiewski,M.M., Mastellos,D., Strey,C.W., Pierson,C.L., Lambris,J.D., Zetoune,F.S., and Ward,P.A., Increased C5a receptor expression in sepsis. J Clin. Invest. 2003. 170:503-507.

50. Stahel,P.F., Kariya,K., Shohami,E., Barnum,S.R., Eugster,H., Trentz,O., Kossmann,T., and Morganti-Kossmann,M.C., Intracerebral complement C5a receptor (CD88) expression is regulated by TNF and lymphotoxin-alpha following closed head injury in mice. J Neuroimmunol. 2000. 109: 164-172.

51. Drouin,S.M., Kildsgaard,J., Haviland,J., Zabner,J., Jia,H.P., McCray,P.B., Jr., Tack,B.F., and Wetsel,R.A., Expression of the complement anaphylatoxin C3a and C5a receptors on bronchial epithelial and smooth muscle cells in models of sepsis and asthma. J Immunol 2001. 166: 2025-2032.

52. Rodgaard,A., Thomsen,B.S., Bendixen,G., and Bendtzen,K., Increased expression of complement receptor type 1 (CR1, CD35) on human peripheral blood T lymphocytes after polyclonal activation in vitro. Immunol Res. 1995. 14: 69-76.

53. Saito,Y., Nakagawa,C., Uchida,H., Sasaki,F., and Sakakibara,H., Adrenomedullin suppresses fMLP-induced upregulation of CD11b of human neutrophils. Inflammation 2001. 25: 197-201.
54. Burg,M., Martin,U., Bock,D., Rheinheimer,C., Kohl,J., Bautsch,W., and Klos,A., Differential regulation of the C3a and C5a receptors (CD88) by IFN- gamma and PMA in U937 cells and related myeloblastic cell lines. J Immunol 1996. 157: 5574-5581.
55. Dempsey,P.W., Allison,M.E.D., Akkaraju,S., Goodnow,C.C., and Fearon,D.T., C3d of complement as a molecular adjuvant: bridging innate and acquired immunity. Science 1996. 271: 348-350.

PART 3

NOVEL REGULATORY ROLES
OF COMPLEMENT
IN HEALTH AND DISEASE

5

Coordination of Adaptive Immune Responses by C3

Anna Erdei[*°], Eszter Molnár[*], Eszter Csomor[*], Zsuzsa Bajtay[*] and József Prechl[°]

[*]Department of Immunology, and [°]Research Group of the Hungarian Academy of Sciences at the Department of Immunology, Eötvös Loránd University, Budapest, Hungary

Abstract: Once triggered, complement activation leads to the generation of various C3 degradation products. Receptors for these fragments are expressed by cells of both the innate and adaptive immune system, enabling complement activation to exert both indirect and direct effects on adaptive immune responses. The anaphylatoxin C3a recruits and primes granulocytes and macrophages and influence lymphocyte functions as well. C3 cleavage fragments covalently linked to the antigen influence its fate on the level of the organism and on the level of the cell as well. C3 receptors present on lymphocytes set the threshold for cellular activation and may thereby also shape the immune repertoire.

Key words: C3-fragments, C3-receptors, CR1, CR2, CR3, CR4, lymphocyte activation, antibody response, local synthesis

1. INTRODUCTION

The complement system provides a major defence mechanism against pathogens and plays an important role in inflammation and regulation of immune responses. The physiological role of complement components, their action on a wide variety of cell types continues to be a major field of interest. Activation of component C3 and consequent generation of various fragments is central and crucial not only in the course of the cascade but for most biological activities exerted by complement. Several of these functions are mediated by various receptors expressed on a wide variety of cell types, including cells of both the innate and adaptive immune systems.

2.   GENERATION OF LIGANDS FOR C3-RECEPTORS

During the cascade, limited proteolysis generates several biologically active fragments of C3. Cleavage of intact C3 produces C3a, a 77 amino acid long peptide, which is released from the amino terminus of the α-chain. The removal of this small molecule induces a conformational change in the larger fragment C3b, leading to the exposure of an internal thiolester-group. This short-lived "nascent" C3b molecule is highly reactive with nucleophiles, such as water, hydroxyl and amino groups. Consequently it may attach covalently to suitable placed acceptor surfaces, or will be hydrolysed in the fluid phase [1]. Covalently fixed C3b may be degraded by factor I in the presence of cofactors, resulting in surface-bound iC3b and further cleavage generates C3dg, and C3d fragments [2]. Thus activation of complement results in cells or particles bearing C3b, iC3b and C3dg/C3d fragments, forming the ligands for various receptors (Fig.1 and Table I). All the receptor-binding sites are localized on the α-chain of C3.

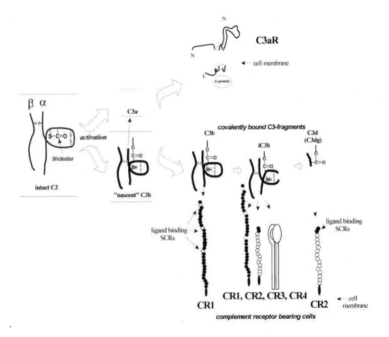

Figure 1. C3 receptors and their ligands; generation of C3-fragments

3.   RECEPTORS FOR C3-DERIVED FRAGMENTS

3.1   Receptor for C3a

The smaller degradation product C3a has the ability to activate serosal type mast cells and basophils, to cause smooth muscle contraction, to enhance vascular permeability, and acts as chemoattractant for macrophages, neutrophils, activated lymphocytes, basophils and mast cells. Understanding the molecular features of the interaction between anaphylatoxins and different cell types was greatly facilitated by cloning the structurally related receptors for C5a (C5aR, CD88) [3] and C3a (C3aR) [4,5,6]. These receptors belong to the family of G_i-protein coupled seven membrane-spanning receptors ("rhodopsin subfamily"), however, human C3aR has unique structural characteristics compared with most other G-protein coupled molecules, since it has glycosylation sites at the N-terminal end and in the large second extracellular loop (Fig.1). Receptors for C3a are found on a wide variety of cell types including neutrophils, basophils, monocytes, T lymphocytes, mast cells, eosinophils and neurons, suggesting an even more diverse function of C3a than previously believed.

3.2   Receptors Interacting with Covalently-Bound C3 Fragments

The larger products of component C3 - such as C3b, iC3b, C3dg (Fig.1) - are involved in several effector functions and regulatory immune processes, including phagocytosis, antibody responses, cytotoxic reactions and immunomodulation. Probably the most important receptor-mediated functions of complement are the activation of various complement receptor bearing cells and uptake and localization of opsonized particles.

3.2.1   Complement Receptor Type 1 (CR1, CD35)

This single-chain protein binds C3b and C4b with high affinity and, as a cell membrane receptor, it is involved in the regulation of complement activation. Like all members of the RCA (Regulators of Complement Activation) family this molecule also contains repeated structures called SCR (Short Consensus Repeats). Human CR1 has four polymorphic forms containing up to 34 SCRs. The extracellular part of the common form of CR1 is composed of 30 tandemly arranged SCR-domains. These repeats are organized into four groups - also called *long homologous repeats* - LHR - (each having seven repetead structures SCRs), with two additional SCRs.

The ligand binding sites are located on the second SCR in the first three LHRs, providing the basis for multivalent interaction with C3b- and C4b-coated cells and particles (Fig.1). As soluble CR1 it also occurs in the plasma and in urine. For summary see [7].

3.2.1.1   The Functions of CR1

CR1 is present on primate erythrocytes, monocytes/macrophages, eosinophils, neutrophils, follicular dendritic cells and on T and B lymphocytes. In addition to its role in controlling complement activation this receptor has several other important functions. On macrophages and polymorphonuclear cells it serves as an opsonin-receptor, providing a major defence mechanisms against systemic bacterial and fungal infections. CR1 found on erythrocytes serves as a vehicle for the transport and clearance of immune complexes. By trapping complement-coated immune complexes, CR1 expressed on FDC in lymph nodes and spleen helps to maintain immunological memory. The role of CD35 in lymphocyte activation will be discussed later in this chapter.

3.2.2   Complement Receptor Type 2 (CR2, CD21)

In humans two isoforms of this single chain glycoprotein have been described: the well-characterized short form of CR2 (CD21) which comprises 15 SCRs and the recently reported long CR2 (CD21L) containing an additional exon (10a); for summary see [8]. The shorter isoform is expressed on B-lymphocytes, activated T-cells cells and epithelial cells, but not on monocytes/macrophages, granulocytes and erythrocytes. The longer CR2 isoform appears to be expressed exclusively on human FDC. The ligand binding site of CD21 resides in the first two SCRs. It binds iC3b, C3dg and C3d with high affinity and also reacts with interferon α, CD23 and the Epstein-Barr virus (EBV). Human and mouse CR1 and CR2 proteins are homologous. However, while human CR1 and CR2 are products of separate genes, in mice these two molecules are formed by the alternative splicing of exons encoding the C3b/C4b binding sites (see more details later).

3.2.2.1   The Functions of CR2

Probably the most important physiological function of CR2 - as it will be discussed later - is its involvement in B-cell activation by the association with CD19 and TAPA-1 on the surface of these cells. Like CR1, CR2 on FDC has been shown to trap immune complexes in germinal centers, most probably playing a role in the development of B-cell memory. CR2 is also the receptor for EBV, enabling the virus to enter B-cells without the involvement of complement. By interacting with CD23, the low affinity receptor for IgE, CR2 may be involved in regulation of IgE production, as well [9].

3.2.3   CD46 (MCP)

The human membrane cofactor protein (MCP) contains 4 SCRs and binds C3b [10]. In addition to its regulatory role it is involved in T cell activation and serves as receptor to several pathogens including measles virus and herpes virus 6 [11].

3.2.4   Murine CR1/2 and Crry

It has to be pointed out that human and mouse receptors CR1 and CR2 are not identical. In contrast to men, where separate genes code for these two cell membrane molecules, in murine systems type 1 and type 2 complement receptors (mCR1/2, CD35/CD21) are encoded by a single gene, mCr2 and alternative splicing gives rise to the two products. In mice type 1 complement receptor (mCR1) comprises 21 SCR, while mCR2 is identical to mCR1 except that it lacks the first 6 SCRs [12;13;14]. Thus it is these N terminal 6 SCRs, which endow mCR1 with activities characteristic of hCR1, namely binding C3b and exerting cofactor activity [15]. Since it is the membrane proximal, transmembrane and intracytoplasmic regions that are shared, the two receptors are likely to associate with the same membrane and cytoplasmic proteins. The C3d binding region is located in the N terminal two SCRs of CR2 [16] while the first two SCR in CR1 are responsible for C3b binding [17].

In mice and rats an additional complement receptor-related gene product, Crry is also expressed. This membrane-bound regulator containing 5 (in mice) or 6-7 (in rats) SCR has similar role to MCP and DAF - as its expression is necessary to resist spontaneous complement attack [18].

3.2.5   Complement Receptor Type 3 (CR3, CD11b/CD18, Mac-1)

CR3 is a heterodimer containing the 165 kD α-chain (CD11b) and the 95 kD β-chain (CD18). The latter polypeptide is identical with the β-chains of LFA-1 and p150.95, the related leukocyte integrins (also named β2-integrins). It is the α-chain of the receptor that posseses the binding site for iC3b and to lesser extent to C3b and C3dg. Binding of the ligands to the integrins is calcium-dependent [19,20].

3.2.5.1   The Functions of CR3

CR3 is expressed on several cell types including all myeloid lineage cells, NK cells some B cells and DCs. Unlike the interaction between C3b and CR1, binding of iC3b to CR3 is sufficient on its own to initiate phagocytosis. In addition to binding iC3b, CR3 is one of the major adhesion molecules expressed by phagocytes. Like LFA-1, it interacts with ICAM-1, as well. It has a lectin-binding capacity and interacts with carbohydrates of other membrane constituents [21]. Triggering of CR3 via its lectin-site results in oxydative burst in phagocytes - a process where CR3 promotes transmembrane signalling by interacting with GPI-anchored membrane glycoproteins such as CD14, CD87 and FcγRIII [22]. By binding to ICAM-1, CR3 enhances the adhesion of monocytes and neutrophils to the endothelium in the absence of complement proteins and facilitates the accumulation of these cells at sites of tissue injury. CR3 on NK cells is involved in cytotoxic reactions by its dual ligation [23].

3.2.6   Complement Receptor Type 4 (CR4, CD11c/CD18)

CR4 is similar in structure to other integrins. It is also a heterodimer, containing the 150 kDa α-chain (CD11c) and the β-chain, which is identical to that of CR3. Its ligand specificity and tissue distribution are similar to those of CR3, i.e. it is expressed mainly on myeloid cells. In addition to iC3b it also has other ligands, and binds to ICAM-1 (Table 1.) Recently CR4+ DC were shown to play an important role in CTL responses to infection with the intracellular bacterium Listeria Monocytogenes [24].

4.   LOCAL SYNTHESIS OF COMPLEMENT C3

The major source of circulating complement is the liver, however many other cells are able to produce some or all of the complement components, leading to higher local concentrations. Several cell types have been shown to synthesize C3, such as monocytes and macrophages, glomerular and tubular cells in the kidney, epithelial cells in the lung and intestine, endothelial cells, fibroblasts, synovial cells, adipocytes, brain cells, keratinocytes, kidney glomerular mesangial cells [25,26,27,28]. Locally produced complement usually exerts a beneficial effect in inflammatory events [29] and may be involved in immunoregulatory processes as well (i.e. in germinal centers). Most of the cells secreting complement proteins can be stimulated via their complement receptors, resulting in a positive feedback that may enhance local immune defence.

Table 1. Complement receptors binding C3 degradation products

Type	Ligand	Structure, Mw	Distribution	Function
CR1 (CD35)	C3b>C4b>iC3b	single chain, 160-260 kDa glycoprotein, 4 allotypes, contains (28-34 SCR)	monocytes, macrophages, neutrophils, eosinophils, primate erythrocytes, podocytes, B-cells, T-cell FDC	immune adherence, phagocytosis, IC clearance, IC localization in germinal centres, control of complement activation, regulation of B cell activation
CR2 (CD21)	C3dg>C3d, iC3b, IFNα EBV, CD23	single chain glycoprotein, two isoforms: *CD21S*:145 kDa, (15 SCR), *CD21L* (16 SCR)	B-cells, activated T-cells, epithelial cells, basophils, mast cells, FDC	B cell activation, IC localization in germinal centres, rescue of germinal center cells
CR1/2 (CD21/35) in mice	C3dg, C3d, C3b, iC3b	single chain glycoproteins, alternative splicing results in CR2, 145 kDa (16 SCR) CR1, 180 kDa (21 SCR)	B-cells, activated T-cells, epithelial cells, basophils, mast cells, FDC	B- and T-cell activation, IC localization in germinal centres, rescue of germinal center cells
CR3 (CD11b/ CD18) (Mac-1, OKM-1,)	iC3b factor X, ICAM-1, fibrinogen, LPS, carbohydrates	heterodimer of glycoproteins α-chain:165 kDa, β-chain:95 kDa	monocytes, macrophages, neutrophils, NK cells, B cells, T_C cells, mast cells, DC, FDC	phagocytosis, adhesion, promoting signal transduction, oxidative burst, NK cytotoxicity
CR4 (CD11c/ CD18) (p150.95)	iC3b, ICAM-1, fibrinogen, denatured proteins	heterodimer of glycoproteins α-chain:150 kDa, β-chain:95 kDa	monocytes, macrophages, neutrophils, NK cells, activated B cells, T_C cells, mast cells, DC	phagocytosis, adhesion, T cell functions,
C3aR	C3a	single chain, 54 kDa, G-protein linked, contains seven transmembrane segments	mast cells, basophils, neutrophils, monocytes lymphocytes, astrocytes, neurons	increasing vascular permeability, triggering serosal type mast cells, recruiting leukocytes, smooth muscle contraction
CD46	C3b/C4b, Measles virus Herpes virus 6, *Streptococcus Neisseria*	4 SCR	all cell types	protection of host cells, T-cell activation
Crry (in mice and rats)	C3b/C4b	4 SCR (mice) 6-7 (rat)	all cell types	protection of host cells

4.1   Macrophages

Several studies have shown the advantages of the local synthesis of C3 and C4 by splenic macrophages. Complement C3 has been shown to play an important role in the process of local opsonization, leading to more efficient phagocytosis of various pathogens [30]. Mice with a disrupted C4 (C4 -/-) or C3 (C3 -/-) locus have an impaired humoral response to T-dependent antigens, characterized by a reduced number and smaller size of germinal centers and by an reduced retention of antigen by FDC. The reconstitution of deficient animals with enriched fraction of wild-type bone marrow-derived macrophages however, led to the rescue of the humoral response [31,32].

4.2   Kidney

Recently many studies have demonstrated that the kidney is a main source of extrahepatic complement [33,34,35]. In the normal human kidney, the expression and the ratio of components of the classical and alternative activation pathways may vary depending on the anatomical site [36]. Factor D and properdin is expressed mainly in the glomeruli, whilst factor B expression localizes in the medulla. C2, C3 and C4 components and the factor H arise predominantly from the cortical tubule-rich region. C1q is similarly expressed in all fractions. Timmerman et al. described that many of these molecules, like C2, C3, C4, factor B and factor H, are present also in fetal human kidneys, suggesting a role during renal development [37].

Recently several publications emphasized the beneficial role of extrahepatic complement synthesis [29]. It is interesting to point out that while the kidney is a major source of complement proteins, the expression of regulatory molecules in the glomerular and tubular cells is very low. This may result in the vulnerability of the kidney and could be one of the causes of renal diseases and allograft rejection [26,34]. Furthermore, it has also been shown that immunecomplexes upregulate the expression of component C3 by human mesangial cells, leading to the encancement of inflammation [38].

The important role of locally synthesized C3 in renal transplantation was demonstrated in experiments where kidneys from C3-negative or C3-positive donors were transplanted. The results showed that transplantation from C3-positive donor into C3-negative recipient leads to acute rejection, while C3-deficient grafts were not acutely rejected. This emphasizes the importance of locally synthesized in contrast to circulating complement [33].

5. INDIRECT EFFECTS OF C3 ON THE ADAPTIVE RESPONSES

5.1 Induction of Cytokine Secretion by Cells of the Innate Immune System Via C3 Receptors

Table 2 lists some of the known effects of C3 on cytokine secretion by monocytes and macrophages. Complement-coated antigens were shown to suppress the production of pro-inflammatory cytokines, IL-6, IL-12 and TNFα by several authors. Bacle et al. reported the induction of IL-1 production by human monocytes upon stimulation by C3b and C3d [39]. Another study using UV-exposed human skin monocytes demonstrated IL-10 production induced by iC3b [40].

Table 2. Effects of C3-derived fragments on cytokine production

Cell type	Ligand	Effect	Reference
Human monocytes	soluble polimerized human C3b and C3d	induction of IL-1 production	[39]
Human peripheral whole blood cells	immune complexes	induction of IL-10 production	[43]
Human UV exposed skin Mo/Mph	iC3b	induction of IL-10 production	[40]
Human UV exposed skin Mo/Mph	iC3b	suppression of IL-12 mRNA and peptide production	[40]
Human monocytes	iC3b, anti-CD11b, anti-CD18	suppression of IL-12 production	[44]
In vivo experiments with mice	anti-CD11b, anti-CD18	suppression of IL-12 production	[44]
Human peripheral whole blood cells	immune complexes	suppression of IC induced TNFα production	[43]

Viruses were also shown to play a role in the anti-inflammatory events mediated by complement receptors. The well-known immunosuppressive effect of measles virus is associated with the decreased IL-12 production of monocytes, macrophages and dendritic cells. This effect is caused by the cross-linking of the C3b- and C4b-binding surface molecule, CD46 (MCP) by the virion. [41]. Epstein-Barr virus (EBV), which binds to CD21 (CR2) down-regulates the production of IL-1, IL-6, IL-12 and TNF-α by macrophages both in vivo and in vitro [42].

5.2   B Cell Response

The importance of complement in immune responses against T cell dependent antigens was proven by certain experiments using mAb-s against complement components or soluble complement receptors [45,46,47]. Immunization of complement-deficient animals confirmed these observations [48,49,50]. Using the model antigen hen egg lysozyme (HEL), fused to murine C3d molecule, lead to increased antigen-specific response and antigens bearing two or three copies of C3d were found to be 1000- and 10000- fold more immunogenic than HEL alone [51]. C3b has also been shown to increase antibody response when coupled to antigen [52]. These data show that complement components covalently bound to the surface of antigens may directly enhance BCR signalling. On the other hand the interaction of complement receptors with activated complement components may facilitate the formation of germinal centres (GC). Antigen uptake, processing and the presentation by antigen-presenting cells (APC) to T cells are required for the development of an efficient immune response. The most effective APC-s are dendritic cells, macrophages and B cells, all of which express high levels of class I and class II MHC molecules, and are able to internalize and present antigens to T cells. Opsonization of antigen by complement fragments leads to targeting to CR1/2 expressing cells, like FDC and capturing the antigen by the latter leads to increased GC formation, even if limited amount of antigen is administered. In mice deficient in CR1/2 or in complement components, fewer and smaller GCs were observed than in normal mice, and less antigen could be detected on the surface of FDCs [48;49]. To separate the effect of CR1/2 on B cells and on FDCs, bone marrow chimeric mice were generated by grafting wild-type bone marrow into sub lethally irradiated Cr2-/- mice. After immunization with a T-dependent antigen the primary and secondary antibody responses were monitored. CR1/2 on FDC proved to be important in follicular trapping of IC and GC formation, in B cell maturation to Ig-secreting or memory B cells, and in the maintenance of long-lasting antibody titers during immune responses [53,54].

Several bacteria and viruses induce B cell response without T cell help. These TI antigens can be divided to two groups; TI-1 antigens, which lead to B cell activation without secondary signals, and TI-2 antigens, which need T-cell help for B cell activation.

The splenic marginal zone is a specialized lymphoid compartment, which plays an important role in initiation of immune response against TI-2 antigens. Marginal zone B cells, which carry high levels of CR1/2, can respond rapidly to blood-borne antigens, generating IgM-producing plasmablasts, because of their multireactivity and low activation threshold [55,56].

Antibody response against Group B Streptococcus was found impaired in mice deficient in C3 or CD21/CD35. When immunized, deficient mice showed impaired antigen localization in marginal zone, lower Ag-specific IgM levels, lack of isotype switch, and decreased uptake of capsular polysaccharide antigens by FDCs as compared to wild-type mice. These data suggest, that the normal immune response requires C3 mediated targeting of antigen to the marginal zone and to FDCs [57].

Production of virus-neutralizing IgM and IgG by marginal zone B cells was studied in C3-/- mice after immunization with live and non-replicating vesicular stomatitis virus, a TI-1 type antigen. The results of these experiments suggest that complement plays a role in targeting antigen to CR3 and CR4 expressing macrophages in the marginal zone, facilitating the T-cell independent activation of marginal zone B cells [58].

5.3   T Cell Response

The role of complement in T cell responses was studied using C3-/- and Cr2-/- mice, infected with influenza virus. Priming of T-helper and T-cytotoxic cells and production of IFN were impaired in C3-deficient, but not in Cr2-deficient mice [59]. Studies carried out with C3-/-, Cr2-/- and wild-type mice immunized with lymphocytic choriomeningitis virus (LCMV) also revealed that C3 activity is required for optimal expansion of the virus specific effector CD8 T cells while it is not dependent upon CR1/2 [60].

6.   DIRECT EFFECTS VIA C3 RECEPTORS ON LYMPHOCYTES

6.1   B Lymphocytes

6.1.1   Role of CD35 on B cells

While CR1 on mouse B cells plays similar role as CR2, in humans CD35 seems to have different function. Our experiments with human B cells and the natural ligand C3 suggest that CR1 clustering mediates inhibition, counteracting with BCR mediated signals [61]. These data suggest that human CR1 provides an additional level of regulation, and depending on the degradation stage of C3 either CR1-mediated inhibition or CR2-mediated enhancement of B-cell proliferation may take place. As CD35 possesses a short cytoplasmic tail its signaling ability probably depends on the clustering of other molecules on the B-cell surface.

6.1.2   The CD21/CD19/CD81 Co-Receptor Complex

CR2 associates with two transmembrane molecules on the surface of both human and murine B cells: CD19 and CD81. The receptor complex so formed has been extensively studied with respect to its ability to positively modulate signaling through the B-cell antigen receptor. This property may be related to the prolonged presence of BCR in lipid rafts when co-ligated with CR2 [62]. Besides this co-receptor function the complex also mediates presentation of the ligands of CR2. Although uptake of antigen via CR2 enhances antigen presentation in vitro, the in vivo relevance and possible outcome of such a process is not known. B cells require the involvement of the BCR in the antigen uptake in order to become activated and potent antigen presenting cells. Uptake of C3d coated antigen is most efficient when it co-ligates BCR and CR2 [63,64].

The role of the co-receptor complex is underlined by the fact that genetic disruption of the respective genes results in abnormal B cell development and maturation. To date three independent clones of CR1/2 deficient mice have been created [48,50,49] all displaying impaired humoral immune responses as a common feature.

6.1.3   The CD21/CD35 Complex

CR2 has been reported to associate with CD35 without CD19 [65]. The role of such a CR1-CR2 complex might be the capture and/or internalization of C3b/iC3b/C3dg coated antigen[66]. CR2 is capable of transducing signals on its own [67,68], thus such complexes may also modulate activation of the B cell.

6.2   T Lymphocytes

Despite the fact, that T cells do not generally carry complement receptors there are several reports showing subpopulations or activation states of T cells with CR expression. In addition to CR1, CR2 and CR3, regulatory receptors like CD46, CD55 and Crry were also shown to modulate T-cell function. Moreover, the small activation fragment C3a had also been reported to effect T cell activity.

6.2.1   Putative Functions of CD21 on T Cells

CR2 was first demonstrated to be present on human T cells and thymocytes (reviewed in [69]). Whether its function and isoform is the same as that of CR2 on B cells is still unknown. Recent studies imply that it may be an intracellular or „occult" antigen [70]. Interestingly the percentage of CR2 positive T cells in umbilical cord blood is significantly higher than that in adult peripheral blood [71].

Recently APCs such as B-lymphocytes and macrophages bearing covalently fixed C3-fragments had been shown to enhance the proliferation of antigen-specific T-cells. The expression of CR1/2 on activated T-cells had been demonstrated and its role in the enhanced proliferation was suggested [72]. More recent studies confirmed that CR2+ T cells appear under pathological conditions like kidney transplantation [33,73].

As T lymphocytes do not express CD19, CR2 on these cells should use other means to signal. Although proteins that associate with CR2 on human T cells have been detected [74], it is more likely that CR2 affects T-cell activation indirectly by promoting adhesion to antigen presenting cells which are covered by C3 split products [72].

6.2.2   Role of Regulatory C3 Receptors (CD46 and Crry) on T Cells

That human CD46, a widely expressed regulatory receptor for C3b, has pro-proliferative signaling properties - besides its pathogen and complement binding function - was suggested by Astier et al. [75]. Interestingly, co-engagement of CD3 and CD46 on human CD4+ T cells in the presence of IL-2 induces a regulatory phenotype with IL-10 production [76]. Transgenic human CD46 isoforms can also modulate murine T-cell function [77]. Crry – a regulatory receptor unique to rodents – was also shown to possess co-stimulatory properties on murine T cells [78] and rat thymocytes [79]. Thus, activation of the complement cascade may directly influence the fate of T cells and thereby help in fine-tuning of the immune response.

7.   THE ROLE OF C3 IN SHAPING THE LYMPHOCYTE REPERTOIRE

Of the maximal theoretical repertoire attainable by recombination of V, D, J segments and hypermutation, lymphocytes in a given individual use a more limited set of antigen receptors. This repertoire of receptors is the result of the combined selection forces determined by the genetic makeup of the individual and environmental factors. The former sets the framework for selecting the clones with the potential of interacting with self cells without injuring them, the latter creates or deletes clones thereby forming an immunological imprint reflecting encounters with various antigens during the lifetime of the individual.

Complement component C3, as discussed above, can influence the activation of B and T lymphocytes by several means. The direct evidence that complement takes part in shaping the B cell repertoire comes from experiments with Cr2-/- mice. The B1 subset of B cells is regarded as a self-replenishing population responsible both for natural and self-reactive antibody production. Genetic disruption of the Cr2 gene has been reported to result in the reduction of the number of B1 cells [48]. This reduction seems to specially affect the subset of cells producing tissue injuring antibodies [80,81]. On the other hand, if transgenic CR2 is expressed prematurely – during the pro-B cell stage instead of the immature stage – B-cell development will be abnormal, with reduced numbers of functional mature B cells [82].

Besides its role in aiding the formation of the normal mature B cell repertoire, C3 is also of crucial importance during the generation of humoral immune responses. Direct evidence that the attachment of C3 split products to the antigen enhances humoral responses comes from experiments with recombinant proteins [83], chemically engineered constructs [84]and naked DNA vaccines [85]. In a similar manner humoral responses can be improved by conjugating antigen to antibodies recognizing CR2 [86]. Antibody dependent enhancement of humoral responses is also dependent on complement and CR2 in the case of IgM and IgG3 [87;88;89].

In summary, complement component C3 exerts its effects on the adaptive immune system from the stage of lymphocyte development through the regulation of expansion to the maintenance of long-term antibody responses. Although the effects of ligand binding to complement receptors have been characterized at the cellular level, and animal studies confirm the importance of an intact complement system for normal immune reactions, there is still a gap in our understanding of several complement-mediated in vivo immunological phenomena. Present and future studies investigating cellular interactions at the level of organs and organisms will allow complement directed genetic and pharmacological interventions in various pathologies.

8.   REFERENCES

1.   Law,S.K. and Dodds,A.W., The internal thioester and the covalent binding properties of the complement proteins C3 and C4. Protein Sci. 1997; 6:263-274.
2.   Ross,G.D., Lambris,J.D., Cain,J.A., and Newman,S.L., Generation of three different fragments of bound C3 with purified factor I or serum. I. Requirements for factor H vs CR1 cofactor activity. J.Immunol. 1982; 129:2051-2060.
3.   Gerard,N.P. and Gerard,C., The chemotactic receptor for human C5a anaphylatoxin. Nature 1991; 349:614-617.
4.   Ames,R.S., Li,Y., Sarau,H.M., Nuthulaganti,P., Foley,J.J., Ellis,C., Zeng,Z., Su,K., Jurewicz,A.J., Hertzberg,R.P., Bergsma,D.J., and Kumar,C., Molecular cloning and characterization of the human anaphylatoxin C3a receptor. J.Biol.Chem. 1996; 271: 20231-20234.
5.   Crass,T., Raffetseder,U., Martin,U., Grove,M., Klos,A., Kohl,J., and Bautsch,W., Expression cloning of the human C3a anaphylatoxin receptor (C3aR) from differentiated U-937 cells. Eur.J.Immunol. 1996;26: 1944-1950.
6.   Ember,J.A. and Hugli,T.E., Complement factors and their receptors. Immunopharmacology 1997; 38: 3-15.
7.   Moreley,B.J. and Walport,M.J., The Complement Facts Book. 2000. 136-145.
8.   Moreley,B.J. and Walport,M.J., The Complement Facts Book. 2000. 146-152.
9.   Bonnefoy,J.Y., Lecoanet-Henchoz,S., Gauchat,J.F., Graber,P., Aubry,J.P., Jeannin,P., and Plater-Zyberk,C., Structure and functions of CD23. Int.Rev.Immunol. 1997; 16: 113-128.
10. Lublin,D.M., Liszewski,M.K., Post,T.W., Arce,M.A., Le Beau,M.M., Rebentisch,M.B., Lemons,L.S., Seya,T., and Atkinson,J.P., Molecular cloning and chromosomal localization of human membrane cofactor protein (MCP). Evidence for inclusion in the multigene family of complement-regulatory proteins. J.Exp.Med. 1988; 168:181-194.
11. Liszewski,M.K., Farries,T.C., Lublin,D.M., Rooney,I.A., and Atkinson,J.P., Control of the complement system. Adv.Immunol. 1996. 61:201-83.: 201-283.
12. Fingeroth,J.D., Benedict,M.A., Levy,D.N., and Strominger,J.L., Identification of murine complement receptor type 2. Proc.Natl.Acad.Sci.U.S.A 1989. 86: 242-246.
13. Kurtz,C.B., O'Toole,E., Christensen,S.M., and Weis,J.H., The murine complement receptor gene family. IV. Alternative splicing of Cr2 gene transcripts predicts two distinct gene products that share homologous domains with both human CR2 and CR1. J.Immunol. 1990. 144: 3581-3591.
14. Molina,H., Kinoshita,T., Inoue,K., Carel,J.C., and Holers,V.M., A molecular and immunochemical characterization of mouse CR2. Evidence for a single gene model of mouse complement receptors 1 and 2. J.Immunol. 1990. 145: 2974-2983.
15. Kinoshita,T., Takeda,J., Hong,K., Kozono,H., Sakai,H., and Inoue,K., Monoclonal antibodies to mouse complement receptor type 1 (CR1). Their use in a distribution study showing that mouse erythrocytes and platelets are CR1-negative. J.Immunol. 1988. 140: 3066-3072.
16. Pramoonjago,P., Takeda,J., Kim,Y.U., Inoue,K., and Kinoshita,T., Ligand specificities of mouse complement receptor types 1 (CR1) and 2 (CR2) purified from spleen cells. Int.Immunol. 1993. 5: 337-343.
17. Molina,H., Kinoshita,T., Webster,C.B., and Holers,V.M., Analysis of C3b/C3d binding sites and factor I cofactor regions within mouse complement receptors 1 and 2. J.Immunol. 1994. 153: 789-795.

18. Miwa,T., Zhou,L., Hilliard,B., Molina,H., and Song,W.C., Crry, but not CD59 and DAF, is indispensable for murine erythrocyte protection in vivo from spontaneous complement attack. Blood 2002. 99: 3707-3716.

19. Lee,J.O., Rieu,P., Arnaout,M.A., and Liddington,R., Crystal structure of the A domain from the alpha subunit of integrin CR3 (CD11b/CD18). Cell 1995. 80: 631-638.

20. Goodman,T.G. and Bajt,M.L., Identifying the putative metal ion-dependent adhesion site in the beta2 (CD18) subunit required for alphaLbeta2 and alphaMbeta2 ligand interactions. J.Biol.Chem. 1996. 271: 23729-23736.

21. Hogg,N., Roll, roll, roll your leucocyte gently down the vein... Immunol.Today 1992. 13: 113-115.

22. Petty,H.R. and Todd,R.F., III, Integrins as promiscuous signal transduction devices. Immunol.Today 1996. 17: 209-212.

23. Thornton,B.P., Vetvicka,V., and Ross,G.D., Function of C3 in a humoral response: iC3b/C3dg bound to an immune complex generated with natural antibody and a primary antigen promotes antigen uptake and the expression of co-stimulatory molecules by all B cells, but only stimulates immunoglobulin synthesis by antigen-specific B cells. Clin.Exp.Immunol. 1996. 104: 531-537.

24. Jung,S., Unutmaz,D., Wong,P., Sano,G., De los,S.K., Sparwasser,T., Wu,S., Vuthoori,S., Ko,K., Zavala,F., Pamer,E.G., Littman,D.R., and Lang,R.A., In vivo depletion of CD11c(+) dendritic cells abrogates priming of CD8(+) T cells by exogenous cell-associated antigens. Immunity. 2002. 17: 211-220.

25. Andrews,P.A., Zhou,W., and Sacks,S.H., Tissue synthesis of complement as an immune regulator. Mol.Med.Today 1995. 1: 202-207.

26. Sacks,S. and Zhou,W., The effect of locally synthesised complement on acute renal allograft rejection. J.Mol.Med. 2003. .:

27. Thomas,A., Gasque,P., Vaudry,D., Gonzalez,B., and Fontaine,M., Expression of a complete and functional complement system by human neuronal cells in vitro. Int.Immunol. 2000. 12: 1015-1023.

28. Marsh,J.E., Zhou,W., and Sacks,S.H., Local tissue complement synthesis--fine tuning a blunt instrument. Arch.Immunol.Ther.Exp.(Warsz.) 2001. 49 Suppl 1:S41-6.: S41-S46.

29. Laufer,J., Katz,Y., and Passwell,J.H., Extrahepatic synthesis of complement proteins in inflammation. Mol.Immunol. 2001. 38: 221-229.

30. Ezekowitz,R.A., Sim,R.B., Hill,M., and Gordon,S., Local opsonization by secreted macrophage complement components. Role of receptors for complement in uptake of zymosan. J.Exp.Med. 1984. 159: 244-260.

31. Gadjeva,M., Verschoor,A., Brockman,M.A., Jezak,H., Shen,L.M., Knipe,D.M., and Carroll,M.C., Macrophage-derived complement component C4 can restore humoral immunity in C4-deficient mice. J.Immunol. 2002. 169: 5489-5495.

32. Fischer,M.B., Ma,M., Hsu,N.C., and Carroll,M.C., Local synthesis of C3 within the splenic lymphoid compartment can reconstitute the impaired immune response in C3-deficient mice. J.Immunol. 1998. 160: 2619-2625.

33. Pratt,J.R., Basheer,S.A., and Sacks,S.H., Local synthesis of complement component C3 regulates acute renal transplant rejection. Nat.Med. 2002. 8: 582-587.

34. Zhou,W., Marsh,J.E., and Sacks,S.H., Intrarenal synthesis of complement. Kidney Int. 2001. 59: 1227-1235.

35. Tang,S., Zhou,W., Sheerin,N.S., Vaughan,R.W., and Sacks,S.H., Contribution of renal secreted complement C3 to the circulating pool in humans. J.Immunol. 1999. 162: 4336-4341.

36. Song,D., Zhou,W., Sheerin,S.H., and Sacks,S.H., Compartmental localization of complement component transcripts in the normal human kidney. Nephron 1998. 78: 15-22.

37. Timmerman,J.J., van der Woude,F.J., Gijlswijk-Janssen,D.J., Verweij,C.L., van Es,L.A., and Daha,M.R., Differential expression of complement components in human fetal and adult kidneys. Kidney Int. 1996. 49: 730-740.

38. Timmerman,J.J., Gijlswijk-Janssen,D.J., Van Der Kooij,S.W., van Es,L.A., and Daha,M.R., Antigen-antibody complexes enhance the production of complement component C3 by human mesangial cells. J.Am.Soc.Nephrol. 1997. 8: 1257-1265.

39. Bacle,F., Haeffner-Cavaillon,N., Laude,M., Couturier,C., and Kazatchkine,M.D., Induction of IL-1 release through stimulation of the C3b/C4b complement receptor type one (CR1, CD35) on human monocytes. J.Immunol. 1990. 144: 147-152.

40. Yoshida,Y., Kang,K., Berger,M., Chen,G., Gilliam,A.C., Moser,A., Wu,L., Hammerberg,C., and Cooper,K.D., Monocyte induction of IL-10 and down-regulation of IL-12 by iC3b deposited in ultraviolet-exposed human skin. J.Immunol. 1998. 161: 5873-5879.

41. Karp,C.L., Measles: immunosuppression, interleukin-12, and complement receptors. Immunol.Rev. 1999. 168: 91-101.

42. D'Addario,M., Ahmad,A., Morgan,A., and Menezes,J., Binding of the Epstein-Barr virus major envelope glycoprotein gp350 results in the upregulation of the TNF-alpha gene expression in monocytic cells via NF-kappaB involving PKC, PI3-K and tyrosine kinases. J.Mol.Biol. 2000. 298: 765-778.

43. Yentis,S.M., Gooding,R.P., and Riches,P.G., The effects of IgG and immune complexes on the endotoxin-induced cytokine response. Cytokine 1994. 6: 247-254.

44. Marth,T. and Kelsall,B.L., Regulation of interleukin-12 by complement receptor 3 signaling. J.Exp.Med. 1997. 185: 1987-1995.

45. Heyman,B., Wiersma,E.J., and Kinoshita,T., In vivo inhibition of the antibody response by a complement receptor- specific monoclonal antibody. J.Exp.Med. 1990. 172: 665-668.

46. Hebell,T., Ahearn,J.M., and Fearon,D.T., Suppression of the immune response by a soluble complement receptor of B lymphocytes. Science 1991. 254: 102-105.

47. Gustavsson,S., Kinoshita,T., and Heyman,B., Antibodies to murine complement receptor 1 and 2 can inhibit the antibody response in vivo without inhibiting T helper cell induction. J.Immunol. 1995. 154: 6524-6528.

48. Ahearn,J.M., Fischer,M.B., Croix,D., Goerg,S., Ma,M., Xia,J., Zhou,X., Howard,R.G., Rothstein,T.L., and Carroll,M.C., Disruption of the Cr2 locus results in a reduction in B-1a cells and in an impaired B cell response to T-dependent antigen. Immunity. 1996. 4: 251-262.

49. Molina,H., Holers,V.M., Li,B., Fung,Y., Mariathasan,S., Goellner,J., Strauss-Schoenberger,J., Karr,R.W., and Chaplin,D.D., Markedly impaired humoral immune response in mice deficient in complement receptors 1 and 2. Proc.Natl.Acad.Sci.U.S.A 1996. 93: 3357-3361.

50. Haas,K.M., Hasegawa,M., Steeber,D.A., Poe,J.C., Zabel,M.D., Bock,C.B., Karp,D.R., Briles,D.E., Weis,J.H., and Tedder,T.F., Complement receptors CD21/35 link innate and protective immunity during Streptococcus pneumoniae infection by regulating IgG3 antibody responses. Immunity. 2002. 17: 713-723.

51. Dempsey,P.W., Allison,M.E., Akkaraju,S., Goodnow,C.C., and Fearon,D.T., C3d of complement as a molecular adjuvant: bridging innate and acquired immunity. Science 1996. %19;271: 348-350.

52. Villiers,M.B., Villiers,C.L., Laharie,A.M., and Marche,P.N., Amplification of the antibody response by C3b complexed to antigen through an ester link. J.Immunol. 1999. 162: 3647-3652.
53. Fang,Y., Xu,C., Fu,Y.X., Holers,V.M., and Molina,H., Expression of complement receptors 1 and 2 on follicular dendritic cells is necessary for the generation of a strong antigen-specific IgG response. J.Immunol. 1998. 160: 5273-5279.
54. Barrington,R.A., Pozdnyakova,O., Zafari,M.R., Benjamin,C.D., and Carroll,M.C., B lymphocyte memory: role of stromal cell complement and FcgammaRIIB receptors. J.Exp.Med. 2002. 196: 1189-1199.
55. Zandvoort,A. and Timens,W., The dual function of the splenic marginal zone: essential for initiation of anti-TI-2 responses but also vital in the general first- line defense against blood-borne antigens. Clin.Exp.Immunol. 2002. 130: 4-11.
56. Martin,F., Oliver,A.M., and Kearney,J.F., Marginal zone and B1 B cells unite in the early response against T- independent blood-borne particulate antigens. Immunity. 2001. 14: 617-629.
57. Pozdnyakova,O., Guttormsen,H.K., Lalani,F.N., Carroll,M.C., and Kasper,D.L., Impaired antibody response to group B streptococcal type III capsular polysaccharide in C3- and complement receptor 2-deficient mice. J.Immunol. 2003. 170: 84-90.
58. Ochsenbein,A.F., Pinschewer,D.D., Odermatt,B., Carroll,M.C., Hengartner,H., and Zinkernagel,R.M., Protective T cell-independent antiviral antibody responses are dependent on complement. J.Exp.Med. 1999. 190: 1165-1174.
59. Kopf,M., Abel,B., Gallimore,A., Carroll,M., and Bachmann,M.F., Complement component C3 promotes T-cell priming and lung migration to control acute influenza virus infection. Nat.Med. 2002. 8: 373-378.
60. Suresh,M., Molina,H., Salvato,M.S., Mastellos,D., Lambris,J.D., and Sandor,M., Complement component 3 is required for optimal expansion of CD8 T cells during a systemic viral infection. J.Immunol. 2003. 170: 788-794.
61. Jozsi,M., Prechl,J., Bajtay,Z., and Erdei,A., Complement receptor type 1 (CD35) mediates inhibitory signals in human B lymphocytes. J.Immunol. 2002. 168: 2782-2788.
62. Cherukuri,A., Cheng,P.C., Sohn,H.W., and Pierce,S.K., The CD19/CD21 complex functions to prolong B cell antigen receptor signaling from lipid rafts. Immunity. 2001. 14: 169-179.
63. Cherukuri,A., Cheng,P.C., and Pierce,S.K., The role of the CD19/CD21 complex in B cell processing and presentation of complement-tagged antigens. J.Immunol. 2001. 167: 163-172.
64. Prechl,J., Baiu,D.C., Horvath,A., and Erdei,A., Modeling the presentation of C3d-coated antigen by B lymphocytes: enhancement by CR1/2-BCR co-ligation is selective for the co-ligating antigen. Int.Immunol. 2002. 14: 241-247.
65. Tuveson,D.A., Ahearn,J.M., Matsumoto,A.K., and Fearon,D.T., Molecular interactions of complement receptors on B lymphocytes: a CR1/CR2 complex distinct from the CR2/CD19 complex. J.Exp.Med. 1991. 173: 1083-1089.
66. Grattone,M.L., Villiers,C.L., Villiers,M.B., Drouet,C., and Marche,P.N., Co-operation between human CR1 (CD35) and CR2 (CD21) in internalization of their C3b and iC3b ligands by murine-transfected fibroblasts. Immunology 1999. 98: 152-157.
67. Barel,M., Le Romancer,M., and Frade,R., Activation of the EBV/C3d receptor (CR2, CD21) on human B lymphocyte surface triggers tyrosine phosphorylation of the 95-kDa nucleolin and its interaction with phosphatidylinositol 3 kinase. J.Immunol. 2001. 166: 3167-3173.

68. Bouillie,S., Barel,M., and Frade,R., Signaling through the EBV/C3d receptor (CR2, CD21) in human B lymphocytes: activation of phosphatidylinositol 3-kinase via a CD19-independent pathway. J.Immunol. 1999. 162: 136-143.

69. Tsoukas,C.D. and Lambris,J.D., Expression of EBV/C3d receptors on T cells: biological significance. Immunol.Today 1993. 14: 56-59.

70. Sandilands,G.P., Hauffe,B., Loudon,E., Marsh,A.G., Gondowidjojo,A., Campbell,C., Ferrier,R.K., and Rodie,M.E., Detection of cytoplasmic CD antigens within normal human peripheral blood leucocytes. Immunology 2003. 108: 329-337.

71. Thornton,C.A., Holloway,J.A., and Warner,J.O., Expression of CD21 and CD23 during human fetal development. Pediatr.Res. 2002. 52: 245-250.

72. Kerekes,K., Prechl,J., Bajtay,Z., Jozsi,M., and Erdei,A., A further link between innate and adaptive immunity: C3 deposition on antigen-presenting cells enhances the proliferation of antigen-specific T cells. Int.Immunol. 1998. 10: 1923-1930.

73. Kaya,Z., Afanasyeva,M., Wang,Y., Dohmen,K.M., Schlichting,J., Tretter,T., Fairweather,D., Holers,V.M., and Rose,N.R., Contribution of the innate immune system to autoimmune myocarditis: a role for complement. Nat.Immunol. 2001. 2: 739-745.

74. Prodinger,W.M., Larcher,C., Schwendinger,M., and Dierich,M.P., Ligation of the functional domain of complement receptor type 2 (CR2, CD21) is relevant for complex formation in T cell lines. J.Immunol. 1996. 156: 2580-2584.

75. Astier,A., Trescol-Biemont,M.C., Azocar,O., Lamouille,B., and Rabourdin-Combe,C., Cutting edge: CD46, a new costimulatory molecule for T cells, that induces p120CBL and LAT phosphorylation. J.Immunol. 2000. 164: 6091-6095.

76. Kemper,C., Chan,A.C., Green,J.M., Brett,K.A., Murphy,K.M., and Atkinson,J.P., Activation of human CD4+ cells with CD3 and CD46 induces a T-regulatory cell 1 phenotype. Nature 2003. 421: 388-392.

77. Marie,J.C., Astier,A.L., Rivailler,P., Rabourdin-Combe,C., Wild,T.F., and Horvat,B., Linking innate and acquired immunity: divergent role of CD46 cytoplasmic domains in T cell induced inflammation. Nat.Immunol. 2002. 3: 659-666.

78. Fernandez-Centeno,E., de Ojeda,G., Rojo,J.M., and Portoles,P., Crry/p65, a membrane complement regulatory protein, has costimulatory properties on mouse T cells. J.Immunol. 2000. 164: 4533-4542.

79. Arsenovic-Ranin,N., Vucevic,D., Okada,N., Dimitrijevic,M., and Colic,M., A monoclonal antibody to the rat Crry/p65 antigen, a complement regulatory membrane protein, stimulates adhesion and proliferation of thymocytes. Immunology 2000. 100: 334-344.

80. Reid,R.R., Woodcock,S., Shimabukuro-Vornhagen,A., Austen,W.G., Jr., Kobzik,L., Zhang,M., Hechtman,H.B., Moore,F.D., Jr., and Carroll,M.C., Functional activity of natural antibody is altered in Cr2-deficient mice. J.Immunol. 2002. 169: 5433-5440.

81. Fleming,S.D., Shea-Donohue,T., Guthridge,J.M., Kulik,L., Waldschmidt,T.J., Gipson,M.G., Tsokos,G.C., and Holers,V.M., Mice deficient in complement receptors 1 and 2 lack a tissue injury-inducing subset of the natural antibody repertoire. J.Immunol. 2002. 169: 2126-2133.

82. Marchbank,K.J., Kulik,L., Gipson,M.G., Morgan,B.P., and Holers,V.M., Expression of human complement receptor type 2 (CD21) in mice during early B cell development results in a reduction in mature B cells and hypogammaglobulinemia. J.Immunol. 2002. 169: 3526-3535.

83. Dempsey,P.W., Allison,M.E., Akkaraju,S., Goodnow,C.C., and Fearon,D.T., C3d of complement as a molecular adjuvant: bridging innate and acquired immunity. Science 1996. %19;271: 348-350.

84. Villiers,M.B., Villiers,C.L., Laharie,A.M., and Marche,P.N., Amplification of the antibody response by C3b complexed to antigen through an ester link. J.Immunol. 1999. 162: 3647-3652.

85. Ross,T.M., Xu,Y., Bright,R.A., and Robinson,H.L., C3d enhancement of antibodies to hemagglutinin accelerates protection against influenza virus challenge. Nat.Immunol. 2000. 1: 127-131.

86. Baiu,D.C., Prechl,J., Tchorbanov,A., Molina,H.D., Erdei,A., Sulica,A., Capel,P.J., and Hazenbos,W.L., Modulation of the humoral immune response by antibody-mediated antigen targeting to complement receptors and Fc receptors. J.Immunol. 1999. 162: 3125-3130.

87. Applequist,S.E., Dahlstrom,J., Jiang,N., Molina,H., and Heyman,B., Antibody production in mice deficient for complement receptors 1 and 2 can be induced by IgG/Ag and IgE/Ag, but not IgM/Ag complexes. J.Immunol. 2000. 165: 2398-2403.

88. Heyman,B., Pilstrom,L., and Shulman,M.J., Complement activation is required for IgM-mediated enhancement of the antibody response. J.Exp.Med. 1988. 167: 1999-2004.

89. Diaz,d.S., Dahlstrom,J., Carroll,M.C., and Heyman,B., A role for complement in feedback enhancement of antibody responses by IgG3. J.Exp.Med. 2003. 197: 1183-1190.

6

Terminal Complement Complex: Regulation of Formation and Pathophysiological Functions

Francesco Tedesco[*], Roberta Bulla[*] and Fabio Fischetti[°]
[*]Department of Physiology and Pathology, University of Trieste, Italy, [°]Department of Medicine and Neurology, University of Trieste, Italy

Abstract: The assembly of the five late components of the complement system leads to the formation of the terminal complement complex (TCC) that inserts into the membrane of the target cells as membrane attack complex causing lysis. However, the cytolytic activity is one of the several functions exhibited by the complex, and probably not the most important one due to the efficient control exerted by several regulators acting both in the fluid phase and on the cell membrane. A wealth of data has been collected over the last two decades indicating that this complex may exhibit non-cytotoxic effects on different cells both in the sublytic and the non cytolytic forms. There is clear evidence that TCC is a potent pro-inflammatory complex acting on endothelial and phagocytic cells. The critical role of the late complement components in the host defense is emphasized by the increased susceptibility of individuals with inherited deficiencies of these components to meningococcal infections. Besides the protective functions, TCC may also contribute to tissue damage in several pathological conditions associated with unrestricted complement activation. Efforts are now being made by several groups to develop therapeutic strategies to control the undesired effects of TCC using neutralizing antibodies against these components.

Key words: TCC, MAC, non-cytoxic effects; synthesis; inherited deficiencies, in vivo effects

1. INTRODUCTION

Activation of the late components of the complement (C) system from C5 to C9 represents the final step of the C cascade leading to the assembly of the Terminal C Complex (TCC). This complex, like the activation products of C3 and C5, exhibits effector function on target cells once they are recognized by the early components of the classical, alternative and lectin pathways. The structural organization of this macromolecular complex proceeds through a common pathway that starts with the cleavage of C5 into

C5a and C5b and ends with the binding of C9 that undergoes a process of polymerisation.

TCC is the only C activation product that has a direct effect on cell target causing cytolysis by inserting as the membrane attack complex (MAC) into the cell membrane. The cytolytic activity was the first function of the C system to be discovered at the end of the 19th century when it was found that serum exhibited a bactericidal activity, which was independent on leukocytes and was related to the presence of heat labile factors in the serum (Nutall, 1988). This initial observation made on bacteria was later confirmed on eucariotic cells, and the lysis of sensitized sheep red blood cells and of rabbit erythrocytes have now become the test system routinely used to measure the function of the classical and of the alternative pathways respectively of C activation.

Further studies on C dependent lysis of various target cells led to the recognition that MAC, despite the ability to bind to cell membrane, does not always exert lytic activity. This is the case, for instance, of gram positive bacteria, but it is also true for nucleated cells, that have been found to use different strategies to avoid the cytolytic destruction by MAC. An important advancement in our understanding of cell resistance to C-dependent lysis was made by the discovery of regulatory proteins that control the assembly of MAC and act both in the fluid phase and more importantly on the cell membrane. These regulatory molecules represent an efficient safeguard against any undesired attack by MAC in view of the fact that C activation products, once formed, do not distinguish between self and non self and may represent a real danger for host cells and tissues in situations of massive C activation. Such an efficient control of C-dependent lysis by regulatory proteins and other mechanisms of cell rescue would suggest that cytolysis is not the only, and probably not the primary function of MAC. Indeed numerous data collected in the last two decades provide supporting evidence that sublytic MAC induces a number of non-lethal effects particularly on nucleated cells.

The picture that is slowly emerging from in vitro and in vivo studies is that MAC has a dual role of protective and destructive complex depending on the type of target that it is able to attack. There is no doubt that MAC represents an important means of defence in infections sustained by gram negative bacteria and this protective function is facilitated by the presence of the late components not only in the circulation but also in the extravascular fluids. The role of MAC is critical in the control of Neisserial infections that occur with high frequency in patients with inherited deficiencies of one of the late components. On the other hand, MAC may be an important vehicle of cell and tissue destruction in situations of chronic inflammatory processes associated with massive C resulting in the release of C activation products including MAC.

2.   ASSEMBLY OF MAC AND REGULATION OF ITS FORMATION

While the early components of the C system serve to recognize a large variety of potential targets and trigger the three activation pathways, the late components are primarily involved in the neutralization of the targets and contribute to form a multimolecular complex that inserts into the cell target as MAC. This is the first perforin that was recognized before the identification of the perforins secreted by CTL and NK cells. The assembly of MAC is a highly sophisticated process that leads five soluble glycoproteins to establish firm interaction through non covalent bonds forming a multimolecular complex. The physicochemical characteristics of the late components and the chromosomal localization of the genes controlling their synthesis are presented in Table 1.

Table 1. Characteristics of the late complement components

Component	Subunit	Chromosomal location	MW (KDa)	Serum Concentration (µg/ml)
C5		9q33	190	75
C6		5p12-14	120	65
C7		5p12-14	121	60
C8			151	67
	α	1p32	64	
	β	1p32	64	
	γ	9q34.3	22	
C9		5p13	71	60

The protein-protein interactions that bring together one molecule of each of the terminal components from C5 to C8 and several molecules of C9 are favoured by the special molecular structure of these proteins that are organized in modules. Some of these modules mediating the interactions are present in other proteins unrelated to the C system and include thrombospondin type 1, low density lipoprotein receptor and epidermal growth factor. Other modules particularly rich in cystein are found in the C regulators factor H and I. Of the five late components only C6, C7, C8 and C9 share this structural organization in modules and are therefore considered members of the same family.

C5 that initiates the membrane attack pathway differs from the other terminal components in that it is structurally related to C3 and C4 and therefore represents a link between the terminal pathway and the early components (Lambris, 1998). Like the two structurally related molecules, C5 undergoes limited proteolysis as a result of complement activation and is cleaved by the C5 convertases of the classical and alternative pathways into a small chemotactic peptide and a major fragment C5b comprising the α^1 and the β chains linked by disulfide bridge. Activation of C5 by cell-bound C5 convertases enables the released C5b to bind to target cells and to expose a transient binding site for C6. C3b on the cell membrane offers a binding site for C5b, which then interacts with C6 to form the stable bimolecular complex C5b6. Marshall and colleagues (1996) have identified in the glycophorin of erythrocytes an additional binding site for C56, which specifically interacts with the sialylated region of this molecules via ionic forces. Binding of C7 to C5b6 leads to the assembly of the more stable trimolecular complex C5b-7 that exposes hydrophobic residues allowing the insertion of the complex into the phospholipid bilayer of the cell membrane (DiScipio 1988). Bound C5b6 that is not stabilized by C7 is released in the fluid phase as a stable complex, which can then interact with C7 exposing a transient binding site for phospholipids. The term, reactive lysis, has been introduced by Lachmann and Thompson in 1970 to indicate that C5b-7 assembling in the fluid phase is still able to attack bystander cells and to cause lysis of the target following completion of the terminal pathway.

With the formation of C5b-7, the assembling terminal complex starts interacting with the membrane phospholipids due to its affinity for lipids, which increases with the binding of C8 to C5b-7 through the C8β subunit resulting in the assembly of C5b-8 complex that penetrates deeper into the cell target causing slow lysis of red cells (Podack, 1979). The ability of C5b-7 to insert into the membrane is shortlived and decays in less than 1 minute. In the absence of a target, the complex becomes inactive and accumulates in the fluid phase as aggregates, though it is still able to bind the remaining late components (Tedesco, 1997). Deep insertion of C5b-8 into the phospholipid bilayer is not sufficient to create a transmembrane pore and it is only after the binding of C9 that a true channel is formed by MAC. This complex has a tubular appearance when viewed by electron microscopy with a inner diameter of approximately 100 Å. C9 is directly responsible for the structural organization of the pore to which it contributes by forming the wall through a unique process of polymerization that starts with the binding of the first molecule of C9 to C5b-8 followed by attachment of several other molecules of this C component (Tschopp, 1984; Bhakdi, 1984).

The spatial position of the individual late component within the terminal complex and their localization across the membrane have to some extent been clarified using various experimental procedures. Trypsin treament of erythrocytes bearing MAC results in the release of C5b while the other late components remain bound to the red cell membrane indicating that C5b is located on the external side of the complex (Bhakdi, 1980). Electron microscopy analysis using gold label to localize the late components confirmed the position of C5b on the external side of the membrane (Tschopp, 1982). Photoreactive glycolipid probes were also employed to identify the late components that were physically associated with the membrane and it was found that C8α-γ and C9 were the most labeled followed by C6 and C7 while C5b and C8β were the least labeled again suggesting that both the β subunit of C8 and C5b were located on the external side of the membrane (Podack, 1981).

The preferential binding of MAC to membrane phospholipid was clearly demonstrated using artificial liposomes that released their trapped marker when exposed to the terminal complex in the reactive lysis system (Lachmann, 1970b). This observation was confirmed using liposomes prepared with lipids extracted from human erythrocytes, which were also found to be susceptible to the reactive lysis. Interestingly, liposomes containing red cell lipids obtained from PNH patients were exquisitely more sensitive than liposomes prepared with lipids from normal red cells (Tedesco, 1981a). The trimolecular complex that does not bind to the cell target is still able to bind C8 and C9 forming a cytolytically inactive terminal complex that circulates in plasma and in other extravascular fluid. The complex that is formed in the fluid phase is controlled by two C regulators, vitronectin and clusterin, that inhibit the cytololytic activity and the ability of the complex to bind to the cell membrane. Vitronectin binds preferentially to C5b-7 to form SC5b-7 (Podack. 1977) and inhibits the polymerization of C9 (Milis, 1993) and the binding of the complex to heparin (Hogasen, 1992). In addition, vitronectin promotes binding of SC5b-9 to the vitronectin receptor on endotelial cells inducing cell adhesion to these cells (Biesecker, 1990). Clusterin is another C regulator that acts at the level of C7 in the complex C5b-7 preventing the insertion of this complex into the cell membrane, but it also binds to C8β and to the b domain of C9, thus inhibiting the polymerization of C9 (Tschopp, 1993). Neither of the two inhibitors, however, interfere with the full assembly of the complex, though the number of C9 molecules detected in the soluble inactive complex is substantially lower than that present in MAC and does not exceed 4 molecules. This complex, like MAC, can be detected using monoclonal antibodies that recognize a neoantigen expressed on polymerized C9 and the complex containing vitronectin and clusterin is regarded as cytolytically inactive.

3.   SYNTHESIS OF THE LATE COMPONENTS

The liver is the major site of synthesis of the components of the C system including the terminal components. The initial information was obtained in the late seventies following the recognition of the structural polymorphism of some of these components at the protein level that provided an invaluable tool to follow their synthesis in the recipients of liver transplants. A switch from recipient to donor allotype was observed for C6 and C8 proving that both these components were produced in the liver (Hobart, 1977; Alper, 1980), although an extrahepatic source of C6 has been shown in C6 deficient rats transplanted with bone marrow from C6 sufficient animals (Brauer, 1994). A similar approach was followed a decade ago by Würzner and colleagues, who used monoclonal antibodies to detect the polymorphic variant C7M and found that less than half of the circulating C7 is of liver origin (Würzner, 1994). Subsequent work revealed that bone marrow was an additional source of C7 contributing to approximately 25 % of the total circulating pool of C7 (Naughton, 1996). The data supporting the conclusion that C5 and C9 are synthesized by the liver are less conclusive, although messages for these components can easily be detected in the liver and both these components, as well as C6, C7 and C8, have been cloned from cDNA libraries prepared from the liver (Haviland, 1991; Wetsel, 1990; Discipio, 1989; Haefliger, 1989; DiScipio, 1988; Rao, 1987; Howard, 1987; Ng, 1987; Haefliger, 1987; DiScipio, 1984; Stanley, 1985).

The finding of donor allotypes in recipients of liver transplant, the detection of messages for the late components and their cloning from liver cDNA libraries do not clarify whether hepatocytes or Kupffer cells are the source of these components. This issue was addressed two decades ago by Morris and coworkers (1982), who analysed the hepatoma cell line HepG2 for their ability to secrete C components measured by hemolytic assays. They were able to measure C5, small amounts of C6, traces of C8, but failed to detect C7 and C9. In a subsequent study our group essentially confirmed these data using sensitive ELISA and, in addition, found that IL-1α, TNFα and IL-6 stimulate the secretion of increased levels of C8, but had only a marginal effect on the secretion of C5, and were totally ineffective on the secretion of the remaining late components (Perissutti, 1994).

Based on the transitory appearance of the donor allotype of C7 in recipients of liver transplant, Würzner and associates (*1994*) suggested that Kupffer cells may be the most likely source of C7 in the liver because these donor phagocytic cells are eventually replaced by the bone marrow derived cells in the recipient. This is in line with previous findings by two different groups that mononuclear phagocytes synthesize all the late components (McPhaden, 1993; Hetland et al., 1986). We have followed the expression and the secretion of these components by monocytes during their maturation into macrophages and found that C6 is the late component most abundantly secreted by monocytes and that the amount produced by macrophages is approximately 5-6 fold higher as opposed to the marginal increase of the other components (Fig. 1 a, b). Synthesis of the late components is unaffected by IL-1β and TNFα, but IL-6, IFN-γ and LPS up-regulates C7 and to some extent also C9.

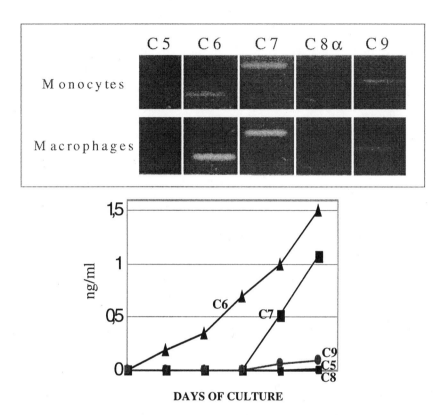

Figure 1. Expression of mRNA and secretion of the late complement components by mononuclear phagocytes as a result of maturation from monocytes to macrophages. The cells were analysed for mRNA at day 1 and day 8 of culture as a source of monocytes and macrophages respectively.

Several other cell types have been shown to express the messages and synthesize the late components in various tissues. Astrocytes in the brain are able to secrete the terminal components as well as components of the classical and alternative pathways providing a local source of TCC that may cause destructive effects on neurons and oligodendrocytes (Gasque, 1995). Renal tubular cells may also contribute to the local production of the terminal component as these cells express messages for these proteins and secrete measurable levels of the late C components (Tedesco et al.

unpublished observations). Whether the locally produced late components may contribute to the tissue damage is not clear, though kidneys from C6 sufficient rats transplanted into C6 deficient recipients failed to restore renal damage in a rat model of antibody-dependent nephritis seem to rule out a major contribution of TCC in this process (Timmerman, 1997). However, local synthesis of C3 seems to play a critical role in graft rejection because kidney from C3 deficient animals transplanted into compatible normal recipients were not rejected unlike the kidney from C sufficient animals (Pratt, 2002).

Besides macrophages, other cells widely distributed in the tissues are able to synthesize the late components and these include fibroblasts and endothelial cells (Garred, 1990; Johnson, 1991). However, although the messages for these components can easily be detected by PCR analysis, the amount of proteins secreted by these cells is very low and is often at the lowest limit of sensitivity of the detection system. This is not the case of C7 secreted by the endothelium, which we regard as the main extrahepatic source of this terminal component considering the large surface area covered by the endothelial cells in the vascular tree (Langeggen, 2000). At any rate, as pointed out by Morgan and Gasque (1997), the limited amount of the terminal components made locally available by tissue cells does not prevent the release of activation products that can be very effective on the surrounding cells.

4.   THE TCC AS A DEFENCE SYSTEM AGAINST BACTERIA

The wide distribution of the terminal components in the circulation and in tissues and the ease with which the terminal complex can assemble following the triggering of C activation through one of the initiating pathways make this complex a potentially powerful defense system against infectious agents, and in particular against bacteria. The ability of MAC to kill bacteria is strictly dependent on the structural organization of their cell wall that makes gram negative bacteria susceptible and gram positive bacteria resistant to C-dependent killing. The thick peptidoglycan layer of gram positive bacteria prevents the productive insertion of MAC into the cell wall despite the physical binding of the complex. On the other hand, gram negative bacteria are not always susceptible to C attack and may use different strategies to evade killing by MAC. One way to become resistant would be to acquire a capsule that forms a protective shield against the insertion of MAC. Alternatively, MAC may bind to the long O polysaccharide chain at some distance from the bacterial wall and it is easily shed (Joiner, 1983; Joiner, 1988). Finally, bacteria may synthesize molecules capable of preventing the assembly of an efficient MAC that requires multimeric C9 for the damage of the inner membrane (Block, 1987). Fernieking et al. (2001) have recently reported the presence of an inhibitor in a strain of Streptococcus that acts at the level of C5b-7 preventing its uptake onto cell membranes. More recently, we have documented a CD59-like molecule on C-resistant strains of Borrelia burgdorferi that inhibits the polymerization of C9 in the C5b-9 complex and is recognized by various antisera to human CD59 (Pausa, 2003). This molecule differs from human CD59 by having a higher molecular weight (~80 kDa) and by interacting preferentially with C8β rather than with C8α beside C9.

Insertion of MAC into the outer membrane leads to the influx of lysozyme that helps to dissolve the peptidoglycan layer (Inoue, 1959). However, lysozyme is not strictly required for bacterial killing because we were able to prove that E.coli O111:B4 can be killed using purified terminal components (Rottini, 1985). This finding was later confirmed by Bloch and associates (1987), who induced C-dependent killing of E. coli J5 not associated with the alteration of the peptidoglycan layer in the absence of lysozyme. The terminal complex causes bacterial killing not only through a direct effect on microorganisms, but also by promoting their intracellar killing. We have shown that E.coli O111:B4 coated by IgM antibodies and by C components up to C7 to form the bacterial intermediate BAC1-7 are easily engulfed by PMN, but survive inside these cells. The bacteria are only killed if they are coated by C8 becoming the target of endocellular cationic proteins (Tedesco; 1981b). Mannion et al. (1990) reported essentially similar results showing that E.coli sensitized with C7 deficient serum were regularly phagocytosed, but not killed and that efficient killing was obtained using sublytic amount of normal human serum to sensitize the bacteria.

5.   INHERITED DEFICIENCIES OF THE LATE COMPLEMENT COMPONENTS

The increased susceptibility of individuals with inherited deficiencies of C components to bacterial infections underscore the critical role played by the C system in the defense against these infectious agents. A sufficient number of patients with selective deficiencies of the late components have now been identified in different parts of the world to allow a clear definition of a close association of these deficiencies with meningococcal disease (MD). Infections occur in these patients with special clinical features that are not fully explained. An observation made originally by Petersen et al (1979) and later confirmed and extended by Densen and colleagues (Ross, 1984;

Figueroa, 1991) was that a large proportion of these patients experience infections caused by Neisseria meningitidis and less frequently by Neisseria gonorrhoea, despite the fact that all gram negative bacteria are potentially susceptible to the bacteridal activity of the C system. This is not due to bias in the selection of patients because screening of patients undergoing infections by a variety of bacteria for C activity did not reveal a significant increase in the late C component deficiencies (LCCD) associated with infections caused by bacteria other than meningococcus. The results of retrospective studies carried out by different groups have disclosed the propensity of these patients to be particularly susceptible to meningococcal disease caused by uncommon serotypes, and in particular Y, and W135 and to lesser extent X (Ross, 1984; Fjien, 1989). Other studies have challenged the conclusion that uncommon serotypes are prevalent among late C components deficient patients documenting the contribution of common serotypes that more frequently infect the general population. In a survey of Italian patients with meningococcal disease ten patients were identified to have selective deficiencies of C8β , C7 and C6, and they were all found be infected by N. meningitidis of serogroup C (D'Amelio, 1992). A similar observation was made by Platonov and co-workers (1993) in a large group of 30 Russian patients with late C components deficiency and meningococcal disease caused by common serogroups (A, B, and C) in 15 out of 18 patients in whom the serogroups of Neisseria meningitides was identified.

Other special features of MD in LCCD patients are the age of occurrence, the low mortality rate of the disease and the increased frequency of recurrent episodes. The first episode of MD in patients with LCCD occurs at an elder age of over 10 years than in C sufficient patients who are more often infected at a the age of 3-5 years. This age difference, which is currently used as one of the diagnostic criteria to suspect an LCCD, has not received a satisfactory explanation. If the absence of protective antibodies accounts for the risk of C sufficient individuals for MD, then it is difficult to understand why this is not true for LCCD patients, who have also the disadvantage of lacking MAC as an important defence system. On the other hand, the increased susceptibility of LCCD patients to MD at an age when the normal population is generally protected cannot be attributed to a reduced antibody response, which has been found to be essentially similar to that observed in patients with normal C activity (Ross, 1984; Potter, 1990; Biselli, 1993). As LCCD patients are unable to use MAC to kill meningocci even in the presence of specific antibodies, promotion of phagocytosis and intracellular killing of these bacteria become the critical means of defense of these patients against Neisserial infections. However, this mechanism of protection may be compromised by an increased incidence of certain

FcγRIIa and IIIb allotypes found by Fijen and co-workers (2000) to be associated with MD as a result of reduced internalization of opsonized meningococci. This represents therefore an additional risk factor for MD in LCCD patients.

A striking feature of MD in LCCD patients is the mild clinical course of infection. We have found that purpura, disseminated intravascular coagulation and hypotension occurred more frequently in C-sufficient than in LCCD patients of our study group (Tedesco, 1993) and Platonov et al (1993) reported similar findings showing that shock and brain edema were less common in their group of LCCD patients. These data suggest that MAC contributes to the development of clinical complications in MD either via direct vascular and pro-coagulant effects or indirectly by inducing the release of endotoxin from meningococci known to exert similar effects. Brandtzaeg and co-workers (1989) have provided evidence for the contribution of SC5b-9 and endotoxin to the onset of multiple organ failure and death showing that the concentration of SC5b-9 in patients with MD was strongly correlated with the level of endotoxin and both were inversely related to the survival of these patients. This concept was further supported by the observation that a C6 deficient patient showed clinical signs of shock and detectable level of endotoxin after receiving fresh frozen plasma for the treatment of severe complications of MD (Lehner, 1992).

Vaccination of LCCD individuals with tetravalent meningoccoccal polysaccharides is currently proposed as an effective measure to prevent the risk of infections in these patients. The goal is to favour the production of opsonizing antibodies that promote intracellular killing of bacteria by phagocytes. Ross and colleagues (1987) have provided in vitro evidence that support the beneficial effect of vaccination showing that the serum obtained form a C8 deficient patients vaccinated with the bivalent A-C meningococcal vaccine was able to promote efficient phagocytic killing of meningococci of different serogroups. LCCD patients have now been vaccinated by several groups with menigococcal capsular polysaccharide vaccine and the data that have been collected indicate the following: 1. the antibody response in these patients is not different from that observed in C-sufficient patients (Andreoni, 1993; Platonov, 1995; Fijen, 1998); 2. the antibody-mediated phagocytic killing of meningococci appears to be the most reliable method to monitor the efficacy of vaccination (Andreoni, 1993; Schlesinger, 1994; Fijen, 1998); 3. the titers of antibodies tend to decline with time and revaccination is required (Fijen, 1998); 4. despite vaccination, MD may still occur in LCCD patients raising the possibilty that additional factors besides the intact C system play an important role in the clearance of meningococci and these include the subclass of the antibodies and the allotype of the FcR.

6.   NON CYTOTOXIC EFFECTS OF TCC

The lytic activity has historically been regarded as the hallmark of the biological functions of the C system and is currently been exploited for the evalation of the functional C activity. However, the ability of TCC to behave as MAC causing transmembrane pores through the phospholipid bilayer of the target cells is restricted by several constraints. Thus, both soluble and membrane-bound regulators neutralize the complex interfering with the polymerization of C9 and reducing in this way the lytic efficiency of the complex (Morgan, 1999). In addition, the complex often fails to form effective pores on nucleated cells and simply causes disruption of membrane phospholipids and, even when regular pores are produced, they may be repaired by a metabolic processes of the cell target (Ohanian, 1981; Carney, 1985) Finally, the cell may react to the insertion of MAC by physically removing the complex from the surface through a process of vesiculation, that has been shown to occur on different cell types including neutrophils, platelets and erythrocytes (Morgan, 1987; Sim, 1986; Iida, 1991).

An important biological effect of sublytic MAC is to promote inflammation through the stimulation of several cell types involved in this process including phagocytes and endothelial cells. One of the key events observed after sublytic attack of phagocytic cell by MAC is the rapid rise in intracellar Ca^{2+} concentration (Morgan, 1985; Carney, 1986) contributed both by extracellular source and also by the release of intracellular stores. External Ca^{2+} that leaks inside the cell through the MAC pore seems to be involved in vesciculation because this process is prevented by the removal of extracellular calcium by means of chelating agents (Morgan, 1985). However, release of Ca^{2+} from intracellular store can also occur in the absence of external calcium as a result of MAC-dependent direct stimulation of phospholipase C, which in turn induces the formation of IP3 (Morgan, 1989).

Arachidonic acid (AA) derivatives including prostaglandins, leukotrienes and thromboxanes represent some of pro-inflammatory products that are released from phagocytes upon stimulation by MAC. Release of these derivatives by phagocytes is dependent, at least in part, on external calcium, and is induced through the activation of phospholipase A2. (Hänsch, 1984; Seeger, 1986; Imagawa, 1987). Other tissue specific cells, such as glomerular mesangial and epitelial cells, have also been shown to release AA derivatives when exposed to sublytic MAC (Lovett, 1987; Hansch, 1988).

Phagocytes stimulated by sublytic MAC may promote inflammation by producing reactive oxygen metabolites (Morgan, 1985; Hansch, 1987) and also proinflammatory cytokines (Hansch.1987). Similar products may be released by other tissue specific cells exposed to sublytic MAC, such as glomerular mesangial cells or synovial cells, contributing in this way to amplify the local development of the inflammatory process (Adler, 1986; Lovett, 1987; Schönermark, 1991).

Endothelial cells lining the microvascular vessels are often exposed and activated by MAC that can be formed both in the circulation and in the extravascular fluid as a result of C activation (Saadi, 1998; Tedesco, 1999). Sublytic MAC assembled on the surface of endothelial cells has been shown to induce the expression of P-selectin (Hattori, 1989), to potentiate the action of TNF-α in promoting the surface appearance of E-selectin and ICAM-1 (Kilgore, 1995), and to stimulate the release of chemokines (Kilgore, 1996) and plalelet-activating factor (Benzaquen, 1994). Sublytic MAC may also exert a procoagulant effect through various mechanisms, that include release of von Willebrand Factor (Hattori, 1989), shedding of membrane vesicles or exposure of membrane phospholipids that promote the assembly of prothrombinase (Hamilton, 1990) and surface expression of tissue factor (Saadi, 1995). Most of these effects are dependent on the production of IL-1α by EC stimulated by MAC, which is also responsible for the release of the vasoconstrictor agent tromboxane A2 (Bustos, 1997), whereas MAC seems to exert a direct effect on the release of the vasodilator prostaglandin I2 by endothelial cells (Suttorp, 1987). Sublytic MAC deposited on EC was also found to promote interaction of plasminogen with C9 of the bound complex that in turn stimulated fibrinolytic activity (Christiansen, 1997). The terminal C complex, even in its cytolyticaly inactive form (iTCC), is also able to bind to endothelial cells and to stimulate these cells to express the adhesion molecules ELAM-1, ICAM-1 and VCAM1 and tissue factor (Tedesco, 1997). More recently, this complex was shown to induce secretion of IL-8 and MCP-1 by endothelial cells and to cause migration of polymorphonuclear leukocytes through a monolayer of endothelial cells in an vitro model of a transwell and through the endothelium of the microvessels of the ileal mesentery in vivo (Dobrina, 2002) (Figure 2).

Binding of sublytic complex or inactive TCC to cells may affect their survival resulting either in increased protection or in promotion of apoptosis depending on the cell type involved. Rus and colleagues (1996) have provided evidence for a distinct role of C5b-9 in rescuing oligodendrocytes from undergoing apoptosis through the mitocondrial pathway when cultured in the absence of serum growth factors. This in vitro observation was later confirmed by the finding that the number of apoptotic Schwann cells in an in vivo model of experimental autoimmune neuritis was reduced when the model was established in C6 deficient rat (Daschiell, 2000).

C5b-9 may have an opposite effect inducing apoptosis of myocardial cells in an experimental model of ischemia reperfusion dependent myocardial damage (Vakeva, 1998) and of endothelial cell in a model of antibody-mediated mesangial glomerulonephritis (Hughes, 2000). The ability of C5b-9 to induce apoptosis was recently shown in an vitro model of rat mesangial cells sensitized with C fixing antibodies and incubated with a source of C (Nauta, 2002). Exposure of phosphatidylserine and fragmentation of nuclei in antibody-sensitized cells were not seen when normal rat serum was replaced by C6 deficient serum. More direct evidence for the role of C5b-9 in causing apoptosis was obtained by exposing mesangial cells to cytolytically inactive complex, which caused increased activity of apoptosis associated caspase 3 (Nauta, 2002).

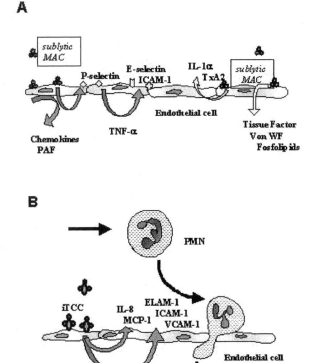

Figure 2. Biological effects of sublytic MAC (A) and cytolytically inactive terminal complement complex on endothelial cells

Attack by sublytic MAC may stimulate cells to elaborate protective mechanims that promote resistance to subsequent attack by the same cytolyticaly active complex. Mason et al. (1999) have clearly shown that endothelial cells exposed to sublytic MAC tend to express increased amounts of DAF that protect the cells from C dependent cytolysis. Reiter and Fishelson (1992) identified a large C induced protein of about 900 kDa that is expressed on the surface of human leukaemia cells following attack by sublytic MAC and is involved in C resistance. Protein synthesis is required for the expression of C resistance.

7.   THE INVOLVEMENT OF TCC IN DISEASE

TCC has been implicated in the onset and progression of several diseases not necessarily immune-mediated that involve various tissue and organs including vasculopathies, connective tissue diseases, neurologic, renal and skin diseases. Indirect evidence supporting the contribution of TCC to tissue damage in these diseases is provided by the finding of soluble TCC in biological fluids (Mollnes, 1986; Sanders,1988) and the detection of TCC deposits at tissue level (Morgan, 1989; Hansch, 1998) in amounts that are related to the level of activity of the disease. In vivo models of C- mediated diseases have been established in animal with selective deficiencies of one of the late components which have proved to be an invaluable tool to assess the in vivo role of TCC in the initiation and the maintenance of these pathological conditions (Frank, 1995). The use of C regulatory proteins or antibodies to late C components to prevent the assembly of MAC has further contributed to define the direct effect of TCC in different experimental conditions. We shall review some of the diseases in which TCC has been implicated on the basis of clinical observations in patients with these diseases and of data obtained from in vitro and in vivo models.

7.1   Renal Disease

The presence of C5b-9 complex has been revealed at tissue level in the kidney of patients with several forms of nephropathies (Biesecker, 1981; Hinglais, 1986; Falk, 1987). In addition, elevated levels of this complex are detected in the urine of patients with membranous nephropathies (Schulze, 1991), focal glomerular sclerosis and diabetic nephropathy (Ogrodowski, 1991) and they seem to correlate with the degree of proteinuria (Ogrodowski, 1991). Local deposits and urinary excretion of C5b-9 have also documented in animal models of inflammatory kidney disease (Koffler, 1983; Schulze, 1989) and the results obtained in animals with selective deficiencies of C6 support the conclusion that C5b-9 is required to cause tissue damage in these models. Thus, Groggel (1983) established an experimental model of membranous nephropathy in rabbits and showed that C6 deficient, unlike C sufficient animals, do not develop proteinuria, although similar elecrondense deposits of Ig and C3 were observed in the two groups of rabbits.

A strain of C6 deficient rats identified by Leenaerts and colleagues (1994) has been employed to demonstrate the role of MAC in various models of experimental C-dependent glomerulonephritis using antibodies directed against mesangial cells (Yamamoto, 1987) or glomerular epithelial or endothelial cells (Couser, 1990; Brandt, 1996; Nangaku, 1997). Evidence accumulating in the last few years suggest that C components filtering in the urine in patients and animal models with non selective proteinuria (Nangaku, 1999) may be activated intraluminally forming the membrane attack complex that is ultimately responsible for tubulointerstitial damage and progressive renal disease (Hsu, 2003)

7.2   Connective Tissue Disease

Elevated levels of C5b-9 have been detected in the synovial fluids of patients with rheumatoid arthritis (Mollnes, 1986; Brodeur, 1991) and deposits of the same complex have been documented on the synovial membrane of these patients (Sanders, 1986) in amounts that are related to the degree of disease activity (Oleesky, 1991; Corvetta, 1992). Evidence has also been provided suggesting that part of this TCC is produced locally in the synovial tissues (Neumann, 2002). The critical role played by TCC in the induction of arthritis is supported by the finding of Wang et al. (2000) that C5-deficient mice are resistant to the induction of collagen-induced arthritis and of Mizuno and colleagues (1997) that neutralization of synovial CD59 in rats by intraarticular injection of specific antibodies results in acute joint inflammation. More recently, using a rabbit model antigen-induced arthritis, Tramontini et al (2002) showed that joint swelling, leukocyte accumulation in the synovial fluid and IL-8 expression in the synovial membrane were all significantly reduced in C6 deficient rabbits than in C6-sufficient animals.

C activation products including TCC are usually found in plasma (Porcel, 1995), biological fluids (Sanders, 1988) and at tissue level, particularly kidney and skin (Biesecker, 1983; Biesecker, 1982) in patients with SLE. The levels of TCC, C3a and C4a increase significantly in these patients, as compared to those observed in patients with stable lupus and normal controls, and correlate with the score of disease activity representing therefore the most useful parameter to monitor the disease activity in terms of sensitivity and specificity (Porcel, 1995) even in the absence of clear changes in the levels of C3 and C4 (Gawryl, 1988; Falk,1985). Increased levels of TCC are detected in the cerebrospinal fluid and serum in patients with Sjogren's syndrome presenting with clinical sign of involvement of the central nervous system (Sanders, 1988).

A role for TCC in the development of muscle damage in the course of dermatomyositis has also been recently suggested by the immunohistochemical detection of MAC on the muscle vessels of patients with this disease (Kissel, 1986; Mascaro, 1995; Goncalves, 2002).

7.3   Neurologic and Neuromuscular Diseases

MAC has been implicated in the progression of lesions in patients with multiple sclerosis, Alzheimer's disease and neurotrauma. Increased levels of TCC are detected in the cerebrospinal fluid of patients with multiple sclerosis (Mollnes, 1987) and they seem to be higher in patients with multiple attacks (Sellebjerg, 1998) with a positive correlation between levels of TCC in the cerebrospinal fluid and neurological disability. TCC is deposited at the site of the lesion in the periventricular area (Compston, 1989) and particularly around the active plaques (Storchet, 1998). An in vivo model of antibody-mediated demyelinating experimental autoimmune encephalomyelitis resembling the human disease has recently been established in both C6-deficient and C6-sufficient rats by Mead and colleagues (2002). The interesting finding was that the C6 deficient rats, that were unable to form MAC, failed to show demyelisation, unlike the control rats and the disease had in general a mild course in the group of C6-deficient rats proving the important contribution of MAC to the onset of demyelination.

MAC is usually localized in senile plaques in patients with Alzheimer's disease (Itagaki, 1994) and is present abundantly in the cortex of these patients associated with neurons containing neurofibrillary tangle, dystrophic neurites within neuritic plaques, and neuropil threads (Webster, 1997). Using a human neuronal cell line, Shen et al. (1998) showed that beta-amyloid peptide is able to induce expression of most C components in these cells and to promote assembly of MAC on their surface following the removal of cell-bound CD59. Along this line, evidence has been provided by Yang et al. (2000) that the expression of CD59 is significantly reduced on the frontal cortex and hippocampus of patients with Alzheimer's disease, unlike that of C9, which is significantly increased.

MAC has been detected on the peripheral nerves of patients suffering from Guillain-Barré syndrome (Koski, 1987; Putzu, 2000), and a relationship has been found between circulating levels of C-fixing anti-myelin antibodies and TCC in these patients (Koski, 1987).

The contribution of MAC deposition to myelin alterations seen in patients with polyneuropathy associated with monoclonal gammopathy was suspected on the basis of co-localization of the monoclonal antibodies directed against the myelin-associated glycoprotein (MAG) and MAC on the altered myelin sheaths (Monaco, 1990). More direct evidence for the role of MAC in causing myelin alterations was obtained in a rabbit model of peripheral neuropathy induced by injecting anti-MAG antibodies into the sciatic nerve, which caused marked demyelisation associated with deposition of MAC (Monaco, 1995). These antibodies had no effect when injected into C6 deficient rabbits.

Data collected over several years suggest that MAC plays an important role in the loss of acetylcholine receptor at the neuromuscular junction in patients with myasthenia gravis (MG). This was initially suspected following the observation that C9 was deposited at the motor end-plate of the MG muscle fibres (Sahashi, 1980). The contribution of MAC to the ultrastructural damage in the postsynaptic membrane of myastenic muscle was further supported by the finding that an experimental model of MG could not be established in C5 deficient mice (Christadoss, 1988) and that treatment of rats with antibodies to C6 prevented the occurrence of the acute manifestation of the disease (Biesecker, 1989). The involvement of C in the induction of experimental model of myasthenia gravis is also proved by the recent finding of Lin and co-workers (2002) who showed that Daf1(-/-) mice were more susceptible to antibody-mediated experimental MG than control Daf1(+/+) mice. We have been able to induce contraction restricted to the endplate area of freshly isolated rat muscle fibres that have been exposed to anti-acetylcholine receptor and fresh human serum as a source of C (Mozrzymas, 1993).

7.4   Cardiovascular Diseases

C inhibition as therapeutic tool to reduce tissue injury induced by ischemia-reperfusion (I/R) phenomena at myocardial level has been investigated both in patients and animal models (Lucchesi, 1997). Endothelial cells are the primary target of C activation products during ischemia/reperfusion (I/R), as indicated by the detection of C1q and MAC deposits along endothelial cell surface (Weiser, 1996). TCC bound to these cells has recently been shown by Dobrina and coworkers (Blood, 2002) to induce PMN emigration through the endothelial wall as assessed by in vitro and in vivo experimental models. The complex was found by Vakeva et al. (1992) to be present in infarcted areas of myocardium and to be associated with decreased expression of CD59 suggesting unrestricted activation of C in hypoxic tissues. Ligation of a coronary artery for a few hours in a rabbit model of I/R myocardial damage, followed by reperfusion, leads to tissue deposition of TCC (Mathey, 1994). The reduced tissue damage observed in C6 deficient animals after myocardial and renal ischemia/reperfusion injury (Ito, 1996; Zhou, 2000) lends support to the involvement of TCC in tissue destruction. Similar results were obtained by Kilgore and coworkers (1998) who also found lower expression of IL-8 in animals undergoing prolonged myocardial I/R. Treatment of pigs (Amsterdam, 1995) and rats (Vakeva, 1998) with anti-C5 antibodies prior to ligation of coronary artery rduces myocardial necrosis, PMN infiltration and cell apoptosis.

TCC seems to be implicated also in the inflammatory process leading to the development of atherosclerosis, as suggested by the detection of C5b-9deposits in atherosclerotic lesions in humans at the level of fibrous plaque and in the intima (Niculescu, 1987). Furthermore, C6 deficient rabbits fed with cholesterol enriched diet exhibit less arterial lesions as compared to C-sufficient animals (Schmiedt, 1998), in which C5b-9 has been shown to co-localize with cholesterol in the sub-endothelium of the aorta. Seifert and colleagues (1989) observed that intimal deposition of C5b-9 precedes monocyte infiltration and foam cell formation.

The endothelium of a xenotransplant is the target of MAC assembled on these cells as a result antibody-dependent C activation (Platt, 1991). The critical role played by TCC in the vascular damage is proved by the finding that xenogenic hearts survive in C6-deficient rats longer than in C-sufficient animals (Brauer, 1995). These data have been confirmed transplanting allogenic lung in C6 sufficient and C6 deficient recipient rats (Nakashima, 2002). Interestingly, this study showed also increase in the number of alveolar macrophages and capillary injury when that lungs were transplanted from C6-sufficient donors to C6-deficient recipients suggesting that locally produced C6 could restore assembly of TCC and contributes to tissue alterations. The contribution of TCC in the development of accelerated graft arteriosclerosis has been recently ascertained also in cardiac transplants (Quian, 2001).

8. THERAPEUTIC CONTROL OF TCC

The findings from in vitro and in vivo experimental models that TCC is involved in cell and tissue damage has prompted an intensive search for therapeutic tools that could effectively neutralize the undesired biological effects of this complex. Peptides competing for the functionally active sites of the late components and monoclonal antibodies inhibiting their functional activities represent two important choices that have a potential application as therapeutic agents in clinical conditions are associated with unrestricted C activation. Low and Ogata (1999) have identified peptides in C5 that inhibit its functional activity on their position in proximity to insertion-deletion structures in the C3/4/5 protein family. Some of them are located at some distances from the cleavage site on the α chain of the molecule by the C5 convertase, suggesting that these molecular portions of C5 offer binding sites to the enzyme prior to its interaction with the cleavage site. We have recently synthesized a peptide of 18 aa corresponding to the cleavage site of C5 and able to inhibit its splitting as a result of activation by the C5 convertase (Marzari, 2002). However, to our knowledge none of these peptides have yet been tested in vivo to control C activation and the limitations to their clinical use are their rapid clearance from the circulation, and in addition their susceptibility to cleavage by peptidases.

Neutralizig monoclonal antibodies (mAb) to late C components appear to be more promising as therapeutic agents and so far mAbs to C5 have proved to be effective in vivo in preventing the onset and progression of collagen-induced arthritis (Wang, 1995), in ameliorating the glomerulonephritis in lupus prone mice (Wang, 1996), in reducing the size of infarct areas and the degree of apoptosis following myocardial ischemia and reperfusion (Vakeva, 1998), and in preventing hyperacute rejection of xenotranplanted organs (Wang, 1999). A humanized scFv anti-human C5 now available for clinical trials has been found to attenuate myocardial damage, cognitive deficits and blood loss in patents undergong ardiopulmonary bypass (Fitch, 1999) and is now being tested in chronic inflammatory diseases including rheumatoid arthritis, glomerulonephritis and other autoimmune diseases together with another variant form (Kaplan, 2002).

We have recently isolated a neutralizing scFv anti-human C5 from a human phage display library (Marzari, 2002). This scFv is directed against the cleavage site of C5 and is able to inhibit the generation of C5a and the assembly of TCC from human C5 as well as from the C5 from other species including mouse, rat and rabbit offering the unique advantage over other anti-human C5 to be tested in animal model prior to its clinical use in man.

9.   REFERENCES

Adler, S., Baker, P.J., Johnson, R.J., Ochi, R.F., Pritzl, P., Couser, W.G. Complement membrane attack complex stimulates production of reactive oxygen metabolites by cultured rat mesangial cells. J Clin Invest 1986; 77: 762-767

Alper, C.A., Raum, D., Awdeh, Z.L., Petersen, B.H., Taylor, P.D., Starzl, T.E. Studies of hepatic synthesis in vivo of plasma proteins, including orosomucoid, transferrin, alpha 1 antitrypsin, C8. and factor B. Clin Immunol Immunopathol 1980; 16:84-89

Amsterdam, E.A., Stahl, G.L., Pan, H.L., Rendig, S.V., Fletcher, M.P., Longhurst, J.C. Limitation of reperfusion injury by a monoclonal antibody to C5a during myocardial infarction in pigs. Am J Physiol 1995; 268:H448-457

Andreoni, J., Käyhty, H., Densen, P. Vaccination and the role of capsular polysaccharide antibody in prevention of recurrent meningococcal disease in late complement component-deficient individuals. J Infect Dis 1993; 168:227-231

Benzaquen, L.R., Nicholson-Weller, A., Halperin, J.A. Terminal complement proteins C5b-9 release basic fibroblast growth factor and platelet-derived growth factor from endothelial cells. J Exp Med 1994; 179: 985-992

Bhakdi, S., Tranum-Jensen, J., Klump, O. The terminal membrane C5b-9 complex of human complement. Evidence for the existence of multiple protease-resistant polypeptides that form the trans-membrane complement channel. J Immunol 1980; 124:2451-2457

Bhakdi, S., Tranum-Jensen, J. On the cause and nature of C9-related heterogeneity of terminal complement complexes generated on target erythrocytes through the action of whole serum. J Immunol 1984; 133:1453-1463

Biesecker, G., Katz, S., Koffler, D. Renal localization of the membrane attack complex in systemic lupus erythematosus nephritis. J Exp Med 1981; 154:1779-1794

Biesecker, G., Lavin, L., Ziskind, M.,Koffler, D. Cutaneous localization of the membrane attack complex in discoid and systemic lupus erythematosus. New Engl J Med 1982; 306:264-270

Biesecker, G., Gomez, C.M. Inhibition of acute passive transfer experimental autoimmune myasthenia gravis with Fab antibody to complement C6. J Immunol 1989; 142:2654-2659

Biesecker, G. The complement SC5b-9 complex mediates cell adhesion through a vitronectin receptor. J. Immunol 1990; 145:209-214

Biselli, R., Casapollo, I., D'Amelio, R., Salvato, S., Matricardi, P.M., Brai, M. Antibody response to meningococcal polysaccharides A and C in patients with complement defects. Scand J Inmmunol 1993; 37: 644-650

Bloch, E.F., Schmetz, M.A., Foulds, J., Hammer, C.H., Frank, M.M., Joiner, K.A. Multimeric C9 within C5b-9 is required for inner membrane damage to Escherichia coli J5 during complement killing. J Immunol. 1987; 138:842-848

Brandt, J., Pippin, J., Schulze, M., Hansch, G.M., Alpers, C.E., Johnson, R.J., Gordon K, Couser WG. Role of the complement membrane attack complex (C5b-9) in mediating experimental mesangioproliferative glomerulonephritis. Kidney Int 1996; 49: 335-343

Brandtzaeg, P., Mollnes, T.E., Kierulf, P. Complement activation and endotoxin levels in systemic meningococcal disease. J Infect Dis 1989; 160:58-65

Brauer, R.B., Baldwin, W.M. 3rd, Wang, D., Horwitz, L.R., Hess, A.D., Klein, A.S., Sanfilippo, F. Hepatic and extrahepatic biosynthesis of complement factor C6 in the rat. J Immunol 1994; 153: 3168-3176

Brauer, R.B., Baldwin, W.M. 3rd, Ibrahim, S., Sanfilippo, F. The contribution of terminal complement components to acute and hyperacute allograft rejection in the rat. Transplantation. 1995; 59:288-293

Brodeur, J.P., Ruddy, S., Schwartz, L.B., Moxley, G. Synovial fluid levels of complement SC5b-9 and fragment Bb are elevated in patients with rheumatoid arthritis. Arthritis Rheum 1991; 34: 1531-1537

Bustos, M., Coffman, T.M., Saadi, S., Platt, J.L. Modulation of eicosanoid metabolism in endothelial cells in a xenograft model. Role of cyclooxygenase-2. J Clin Invest 1997; 100:1150-1158

Carney, D.F, Koski, C.L., Shin, M.L. Elimination of terminal complement intermediates from the plasma membrane of nucleated cells: the rate of disappearance differs for cells carrying C5b-7 and C5b-8 or a mixture of C5b-8 with a limited number of C5b-9. J Immunol 1985; 134:1804-1809

Carney, D.F., Hammer, C.H., Shin, M.L. Elimination of terminal complement complexes in the plasma membrane of nucleated cells: influence of extracellular Ca^{2+} and association with cellular Ca^{2+}. J Immunol 1986; 137:263-270

Christadoss, P. C5 gene influences the development of murine myasthenia gravis. J Immunol 1988; 140:2589-2592

Christiansen, V.J., Sims, P.J., Hamilton, K.K. Complement C5b-9 increases plasminogen binding and activation on human endothelial cells. Arterioscler Thromb Vasc Biol. 1997:17: 164-171

Compston, D. A., Morgan, B. P., Campbell, A. K., Wilkins, P., Cole, G., Thomas, N. D., Jasani, B. Immunocytochemical localization of the terminal complement complex in multiple sclerosis. Neuropathol Appl Neurobiol 1989; 15:307-316

Corvetta, A., Pomponio, G., Rinaldi, N., Luchetti, M.M., Di Loreto, C., Stramazzotti, D. Terminal complement complex in synovial tissue from patients affected by rheumatoid arthritis, osteoarthritis and acute joint trauma. Clin Exp Rheumatol 1992; 10: 433-438

Couser, W.G. Mediation of immune glomerular injury. J Am Soc Nephrol 1990; 1:13-29

D'Amelio, R., Agostoni, A., Biselli, R., Brai, M., Caruso, G., Cicardi, M., Corvetta, A., Fontana, L., Misiano, G., Perricone, R., Quinti, I., Schena, F.P., Stroffolini, T., Tedesco, F. Complement deficiency and antibody profile in survivors of meningococcal meningitis due to common serogrops in Italy. Scand J Immunol 1992; 35:589-595

Dashiell, S.M., Rus, H., Koski, C.L. Terminal complement complexes concomitantly stimulate proliferation and rescue of Schwann cells from apoptosis. Glia 2000; 30:187-198

DiScipio, R.G., Gehring, M.R., Podack, E.R., Kan, C.C., Hugli, T.E., Fey, G.H. Nucleotide sequence of cDNA and derived amino acid sequence of human complement component C9. Proc Natl Acad Sci U S A 1984; 81:7298-7302

DiScipio, R.G., Chakravarti, D.N., Muller-Eberhard, H.J., Fey, G.H. The structure of human complement component C7 and the C5b-7 complex. J Biol Chem. 1988; 263:549-560

DiScipio, R.G., Hugli, T.E. The molecular architecture of human complement component C6. J Biol Chem 1989; 264:16197-16206

Dobrina, A. Pausa, M., Fischetti, F., Bulla, R., Vecile, E., Ferrero, E., Mantovani, A., Tedesco, F. Cytolytically inactive terminal complement complex causes transendothelial migration of polymorphonuclear leukocytes in vitro and in vivo. Blood 2002; 99:185-192

Falk, R.J., Dalmasso, A.P., Kim, Y., Lam, S., Michael, A. Radioimmunoassay of the attack complex of complement in serum from patients with systemic lupus erythematosus. N Engl J Med 1985; 312:1594-1599

Falk, R.J., Podack, E., Dalmasso, A.P., Jennette, J.C. Localization of S protein and its relationship to the membrane attack complex of complement in renal tissue. Am J Pathol 1987; 127:182-190

Fernie-King, B.A., Seilly, D.J., Willers, C., Wurzner, R., Davies, A., Lachmann, P.J. Streptococcal inhibitor of complement (SIC) inhibits the membrane attack complex by preventing uptake of C567 onto cell membranes. Immunology 2001; 103:390-398

Figueroa J. E., Densen P. Infectious diseases associated with complement deficiencies. Clin Microbiol Rev 1991; 4:359-395

Fijen, C.A., Bredius, R.G., Kuijper, E.J., Out, T.A., De Haas, M., De Wit, A.P., Daha, M.R., De Winkel, J.G. The role of Fcgamma receptor polymorphisms and C3 in the immune defence against Neisseria meningitidis in complement-deficient individuals. Clin Exp Immunol 2000; 120:338-345

Fijen, C.A., Kuijper, E.J., Hannema, A.J., Sjöholm, A.G., van Putten, J.P.M Complement deficiencies in patients over ten years old with meningococcal disease due to uncommon serogroups. Lancet 1989; ii:585-588

Fijen, C.A., Kuijper E.J., Drogari-Apiranthitou, M., van Leeuwen, Y., Daha, M.R., Dankert J. Protection against meningococcal serogroup ACYW disease in complement-deficient individuals vaccinated with the tetravalent meningococcal capsular polysaccharide vaccine. Clin Exp Immunol 1998; 114:362-369

Fitch, J.C., Rollins, S., Matis, L., Alford, B., Aranki, S., Collard, C.D., Dewar, M., Elefteriades, J., Hines, R., Kopf, G., Kraker, P., Li, L., O'Hara, R., Rinder, C., Rinder, H.,

Shaw, R., Smith, B., Stahl, G., Shernan, S.K. Pharmacology and biological efficacy of a recombinant, humanized, single-chain antibody C5 complement inhibitor in patients undergoing coronary artery bypass graft surgery with cardiopulmonary bypass. Circulation 1999; 100:2499-2506

Frank, MM. Animal models for complement deficiencies. J Clin Immunol 1995; 15:113S-121S

Garred, P., Hetland, G., Mollnes, T.E., Stoervold, G. Synthesis of C3, C5, C6, C8 and C9 by human fibroblasts. Scand J Immunol 1990; 32:555-560

Gasque, P., Fontaine, M., Morgan, B.P. Complement expression in human brain: biosynthesis of terminal pathway components and regulators in human glial cells and cell lines. J Immunol 1995; 154:4726-4733

Gawryl, M.S., Chudwin, D.S., Langlois, P.F., Lint, T.F. The terminal complement complex, C5b-9, a marker of disease activity in patients with systemic lupus erythematosus. Arthritis Rheum 1988; 31:188-195

Goncalves, F.G., Chimelli, L., Sallum, A.M., Marie, S.K., Kiss, M.H., Ferriani, V.P. Immunohistological analysis of CD59 and membrane attack complex of complement in muscle in juvenile dermatomyositis. J Rheumatol 2002; 29:1301-1307

Groggel, G.C., Adler, S., Rennke, H.G., Couser, W.G., Salant, D.J. Role of the terminal complement pathway in experimental membranous nephropathy in the rabbit. J Clin Invest 1983; 72:1948-1957

Haefliger, J.A., Jenne, D., Stanley, K.K., Tschopp, J. Structural homology of human complement component C8 gamma and plasma protein HC: identity of the cysteine bond pattern. Biochem Biophys Res Commun 1987; 149:750-754

Haefliger, J.A., Tschopp, J., Vial, N., Jenne, D.E. Complete primary structure and functional characterization of the sixth component of the human complement system. Identification of the C5b-binding domain in complement C6. J Biol Chem. 1989; 264:18041-18051

Hamilton, K.K., Hattori, R., Esmon, C.T., Sims, P.J. Complement proteins C5b-9 induce vesiculation of the endothelial plasma membrane and expose catalytic surface for assembly of the prothrombinase enzyme complex. J Biol Chem 1990; 265:3809-3814

Hänsch, G.M., Seitz, M., Martinotti, G., Betz, M., Rauterberg, E.W., Gemsa, D. Macrophages release arachidonic acid, prostaglandin E_2, and thromboxane in response to late complement components. J Immunol 1984; 133:2145-2150

Hänsch, G.M., Seitz, M., Betz, M. Effect of the late complement components C5b-9 on human monocytes: release of prostanoids, oxygen radicals and of a factor inducing cell proliferation. Int Arch Allegy Appl Immunol 1987; 82:317-320

Hänsch, G.M., Betz, M., Gunther, J., Rother, K.O., Sterzel, B. The complement membrane attack complex stimulates the prostanoid production of cultured glomerular epithelial cells. Int Arch Allergy Appl Immunol 1988; 85: 87-93

Hänsch, G.M., Shin, M.L. "Complement attack phase". In *The complement system*, Rother, K., Till, G.O., Hänsch, G.M eds, Springer-Verlag, Berlin, 1998

Hattori, R., Hamilton, K.K., McEver, R.P., Sims, P.J. Complement proteins C5b-9 induce secretion of high molecular weight multimers of endothelial von Willebrand factor and translocation of granule membrane protein GMP-140 to the cell surface. J Biol Chem 1989; 264: 9053-9060

Haviland, D.L., Haviland, J.C., Fleischer, D.T., Hunt, A., Wetsel, R.A. Complete cDNA sequence of human complement pro-C5. Evidence of truncated transcripts derived from a single copy gene. J Immunol 1991; 146:362-368

Hetland, G., Johnson, E., Falk, R., Eskeland, T. Synthesis of complement components C5, C6, C7, C8 and C9 in vitro by human monocytes and assembly of the terminal complement complex . Scand J Immunol 1986; 24:421-428

Hinglais, N., Kazatchkine, M.D., Bhakdi, S., Appay, M.D., Mandet, C., Grossetete, J., Bariety, J. Immunohistochemical study of the C5b-9 complex of complement in human kidneys. Kidney Int 1986; 30:399-410

Hobart, M.J., Lachmann, P.J., Calne, R.Y. C6: Synthesis by the liver in vivo. J Exp Med 1977; 146:629-630

Hogasen, K., Mollnes, T.E., Harboe, M. Heparin-binding properties of vitronectin are linked to complex formation as illustrated by in vitro polymerization and binding to the terminal complement complex. J Biol Chem 1992; 267:23076-23082

Howard, O.M., Rao, A.G., Sodetz, J.M. Complementary DNA and derived amino acid sequence of the beta subunit of human complement protein C8: identification of a close structural and ancestral relationship to the alpha subunit and C9. Biochemistry 1987; 26:3565-3570

Hsu, S.I., Couser, W.G. Chronic progression of tubulointerstitial damage in proteinuric renal disease is mediated by complement activation: a therapeutic role for complement inhibitors? J Am Soc Nephrol 2003; 14:S186-191

Hughes, J., Nangaku, M., Alpers, C.E., Shankland, S.J., Couser, W.G., Johnson, R.J. C5b-9 membrane attack complex mediates endothelial cell apoptosis in experimental glomerulonephritis. Am J Physiol Renal Physiol 2000; 278:F747-F757

Iida, K., Whitlow, M., Nussezweig, V. Membrane vesiculation protects erythrocytes from destruction by complement. J Immunol 1991; 147: 2638-2642

Imagawa, D.K., Barbour, S.E., Morgan, B.P., Wright, T.M., Shin, H.S., Ramm, L.E. Role of complement C9 and calcium in the generation of arachidonic acid and its metabolites from rat polymorphonuclear leukocytes. Mol Immunol 1987; 24:1263-1271

Inoue, K., Tanigawa, Y., Takubo, M., Satani, M., Amano, T. Quantitative studies on immune bacteriolysis. II. The role of lysozyme in immune bacteriolysis. Biken J. 1959; 2:1-20

Itagaki, S., Akiyama, H., Saito, H., McGeer, P.L. Ultrastructural localization of complement membrane attack complex (MAC)-like immunoreactivity in brains of patients with Alzheimer's disease. Brain Res 1994; 645:78-84

Ito, W., Schafer, H.J., Bhakdi, S., Klask, R., Hansen, S., Schaarschmidt, S., Schofer, J., Hugo, F., Hamdoch, T., Mathey, D. Influence of the terminal complement-complex on reperfusion injury, no-reflow and arrhythmias: a comparison between C6-competent and C6-deficient rabbits. Cardiovasc Res 1996; 32:294-305

Johnson, E., Hetland, G. Human umbilical vein endothelial cells synthesize functional C3, C5, C6, C8 and C9 in vitro. Scand J Immunol 1991; 33:667-671

Joiner, K.A., Warren, K.A., Brown, E.J., Swanson, J., Frank, M.M. Studies on the mechanism of bacterial resistance to complement-mediated killing. IV. C5b-9 forms high molecular weight complexes with bacterial outer membrane constituents on serum-resistant but not on serum-sensitive Neisseria gonorrhoeae. J Immunol 1983; 131:1443-1451

Joiner, K.A. Complement evasion by bacteria and parasites. Ann Rev Microbiol 1988; 42: 201-230

Kaplan, M. Eculizumab, (Alexion). Curr Opin Investig Drugs 2002 Jul; 3:1017-1023

Kilgore, K.S., Flory, C.M., Miller, B.F., Evans, V.M., Warren, J.S. The membrane attack complex of complement induces interleukin-8 and monocyte chemoattractant protein-1 secretion from human umbilical vein endothelial cells. Am J Pathol 1996; 149:953-961

Kilgore, K.S., Shen, J.P., Miller, B.F., Ward, P.A., Warren, J.S. Enhancement by the complement membrane attack complex of tumor necrosis factor-α-induced endothelial cell expression of E-selectin and ICAM-1. J. Immunol. 1995; 155: 1434-1441

Kilgore, K.S., Park, J.L., Tanhehco, E.J., Booth, E.A., Marks, R.M., Lucchesi, B.R. Attenuation of interleukin-8 expression in C6-deficient rabbits after myocardial ischemia/reperfusion. J Mol Cell Cardiol 1998; 30:75-85

Kissel, J.T., Mendell, J.R., Rammohan, K.W. Microvascular deposition of complement membrane attack complex in dermatomyositis. New Engl J Med 1986; 314: 329-334

Koffler, D., Biesecker, G., Noble, B., Andres, G.A., Martinez-Hernandez, A. Localization of the membrane attack complex (MAC) in experimental immune complex glomerulonephritis. J Exp Med 1983; 157:1885-1905

Koski, C.L., Sanders, M.E., Swoveland, P.T., Lawley, T.J., Shin, M.L., Frank, M.M., Joiner, K.A. Activation of terminal components of complement in patients with Guillain-Barre syndrome and other demyelinating neuropathies. J Clin Invest 1987; 80:1492-1497

Lachmann, P.J., Thompson, R.A. Reactive lysis: the complement-mediated lysis of unsensitized cells. II. The characterization of activated reactor as C56 and the participation of C8 and C9. J Exp Med 1970a; 131:643-657

Lachmann, P.J., Munn, E.A.,Weissmann, G. Complement mediated lysis of liposomes produced by the reactive lysis procedure. Immunology 1970b; 19:983-986

Lambris, J.D., Sahu, A., Wetsel, R.A. "The chemistry and biology of C3, C4 and C5". In *The human complement system in health and disease*, John E Volanakis and Michael M Frank eds., Marcel Dekker, Inc. New York, 1998

Langeggen, H., Pausa, M., Johnson, E., Casarsa, C., Tedesco, F., The endothelium is an extrahepatic site of synthesis of the seventh component of the complement system. Clin. Exp Immunol 2000; 121:69-76

Leenaerts, P.L., Stad, R.K., Hall, B.M., Van Damme, B.J., Vanrenterghem, Y., Daha, M.R. Hereditary C6 deficiency in a strain of PVG/c rats. Clin Exp Immunol 1994; 97:478-482

Lehner, P.J., Davies, K.A., Walport, M.J., Cope, A.P., Würzner, R., Orren, A., Morgan, B.P., Cohen, J. Meningococcal septicaemia in a C6-deficient patient and effects of plasma transfusion on lipopolysaccharide release. Lancet 1992; 340:1379-1381

Lin, F., Kaminski, H.J., Conti-Fine, B.M., Wang, W., Richmonds, C., Medof, M.E. Markedly enhanced susceptibility to experimental autoimmune myasthenia gravis in the absence of decay-accelerating factor protection. J Clin Invest 2002; 110:1269-1274

Lovett, D.H., Hänsch, G.M., Goppelt, M., Resch, K., Gemsa, D. Activation of glomerular mesangial cells by the terminal membrane attack complex of complement. J Immunol 1987; 138:2473-2480

Low, P.J., Ai, R., Ogata, R.T. Active sites in complement components C5 and C3 identified by proximity to indels in the C3/4/5 protein family. J Immunol 1999; 162:6580-6588

Lucchesi, B.R., Kilgore, K.S. Complement inhibitors in myocardial ischemia/reperfusion injury. Immunopharmacology. 1997; 38:27-42

Mannion, B.A., Weiss, J., Elsbach, P. Separation of sublethal and lethal effects of polymorphonuclear leukocytes on Escherichia coli. J Clin Invest 1990; 86: 631-641

Marshall, P., Hasegawa, A., Davidson, E.A., Nussenzweig, V., Whitlow, M. Interaction between complement proteins C5b-7 and erythrocyte membrane sialic acid. J Exp Med 1996; 184:1225-1232

Marzari, R., Sblattero, D., Macor, P., Fischetti, F., Gennaro, R., Marks, J.D., Bradbury, A., Tedesco F. The cleavage site of C5 from man and animals as a common target for neutralizing human monoclonal antibodies: in vitro and in vivo studies. Eur J Immunol 2002 ; 32:2773-2782

Mascaro, J.M. Jr., Hausmann, G., Herrero, C., Grau, J.M., Cid, M.C., Palou, J., Mascaro, J.M. Membrane attack complex deposits in cutaneous lesions of dermatomyositis. Arch Dermatol 1995; 131:1386-1392

Mason, J.C., Yarwood, H., Sugars, K., Morgan, B.P., Davies, K.A., Haskard, D.O. Induction of decay-accelerating factor by cytokines or the membrane-attack complex protects vascular endothelial cells against complement deposition. Blood 1999; 94:1673-82

Mathey, D., Schofer, J., Schafer, H.J., Hamdoch, T., Joachim, H.C., Ritgen, A., Hugo, F., Bhakdi, S. Early accumulation of the terminal complement-complex in the ischaemic myocardium after reperfusion. Eur Heart J 1994; 15:418-423

McPhaden, A.R., Whaley, K. Complement biosynthesis by mononuclear phagocytes. Immunol Res 1993; 12:213-232

Mead, R.J., Singhrao, S.K., Neal, J.W., Lassmann, H., Morgan, B.P. The membrane attack complex of complement causes severe demyelination associated with acute axonal injury. J Immunol 2002; 168:458-465

Milis, L., Morris, C.A., Sheehan, M.C., Charlesworth, J.A., Pussell, B.A. Vitronectin-mediated inhibition of complement: evidence for different binding sites for C5b-7 and C9. Clin Exp Immunol 1993; 92:114-119

Mizuno, M., Nishikawa, K., Goodfellow, R.M., Piddlesden, S.J., Morgan, B.P., Matsuo, S. The effects of functional suppression of a membrane-bound complement regulatory protein, CD59, in the synovial tissue in rats. Arthritis Rheum 1997; 40: 527-533

Mollnes, T.E., Lea, T., Mellbye, O.J., Pale, J., Grand , O., Harboe, M. Complement activation in rheumatoid arthritis evaluated by C3dg and the terminal complement complex. Arthritis Rheum. 1986; 29:715-721

Mollnes, T.E., Vandvik, B., Lea, T., Vartdal, F. Intrathecal complement activation in neurological diseases evaluated by analysis of the terminal complement complex. J Neurol Sci 1987; 78:17-28

Monaco, S., Bonetti, B., Ferrari, S., Moretto, G., Nardelli, E., Tedesco, F., Mollnes, T.E., Nobile-Orazio, E., Manfredini, E., Bonazzi, L., Rizzato, N. Complement-mediated demyelination in patients with IgM monoclonal gammopathy and polyneuropathy. N Engl J Med 1990; 322:649-652

Monaco, S., Ferrari, S., Bonetti, B., Moretto, G., Kirshfink, M., Nardelli, E., Nobile-Orazio, E., Zanusso, G., Rizzuto, N., Tedesco, F. Experimental induction of myelin changes by anti-MAG antibodies and terminal complement complex. J Neuropathol Exp Neurol 1995; 54:96-104

Morgan, P.B. and Harris, CL. *Complement regulatory proteins.* San Diego: Academic Press, 1999

Morgan, B.P., Campbell, A.K. The recovery of human polymorphonuclear leukocytes from sublytic complement attack is mediated by changes in intracellular free calcium. Biochem J 1985; 231:205-208

Morgan, B.P. Dankert, J.R, Esser, A.F. Recovery of human neutrophils from complement attack: removal of the membrane attack complex by endocytosis and exocytosis. J Immunol 1987; 138:246-253

Morgan, B.P. Complement membrane attack on nucleated cells: resistance, recovery and non-lethal effects. Biochem J 1989; 264: 1-14

Morgan, B.P., Gasque, P. Extrahepatic biosynthesis: where, when and why? Clin Exp Immunol 1997; 107:1-7

Morris, K.M., Aden, D.P., Knowles, B.B., Colten, H.R. Complement biosynthesis by the human hepatoma cell line HepG2. J Clin Invest 1982; 70:906-913

Mozrzymas, J.W., Lorenzon, P., Riviera, A.P., Tedesco, F., Ruzzier, F. An electrophysiological study of the effects of myasthenia gravis sera and complement on rat isolated muscle fibres. J Neuroimmunol 1993; 45:155-162

Nakashima, S., Qian, Z., Rahimi, S., Wasowska, B.A., Baldwin, W.M. 3rd. Membrane attack complex contributes to destruction of vascular integrity in acute lung allograft rejection. J Immunol 2002; 169:4620-4627

Nangaku, M., Alpers, C.E., Pippin, J., Shankland, S.J., Kurokawa K., Adler S, Johnson, R.J., Couser, W.G. Renal microvascular injury induced by antibody to glomerular endothelial cells is mediated by C5b-9. Kidney Int 1997; 52:1570-1578.

Nangaku, M., Pippin, J., Couser, W.G. Complement membrane attack complex (C5b-9) mediates interstitial disease in experimental nephrotic syndrome. J Am Soc Nephrol 1999; 10:2323-2331

Naughton, M.A., Walport, M.J., Wurzner, R., Carter, M.J., Alexander, G.J., Goldman, J.M., Botto, M. Organ-specific contribution to circulating C7 levels by the bone marrow and liver in humans. Eur J Immunol 1996; 26:2108-2112

Nauta, A.J., Daha, M.R., Tijsma, O., van de Water, B., Tedesco, F., Roos, A. The membrane attack complex of complement induces caspase activation and apoptosis. Eur J Immunol 2002; 32:783-792

Neumann, E., Barnum, S.R., Tarner, I.H., Echols, J., Fleck, M., Judex, M., Kullmann, F., Mountz, J.D., Scholmerich, J., Gay, S., Muller-Ladner, U. Local production of complement proteins in rheumatoid arthritis synovium. Arthritis Rheum 2002; 46: 934-945

Ng, S.C., Rao, A.G., Howard, O.M., Sodetz , J.M. The eighth component of human complement: evidence that it is an oligomeric serum protein assembled from products of three different genes. Biochemistry 1987; 26:5229-5233

Niculescu, F., Hugo, F., Rus, H.G., Vlaicu, R., Bhakdi, S. Quantitative evaluation of the terminal C5b-9 complement complex by ELISA in human atherosclerotic arteries. Clin Exp Immunol 1987; 69:477-483.

Nutall, G. Experimente über die bakterienfeindlichen Einflüsse des tierischen Körpers. Z Hyg Infektionskr 1988; 4:353-394

Ogrodowski, J.L., Hebert, L.A., Sedmak, D., Cosio, F.G., Tamerius, J., Kolb, W. Measurement of SC5b-9 in urine patients with the nephrotic syndrome. Kidney Int 1991, 40:1141-1147

Ohanian, S.H., Schlager, S.I. Humoral immune killing of nucleated cells: mechanisms of complement-mediated attack and target cell defense. Crit Rev Immunol 1981; 1:165-209

Oleesky, D.A., Daniels, R.H., Williams, B.D., Amos, N., Morgan, B.P. Terminal complement complexes and C1/C1 inhibitor complexes in rheumatoid arthritis and other arthritic conditions. Clin Exp Immunol 1991; 84:250-255

Pausa, M., Pellis, V., Cinco, M., Giulianini, P.G., Presani, G., Perticarari, S., Murgia R., Tedesco, F. Serum-resistant strains of *Borrelia burgdorferi* evade complement-mediated killing by expressing a CD59-like complement inhibitory molecule. J Immunol 2003; 170:3214-3222

Perissutti, S., Tedesco, F. Effect of cytokines on the secretion of the fifth and the eighth complement components by HepG2 cells. Int J Clin Lab Res 1994; 24:45-48

Petersen, B.H., Lee T.J., Snyderman, R., Brooks, G.F. Neisseria menngitidis and Neisseria gonorrhoeae bacteriemia associated with C6, C7, or C8 defeciency. Ann Intern Med 1979; 90:917-920

Platonov, A.E., Belobodorov, V.B., Vershinina, I.V. Meningococcal disease in patients with late complement component deficiency: studies in the U.S.S.R. Medicine 1993; 72:374-392

Platonov, A.E., Beloborodov, V.B., Pavlova, L.I., Vershinina, I.V., Kayhty, H. Vaccination of patients deficient in a late complement component with tetravalent meningococcal capsular polysaccharide vaccine. Clin Exp Immunol 1995; 100:32-39

Platt, J.L., Bach, F.H. The barrier to xenotransplantation. Transplantation. 1991; 52:937-947

Podack, E.R., Kolb, W.P., Muller-Eberhard, H.J. The SC5b-7 complex: formation, isolation, properties, and subunit composition. J Immunol 1977; 119:2024-2029

Podack, E.R., Biesecker, G., Muller-Eberhard, H.J. Membrane attack complex of complement: generation of high-affinity phospholipid binding sites by fusion of five hydrophilic plasma proteins. Proc Natl Acad Sci U S A 1979;76:897-901

Podack, E.R., Stoffel, W., Esser, A.F., Muller-Eberhard, H.J. Membrane attack complex of complement: distribution of subunits between the hydrocarbon phase of target membranes and water. Proc Natl Acad Sci U S A 1981; 78:4544-4548

Porcel, J.M., Ordi, J., Castro-Salomo, A., Vilardell, M., Rodrigo, M.J., Gene, T., Warburton, F., Kraus, M., Vergani, D. The value of complement activation products in the assessment of systemic lupus erythematosus flares. Clin Immunol Immunopathol 1995; 74:283-288

Potter, P.C., Frasch, C.E., van der Sande, W.J., Cooper, R.C., Patel, Y., Orren, A. Prophylaxis against *Neisseria meningitidis* infections and antibody responses in patients with deficiency of the sixth component of complement. J Infect Dis 1990; 161:932-937.

Pratt, J.R., Basheer, S.A., Sacks, S.H. Local synthesis of complement component C3 regulates acute renal transplant rejection. Nat Med 2002; 8:582-587

Putzu, G.A., Figarella-Branger, D., Bouvier-Labit, C., Liprandi, A., Bianco, N., Pellissier, J.F. Immunohistochemical localization of cytokines, C5b-9 and ICAM-1 in peripheral nerve of Guillain-Barre syndrome. J Neurol Sci 2000; 174:16-21

Qian, Z,, Hu, W., Liu, J., Sanfilippo, F., Hruban, R., Baldwin, W.M. Terminal complement proteins in mediating processes of accelerated graft arteriosclerosis in cardiac transplants. Transplant Proc 2001; 33:370-371

Rao, A.G., Howard, O.M., Ng, S.C., Whitehead, A.S., Colten, H.R., Sodetz, J.M. Complementary DNA and derived amino acid sequence of the alpha subunit of human complement protein C8: evidence for the existence of a separate alpha subunit messenger RNA. Biochemistry 1987; 26:3556-3564

Reiter, Y., Fishelson., Z. Complement membrane attack complexes induce in human leukemic cells rapid expression of large proteins (L-CIP). Mol Immunol 1992; 29:771-781

Ross, S.C., Densen, P. Complement deficiency states and infections: epidemiology, pathogenesis and consequences of Neisseria and other infections in an immune deficiency. Medicine 1984; 63:243-273

Ross, S.C., Rosenthal, P.J., Berberich, H.M., Densen, P. Killing of *Neisseria meningitidis* by human neutrophils: implications for normal and complement-deficient individuals. J Infect Dis 1987; 155:1266-1275

Rottini, G., Tedesco, F., Basaglia, M., Roncelli, L., Patriarca, P. Kinetics of assembly and decay of complement components on Escherichia coli O111:B4 preparation of stable intermediates. Infect Immun 1985; 49:402-406

Rus, H.G., Niculescu, F., Shin, M.L. Sublytic complement attack induces cell cycle in oligodendrocytes. J.Immunol 1996; 156: 4892-4900

Saadi, S., Holzknecht, R.A., Patte, C.P., Stern, D.M., Platt, J.L. Complement-mediated regulation of tissue factor activity in endothelium. J Exp Med 1995; 182:1807-1814

Saadi, S., Platt, J.L. "Endothelial cell response to complement activation." In *The human complement system in health and disease*, Volanakis, J.E., Frank, M.M. eds, Marcel Dekker, Inc. New York, 1998

Sahashi, K., Engel, A.G., Lambert, E.H., Howard, F.M.Jr. Ultrastructural localization of the terminal and lytic ninth complement component (C9) at the motor end-plate in myasthenia gravis. J Neuropathol Exp Neurol 1980; 39:160-172

Sanders, M.E., Kopicky, J.A., Wigley, F.M., Shin, M.L., Frank, M.M., Joiner, K.A. Membrane attack complex of complement in rheumatoid synovial tissue demonstrated by immunofluorescent microscopy. J Rheumatol 1986; 13:1028-1034

Sanders, M.E., Alexanders, E.L., Koski, C.L., Shin, M.L., Sano, Y., Frank, M.M., Joiner, K.A. Terminal complement complexes (SC5b-9) in cerebrospinal fluid in autoimmune nervous system diseases. Ann N Y Acad Sci 1988; 540:387-388

Schlesinger, M., Greenberg, R., Levy, J., Kayhty, H., Levy, R. Killing of meningococci by neutrophils: effect of vaccination on patients with complement deficiency. J Infect Dis 1994; 170:449-453

Schmiedt, W., Kinscherf, R., Deigner, H.P., Kamencic, H., Nauen, O., Kilo, J., Oelert, H., Metz, J., Bhakdi, S. Complement C6 deficiency protects against diet-induced atherosclerosis in rabbits. Arterioscler Thromb Vasc Biol 1998; 18:1790-1795

Schönermark, M., Deppisch, R., Riedasch, G., Rother, K., Hänsch, G.M. Induction of mediator release from human glomerular mesangial cells by the terminal complement components C5b-9. Int Arch Allergy Appl Immunol 1991; 96:331-337

Schulze, M., Baker, P.J., Perkinson, D.T., Johnson, R.J., Ochi, R.F., Stahl, R.A., Couser, W.G. Increased urinary excretion of C5b-9 distinguishes passive Heymann nephritis in the rat. Kidney Int 1989; 35:60-68

Schulze, M., Donadio, J.V., Pruchno, C.J., Baker, P.J, Johnson, R.J., Stahl, R.A.K., Watkins, S., Martin, D.C., Wurzner, R., Gotze, O., Couser, W.G. Elevated urinary excretion of the C5b-9 complex in membranous nephropathy. Kidney Int 1991; 40:533-538

Seeger, W., Suttorp, N., Hellwig, A., Bhakdi, S. Noncytolytic complement complexes may serve as calcium gates to elicit leukotriene B4 generation in human polymorphonuclear leukocytes. J Immunol 1986; 137:1286-1293

Seifert, P.S., Hugo, F., Hansson, G.K., Bhakdi, S. Prelesional complement activation in experimental atherosclerosis. Terminal C5b-9 complement deposition coincides with cholesterol accumulation in the aortic intima of hypercholesterolemic rabbits. Lab Invest 1989; 60:747-754

Sellebjerg, F., Jaliashvili, I., Christiansen, M., Garred, P. Intrathecal activation of the complement system and disability in multiple sclerosis. J Neurol Sci 1998; 157:168-174

Shen, Y., Sullivan, T., Lee, C.M., Meri, S., Shiosaki, K., Lin, C.W. Induced expression of neuronal membrane attack complex and cell death by Alzheimer's beta-amyloid peptide. Brain Res 1998; 796:187-197

Sims, P.J., Wiedmer, T. Repolarization of the membrane potential of blood platelets after complement damage: evidence for a Ca++ - dependent exocytotic elimination of C5b-9 pores. Blood 1986; 68:556-561

Stanley, K.K., Kocher, H.P., Luzio, J.P., Jackson, P., Tschopp, J. The sequence and topology of human complement component C9. EMBO J 1985; 4:375-382

Storch, MK., Piddlesden, S., Haltia, M., Iivanainen, M., Morgan, P., Lassman, H. Multiple sclerosis: in situ evidence for antibody- and complement-mediated demyelination. Ann Neurol 1998; 43:465-471

Suttorp, N., Seeger, W., Zinsky, S., Bhakdi, S. Complement complex C5b-8 induces PGI$_2$ formation in cultured endothelial cells. Am J Physiol 1987; 253: C13-C21

Tedesco, F., Kahane, I., Zanella, A., Giovanetti, A.M., Sirchia, G. Functional study of lipids of PNH red cell membranes: susceptibility of liposomes to reactive lysis. Blood 1981a; 57:900-905

Tedesco, F., Rottini, G.D., Patriarca, P. Modulating effect of the late-acting components of the complement system on the bactericidal activity of human polymorphonuclear leukocytes on E. coli O111:B4. J Immunol 1981b; 127:1910-1915

Tedesco, F., Nürnberger, W., Perissutti, S. Inherited deficiencies of the terminal complement components. Intern Rev Immunol 1993; 10:51-64

Tedesco, F., Pausa, M. Nardon, E., Introna, M., Mantovani,A., Dobrina, A. The cytolytically inactive terminal complement complex activates endothelial cells to express adhesion molecules and tissue factor procoagulant activity. J Exp Med 1997; 185:1619-1627

Tedesco, F., Fischetti, F., Pausa, M., Dobrina, A., Sim, R.B., Daha, M.R. Complement-endothelial cell interactions: pathophysiological implications. Mol Immunol 1999; 36:261-268

Timmerman, J.J., van Dixhoorn, M.G., Schraa, E.O., van Gijlswiijk-Janssen, D.J., Muizert, Y., Van Es, L.A., Daha, M.R. Extrahepatic C6 is as effective as hepatic C6 in the generation of renal C5b-9 complexes. Kidney Int 1997; 51:1788-1796

Tramontini, N.L., Kuipers, P.J., Huber, C.M., Murphy, K., Naylor, K.B., Broady, A.J., Kilgore, K.S. Modulation of leukocyte recruitment and IL-8 expression by the membrane attack complex of complement (C5b-9) in a rabbit model of antigen-induced arthritis. Inflammation 2002; 26: 311-319

Tschopp, J., Podack, E.R., Muller-Eberhard, H.J. Ultrastructure of the membrane attack complex of complement: detection of the tetramolecular C9-polymerizing complex C5b-8. Proc Natl Acad Sci U S A 1982; 79:7474-7478

Tschopp, J. Ultrastructure of the membrane attack complex of complement. Heterogeneity of the complex caused by different degree of C9 polymerization. J Biol Chem 1984; 259:7857-7863.

Tschopp, J., Chonn, A., Hertig, S. Clusterin, the human apolipoprotein and complement inhibitor, binds to complement C7, C8 beta, and the b domain of C9. J. Immunol 1993; 151:2159-2165

Vakeva, A., Laurila, P., Meri, S. Loss of expression of protectin (CD59) is associated with complement membrane attack complex deposition in myocardial infarction. Lab Invest 1992; 67:608-616

Väkevä, A.P., Agah, A., Rollins, S.A., Matis, L.A., Li, L., Stahl, G.L. Myocardial infarction and apoptosis after myocardial ischemia and reperfusion: role of the terminal complement components and inhibition by anti-C5 therapy. Circulation 1998; 97:2259-2267

Wang, H., Rollins, S.A., Gao, Z., Garcia, B., Zhang, Z., Xing, J., Li, L., Kellersmann, R., Matis, L.A., Zhong, R. Complement inhibition with an anti-C5 monoclonal antibody prevents hyperacute rejection in a xenograft heart transplantation model. Transplantation 1999; 68:1643-1651

Wang, Y., Rollins, S.A., Madri, J.A., Matis, L.A. Anti-C5 monoclonal antibody therapy prevents collagen-induced arthritis and ameliorates established disease. Proc Natl Acad Sci U S A 1995; 92:8955-8959

Wang, Y., Hu, Q., Madri, J.A., Rollins, S.A., Chodera, A., Matis, L.A. Amelioration of lupus-like autoimmune disease in NZB/WF1 mice after treatment with a blocking monoclonal antibody specific for complement component C5. Proc Natl Acad Sci U S A 1996; 93:8563-8568

Wang, Y., Kristan, J., Hao, L., Lenkoski, C.S., Shen, Y., Matis, L.A. A role for complement in antibody-mediated inflammation: C5-deficient DBA/1 mice are resistant to collagen-induced arthritis. J Immunol 2000; 164: 4340-4347

Webster, S., Lue, L.F., Brachova, L., Tenner, A.J., McGeer, P,L., Terai, K., Walker, D.G., Bradt, B., Cooper, N.R., Rogers, J. Molecular and cellular characterization of the membrane attack complex, C5b-9, in Alzheimer's disease. Neurobiol Aging 1997; 18:415-421

Weiser, M.R., Williams, J.P., Moore, F.D.Jr., Kobzik, L., Ma, M., Hechtman, H.B., Carroll, M.C. Reperfusion injury of ischemic skeletal muscle is mediated by natural antibody and complement. J Exp Med 1996; 183:2343-2348

Wetsel, R.A., Fleischer, D.T., Haviland, D.L. Deficiency of the murine fifth complement component (C5). A 2-base pair gene deletion in a 5'-exon. J Biol Chem 1990; 265:2435-2440

Würzner, R., Joysey, V.C., Lachmann, P.J. Complement component C7. Assessment of in vivo synthesis after liver transplantation reveals that hepatocytes do not synthesize the majority of human C7. J Immunol 1994; 152:4624-4629

Yamamoto, T., Wilson, C.B. Complement dependence of antibody-induced mesangial cell injury in the rat. J Immunol 1987; 138: 3758-3765

Yang, L.B., Li, R., Meri, S., Rogers, J., Shen, Y. Deficiency of complement defense protein CD59 may contribute to neurodegeneration in Alzheimer's disease. J Neurosci 2000; 20:7505-7509

Zhou, W., Farrar, C.A., Abe, K., Pratt, J.R., Marsh, J.E., Wang, Y., Stahl, G.L., Sacks, S.H. Predominant role for C5b-9 in renal ischemia/reperfusion injury. J Clin Invest 2000; 105:1363-1371

7

The Many Faces of the Membrane Regulators of Complement

Claire L. Harris and B. Paul Morgan
Department of Medical Biochemistry and Immunology, University of Wales College of Medicine, Heath Park, Cardiff, CF14 4XN, UK

Abstract: The complement-inhibitory activities of the membrane complement regulators, decay accelerating factor (DAF), membrane cofactor protein (MCP), CD59 and complement receptor 1 (CR1), and their role in protection of "self" from the damaging effects of complement have long been understood. In recent years it has become clear that these proteins have additional roles and functions in health and disease. Some of these are to the host's benefit, whereas others are detrimental. These membrane proteins are abused by a multitude of pathogens, which use them as receptors to bind and enter host cells. Ligand binding to the regulator can trigger signaling cascades in diverse cell types resulting in cellular responses ranging from proliferation to apoptosis. Some may even play a role in the reproductive process. These recently described novel functions form the focus of this chapter. It is likely that this story is far from complete and other unexpected roles of membrane complement regulatory proteins will emerge in the near future.

Key words: decay accelerating factor, CD55, membrane cofactor protein, CD46, complement receptor 1, CD35, CD59

1   INTRODUCTION

Numerous complement (C) regulatory proteins (CReg) have evolved to meet the need to protect "self" from the potentially destructive effects of C. These proteins, present both in biological fluids and on cell membranes, police the body, preventing uncontrolled C activation in the fluid phase and rapidly inactivating any foci of activation on membranes. The CReg belong to three structurally and functionally distinct families of proteins: the serine protease inhibitors (SERPINs; C1inhibitor; C1inh), the "regulators of C activation" (RCA) family and the Ly-6 superfamily (CD59). Their task is to focus C activation on the membranes of genuine targets, to destroy active components that have "drifted" from the site of activation, and to prevent amplification of any nidus of activated C on self cells. The various CReg proteins collaborate to control the three activation pathways, classical (CP), alternative (AP) and lectin (LP) by regulating the amplification enzymes in these pathways. The regulators of the terminal pathways bind to the components of the forming membrane attack complex (MAC), thereby preventing the polymerisation of C9 and formation of the MAC pore.

The CReg are, as the name implies, best known for their roles in regulating C activation. These roles are briefly summarised here:

C1inh is a soluble protein that functions at the earliest stages of the C cascade. It inactivates the active C1 complex by covalently binding to the serine proteases C1r and C1s and removing them from the activated complex, switching off CP activation. C1inh also regulates the lectin pathway by binding to the MBL-associated proteases (MASPs).

The RCA-encoded CReg comprise *factor H* (fH), *C4b binding protein* (C4bp), *decay accelerating factor* (DAF; CD55), *membrane cofactor protein* (MCP; CD46) and *complement receptor 1* (CR1; CD35). The genes for these proteins, and several structurally related proteins playing other non-regulatory roles in C, are found in the RCA gene cluster on chromosome 1. All contain a structural module termed the short consensus repeat (SCR), a domain comprising approximately 60 amino acids that confers C3b/C4b binding affinity to the proteins and contains the regulatory function of the molecule. The number of domains varies from 4 (in MCP, DAF) to 37 (CR1, "B" isoform). C4bp and fH are soluble proteins whereas MCP, DAF and CR1 are expressed on the membrane. All function by inactivating the C3 and C5 convertase enzymes, either through "cofactor" or "decay accelerating" activity (Figure 1). Binding of a cofactor to either C3b or C4b enables a plasma serine protease, *factor I* (fI), to proteolytically cleave the active component and irreversibly inactivate the enzymes. The complementary activity, decay acceleration, is characterised by the ability of the regulator to destabilise the association between the enzyme components leading to their decay. CR1, fH (in the AP) and C4bp (in the CP) have both activities, MCP has cofactor activity and DAF has decay accelerating activity.

CD59 is a small molecule (~20kDa) associated with the plasma membrane through a GPI anchor. It blocks formation of the MAC by binding C8 within the C5b-8 complex, preventing unfolding and polymerisation of the final component, C9 (Figure 1).

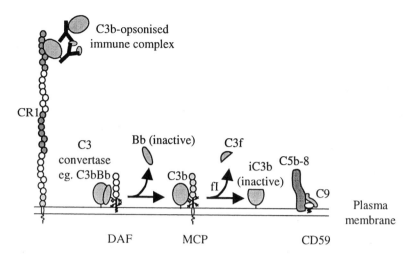

Figure 1. 'Conventional' roles of the membrane complement regulatory proteins. DAF binds to the convertases formed during all activation pathways and accelerates 'decay' of the subunits whereas MCP displays 'cofactor' activity enabling a plasma serine protease, factor I (fI), to irreversibly inactivate the major convertase subunits, C3b and/or C4b. CR1 has 'extrinsic' activity and functions in the extracellular milieu to bind C3b-opsonised particles, it has both decay and cofactor activity. If the activation pathway regulators fail to prevent C5b-8 formation, or if these components accidentally deposit on an 'innocent bystander' cell, CD59 prevents C9 unfolding correctly and polymerising to form the MAC.

The C-inhibitory roles of the CRegs have long been understood. The activity ascribed to C1inh was described as early as 1957, the regulatory functions of fH, C4bp and CR1 were described in the late 1970's and those of DAF, MCP and CD59 in the mid to late 1980's. Clearance of pathogens and infected cells has been perceived as the major role of C in the body, and the role of the CReg has been viewed simply as protection of host cells from "bystander lysis". The mechanisms by which C is activated, MAC is assembled and the ways in which CReg function to inactivate C complexes are all well defined. It is becoming increasingly clear, however, that C and its regulators have many other roles and functions in health and disease. Due to the widespread distribution of CReg, pathogens such as viruses and bacteria have adapted to use these molecules as receptors to aid infection. In addition CReg are usurped by these and other microorganisms in order to aid survival of the pathogen in the host. Other roles have come to light, for example, the potential role of MCP in fertilisation and reproduction is a current focus of investigation. The roles of the membrane-associated CReg in cell activation events have also been highlighted. Crosslinking of membrane CReg can result in a diverse range of biological responses such as activation of T cells and monocytes, triggering of endothelial cell proliferation or even triggering of apoptosis in various cell types. These, and other "alternative" roles of the human membrane-associated CReg (DAF, MCP, CR1 and CD59) will form the focus of this chapter.

2   USE AND ABUSE OF MEMBRANE COMPLEMENT REGULATORS BY PATHOGENS

Membrane CReg are widely and abundantly distributed throughout the body, on the surfaces of diverse cell types. Perhaps because of this wide distribution, many pathogens have evolved to manipulate host CReg in several different ways. First, many pathogens use these widely-expressed molecules as receptors to aid infection, either through direct binding interactions or via a C-derived opsonin, such as C3b or C3dg. Others have hijacked host CReg either by binding of fluid-phase regulators to the pathogen surface or by budding from CReg-rich areas of the cell membrane, in each case acquiring a protective coating of host CReg. Finally, some pathogens have taken to mimicry evolving their own CReg in order to circumvent attack by host C. These latter two areas, while generating an enormous amount of recent interest (reviewed in ref. 1), are beyond the scope of the current review. Here we will focus on the novel role, subversion of CReg as pathogen receptors.

2.1   DAF as a Pathogen Receptor

DAF has been implicated as a receptor for several pathogens, including uropathogenic strains of *Escherichia coli* and some enteroviruses of the Picornavirus family (Figure 2). DAF was first identified as a receptor for the enterovirus subgroup, echovirus, in 1994. Echoviruses cause a wide range of clinical conditions including rashes, diarrhoea, aseptic meningitis and respiratory disease. These viruses were known to agglutinate erythrocytes, and this activity was found to involve binding of DAF on the erythrocyte surface (2). Characterisation of the antigen-specificities of antibodies that protected from viral infection identified DAF as a receptor for echovirus 7 (EV7) and various other serotypes (including 6, 11, 12, 20 and 21) (3). DAF-binding by EV7 was confirmed independently in the same year using CELICS (cloning by enzyme-linked immuno-colour screening) methodology, a technology that identified many more DAF-binding serotypes (2,4). Not all echoviruses utilise DAF as a receptor, and some serotypes interact with more than one cellular receptor, possibly adapting to use predominantly one receptor in different clinical conditions or in laboratory cultures (2,5).

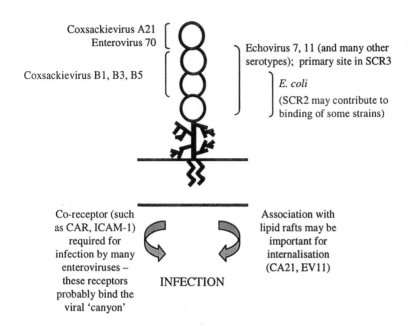

Figure 2. DAF as a pathogen receptor. DAF acts as a cellular receptor for various subgroups of the Picornavirus family, including many echoviruses, several coxsackieviruses and enterovirus 70. The various viruses bind to different domains on DAF implicating independent evolution in the selection of an efficient receptor (brackets indicate binding sites). The physical association of DAF with lipid rafts may contribute to infection, however, DAF probably acts to sequester virus to the cell surface by multiple low affinity interactions whilst productive infection is mediated by a co-receptor such as CAR (coxsackieviruses). DAF also aids anchorage of the uropathogenic bacterium *E. coli.* to epithelial cells. SCR domains are indicated as circles, the region between the fourth SCR domain and the GPI anchor is heavily glycosylated and is known as the ST (serine/threonine)-rich region.

The structural requirements for binding between DAF and various echovirus serotypes have been extensively characterised (6). By using SCR-deletion mutants of DAF, binding of EV7 has been shown to require SCR2, SCR3 and SCR4, and antibodies to the critical domain, SCR3, block binding (2,7). Binding to DAF is not dependent on the glycolipid (GPI) anchor as transmembrane forms can also mediate binding, although the GPI-dependent association of DAF with lipid rafts is essential for internalisation and infection of echovirus 11 (EV11) (2,7,8). Surface plasmon resonance (SPR) analysis of the DAF/EV11 interaction confirms that most binding is mediated via SCR3 with small contributions from SCR2 and SCR4 (7,8). The binding is of low affinity ($K_D \sim 3\mu M$), although overall avidity of binding may be higher due to the multiple binding sites per virion. Modeling of other Picornavirus-receptor interactions has indicated that in many cases the tip of the receptor interacts with a depression or "canyon" on the virus surface. This "canyon hypothesis" suggests that receptor-binding domains are buried in the canyon, sequestered from antibody-mediated immune surveillance, whereas the exposed surface contains domains in which mutations must occur rapidly to present an ever-changing face to the immune system (9). Binding of SCR3, in the middle of the DAF molecule, suggests a different mode of interaction with the echovirus. Indeed, analysis of mutant EV11 binding to DAF, and cryo-electron microscopy reconstructions of the DAF-EV7 interaction indicate that DAF binds well away from the canyon (10,11). Several modes of echovirus interaction with the cell may co-exist. Non-DAF-binding variants bind a high affinity receptor that inserts into the canyon in the mode of a "classical" enterovirus receptor, promoting uncoating and infection. The mode of entry of DAF-binding variants, however, is the subject of much debate. On the one hand DAF may sequester virus on the cell surface by multiple, low affinity interactions, tethering the virus to the cell surface and enabling interaction with the "true" internalisation receptor. The demonstration that soluble forms of DAF bind virus but do not mediate changes in the viral capsid structure that normally accompany infection implicates other cellular proteins in the infection process (9). On the other hand, DAF may sequester virus into the specialised membrane domains in which it is located (lipid rafts) and directly initiate internalisation. Uncoating of the virus may occur within the cell by interaction with an additional, as yet unidentified, intracellular factor (8,10). In this case, DAF acts as a functional uptake and internalisation receptor, rather than solely as a sequestration receptor.

It is significant that the various enteroviruses bind different domains in DAF. Binding to different structural domains on DAF suggests independent, yet repeating, evolution. More evidence is provided by the demonstration that DAF binding to EV7 and EV11 localises to slightly different regions on the virus. Other enteroviruses that bind DAF, such as Coxsackieviruses A21, B1, B3, B5 and enterovirus 70, also demonstrate independent evolution of binding. DAF binding of Coxsackievirus B3 (CB3), a virus implicated in infectious myocarditis, was shown in 1995; an antibody that blocked EV6-DAF interaction also prevented CB3 binding (12). It was soon confirmed that CB1 and CB5 could also bind DAF and the likely binding site was located to SCR2 and SCR3 using SCR-deletion mutants and blocking antibodies (12,13). The precise role of DAF has been unclear as alone it does not mediate CB infection of cells. As with the echoviruses discussed above, it was initially thought that DAF functioned to enhance infection by tethering virus to the cell surface, enabling interaction with high-affinity receptors such as coxsackie-adenovirus receptor (CAR). CAR expression alone in transfected cells is sufficient to permit infection by all CB viruses (14,15). However, recent studies have localised CAR to relatively virus-inaccessible intercellular tight junctions in polarised cells, such as respiratory and intestinal epithelial cells, barriers that the virus must cross in order to infect (16). CB3 cannot infect polarised colonic epithelial cells expressing CAR unless the tight junctions are disrupted. DAF, however, is abundant on the apical surface of such cells and facilitates infection by DAF-binding isolates of CB viruses. Presumably, DAF acts to "shuttle" the virus from the exposed apical surface to CAR.

In contrast to the SCR3 binders described above, coxsackievirus A21 (CA21) and enterovirus 70 (EV70) bind the first SCR in DAF. EV70 is responsible for acute hemorrhagic conjunctivitis in humans, and DAF is expressed at high levels on the conjunctival epithelium (17). The interaction of DAF and EV70 is not as well characterised as for the enteroviruses described above, although DAF clearly binds virus and expression of DAF in NIH 3T3 cells permits virus replication. Whether a co-receptor is involved is unclear. Early studies indicated that EV70-mediated haemagglutination was sensitive to removal of sialic acid from the erythrocyte surface, implicating surface receptors other than DAF (18,19). The co-receptor for the other SCR1-binding virus, CA21, is ICAM-1 (CD54); both DAF and ICAM-1 bind virus, but only binding to ICAM-1 can trigger uncoating and infection (20). However, a fascinating parallel exists for DAF-mediated CA21 infection and EV11 infection in that cross-linking of DAF in lipid rafts appears sufficient to mediate internalisation, with uncoating likely to be an intracellular event (21). A lytic infection of ICAM-1-negative rhabdomyosarcoma cells can be achieved if DAF is cross-linked by antibody to SCR3 prior to incubation with the virus. Although a lytic infection is established, there is no evidence of capsid conformational change in the virus, and the infection is much slower than when the cells are transfected with ICAM-1. It is unclear whether this mode of infection has significance *in vivo*, as effective cross-linking of DAF would be required for internalisation, and virus alone does not effect this. DAF and ICAM-1 may interact on the cell surface through SCR3 on DAF, and this may provide the means for crosslinking DAF prior to internalisation and infection (22).

Picornaviruses are not the only pathogens to have utilised DAF as an attachment receptor. Uropathogenic *E. coli* also bind DAF as a means to infect epithelia. *E. coli* and other gram-negative bacteria are coated with fimbriae, short, hair-like structures which project from the cell surface and express adhesin proteins that enable attachment to target cells. Tethering at multiple sites through these adhesins locks the bacterium on the target surface, preventing its removal as the surface is flushed by fluids such as blood or urine. Various *E. coli* strains haemagglutinated erythrocytes and the erythrocyte antigen mediating adhesion was shown from analyses of cells expressing different blood group antigens to be the Dr(a) antigen of the Cromer blood group, located on DAF (23). The bacterial adhesins mediating the interaction were named Dr adhesins in recognition of this activity. Members of the Dr family of adhesins include the fimbrial Dr haemagglutinin and F1845, and the afimbrial adhesins, AFA.

The majority of Dr adhesins bind SCR3 in DAF, corresponding to the location of the amino acid mutation (Ser165 to Leu) associated with the Dr(a) antigen, although other mutations in SCR3 can prevent binding (24-26). Differences in ligand binding are probably due to differences in the genetic make-up of the adhesins, which are composed of multiple protein subunits. The major structural subunits of the Dr haemagglutinin and F1845 fimbriae, DraE and DaaE respectively, are the DAF-binding domains and are responsible for the binding phenotype of the whole fimbria (27). Other adhesins, termed "X-adhesins", bind DAF but not the Dr(a) functional epitope, strains bearing these adhesins bind other regions on SCR3 or SCR4 (24-26). A recombinant model, based on the ability of CHO cells expressing DAF or DAF mutants to internalise Dr$^+$ and Dr$^-$ strains of *E. coli* has been developed and used to assess the structural requirements for the adhesin/DAF interaction (24,28). This work confirmed the importance of SCR3 in mediating internalisation and also implicated SCR2 in binding some Dr adhesins. The GPI anchor was important for infection, cells expressing transmembrane (TM) forms of DAF were able to bind bacteria efficiently, but had reduced or absent ability to internalise (28). Transmission electron microscopy of bacteria internalised on GPI- or TM-anchored DAF demonstrated that the bacteria were directed to morphologically distinct vacuoles. The different uptake pathways might reflect triggering of distinct events within the cell. It has been shown that adhesin binding to DAF results in intracellular signalling (29), and that DAF clustering and cytoskeletal rearrangements occur around bound bacteria (30). Engagement of host signaling pathways is likely a requirement for bacterial uptake. Even isolated fimbriae or fimbriae bound to latex beads can trigger uptake and internalisation in DAF-transfected CHO cells, suggesting that clustering or cross-linking of DAF by multiple adhesins is sufficient to trigger signaling for internalisation (28).

2.2   MCP as a Pathogen Receptor

Like DAF, the broadly expressed regulator MCP has been exploited by various pathogens as a receptor (Figure 3). The interaction that has received most attention is with the measles virus (MV), an enveloped negative-strand RNA virus of the Morbillivirus genus in the Paramyxoviridae family. MV is responsible for between 1 and 2 million deaths every year, particularly in children. Infection can lead to CNS infection or to suppression of cell-mediated immunity, predisposing to secondary infections such as pneumonia and diarrhoea. MCP was identified as a measles virus receptor independently by two groups in 1993. One group identified MCP as the antigen recognised by an antibody that blocked MV binding to cells, whilst the second group used somatic cell hybrids initially to identify the chromosome conferring MV sensitivity (31,32). MV infection of primary human monocytes resulted in down-regulation of IL-12 production, an effect that was replicated by antibody cross-linking of MCP, confirming the role of MCP as receptor and providing an explanation for the immunosuppression associated with MV infection (33). The MV binding site was located to SCR1 and SCR2 using MCP SCR deletion and chimeric SCR swap mutants (34-36). Various studies have pinpointed the individual residues on MCP involved in the interaction with MV (37-39). The viral recognition surface extends the length of the two SCRs, making it likely that a large area of the virus surface is involved, as discussed above for the DAF/enterovirus interactions (39). The carbohydrate on SCR2 may also be involved and, whilst the extracellular domains of MCP appear sufficient for the initial binding event, the transmembrane domain is necessary for efficient entry and viral replication (40-42).

In the late 1990s, the observation that the common Edmonston (Edm) laboratory strain of MV could not agglutinate erythrocytes of New World monkeys led to the characterisation of an unusual form of MCP lacking the first SCR in these primates (43). Surprisingly, wild-type (WT) virus did not agglutinate erythrocytes from African green monkeys (whose MCP retains SCR1) and New World monkeys were productively infected by (WT) virus (44). These findings strongly suggested the existence of a second receptor, subsequently confirmed by several laboratories (45). MV binds its receptor via the haemagglutinin (HA) protein. Binding assays using recombinant forms of this protein from WT and Edm strains of MV demonstrated that only the laboratory strain HA bound MCP (46). WT virus failed to downregulate MCP on infected cells, a characteristic of Edm MV, and alteration of just a few amino acids in either HA protein could reverse the down-regulating capacity of the virus, presumably by changing its binding characteristics (47,48).   These differences in the binding of WT and laboratory or vaccine strains of MV raised the possibility that MCP was not the relevant receptor in clinical measles infection (49).   By studying the binding characteristics of different virus isolates and analysing their passage history, it has been shown that receptor-binding characteristics of MV were determined by the cell type in which it was passaged. The popular Edm laboratory strain of virus was first isolated from a throat swab in 1954, initially passaged in human kidney cells and subsequently in African green monkey kidney (Vero) cells. These cells express MCP with all four SCR and as a consequence Edm MV can efficiently use this receptor.   In 1990, it was demonstrated that it was easier to isolate virus from the marmoset EBV-transformed B cell line, B95a (50).   These cells express MCP lacking the first SCR essential for binding Edm strain MV, and passage thus favoured usage of a different receptor. The MV receptor in these cells was identified in 2000 using functional expression cloning, and shown to be the marmoset homolog of the signaling lymphocytic activation molecule (SLAM; CD150) (51,52).   The distribution of SLAM is more restricted than MCP; it is primarily located on lymphoid cells, although it is also found on activated monocytes.   These sites of expression mirror the major sites of MV replication *in vivo* and correlate with MV-induced pathogenesis.

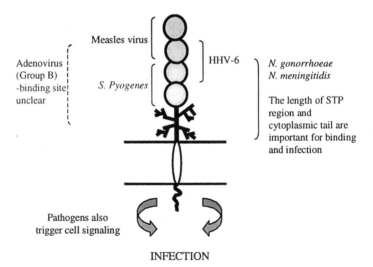

INFECTION

Figure 3. MCP as a pathogen receptor. MCP is a cellular receptor for measles virus, HHV-6, some serotypes of adenovirus and several different bacteria. Binding sites are different and are distributed throughout the protein (brackets indicate binding sites). SCR domains are indicated as circles, the region between the fourth SCR domain and the transmembrane domain is known as the ST (serine/threonine)-rich region. MCP exists as several isoforms with one of two different cytoplasmic tails, termed CYT-1 and CYT-2.

The emergence of SLAM as a candidate pathological receptor *in vivo* focused attention on receptor usage by recent clinical isolates of MV which had not undergone the altered receptor usage typical of laboratory strains. All MV isolates analysed to date used SLAM as a receptor; in fact, most isolates only used SLAM and did not bind MCP (53). However, some isolates were capable of using MCP as a receptor, albeit at a lower efficiency; as might be expected, laboratory strains and Vero-adapted strains used MCP in addition to SLAM (54-56). The evidence indicates that SLAM is the primary MV receptor *in vivo*; however, MCP is much more broadly expressed and it cannot be ruled out that MV may adapt and alter its receptor usage to MCP subsequent to the initial infection. This might be particularly relevant to the brain where SLAM is absent but MCP is expressed at various sites within the brain, including neurones, cerebral endothelium, ependymal cells and oligodendrocytes (57,58). A single amino acid difference (Asn481 to Tyr) in the HA protein is sufficient to confer high affinity MCP-binding to the virus (46). SPR analysis of the kinetics of binding to the Edm HA protein indicated that the association rate for SLAM binding was 20-fold lower than that of MCP; however the subsequent binding was tighter as the dissociation rate was much lower (5-fold) (59). Competition studies indicated that the receptor binding sites on the HA protein were overlapping. It will be interesting to similarly analyse the effect of mutation in other HA proteins on binding to the receptors. Two recent reports demonstrate MV infection of cells which express neither SLAM or MCP, suggesting that yet more MV receptors remain to be identified (60,61).

In 1999, MCP was also implicated as a receptor for herpesvirus 6 (HHV-6), a dsDNA enveloped virus of the β-herpesvirus subfamily (62). HHV-6 primarily infects CD4$^+$ T cells, although it can infect other human cell types. It is virtually ubiquitous in the adult population, with primary infection usually occurring within the first year of life. Re-activation of the latent virus occurs under certain conditions such as immunosuppression and HHV-6 infection may accelerate human immunodeficiency virus (HIV) disease progression; HHV-6 infection is also tentatively linked to multiple sclerosis (63,64). Both major variants of HHV-6 (HHV-6A and HHV-6B) bind MCP (62), binding of the A variant can trigger syncitium formation in human cells in an MCP-dependent manner (65). The molecular details of the interaction between MCP and HHV-6 are incompletely understood. Using SCR-deletion and SCR-substitution the binding site has been localised on MCP and involves SCR2 and SCR3. In sharp contrast to MV binding, SCR1 is dispensable (66). The binding site on the virus is located on a complex of viral proteins comprising glycoprotein H, glycoprotein L and glycoprotein Q (67). The interaction between MCP and HHV-6 and the mechanism of infection requires further attention.

Whilst the interaction of MCP with MV and HHV-6 has been recognised for some time, recent data bring to light the interaction of MCP with one further group of viruses, group B adenoviruses. Adenoviruses are classified into 6 subgroups (A-F) and comprise over 50 serotypes. The majority of these viruses use CAR as their primary attachment receptor; however, a number of the group B adenoviruses utilise MCP as a cellular receptor (68,69). *In vitro* binding of group B adenoviruses to MCP-transfected cells was demonstrated in several studies, and competition with soluble MCP or with a soluble form of the viral fiber knob domain that mediates attachment to the cellular receptor were shown to inhibit infection. Similarly, antibodies to MCP inhibit virus binding, particularly those that bind to the carboxy-terminal SCR domains in MCP. Use of MCP as a receptor *in vivo* was confirmed using human MCP transgenic mice, these animals had virus in all organs three days following injection of virus into the tail vein, while control animals had almost none. The broad distribution of MCP, compared to the limited distribution of CAR, may explain the broad tissue tropism of group B adenoviruses demonstrated *in vitro* and the diverse clinical manifestations seen *in vivo*. It may be possible to take advantage of the receptor differences in the adenovirus subgroups for gene therapy to enable infection of target cells that are normally refractory to infection by CAR-binding viruses.

The number of different viruses that bind to membrane-associated members of the RCA family and utilise them as cellular receptors is ever increasing. Measles virus, HHV-6 and adenovirus subgroups bind MCP, various echoviruses and coxsackieviruses bind DAF and, although not discussed above, Epstein-Barr virus has long been known to bind another member of this family, CR2. The common structural feature of these RCA proteins is the SCR domain, these form a linear array of structural domains that project away from the cell membrane and are ideally placed for exploitation by viruses. DAF and MCP are widely expressed in tissues, including on epithelial cells at mucosal surfaces, these are likely to be the first cells a virus will encounter following entry into the body. In addition these receptors, CR2 included, can initiate signaling cascades and cell activation subsequent to virus binding may be important for infectivity. Given these facts, it may not be surprising that so many viruses have followed a common evolutionary path to exploit these SCR-containing molecules as cellular receptors.

Like DAF, MCP can bind adhesins of various bacteria, including *Neisseria gonorrhoeae* and *Neisseria meningitidis*. In these organisms, adhesins are expressed on cell projections termed pili. The type IV pilus, expressed on the surface of the bacterium, mediates the initial contact with the host cell membrane, facilitating uptake and invasion. The distribution of MCP is broad and includes epithelial cells of the respiratory tract and cells at the blood-brain barrier (70). It is likely that expression at these sites facilitates development of bacterial meningitis. Indeed, recent studies using human MCP transgenic mice confirm the role of MCP in the dissemination of *N. meningitidis* from the airways to the blood and cerebrospinal fluid (71). The interaction between MCP and the *Neisseria* pilus was discovered when it was shown that purified pili bound to 55-60 kDa doublet on blots of SDS PAGE separated epithelial cell lysates. Subsequent transfection and blocking studies confirmed that the pili bound to MCP (72). The length of the ST (serine/threonine-rich) region in MCP has a profound effect on adherence, with the longest BC isoforms mediating best attachment; SCR3 and the N-linked carbohydrate on SCR4 also contribute to binding (73). Signaling events play a role in strengthening the bacterium/cell interaction, ligation of the MCP isoform bearing the cytoplasmic tail termed CYT-2 (see below) appears particularly important in infection. Of note, this isoform of MCP predominates in the CNS and may be of relevance to infection with *N. meningitidis* at this site. Inhibitors of the Src family tyrosine kinases, enzymes known to phosphorylate the cytoplasmic tails of MCP (see below), inhibit bacterial adherence and a candidate enzyme, c-Yes, has been identified (74).

The bacterium *Streptococcus pyogenes* (group A streptococcus), commonly responsible for suppurative and inflammatory infections of the skin, also exploits the C system in several different ways. In addition to sequestering fluid phase C regulators such as fH and C4bp to their surface to prevent C activation and opsonisation, *S. pyogenes* uses MCP as an adherence receptor on keratinocytes (75). The binding site is again located in SCR3 and SCR4. Binding of the bacterium is not competitive with C3b binding, raising the possibility that *S. pyogenes* could usurp the C-regulatory ability of MCP, as it does with fH and C4bp (76). Alternatively binding between C3b on the bacterial surface and MCP could strengthen the bond between the pathogen and the cell surface.

2.3 CD59 as a Pathogen Receptor

There is very little evidence that the broadly expressed GPI-anchored MAC inhibitor, CD59, plays significant roles as a receptor for pathogens.

Antisera against CD59 were recently shown to inhibit infection of rhabdomyosarcoma cells with echoviruses, including strains known to bind DAF (77). The relative roles of DAF and CD59 in these interactions remain unclear. *Aeromonas hydrophila*, a human pathogen that produces deep wound infections and gastroenteritis, secretes a pore-forming toxin, aerolysin, that causes cytolysis of targets (78). A curious observation was that erythrocytes from patients with paroxysmal nocturnal hemoglobinuria (PNH) were resistant to lysis by aerolysin; indeed, this phenomenon has been mooted as a diagnostic test for the condition (79). Loss of sensitivity to lysis correlated with loss of CD59 expression but there is no experimental evidence to support the suggestion that the toxin actually binds CD59.

2.4   CR1 and Binding of HIV

While CR1 has not yet been identified as the primary receptor for any pathogen, it can enhance infection of various cell types by HIV (80,81). Enhancement is due to its capacity to bind C3b and iC3b on C-opsonised virions, not precisely a novel role as it is acting as a C3b receptor. However, this native activity of CR1 has been exploited by HIV, and in these circumstances the binding to C3 activation products on the viral surface is deleterious to the host. HIV virions activate C via both the AP and CP, depositing C3b on the virion surface. However, the virus has strong intrinsic resistance to lysis by C, partly due to the presence of membrane CReg, such as CD59 and DAF, which have been hijacked during budding from the host cell and incorporated into the viral envelope. Binding of soluble CReg, particularly fH, also contributes to a protective coating which degrades C3b to downstream inactive products. Recruitment of the C3 fragment receptors CR1, CR2 and CR3 can enhance infection of cells with HIV, sometimes in a CD4-independent manner (Figure 4) (82,83-87).

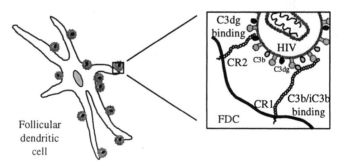

Figure 4. CR1 as a pathogen receptor. Various complement receptors on follicular dendritic cells, including CR1, bind opsonised HIV thereby localising and concentrating virus in an ideal environment for infection of cells within the lymphoid follicles.

These receptors enhance infection by activation of cells following cross-linking of the receptor, targeting C-opsonised HIV to B and T cells and, perhaps most importantly, localising virus to germinal centres in lymphoid tissue enabling prolonged and efficient infection of lymphocytes (81). Both CR1 and CR2 are involved - antibodies to either receptor or soluble forms of these molecules can inhibit infection. It is likely that CR2 plays the major role *in vivo* as it binds C3dg, the final breakdown product of C3b and the form most likely to predominate on the virion (88). Concentration of virus in germinal centres and localisation to follicular dendritic cells (FDCs) is a major feature of HIV pathogenesis. The immune response probably deals with the initial burst of viraemia subsequent to primary infection, but apparent clearance of virus is largely due to sequestration by FDCs which bind opsonised virus via C receptors. Extracellular association of virions with the processes of FDCs, which surround and intimately associate with lymphocytes, has been demonstrated in many studies and provides an efficient means for transmission of infection to cells as they migrate through the lymphoid follicles (89-93).

3   ROLE OF COMPLEMENT REGULATORS IN CELL ACTIVATION

C activates surrounding cells in many different ways. Best described are the soluble C activation products, C5a and C3a, which interact with specific receptors on the cell surface to trigger cellular responses. However, the CReg, present on the membrane to protect from C attack, can themselves trigger cell activation when cross-linked by antibody or ligand. MCP is a transmembrane protein and ligation results in signal transduction via its cytoplasmic tail. CD59 and DAF are GPI-anchored and cannot directly trigger cell activation. These GPI-anchored CReg are located in detergent-insoluble, cholesterol-rich areas of the membrane termed lipid rafts, enriched in molecules that play a role in the innate immune response (94,95). The lipid rafts contain palmitoylated transmembrane adaptor proteins, such as LAT (linker for activation of T cells) and PAG (phosphoprotein associated with glycosphingolipid-enriched microdomains), and a multitude of intracellular signaling molecules such as Src family kinases and G-proteins (96-100). GPI-anchored molecules acquire signaling capacity by associating with adaptor proteins that couple the signal triggered at the cell surface with more distal signaling pathways.

3.1   Signaling Through DAF

Almost all studies of the signaling capability of DAF have utilised antibodies to cross-link the molecule on the surface of cells. Initial work over 10 years ago demonstrated that antibody-mediated cross-linking of DAF on neutrophils resulted in release of Ca^{2+} stores, activation of tyrosine kinases and activation of the oxidase response; in addition monocytes demonstrated enhanced phagocytic activity when activated by DAF (101,102). There has been little follow-up to these initial studies, although a potential role of DAF in T cell activation has been described (103), and recruitment of signal transduction molecules in intestinal epithelial cells following ligation of DAF by *E. coli* adhesin has also been demonstrated (Figure 5) (29).

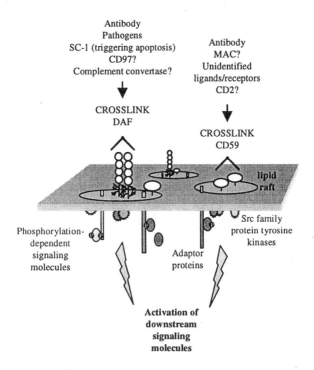

Figure 5. DAF and CD59 in signaling and cell activation. DAF and CD59 are located in detergent-insoluble, cholesterol-rich areas of the membrane termed lipid rafts. Transmembrane adaptor proteins and multiple intracellular signaling molecules, including Src family protein tyrosine kinases, are enriched in these specialised areas of the membrane. Crosslinking of DAF or CD59 with many different ligands, either within or possibly between lipid rafts, results in diverse cellular responses.

Several recent reports suggest that DAF may be a component of the LPS receptor complex, contributing to LPS-induced activation of cells (104-106). Fluorescence resonance energy transfer (FRET) analysis confirmed that the LPS receptor, CD14, is clustered with DAF in lipid rafts in monocytes, along with other receptors such as CD32, CD64 and CD47 (107). Following stimuation with LPS, other receptors, including Toll-like receptor 4 (TLR4), CD11b and CD81 are recruited to these rafts, whilst some, including CD47, are lost from the cluster. DAF remains in the cluster but its role in transducing the LPS signal remains to be clarified. DAF is associated with protein tyrosine kinases within the cell and a putative adaptor protein has been identified, suggesting that DAF may directly mediate signaling events (103,108,109). Whether the C-derived DAF ligands, the convertase components, can themselves trigger signaling via DAF is unknown.

Several other intriguing stories implicating DAF in signaling have emerged. DAF has been identified as a ligand for CD97, a member of the seven-span transmembrane (TM7) protein family, with its extracellular domain comprising epidermal growth factor (EGF) repeats (110,111). CD97 is expressed on monocytes and granulocytes and is upregulated on activated B and T cells. The interaction between DAF and CD97 is of low affinity ($K_D \sim 90\mu M$) and appears to involve the first SCR of DAF, a domain with no clear role in C regulation (112-114). The biological significance of this interaction is as yet unclear but it may be involved in cell activation, migration and/or adhesion in inflammatory conditions. Upregulation of DAF concomitant with increased expression of CD97 on leukocytes at sites of inflammation has been demonstrated in inflammatory diseases, such as arthritis and multiple sclerosis (115,116).

Intriguingly, DAF appears to be over-expressed in certain tumour types, particularly those of colorectal origin; antibody specific for DAF has been used for tumour imaging in these diseases and shed or soluble DAF is excreted at high levels from patients with colorectal cancer (117-119). It appears that a major proportion of the expressed DAF in these tumours is secreted or deposited in the extracellular matrix (ECM) around the tumour cells, this ECM deposition is also seen in some normal tissues (120). Interestingly, CD97, the expression of which is normally limited, has been identified at high levels on tumour cells of various origins, including colorectal cancer (121,122). The high level of expression correlates with high levels of tumour migration and invasion; whether DAF is present at increased levels to protect tumour cells from attack by the C system, or whether it plays a role in cell adhesion and migration, is still a matter of debate. One further twist in the story relates to the expression of a highly glycosylated form of DAF on diffuse- and intestinal-type adenocarcinomas. When DAF is ligated *in vitro* and *in vivo* by a therapeutic anti-DAF antibody, SC-1, rapid tyrosine phosphorylation of intracellular proteins results and caspases-3, -6 and -8 are activated, triggering apoptosis, thus providing a potential anti-cancer therapy (123,124). The tumour cells express two forms of DAF, the normally glycosylated protein and the highly glycosylated form which alone is recognised by SC-1 (125). The mechanics of expression of this highly glycosylated DAF is unknown, and the pathways leading to cell death are unclear. Nevertheless, the capacity of the DAF-binding antibody to efficiently induce tumor cell apoptosis is clearly of major significance for cancer therapy.

3.2 Signaling Through MCP

Although the signaling roles of MCP have been recognised more recently, they have been analysed more extensively than those of DAF. MCP exists on the cell surface in various isoforms resulting from alternative splicing of one gene. All comprise four invariant SCRs, an ST-region of varying length, a transmembrane domain and one of two different cytoplasmic tails, CYT-1 and CYT-2. The first indications that MCP might be involved in modulation of cellular responses came from studies with pathogens, described above, that use MCP as receptor. Ligation of MCP with *N. gonorrhoeae* pili resulted in a Ca^{2+} flux in epithelial cells, and ligation with measles virus (MV) caused a decreased ability of monocytes and dendritic cells to produce IL-12 in response to LPS (33,126,127). Since these early reports, a rapidly expanding literature has implicated MCP in a multitude of cellular responses, including enhancement of NO production from macrophages (128,129), increased production of IL-6 from astrocytes (130), enhancement of IgE class-switching in B cells (131) and activation of T cells (Figure 6) (132-135).

Both MCP cytoplasmic tails are involved in cell signaling events but may have dramatically different effects on the cell. For example, ligation of the CYT-1 isoform of MCP with antibody or MV resulted in enhanced production of NO from macrophages (128,136). In contrast, ligation of the CYT-2 isoform had little effect on the cell. Both tails associate, directly or indirectly, with intracellular kinases. In macrophage this has been demonstrated by expressing either MCP tail as a fusion protein with GST and using these constructs to affinity isolate cytoplasmic proteins from cell lysates (137). Both MCP tail constructs were phosphorylated on tyrosine, as were other co-purifying proteins. The membrane-proximal sequence Tyr-Arg-Tyr-Leu, which is common to both isoforms, appears to have a role in these associations as mutation in this region abolished much of the phosphorylation. However, tyrosine-phosphorylation of CYT-2 was not inhibited to the same extent in these mutants, implicating other phosphorylation targets within this cytoplasmic tail. Subsequent studies have demonstrated tail-specific phosphorylation of CYT-2 by Src family kinases, possibly via phosphorylation of a downstream tyrosine (probably Tyr 354) (74,138).

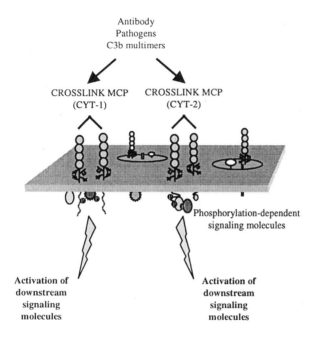

Figure 6. MCP in signaling and cell activation. MCP exists in various isoforms, all are transmembrane with one of two different cytoplasmic tails (CYT-1 and CYT-2). Crosslinking of MCP with various ligands results in phosphorylation of the cytoplasmic domain and other signaling molecules and can have profound activation effects on the cell. The cellular response depends on the cytoplasmic tail expressed and crosslinked. It is unclear whether MCP associates with transmembrane adaptor molecules or even with components of the lipid rafts.

The role of MCP in T cell activation has been the centre of much attention and the signaling pathways involved are some way to being dissected. Co-ordinate ligation of MCP and CD3 on T cells strongly promotes T cell proliferation and can trigger dramatic morphological changes and actin relocalization, cellular responses that may be important for migration and homing of T cells, interaction with antigen presenting cells and formation of the immunological synapse. Cross-linking of MCP on primary human T cells induces phosphorylation of the adaptor proteins p120^{CBL} and LAT (132), and the GTP/GDP exchange factor Vav, which is enhanced if cells are co-stimulated via CD3 (133). Vav is known to play a role in T cell activation-induced actin cytoskeletal rearrangements. Co-stimulation also results in activation of the GTPase Rac, and of extracellular signal-related kinase mitogen-activated protein kinase (Erk MAPK). An elegant study analysed the differential effects of the cytoplasmic tails expressed on T cells on the inflammatory response in the contact hypersensitivity (CHS) reaction to the hapten dinitrofluorobenzene (DNFB) *in vivo* (134). Transgenic mice were generated that expressed either isoform of MCP, and UV-inactivated recombinant vesicular stomatitis virus (VSV) expressing the measles virus hemagglutinin was used to cross-link MCP *in vivo* just prior to sensitisation with DNFB. Following a subsequent challenge with DNFB some days later, mice expressing the CYT-2 isoform showed an enhanced inflammatory response, whereas those with CYT-1 had less inflammation. The effect of CYT-1 appeared to be dominant in that mice expressing both isoforms had the CYT-1 phenotype. The effect was T cell dependent and involved both CD4$^+$ and CD8$^+$ cells. CTL activity in hapten-sensitised CYT-1 mice was impaired whilst CTL in CYT-2 mice showed enhanced cytotoxic actvity. In addition, secretion of CD4$^+$ T cell-derived cytokines, such as IL-10, was differentially modulated with reduced secretion of IL-10 in CYT-2 mice. *In vitro* proliferation assays demonstrated increased proliferation of CD4$^+$ T cells derived from CYT-1 mice and decreased proliferation from CYT-2 mice when co-stimulated with anti-CD3 antibodies. As noted in other studies, T cell morphology was dramatically affected by the stimulation, but only in cells expressing the CYT-1 tail; Vav was phosphorylated and is presumably one of the downstream mediators of this MCP-triggered cellular response. A complementary study using human CD4$^+$ T cells also demonstrated a dramatic effect of CD3/MCP co-stimulation (135). In this case, purified T cells stimulated in the presence of IL-2 acquired a cytokine profile characteristic of T-regulatory cells (Tr1) and phenotypic features expected in memory T cells. It is not clear whether the effects reported in this study are dependent on a specific isoform of MCP on T cells.

An early report of MCP signaling suggested that the natural ligand, C3b, could when dimerised trigger cell activation through MCP (33). No further reports of MCP signaling using natural ligands emerged until the recent demonstration that the T cell activating events *in vivo* and *in vitro* described above were also triggered by C3b oligomers (134-136). In these studies, the effect of C3b was subtly different to that obtained following cross-linking of

MCP with antibody or MV, suggesting that the nature of the ligand or combination of ligands may influence the cellular responses. The ability of MCP, and possibly also of DAF, to signal following ligation with C-derived products, such as C3b or the convertase, throws a new light on the role of the activation pathway regulators in innate and adaptive immunity. In a localised inflammatory reaction, a target cell or pathogen becomes coated in C-derived opsonins, and quite possibly "innocent bystander" cells undergo a limited C attack, which is rapidly controlled by CRegs as described above. Under physiological conditions, production of C3a, C5a and low-level deposition of C3b and consequent ligation of CReg such as MCP may be the only sign of a localised inflammatory reaction. Ligation of CReg on host cells, such as endothelial cells, may stimulate those cells to respond to the local environment by synthesising proteins required either for protection in the face of inflammation and/or for facilitation of an efficient inflammatory response. Leukocytes recruited to the inflammatory site by chemotactic molecules such as C5a, or stimulated by antigen presenting cells, may be activated by various ligands, including C3b interacting with MCP, to respond in an appropriate way. The striking examples of cell activation described above clearly illustrate the potential role of CReg, such as MCP, in bridging innate and T cell-mediated immunity, a fascinating parallel to the role of CR1/CR2 in bridging innate and B cell-mediated immunity as discussed below.

3.3 Signaling Through CD59

CD59, like DAF and other GPI-anchored molecules, signals because of its association in lipid rafts with adaptor molecules and intracellular kinases (Figure 5) (139). Antibody cross-linking of CD59 on human neutrophils was shown rapidly to trigger calcium flux and an oxidase response via activation of tyrosine kinases (102,140). Binding of bivalent mAb alone was not sufficient to trigger these events; further cross-linking with a polyclonal secondary antibody was required, implying that aggregation was an essential prelude to signaling. The requirement for association in lipid rafts was vividly demonstrated by incorporating purified GPI-anchored CD59 into a CD59-negative cell line (141). CD59, at first distributed homogeneously over the cell surface, became clustered in rafts in a time-dependent manner and contemporaneously acquired the capacity to signal upon cross-linking. In lymphocytes, it is apparent that CD59 within lipid rafts interacts with adaptor proteins that link through to intracellular kinases (99,100). The details of signaling are much less clear in other cell types but are likely to involve similar chains of molecules. In HeLa cells, dimerisation of CD59 has been reported to be essential for acquisition of signaling capacity (142).

Whether this is unique to HeLa or a general phenomenon related to association with adaptors has yet to be examined. A recent study reports the intriguing observation that CD59 is involved in LPS signal transduction in oral keratinocytes, cells which do not naturally express CD14 (143). LPS binding to cells resulted in nuclear translocation of NF-κB and induction of granulocyte-macrophage colony-stimulating factor, interleukin-6 and tumour necrosis factor-alpha. Treatment of cells with PI-PLC, anti-CD59 antibodies or with CD59 antisense oligonucleotides inhibited these effects and implicated CD59 in the signal transduction process. The adaptors and downstream signaling molecules, however, were not identified.

The realisation that CD59 signaled triggered a search for natural ligands that bound CD59 to cause cell activation. Several early studies implicated CD59 as a second partner for the T cell surface molecule CD2, already known to bind CD58 (144,145). CHO cells expressing CD59 formed rosettes with T cells and this rosetting was blocked by anti-CD2 mAb. These observations were later extended to show that CD59 interaction with CD2 delivered a co-stimulatory signal for T cell activation (146). A related recent study described activation of cytokine secretion in skin fibroblasts exposed to CD2-expressing HL60 cells (147). Activation was dependent on HL60 expression of CD2 and closely mirrored that caused by cross-linking of CD59 on the fibroblasts. Despite all this evidence, analyses of the interaction of CD59 and CD2 using recombinant soluble proteins and SPR failed to demonstrate any binding (148). These contradictory results imply that a second molecule on T lymphocytes is necessary either as co-ligand or as the primary ligand for CD59. What is not in doubt is that CD59 acts as a co-stimulatory molecule for T cell activation (147,149). A second line of evidence suggesting that cells expressed receptors for CD59 that triggered activation events came from studies of urine-derived factors triggering fibroblast proliferation. A protein component of normal urine induced proliferation of synovial fibroblasts and sequencing of this protein revealed identity at the amino terminus with CD59 (150). No formal evidence that CD59 was responsible for the observed proliferation was obtained and no search for receptors for CD59 was undertaken.

An obvious candidate ligand for CD59 is the MAC or its component proteins. The component proteins of the MAC may bind CD59 under certain circumstances. A recent report described cell activation in THP-1 and U937 cells incubated with C8 that mimicked the effects of antibody cross-linking CD59 in these cells (151). This result is difficult to reconcile with the fact that blood cells and endothelia are continuously exposed to plasma C8 *in vivo*; perhaps denatured or aggregated C8 in the commercial preparation used was responsible for the effects observed. CD59 binds the forming MAC at the C5b-8 stage and inhibits formation of the lytic lesion (152). It has been suggested that binding of CD59 into clusters of forming MAC triggers signaling events that aid clearance of the complex (153). Although the clearance process is well-documented (154,155), involvement of CD59 has yet to be formally tested, primarily because it is difficult to dissociate the effects of the MAC itself from those that might be induced by ligation of CD59.

A recent report described the induction of apoptosis in T cell lines following CD59 cross-linking (156). This study showed that CD59-triggered apoptosis was caused by release of the TNF family member APO2 ligand, and supernatants from such cells caused apotosis in naïve T cells. The physiological relevance of these findings cannot be known until the natural ligands for CD59 are identified.

These two situations, activation by CD59 of cells expressing an unidentified receptor and activation of cells expressing CD59 upon interaction with an unknown ligand are two sides of the same coin. Together they strongly imply that CD59 binds one or more ligand/receptor with consequences both for the cell expressing CD59 and for that expressing the ligand/receptor. Identification of natural ligands/receptors for CD59 is now urgently required.

4 COMPLEMENT REGULATORS AND REPRODUCTION

CReg are essential for successful reproduction, they protect the sperm on its arduous journey to the egg, and the foetus as it develops in the uterus. Sperm in the female genital tract are targets for attack from C, present in abundance in the secretions that lubricate the mucosa (157-159). Protection is provided by membrane CReg, DAF and CD59, expressed on the sperm (160-162), and by seminal fluid which contains soluble CReg such as clusterin and S-protein. Seminal plasma also contains prostasomes, small vesicles derived from prostatic epithelium which have DAF, MCP and CD59 on their surfaces (163,164). *In vitro* experiments demonstrate that the CReg on prostasomes can transfer to membranes of cells in their vicinity, including sperm, hence providing additional protection against C in the genital tract (165-167). The membrane CReg are expressed in abundance on the trophoblast throughout pregnancy, providing protection from maternal C at the interface between mother and foetus (168-170). The critical role of

CReg at this site has been elegantly demonstrated in mice engineered to delete Crry, a ubiquitously expressed homologue of MCP and DAF (171). The embryos of Crry-knockout mice die in utero due to C activation and inflammation in the placenta, however, breeding to C3 knockout mice rescued the embryos, demonstrating the crucial role for C in foetal destruction.

It is not surprising or novel to discover that CReg expressed on the surface of sperm and on the trophoblast function to protect these cells from C attack. However, a surprising alternative role for MCP in fertilisation and reproduction has come to light. It has been known for some time that MCP is found at high levels in the reproductive system; in fact, even before its characterisation as a regulator of the C system, MCP was identified by several different groups as an antigen found on the acrosomal region of sperm (172-174). MCP was localised to the inner acrosomal membrane and was only exposed to extracellular fluid following the acrosome reaction, an essential prelude to fertilisation. The cryptic site of expression suggested a role other than C regulation, possibly in the fertilisation process itself. This notion was supported by observations of abnormal MCP on the sperm of infertile men and by studies demonstrating that antibodies to the first SCR in MCP inhibited sperm/egg interaction (175-177). One report demonstrated an involvement of C3b in the penetration of the egg by sperm, raising the possibility that the MCP/C3b interaction itself might be involved in fertilisation. It may be of relevance that MCP on human sperm is truncated and hypo-glycosylated, and cDNAs for several novel isoforms of MCP, differing in their transmembrane and cytoplasmic regions, have been detected in the testis (161,178-181). Yet more compelling evidence for a role of MCP in the fertilisation process has come from studies in New World monkeys. MCP in these monkeys lacks the first SCR, perhaps due to selective pressure from the measles virus[43]. In testis and on sperm, however, an isoform of MCP that retains the first SCR has been found, strengthening the case for a specific role for MCP in this location (181). It is interesting also that rodents express MCP preferentially or exclusively in the testis (182,183). We have recently found that rat MCP is expressed only on the inner acrosomal membrane of spermatozoa, further implicating the molecule in sperm-egg interactions (184). These accumulating data all point towards a facilitating role for MCP in the reproductive process. The recent generation of an MCP knock-out, however, has muddied the water (185). Instead of the anticipated infertility, litter sizes sired by MCP-/- males were normal or higher than those by wild-type males and the MCP-/- sperm demonstrated an accelerated spontaneous acrosome reaction. These data are difficult to explain but might suggest that MCP on the inner acrosomal membrane stabilises the acrosome by interacting with unidentified components, thereby delaying the spontaneous acrosome reaction. The normal reproductive capacity of C3 knockout mice supports this hypothesis as clearly the interaction of MCP with its complement ligand, C3b, is not a prerequisite for successful fertilisation.

5 CR1 AND CR2: BRIDGING INNATE AND ADAPTIVE IMMUNITY

No review of novel roles of CReg would be complete without a brief description of the crucial part played by CR1 in collaboration with CR2, linking innate and adaptive immunity. The well-known function of CR1 is to act as a receptor for C3b and catalyse its cleavage, allowing CR1 to regulate C activation and play a major role in immune complex handling. On the surface of B cells, these activities are channelled to a different end. CR1 sits in a complex with the C receptor 2 (CR2; CD21) and a number of other proteins, including the B cell receptor (BCR), CD79, CD19, and CD81 (186-188). CR1 binds C3b-coated immune complexes and catalyses cleavage of C3b to C3dg, releasing the complex and enabling it simultaneously to engage CR2 via C3dg, and BCR via antigen. This cross-linking event markedly lowers the threshold required for antigen-mediated signaling through the BCR and subsequent activation of the B cell (189,190). CR2 signaling and its role in the response to antigen has attracted an enormous amount of interest over the past few years, but is beyond the scope of this review. However, it should be emphasised that CR1 plays an essential role, fishing the extracellular milieu for C3b-opsonised complexes and catalysing the generation of C3dg which can then act as a "natural adjuvant" by enabling the immune complex to cross-link CR2 and BCR.

A recent report describes a different role for CR1 on B cells. Multimeric C3b-like complexes were generated and used to cross-link CR1 in isolation (191). This inhibited B cell proliferation in response to BCR ligation even in the presence of co-stimulatory cytokines. The data suggest that CR1 directly or indirectly plays a negative regulatory role in B cell activation. The physiological relevance of this observation *in vitro* remains to be proven.

6 CONCLUDING REMARKS

Because of the enormous potential for C activation to cause damage to self, the famous "double edged sword", numerous CReg evolved to provide protection. These CReg, widely distributed on cell membranes and in biological fluids, have been put to other uses both by the host and by invaders. In this review we have sought to highlight some of the ingenious ways in which the membrane CReg perform multiple tasks, some of benefit to the host, some benefiting only the invader. There are examples both of parsimony, the host using the same molecule to perform multiple roles in immunity, and piracy, pathogens taking advantage of the necessary breadth and abundance of expression of CReg to bind and enter host cells. Many more examples of such multitasking in the CReg are likely to emerge in this active and fast-moving field over the coming years.

Acknowledgements: We thank The Wellcome Trust for financial support.

7 REFERENCES

1. Favoreel, H.W., Van de Walle, G.R., Nauwynck, H.J. , Pensaert, M.B. Virus complement evasion strategies. J Gen Virol 2003; 84: 1-15.
2. Powell, R.M., Schmitt, V., Ward, T., Goodfellow, I., Evans, D.J. , Almond, J.W. Characterization of echoviruses that bind decay accelerating factor (CD55): evidence that some haemagglutinating strains use more than one cellular receptor. J Gen Virol 1998; 79: 1707-1713.
3. Bergelson, J.M., Chan, M., Solomon, K.R., St. John, N.F., Lin, H. , Finberg, R.W. Decay-accelerating factor (CD55), a glycosylphosphatidylinositol-anchored complement regulatory protein, is a receptor for several echoviruses. Proc Natl Acad Sci USA 1994; 91: 6245-6249
4. Ward, T., Pipkin, P.A., Clarkson, N.A., Stone, D.M., Minor, P.D. , Almond, J.W. Decay-accelerating factor CD55 is identified as the receptor for echovirus 7 using CELICS, a rapid immuno-focal cloning method. EMBO J 1994; 13: 5070-5074
5. Powell, R.M., Ward, T., Evans, D.J. , Almond, J.W. Interaction between echovirus 7 and its receptor, decay-accelerating factor (CD55): evidence for a secondary cellular factor in A-particle formation. J Virol 1997; 71: 9306-9312.
6. Powell, R.M., Ward, T., Evans, D.J. , Almond, J.W. Interaction between echovirus 7 and its receptor, decay-accelerating factor (CD55): Evidence for a secondary cellular factor in A-particle formation. J Virol 1997; 71: 9306-9312
7. Clarkson, N.A., Kaufman, R., Lublin, D.M., Ward, T., Pipkin, P.A., Minor, P.D., Evans, D.J. , Almond, J.W. Characterization of the echovirus 7 receptor: domains of CD55 critical for virus binding. J Virol 1995; 69: 5497-5501
8. Stuart, A.D., Eustace, H.E., McKee, T.A. , Brown, T.D. A novel cell entry pathway for a DAF-using human enterovirus is dependent on lipid rafts. J Virol 2002; 76: 9307-9322.
9. Lea, S.M., Powell, R.M., McKee, T., Evans, D.J., Brown, D., Stuart, D.I. , van der Merwe, P.A. Determination of the affinity and kinetic constants for the interaction between the human virus echovirus 11 and its cellular receptor, CD55. J Biol Chem 1998; 273: 30443-30447.
10. Stuart, A.D., McKee, T.A., Williams, P.A., Harley, C., Shen, S., Stuart, D.I., Brown, T.D., Lea, S.M. Determination of the structure of a decay accelerating factor-binding

clinical isolate of echovirus 11 allows mapping of mutants with altered receptor requirements for infection. J Virol 2002; 76: 7694-7704.

11. He, Y., Lin, F., Chipman, P.R., Bator, C.M., Baker, T.S., Shoham, M., Kuhn, R.J., Medof, M.E. , Rossmann, M.G. Structure of decay-accelerating factor bound to echovirus 7: a virus-receptor complex. Proc Natl Acad Sci U S A 2002; 99: 10325-10329.

12. Bergelson, J.M., Mohanty, J.G., Crowell, R.L., St. John, N.F., Lublin, D.M. , Finberg, R.W. Coxsackievirus B3 adapted to growth in RD cells binds to decay-accelerating factor (CD55). J Virol 1995; 69: 1903-1906

13. Shafren, D.R., Bates, R.C., Agrez, M.V., Herd, R.L., Burns, G.F. , Barry, R.D. Coxsackieviruses B1, B3, and B5 use decay accelerating factor as a receptor for cell attachment. J Virol 1995; 69: 3873-3877

14. Bergelson, J.M., Cunningham, J.A., Droguett, G., Kurt-Jones, E.A., Krithivas, A., Hong, J.S., Horwitz, M.S., Crowell, R.L. , Finberg, R.W. Isolation of a common receptor for coxsackie B viruses and adenoviruses 2 and 5. Science 1997; 275: 1320-1323

15. Shafren, D.R., Williams, D.T. , Barry, R.D. A decay-accelerating factor-binding strain of coxsackievirus B3 requires the coxsackievirus-adenovirus receptor protein to mediate lytic infection of rhabdomyosarcoma cells. J Virol 1997; 71: 9844-9848

16. Cohen, C.J., Shieh, J.T., Pickles, R.J., Okegawa, T., Hsieh, J.T. , Bergelson, J.M. The coxsackievirus and adenovirus receptor is a transmembrane component of the tight junction. Proc Natl Acad Sci U S A 2001; 98: 15191-15196.

17. Lass, J.H., Walter, E.I., Burris, T.E., Grossniklaus, H.E., Roat, M.I., Skelnik, D.L., Needham, L., Singer, M. , Medof, M.E. Expression of two molecular forms of the complement decay-accelerating factor in the eye and lacrimal gland. Invest Ophth Vis Sci 1990; 31: 1136-1148

18. Utagawa, E.T., Miyamura, K., Mukoyama, A. , Kono, R. Neuraminidase-sensitive erythrocyte receptor for enterovirus type 70. J Gen Virol 1982; 63: 141-148.

19. Alexander, D.A. , Dimock, K. Sialic acid functions in enterovirus 70 binding and infection. J Virol 2002; 76: 11265-11272.

20. Shafren, D.R., Dorahy, D.J., Ingham, R.A., Burns, G.F. , Barry, R.D. Coxsackievirus A21 binds to decay-accelerating factor but requires intercellular adhesion molecule 1 for cell entry. J Virol 1997; 71: 4736-4743

21. Shafren, D.R. Viral cell entry induced by cross-linked decay-accelerating factor. J Virol 1998; 72: 9407-9412.

22. Shafren, D.R., Dorahy, D.J., Thorne, R.F. , Barry, R.D. Cytoplasmic interactions between decay-accelerating factor and intercellular adhesion molecule-1 are not required for coxsackievirus A21 cell infection. J Gen Virol 2000; 81: 889-894.

23. Nowicki, B., Moulds, J., Hull, R. , Hull, S. A hemagglutinin of uropathogenic Escherichia coli recognizes the Dr blood group antigen. Infect Immun 1988; 56: 1057-1060.

24. Nowicki, B., Hart, A., Coyne, K.E., Lublin, D.M. , Nowicki, S. Short consensus repeat-3 domain of recombinant decay-accelerating factor is recognized by Escherichia coli recombinant Dr adhesin in a model of a cell-cell interaction. J Exp Med 1993; 178: 2115-2121

25. Pham, T., Kaul, A., Hart, A., Goluszko, P., Moulds, J., Nowicki, S., Lublin, D.M. , Nowicki, B.J. dra-related X adhesins of gestational pyelonephritis-associated Escherichia coli recognize Scr-3 and Scr-4 domains of recombinant decay-accelerating factor. Infect Immun 1995; 63: 1663-1668

26. Hasan, R.J., Pawelczyk, E., Urvil, P.T., Venkatarajan, M.S., Goluszko, P., Kur, J., Selvarangan, R., Nowicki, S., Braun, W.A. , Nowicki, B.J. Structure-function analysis of decay-accelerating factor: identification of residues important for binding of the Escherichia coli Dr adhesin and complement regulation. Infect Immun 2002; 70: 4485-4493.

27. Van Loy, C.P., Sokurenko, E.V., Moseley, S.L. The major structural subunits of Dr and F1845 fimbriae are adhesins. Infect Immun 2002; 70: 1694-1702.

28. Selvarangan, R., Goluszko, P., Popov, V., Singhal, J., Pham, T., Lublin, D.M., Nowicki, S., Nowicki, B. Role of decay-accelerating factor domains and anchorage in internalization of Dr-fimbriated Escherichia coli. Infect Immun 2000; 68: 1391-1399.

29. Peiffer, I., Servin, A.L. , Bernet-Camard, M.F. Piracy of decay-accelerating factor (CD55) signal transduction by the diffusely adhering strain Escherichia coli C1845 promotes cytoskeletal F-actin rearrangements in cultured human intestinal INT407 cells. Infect Immun 1998; 66: 4036-4042.

30. Goluszko, P., Selvarangan, R., Popov, V., Pham, T., Wen, J.W. , Singhal, J. Decay-accelerating factor and cytoskeleton redistribution pattern in HeLa cells infected with recombinant Escherichia coli strains expressing Dr family of adhesins. Infect Immun 1999; 67: 3989-3997

31. Naniche, D., Varior-Krishnan, G., Cervoni, F., Wild, T.F., Rossi, B., Rabourdin-Combe, C. , Gerlier, D. Human membrane cofactor protein (CD46) acts as a cellular receptor for measles virus. J Virol 1993; 67: 6025-6032

32. Dorig, R.E., Marcil, A., Chopra, A. , Richardson, C.D. The human CD46 molecule is a receptor for measles virus (Edmonston strain). Cell 1993; 75: 295-305

33. Karp, C.L., Wysocka, M., Wahl, L.M., Ahearn, J.M., Cuomo, P.J., Sherry, B., Trinchieri, G. , Griffin, D.E. Mechanism of suppression of cell-mediated immunity by measles virus. Science 1996; 273: 228-231

34. Manchester, M., Valsamakis, A., Kaufman, R., Liszewski, M.K., Alvarez, J., Atkinson, J.P., Lublin, D.M. , Oldstone, M.B. Measles virus and C3 binding sites are distinct on membrane cofactor protein (CD46). Proc Natl Acad Sci USA 1995; 92: 2303-2307

35. Buchholz, C.J., Schneider, U., Devaux, P., Gerlier, D. , Cattaneo, R. Cell entry by measles virus: long hybrid receptors uncouple binding from membrane fusion. J Virol 1996; 70: 3716-3723

36. Iwata, K., Seya, T., Yanagi, Y., Pesando, J.M., Johnson, P.M., Okabe, M., Ueda, S., Ariga, H. , Nagasawa, S. Diversity of sites for measles virus binding and for inactivation of complement C3b and C4b on membrane cofactor protein CD46. J Biol Chem 1995; 270: 15148-15152

37. Buchholz, C.J., Koller, D., Devaux, P., Mumenthaler, C., Schneider-Schaulies, J., Braun, W., Gerlier, D. , Cattaneo, R. Mapping of the primary binding site of measles virus to its receptor CD46. J Biol Chem 1997; 272: 22072-22079.

38. Manchester, M., Gairin, J.E., Patterson, J.B., Alvarez, J., Liszewski, M.K., Eto, D.S., Atkinson, J.P. , Oldstone, M.B. Measles virus recognizes its receptor, CD46, via two distinct binding domains within SCR1-2. Virology 1997; 233: 174-184

39. Manchester, M., Naniche, D. , Stehle, T. CD46 as a measles receptor: form follows function. Virology 2000; 274: 5-10.

40. Maisner, A., Schneider-Schaulies, J., Liszewski, M.K., Atkinson, J.P. , Herrler, G. Binding of measles virus to membrane cofactor protein (CD46): importance of disulfide bonds and N-glycans for the receptor function. J Virol 1994; 68: 6299-6304

41. Maisner, A. , Herrler, G. Membrane cofactor protein with different types of N-glycans can serve as measles virus receptor. Virology 1995; 210: 479-481

42. Seya, T., Kurita, M., Iwata, K., Yanagi, Y., Tanaka, K., Shida, K., Hatanaka, M., Matsumoto, M., Jun, S., Hirano, A., Ueda, S. , Nagasawa, S. The CD46 transmembrane domain is required for efficient formation of measles-virus-mediated syncytium. Biochem J 1997; 322: 135-144

43. Hsu, E.C., Dorig, R.E., Sarangi, F., Marcil, A., Iorio, C. , Richardson, C.D. Artificial mutations and natural variations in the CD46 molecules from human and monkey cells define regions important for measles virus binding. J Virol 1997; 71: 6144-6154

44. Kobune, F., Takahashi, H., Terao, K., Ohkawa, T., Ami, Y., Suzaki, Y., Nagata, N., Sakata, H., Yamanouchi, K. , Kai, C. Nonhuman primate models of measles. Lab Anim Sci 1996; 46: 315-320.

45. Buckland, R. , Wild, T.F. Is CD46 the cellular receptor for measles virus? Virus Research 1997; 48: 1-9

46. Hsu, E.C., Sarangi, F., Iorio, C., Sidhu, M.S., Udem, S.A., Dillehay, D.L., Xu, W., Rota, P.A., Bellini, W.J. , Richardson, C.D. A single amino acid change in the hemagglutinin protein of measles virus determines its ability to bind CD46 and reveals another receptor on marmoset B cells. J Virol 1998; 72: 2905-2916

47. Schneider-Schaulies, J., Schnorr, J.J., Brinckmann, U., Dunster, L.M., Baczko, K., Liebert, U.G., Schneider-Schaulies, S. , ter Meulen, V. Receptor usage and differential downregulation of CD46 by measles virus wild-type and vaccine strains. Proc Natl Acad Sci USA 1995; 92: 3943-3947

48. Lecouturier, V., Fayolle, J., Caballero, M., Carabana, J., Celma, M.L., Fernandez-Munoz, R., Wild, T.F. , Buckland, R. Identification of two amino acids in the hemagglutinin glycoprotein of measles virus (MV) that govern hemadsorption, HeLa cell fusion, and CD46 downregulation: phenotypic markers that differentiate vaccine and wild-type MV strains. J Virol 1996; 70: 4200-4204

49. Bartz, R., Firsching, R., Rima, B., Ter Meulen, V. , Schneider-Schaulies, J. Differential receptor usage by measles virus strains. J Gen Virol 1998; 79: 1015-1025

50. Kobune, F., Sakata, H. , Sugiura, A. Marmoset lymphoblastoid cells as a sensitive host for isolation of measles virus. J Virol 1990; 64: 700-705.

51. Tatsuo, H., Ono, N., Tanaka, K. , Yanagi, Y. SLAM (CDw150) is a cellular receptor for measles virus. Nature 2000; 406: 893-897.

52. Cocks, B.G., Chang, C.C., Carballido, J.M., Yssel, H., de Vries, J.E. , Aversa, G. A novel receptor involved in T-cell activation. Nature 1995; 376: 260-263.

53. Ono, N., Tatsuo, H., Hidaka, Y., Aoki, T., Minagawa, H. , Yanagi, Y. Measles viruses on throat swabs from measles patients use signaling lymphocytic activation molecule (CDw150) but not CD46 as a cellular receptor. J Virol 2001; 75: 4399-4401.

54. Manchester, M., Eto, D.S., Valsamakis, A., Liton, P.B., Fernandez-Munoz, R., Rota, P.A., Bellini, W.J., Forthal, D.N. , Oldstone, M.B. Clinical isolates of measles virus use CD46 as a cellular receptor. J Virol 2000; 74: 3967-3974.

55. Erlenhofer, C., Duprex, W.P., Rima, B.K., ter Meulen, V. , Schneider-Schaulies, J. Analysis of receptor (CD46, CD150) usage by measles virus. J Gen Virol 2002; 83: 1431-1436.

56. Yanagi, Y., Ono, N., Tatsuo, H., Hashimoto, K. , Minagawa, H. Measles virus receptor SLAM (CD150). Virology 2002; 299: 155-161.

57. Singhrao, S.K., Neal, J.W., Rushmere, N.K., Morgan, B.P. , Gasque, P. Spontaneous classical pathway activation and deficiency of membrane regulators render human neurons susceptible to complement lysis. Am J Pathol 2000; 157: 905-918.

58. McQuaid, S. , Cosby, S.L. An immunohistochemical study of the distribution of the measles virus receptors, CD46 and SLAM, in normal human tissues and subacute sclerosing panencephalitis. Lab Invest 2002; 82: 403-409.

59. Santiago, C., Bjorling, E., Stehle, T. , Casasnovas, J.M. Distinct kinetics for binding of the CD46 and SLAM receptors to overlapping sites in the measles virus hemagglutinin protein. J Biol Chem 2002; 277: 32294-32301.
60. Kouomou, D.W. , Wild, T.F. Adaptation of wild-type measles virus to tissue culture. J Virol 2002; 76: 1505-1509.
61. Hashimoto, K., Ono, N., Tatsuo, H., Minagawa, H., Takeda, M., Takeuchi, K. , Yanagi, Y. SLAM (CD150)-independent measles virus entry as revealed by recombinant virus expressing green fluorescent protein. J Virol 2002; 76: 6743-6749.
62. Santoro, F., Kennedy, P.E., Locatelli, G., Malnati, M.S., Berger, E.A. , Lusso, P. CD46 is a cellular receptor for human herpesvirus 6. Cell 1999; 99: 817-827.
63. Tejada-Simon, M.V., Zang, Y.C., Hong, J., Rivera, V.M., Killian, J.M. , Zhang, J.Z. Detection of viral DNA and immune responses to the human herpesvirus 6 101-kilodalton virion protein in patients with multiple sclerosis and in controls. J Virol 2002; 76: 6147-6154.
64. Swanborg, R.H., Whittum-Hudson, J.A. , Hudson, A.P. Infectious agents and multiple sclerosis-are Chlamydia pneumoniae and human herpes virus 6 involved? J Neuroimmunol 2003; 136: 1-8.
65. Mori, Y., Seya, T., Huang, H.L., Akkapaiboon, P., Dhepakson, P. , Yamanishi, K. Human herpesvirus 6 variant A but not variant B induces fusion from without in a variety of human cells through a human herpesvirus 6 entry receptor, CD46. J Virol 2002; 76: 6750-6761.
66. Greenstone, H.L., Santoro, F., Lusso, P. , Berger, E.A. Human Herpesvirus 6 and Measles Virus Employ Distinct CD46 Domains for Receptor Function. J Biol Chem 2002; 277: 39112-39118.
67. Mori, Y., Yang, X., Akkapaiboon, P., Okuno, T. , Yamanishi, K. Human Herpesvirus 6 Variant A Glycoprotein H-Glycoprotein L-Glycoprotein Q Complex Associates with Human CD46. J Virol 2003; 77: 4992-4999.
68. Segerman, A., Atkinson, J.P., Marttila, M., Dennerquist, V., Wadell, G. , Arnberg, N. Adenovirus type 11 uses CD46 as a cellular receptor. J Virol 2003; 77: 9183-9191.
69. Gaggar, A., Shayakhmetov, D.M. , Lieber, A. CD46 is a cellular receptor for group B adenoviruses. Nat Med 2003; 9: 1408-1412.
70. Shusta, E.V., Zhu, C., Boado, R.J. , Pardridge, W.M. Subtractive expression cloning reveals high expression of CD46 at the blood-brain barrier. J Neuropathol Exp Neurol 2002; 61: 597-604.
71. Johansson, L., Rytkonen, A., Bergman, P., Albiger, B., Kallstrom, H., Hokfelt, T., Agerberth, B., Cattaneo, R. , Jonsson, A.B. CD46 in meningococcal disease. Science 2003; 301: 373-375.
72. Kallstrom, H., Liszewski, M.K., Atkinson, J.P. , Jonsson, A.B. Membrane cofactor protein (MCP or CD46) is a cellular pilus receptor for pathogenic Neisseria. Mol Microbiol 1997; 25: 639-647.
73. Kallstrom, H., Blackmer Gill, D., Albiger, B., Liszewski, M.K., Atkinson, J.P. , Jonsson, A.B. Attachment of Neisseria gonorrhoeae to the cellular pilus receptor CD46: identification of domains important for bacterial adherence. Cell Microbiol 2001; 3: 133-143.
74. Lee, S.W., Bonnah, R.A., Higashi, D.L., Atkinson, J.P., Milgram, S.L. , So, M. CD46 is phosphorylated at tyrosine 354 upon infection of epithelial cells by Neisseria gonorrhoeae. J Cell Biol 2002; 156: 951-957.
75. Okada, N., Liszewski, M.K., Atkinson, J.P. , Caparon, M. Membrane cofactor protein (CD46) is a keratinocyte receptor for the M protein of the group A streptococcus. Proc Natl Acad Sci USA 1995; 92: 2489-2493

76. Giannakis, E., Jokiranta, T.S., Ormsby, R.J., Duthy, T.G., Male, D.A., Christiansen, D., Fischetti, V.A., Bagley, C., Loveland, B.E. , Gordon, D.L. Identification of the streptococcal M protein binding site on membrane cofactor protein (CD46). J Immunol 2002; 168: 4585-4592.

77. Goodfellow, I.G., Powell, R.M., Ward, T., Spiller, O.B., Almond, J.W. , Evans, D.J. Echovirus infection of rhabdomyosarcoma cells is inhibited by antiserum to the complement control protein CD59. J Gen Virol 2000; 81: 1393-1401.

78. Abrami, L., Fivaz, M., Glauser, P.E., Parton, R.G. , van der Goot, F.G. A pore-forming toxin interacts with a GPI-anchored protein and causes vacuolation of the endoplasmic reticulum. J Cell Biol 1998; 140: 525-540.

79. Brodsky, R.A., Mukhina, G.L., Nelson, K.L., Lawrence, T.S., Jones, R.J. , Buckley, J.T. Resistance of paroxysmal nocturnal hemoglobinuria cells to the glycosylphosphatidylinositol-binding toxin aerolysin. Blood 1999; 93: 1749-1756.

80. Stoiber, H., Clivio, A. , Dierich, M.P. Role of complement in HIV infection. Annu Rev Immunol 1997; 15: 649-674

81. Speth, C., Kacani, L. , Dierich, M.P. Complement receptors in HIV infection. Immunol Rev 1997; 159: 49-67

82. Soelder, B.M., Reisinger, E.C., Koefler, D., Bitterlich, G., Wachter, H. , Dierich, M.P. Complement receptors: another port of entry for HIV. Lancet 1989; 2: 271-272.

83. Boyer, V., Desgranges, C., Trabaud, M.A., Fischer, E. , Kazatchkine, M.D. Complement mediates human immunodeficiency virus type 1 infection of a human T cell line in a CD4- and antibody-independent fashion. J Exp Med 1991; 173: 1151-1158

84. Gras, G., Richard, Y., Roques, P., Olivier, R. , Dormont, D. Complement and virus-specific antibody-dependent infection of normal B lymphocytes by human immunodeficiency virus type 1. Blood 1993; 81: 1808-1818

85. Delibrias, C.C., Kazatchkine, M.D. , Fischer, E. Evidence for the role of CR1 (CD35), in addition to CR2 (CD21), in facilitating infection of human T cells with opsonized HIV. Scand J Immunol 1993; 38: 183-189

86. Delibrias, C.C., Mouhoub, A., Fischer, E. , Kazatchkine, M.D. CR1(CD35) and CR2(CD21) complement C3 receptors are expressed on normal human thymocytes and mediate infection of thymocytes with opsonized human immunodeficiency virus. Eur J Immunol 1994; 24: 2784-2788

87. Mouhoub, A., Delibrias, C.C., Fischer, E., Boyer, V. , Kazatchkine, M.D. Ligation of CR1 (C3b receptor, CD35) on CD4+ T lymphocytes enhances viral replication in HIV-infected cells. Clin Exp Immunol 1996; 106: 297-303

88. Kacani, L., Prodinger, W.M., Sprinzl, G.M., Schwendinger, M.G., Spruth, M., Stoiber, H., Dopper, S., Steinhuber, S., Steindl, F. , Dierich, M.P. Detachment of human immunodeficiency virus type 1 from germinal centers by blocking complement receptor type 2. J Virol 2000; 74: 7997-8002.

89. Pantaleo, G., Graziosi, C., Butini, L., Pizzo, P.A., Schnittman, S.M., Kotler, D.P. , Fauci, A.S. Lymphoid organs function as major reservoirs for human immunodeficiency virus. Proc Natl Acad Sci USA 1991; 88: 9838-9842

90. Pantaleo, G., Graziosi, C., Demarest, J.F., Butini, L., Montroni, M., Fox, C.H., Orenstein, J.M., Kotler, D.P. , Fauci, A.S. HIV infection is active and progressive in lymphoid tissue during the clinically latent stage of disease. Nature 1993; 362: 355-358

91. Joling, P., Bakker, L.J., Van Strijp, J.A., Meerloo, T., de Graaf, L., Dekker, M.E., Goudsmit, J., Verhoef, J. , Schuurman, H.J. Binding of human immunodeficiency virus

type-1 to follicular dendritic cells in vitro is complement dependent. J Immunol 1993; 150: 1065-1073

92. Embretson, J., Zupancic, M., Ribas, J.L., Burke, A., Racz, P., Tenner-Racz, K. , Haase, A.T. Massive covert infection of helper T lymphocytes and macrophages by HIV during the incubation period of AIDS. Nature 1993; 362: 359-362

93. Pantaleo, G., Cohen, O.J., Schacker, T., Vaccarezza, M., Graziosi, C., Rizzardi, G.P., Kahn, J., Fox, C.H., Schnittman, S.M., Schwartz, D.H., Corey, L. , Fauci, A.S. Evolutionary pattern of human immunodeficiency virus (HIV) replication and distribution in lymph nodes following primary infection: implications for antiviral therapy. Nat Med 1998; 4: 341-345.

94. Simons, K. , Ikonen, E. Functional rafts in cell membranes. Nature 1997; 387: 569-572.

95. Friedrichson, T. , Kurzchalia, T.V. Microdomains of GPI-anchored proteins in living cells revealed by crosslinking. Nature 1998; 394: 802-805.

96. Stefanova, I., Horejsi, V., Ansotegui, I.J., Knapp, W. , Stockinger, H. GPI-anchored cell-surface molecules complexed to protein tyrosine kinases. Science 1991; 254: 1016-1019

97. Brdicka, T., Cerny, J. , Horejsi, V. T cell receptor signalling results in rapid tyrosine phosphorylation of the linker protein LAT present in detergent-resistant membrane microdomains. Biochem Biophys Res Commun 1998; 248: 356-360.

98. Horejsi, V., Drbal, K., Cebecauer, M., Cerny, J., Brdicka, T., Angelisova, P. , Stockinger, H. GPI-microdomains: a role in signalling via immunoreceptors. Immunol Today 1999; 20: 356-361.

99. Brdicka, T., Pavlistova, D., Leo, A., Bruyns, E., Korinek, V., Angelisova, P., Scherer, J., Shevchenko, A., Hilgert, I., Cerny, J., Drbal, K., Kuramitsu, Y., Kornacker, B., Horejsi, V., Schraven, B. Phosphoprotein associated with glycosphingolipid-enriched microdomains (PAG), a novel ubiquitously expressed transmembrane adaptor protein, binds the protein tyrosine kinase csk and is involved in regulation of T cell activation. J Exp Med 2000; 191: 1591-1604.

100. Leo, A., Wienands, J., Baier, G., Horejsi, V. , Schraven, B. Adapters in lymphocyte signaling. J Clin Invest 2002; 109: 301-309.

101. Shibuya, K., Abe, T. , Fujita, T. Decay-accelerating factor functions as a signal transducing molecule for human monocytes. J Immunol 1992; 149: 1758-1762

102. Morgan, B.P., van den Berg, C.W., Davies, E.V., Hallett, M.B. , Horejsi, V. Cross-linking of CD59 and of other glycosyl phosphatidylinositol-anchored molecules on neutrophils triggers cell activation via tyrosine kinase. Eur J Immunol 1993; 23: 2841-2850

103. Tosello, A.C., Mary, F., Amiot, M., Bernard, A. , Mary, D. Activation of T cells via CD55: recruitment of early components of the CD3-TCR pathway is required for IL-2 secretion. J Inflamm 1998; 48: 13-27.

104. el-Samalouti, V.T., Schletter, J., Chyla, I., Lentschat, A., Mamat, U., Brade, L., Flad, H.D., Ulmer, A.J. , Hamann, L. Identification of the 80-kDa LPS-binding protein (LMP80) as decay-accelerating factor (DAF, CD55). FEMS Immunol Med Microbiol 1999; 23: 259-269.

105. Heine, H., Ulmer, A.J., El-Samalouti, V.T., Lentschat, A. , Hamann, L. Decay-accelerating factor (DAF/CD55) is a functional active element of the LPS receptor complex. J Endotoxin Res 2001; 7: 227-231.

106. Triantafilou, M. , Triantafilou, K. Lipopolysaccharide recognition: CD14, TLRs and the LPS-activation cluster. Trends Immunol 2002; 23: 301-304.

107. Pfeiffer, A., Bottcher, A., Orso, E., Kapinsky, M., Nagy, P., Bodnar, A., Spreitzer, I., Liebisch, G., Drobnik, W., Gempel, K., Horn, M., Holmer, S., Hartung, T., Multhoff, G., Schutz, G., Schindler, H., Ulmer, A.J., Heine, H., Stelter, F., Schutt, C., Rothe, G., Szollosi, J., Damjanovich, S. , Schmitz, G. Lipopolysaccharide and ceramide docking to CD14 provokes ligand-specific receptor clustering in rafts. Eur J Immunol 2001; 31: 3153-3164.

108. Shenoy-Scaria, A.M., Gauen, L.K., Kwong, J., Shaw, A.S. , Lublin, D.M. Palmitylation of an amino-terminal cysteine motif of protein tyrosine kinases p56lck and p59fyn mediates interaction with glycosyl-phosphatidylinositol-anchored proteins. Mol Cell Biol 1993; 13: 6385-6392

109. Kuraya, M. , Fujita, T. Signal transduction via a protein associated with a glycosylphosphatidylinositol-anchored protein, decay-accelerating factor (DAF/CD55). Int Immunol 1998; 10: 473-480

110. Hamann, J., Vogel, B., van Schijndel, G.M. , van Lier, R.A. The seven-span transmembrane receptor CD97 has a cellular ligand (CD55, DAF). J Exp Med 1996; 184: 1185-1189

111. Hamann, J., Eichler, W., Hamann, D., Kerstens, H.M.J., Poddighe, P.J., Hoovers, J.M.N., Hartmann, E., Strauss, M. , van Lier, R.A.W. Expression cloning and chromosomal mapping of the leucocyte activation antigen CD97, a new seven-span transmembrane molecule of the secretin receptor superfamily with an unusual extracellular domain. J Immunol 1995; 155: 1942-1950

112. Hamann, J., Stortelers, C., Kiss-Toth, E., Vogel, B., Eichler, W. , van Lier, R.A. Characterization of the CD55 (DAF)-binding site on the seven-span transmembrane receptor CD97. Eur J Immunol 1998; 28: 1701-1707.

113. Lin, H.H., Stacey, M., Saxby, C., Knott, V., Chaudhry, Y., Evans, D., Gordon, S., McKnight, A.J., Handford, P. , Lea, S. Molecular analysis of the epidermal growth factor-like short consensus repeat domain-mediated protein-protein interactions: dissection of the CD97-CD55 complex. J Biol Chem 2001; 276: 24160-24169.

114. Brodbeck, W.G., Liu, D., Sperry, J., Mold, C. , Medof, M.E. Localization of classical and alternative pathway regulatory activity within the decay-accelerating factor. J Immunol 1996; 156: 2528-2533

115. Hamann, J., Wishaupt, J.O., van Lier, R.A., Smeets, T.J., Breedveld, F.C. , Tak, P.P. Expression of the activation antigen CD97 and its ligand CD55 in rheumatoid synovial tissue. Arthritis Rheum 1999; 42: 650-658.

116. Visser, L., de Vos, A.F., Hamann, J., Melief, M.J., van Meurs, M., van Lier, R.A., Laman, J.D. , Hintzen, R.Q. Expression of the EGF-TM7 receptor CD97 and its ligand CD55 (DAF) in multiple sclerosis. J Neuroimmunol 2002; 132: 156-163.

117. Li, L., Spendlove, I., Morgan, J. , Durrant, L.G. CD55 is over-expressed in the tumour environment. Br J Cancer 2001; 84: 80-86.

118. Spendlove, I., Li, L., Carmichael, J. , Durrant, L.G. Decay accelerating factor (CD55): a target for cancer vaccines? Cancer Res 1999; 59: 2282-2286.

119. Mizuno, M., Nakagawa, M., Uesu, T., Inoue, H., Inaba, T., Ueki, T., Nasu, J., Okada, H., Fujita, T. , Tsuji, T. Detection of decay-accelerating factor in stool specimens of patients with colorectal cancer. Gastroenterology 1995; 109: 826-831

120. Morgan, J., Spendlove, I. , Durrant, L.G. The role of CD55 in protecting the tumour environment from complement attack. Tissue Antigens 2002; 60: 213-223.

121. Steinert, M., Wobus, M., Boltze, C., Schutz, A., Wahlbuhl, M., Hamann, J. , Aust, G. Expression and regulation of CD97 in colorectal carcinoma cell lines and tumor tissues. Am J Pathol 2002; 161: 1657-1667.

122. Aust, G., Steinert, M., Schutz, A., Boltze, C., Wahlbuhl, M., Hamann, J. , Wobus, M. CD97, but not its closely related EGF-TM7 family member EMR2, is expressed on gastric, pancreatic, and esophageal carcinomas. Am J Clin Pathol 2002; 118: 699-707.
123. Vollmers, H.P., Zimmermann, U., Krenn, V., Timmermann, W., Illert, B., Hensel, F., Hermann, R., Thiede, A., Wilhelm, M., Ruckle-Lanz, H., Reindl, L. , Muller-Hermelink, H.K. Adjuvant therapy for gastric adenocarcinoma with the apoptosis-inducing human monoclonal antibody SC-1: first clinical and histopathological results. Oncol Rep 1998; 5: 549-552.
124. Hensel, F., Hermann, R., Schubert, C., Abe, N., Schmidt, K., Franke, A., Shevchenko, A., Mann, M., Muller-Hermelink, H.K. , Vollmers, H.P. Characterization of glycosylphosphatidylinositol-linked molecule CD55/decay-accelerating factor as the receptor for antibody SC-1-induced apoptosis. Cancer Res 1999; 59: 5299-5306.
125. Hensel, F., Hermann, R., Brandlein, S., Krenn, V., Schmausser, B., Geis, S., Muller-Hermelink, H.K. , Vollmers, H.P. Regulation of the new coexpressed CD55 (decay-accelerating factor) receptor on stomach carcinoma cells involved in antibody SC-1-induced apoptosis. Lab Invest 2001; 81: 1553-1563.
126. Fugier-Vivier, I., Servet-Delprat, C., Rivailler, P., Rissoan, M.C., Liu, Y.J. , Rabourdin-Combe, C. Measles virus suppresses cell-mediated immunity by interfering with the survival and functions of dendritic and T cells. J Exp Med 1997; 186: 813-823.
127. Kallstrom, H., Islam, M.S., Berggren, P.O. , Jonsson, A.B. Cell signaling by the type IV pili of pathogenic Neisseria. J Biol Chem 1998; 273: 21777-21782.
128. Hirano, A., Yang, Z., Katayama, Y., Korte-Sarfaty, J. , Wong, T.C. Human CD46 enhances nitric oxide production in mouse macrophages in response to measles virus infection in the presence of gamma interferon: dependence on the CD46 cytoplasmic domains. J Virol 1999; 73: 4776-4785.
129. Kurita-Taniguchi, M., Fukui, A., Hazeki, K., Hirano, A., Tsuji, S., Matsumoto, M., Watanabe, M., Ueda, S. , Seya, T. Functional modulation of human macrophages through CD46 (measles virus receptor): production of IL-12 p40 and nitric oxide in association with recruitment of protein-tyrosine phosphatase SHP-1 to CD46. J Immunol 2000; 165: 5143-5152.
130. Ghali, M. , Schneider-Schaulies, J. Receptor (CD46)- and replication-mediated interleukin-6 induction by measles virus in human astrocytoma cells. J Neurovirol 1998; 4: 521-530.
131. Imani, F., Proud, D. , Griffin, D.E. Measles virus infection synergizes with IL-4 in IgE class switching. J Immunol 1999; 162: 1597-1602.
132. Astier, A., Trescol-Biemont, M.C., Azocar, O., Lamouille, B. , Rabourdin-Combe, C. Cutting edge: CD46, a new costimulatory molecule for T cells, that induces p120CBL and LAT phosphorylation. J Immunol 2000; 164: 6091-6095.
133. Zaffran, Y., Destaing, O., Roux, A., Ory, S., Nheu, T., Jurdic, P., Rabourdin-Combe, C. , Astier, A.L. CD46/CD3 costimulation induces morphological changes of human T cells and activation of Vav, Rac, and extracellular signal-regulated kinase mitogen-activated protein kinase. J Immunol 2001; 167: 6780-6785.
134. Marie, J.C., Astier, A.L., Rivailler, P., Rabourdin-Combe, C., Wild, T.F. , Horvat, B. Linking innate and acquired immunity: divergent role of CD46 cytoplasmic domains in T cell induced inflammation. Nat Immunol 2002; 3: 659-666.
135. Kemper, C., Chan, A.C., Green, J.M., Brett, K.A., Murphy, K.M. , Atkinson, J.P. Activation of human CD4(+) cells with CD3 and CD46 induces a T-regulatory cell 1 phenotype. Nature 2003; 421: 388-392.

136. Hirano, A., Kurita-Taniguchi, M., Katayama, Y., Matsumoto, M., Wong, T.C. , Seya, T. Ligation of human CD46 with purified complement C3b or F(ab')(2) of monoclonal antibodies enhances isoform-specific interferon gamma-dependent nitric oxide production in macrophages. J Biochem (Tokyo) 2002; 132: 83-91.

137. Wong, T.C., Yant, S., Harder, B.J., KorteSarfaty, J. , Hirano, A. The cytoplasmic domains of complement regulatory protein CD46 interact with multiple kinases in macrophages. J Leuk Biol 1997; 62: 892-900

138. Wang, G., Liszewski, M.K., Chan, A.C. , Atkinson, J.P. Membrane cofactor protein (MCP; CD46): isoform-specific tyrosine phosphorylation. J Immunol 2000; 164: 1839-1846.

139. Stefanova, I. , Horejsi, V. Association of the CD59 and CD55 cell surface glycoproteins with other membrane molecules. J Immunol 1991; 147: 1587-1592

140. Lund-Johansen, F., Olweus, J., Symington, F.W., Arli, A., Thompson, J.S., Vilella, R., Skubitz, K. , Horejsi, V. Activation of human monocytes and granulocytes by monoclonal antibodies to glycosylphosphatidylinositol-anchored antigens. Eur J Immunol 1993; 23: 2782-2791

141. van den Berg, C.W., Cinek, T., Hallett, M.B., Horejsi, V. , Morgan, B.P. Exogenous CD59 incorporated into U937 cells through its glycosyl phosphatidylinositol anchor becomes associated with signalling molecules in a time dependent manner. Biochem Soc Trans 1995; 23: 269S

142. Hatanaka, M., Seya, T., Miyagawa, S., Matsumoto, M., Hara, T., Tanaka, K. , Shimizu, A. Cellular distribution of a GPI-Anchored complement regulatory protein CD59: Homodimerization on the surface of HeLa and CD59-Transfected CHO cells. J Biochem -Tokyo 1998; 123: 579-586

143. Yamamoto, T., Nakane, T., Doi, S. , Osaki, T. Lipopolysaccharide signal transduction in oral keratinocytes--involvement of CD59 but not CD14. Cell Signal 2003; 15: 861-869.

144. Deckert, M., Kubar, J., Zoccola, D., Bernard-Pomier, G., Angelisova, P., Horejsi, V. , Bernard, A. CD59 molecule: a second ligand for CD2 in T cell adhesion. Eur J Immunol 1992; 22: 2943-2947

145. Hahn, W.C., Menu, E., Bothwell, A.L., Sims, P.J. , Bierer, B.E. Overlapping but nonidentical binding sites on CD2 for CD58 and a second ligand CD59. Science 1992; 256: 1805-1807

146. Menu, E., Tsai, B.C., Bothwell, A.L., Sims, P.J. , Bierer, B.E. CD59 costimulation of T cell activation. CD58 dependence and requirement for glycosylation. J Immunol 1994; 153: 2444-2456

147. Naderi, S., Hofmann, P., Seiter, S., Tilgen, W., Abken, H. , Reinhold, U. CD2-mediated CD59 stimulation in keratinocytes results in secretion of IL-1alpha, IL-6, and GM-CSF: implications for the interaction of keratinocytes with intraepidermal T lymphocytes. Int J Mol Med 1999; 3: 609-614.

148. van der Merwe, P.A., Barclay, A.N., Mason, D.W., Davies, E.A., Morgan, B.P., Tone, M., Krishnam, A.K., Ianelli, C. , Davis, S.J. Human cell-adhesion molecule CD2 binds CD58 (LFA-3) with a very low affinity and an extremely fast dissociation rate but does not bind CD48 or CD59. Biochemistry 1994; 33: 10149-10160

149. Millan, J., Qaidi, M. , Alonso, M.A. Segregation of co-stimulatory components into specific T cell surface lipid rafts. Eur J Immunol 2001; 31: 467-473.

150. Cabral, A.R. , Castor, C.W. Connective tissue activating peptide-V and CD59: a molecule in search of a job [editorial]. J Rheumatol 1996; 23: 1126-1129

151. Murray, E.W. , Robbins, S.M. Antibody cross-linking of the glycosylphosphatidylinositol-linked protein CD59 on hematopoietic cells induces

signaling pathways resembling activation by complement. J Biol Chem 1998; 273: 25279-25284.

152. Meri, S., Morgan, B.P., Davies, A., Daniels, R.H., Olavesen, M.G., Waldmann, H. , Lachmann, P.J. Human protectin (CD59), an 18,000-20,000 MW complement lysis restricting factor, inhibits C5b-8 catalysed insertion of C9 into lipid bilayers. Immunology 1990; 71: 1-9

153. Morgan, B.P. , Harris, C.L. (1999) *Complement regulatory proteins*. Academic Press, London.

154. Morgan, B.P., Dankert, J.R. , Esser, A.F. Recovery of human neutrophils from complement attack: removal of the membrane attack complex by endocytosis and exocytosis. J Immunol 1987; 138: 246-253

155. Scolding, N.J., Morgan, B.P., Houston, W.A., Linington, C., Campbell, A.K. , Compston, D.A. Vesicular removal by oligodendrocytes of membrane attack complexes formed by activated complement. Nature 1989; 339: 620-622

156. Monleon, I., Martinez-Lorenzo, M.J., Anel, A., Lasierra, P., Larrad, L., Pineiro, A., Naval, J. , Alava, M.A. CD59 cross-linking induces secretion of APO2 ligand in overactivated human T cells. Eur J Immunol 2000; 30: 1078-1087.

157. Price, R.J. , Boettcher, B. The presence of complement in human cervical mucus and its possible relevance to infertility in women with complement-dependent sperm-immobilizing antibodies. Fertil Steril 1979; 32: 61-66

158. Perricone, R., Pasetto, N., De Carolis, C., Vaquero, E., Piccione, E., Baschieri, L. , Fontana, L. Functionally active complement is present in human ovarian follicular fluid and can be activated by seminal plasma. Clin Exp Immunol 1992; 89: 154-157

159. D' Cruz, O.J., Haas, G.G., Jr. , Lambert, H. Evaluation of antisperm complement-dependent immune mediators in human ovarian follicular fluid. J Immunol 1990; 144: 3841-3848

160. Rooney, I.A., Davies, A. , Morgan, B.P. Membrane attack complex (MAC)-mediated damage to spermatozoa: protection of the cells by the presence on their membranes of MAC inhibitory proteins. Immunology 1992; 75: 499-506

161. Simpson, K.L. , Holmes, C.H. Differential expression of complement regulatory proteins decay-accelerating factor (CD55), membrane cofactor protein (CD46) and CD59 during human spermatogenesis. Immunology 1994; 81: 452-461

162. Cervoni, F., Oglesby, T.J., Fenichel, P., Dohr, G., Rossi, B., Atkinson, J.P. , Hsi, B.L. Expression of decay-accelerating factor (CD55) of the complement system on human spermatozoa. J Immunol 1993; 151: 939-948

163. Jenne, D.E. , Tschopp, J. Molecular structure and functional characterization of a human complement cytolysis inhibitor found in blood and seminal plasma: identity to sulfated glycoprotein 2, a constituent of rat testis fluid. Proc Natl Acad Sci USA 1989; 86: 7123-7127

164. Bronson, R.A. , Preissner, K.T. Measurement of vitronectin content of human spermatozoa and vitronectin concentration within seminal fluid. Fertil Steril 1997; 68: 709-713

165. Rooney, I.A., Atkinson, J.P., Krul, E.S., Schonfeld, G., Polakoski, K., Saffitz, J.E. , Morgan, B.P. Physiologic relevance of the membrane attack complex inhibitory protein CD59 in human seminal plasma: CD59 is present on extracellular organelles (prostasomes), binds cell membranes, and inhibits complement-mediated lysis. J Exp Med 1993; 177: 1409-1420

166. Kitamura, M., Namiki, M., Matsumiya, K., Tanaka, K., Matsumoto, M., Hara, T., Kiyohara, H., Okabe, M., Okuyama, A. , Seya, T. Membrane cofactor protein (CD46)

in seminal plasma is a prostasome-bound form with complement regulatory activity and measles virus neutralizing activity. Immunology 1995; 84: 626-632

167. Rooney, I.A., Heuser, J.E. , Atkinson, J.P. GPI-anchored complement regulatory proteins in seminal plasma. An analysis of their physical condition and the mechanisms of their binding to exogenous cells. J Clin Invest 1996; 97: 1675-1686

168. Holmes, C.H., Simpson, K.L., Wainwright, S.D., Tate, C.G., Houlihan, J.M., Sawyer, I.H., Rogers, I.P., Spring, F.A., Anstee, D.J. , Tanner, M.J. Preferential expression of the complement regulatory protein decay accelerating factor at the fetomaternal interface during human pregnancy. J Immunol 1990; 144: 3099-3105

169. Hsi, B.L., Hunt, J.S. , Atkinson, J.P. Differential expression of complement regulatory proteins on subpopulations of human trophoblast cells. J Reprod Immunol 1991; 19: 209-223

170. Holmes, C.H., Simpson, K.L., Okada, H., Okada, N., Wainwright, S.D., Purcell, D.F. , Houlihan, J.M. Complement regulatory proteins at the feto-maternal interface during human placental development: distribution of CD59 by comparison with membrane cofactor protein (CD46) and decay accelerating factor (CD55). Eur J Immunol 1992; 22: 1579-1585

171. Xu, C., Mao, D., Holers, V.M., Palanca, B., Cheng, A.M. , Molina, H. A critical role for murine complement regulator crry in fetomaternal tolerance. Science 2000; 287: 498-501.

172. Fenichel, P., Hsi, B.L., Farahifar, D., Donzeau, M., Barrier-Delpech, D. , Yehy, C.J. Evaluation of the human sperm acrosome reaction using a monoclonal antibody, GB24, and fluorescence-activated cell sorter. J Reprod Fertil 1989; 87: 699-706

173. Anderson, D.J., Michaelson, J.S. , Johnson, P.M. Trophoblast/leukocyte-common antigen is expressed by human testicular germ cells and appears on the surface of acrosome-reacted sperm. Biol Reprod 1989; 41: 285-293

174. Fenichel, P., Dohr, G., Grivaux, C., Cervoni, F., Donzeau, M. , Hsi, B.L. Localization and characterization of the acrosomal antigen recognized by GB24 on human spermatozoa. Mol Reprod Dev 1990; 27: 173-178

175. Kitamura, M., Matsumiya, K., Yamanaka, M., Takahara, S., Hara, T., Matsumoto, M., Namiki, M., Okuyama, A. , Seya, T. Possible association of infertility with sperm-specific abnormality of CD46. J Reprod Immunol 1997; 33: 83-88

176. Anderson, D.J., Abbott, A.F. , Jack, R.M. The role of complement component C3b and its receptors in sperm-oocyte interaction. Proc Natl Acad Sci USA 1993; 90: 10051-10055

177. Taylor, C.T., Biljan, M.M., Kingsland, C.R. , Johnson, P.M. Inhibition of human spermatozoon-oocyte interaction in vitro by monoclonal antibodies to CD46 (membrane cofactor protein). Hum Reprod 1994; 9: 907-911

178. Cervoni, F., Oglesby, T.J., Adams, E.M., Milesifluet, C., Nickells, M., Fenichel, P., Atkinson, J.P. , Hsi, B.L. Identification and characterization of membrane cofactor protein of human spermatozoa. J Immunol 1992; 148: 1431-1437

179. Cervoni, F., Fenichel, P., Akhoundi, C., Hsi, B.L. , Rossi, B. Characterization of a cDNA clone coding for human testis membrane cofactor protein (MCP, CD46). Mol Reprod Dev 1993; 34: 107-113

180. Hara, T., Suzuki, Y., Nakazawa, T., Nishimura, H., Nagasawa, S., Nishiguchi, M., Matsumoto, M., Hatanaka, M., Kitamura, M. , Seya, T. Post-translational modification and intracellular localization of a splice product of CD46 cloned from human testis: role of the intracellular domains in O-glycosylation. Immunology 1998; 93: 546-555

181. Riley, R.C., Tannenbaum, P.L., Abbott, D.H. , Atkinson, J.P. Cutting edge: inhibiting measles virus infection but promoting reproduction: an explanation for splicing and tissue-specific expression of CD46. J Immunol 2002; 169: 5405-5409.

182. Miwa, T., Nonaka, M., Okada, N., Wakana, S., Shiroishi, T. , Okada, H. Molecular cloning of rat and mouse membrane cofactor protein (MCP, CD46): preferential expression in testis and close linkage between the mouse Mcp and Cr2 genes on distal chromosome 1. Immunogenetics 1998; 48: 363-371.

183. Mead, R., Hinchliffe, S.J. , Morgan, B.P. Molecular cloning, expression and characterization of the rat analogue of human membrane cofactor protein (MCP/CD46). Immunology 1999; 98: 137-143.

184. Mizuno, M., Harris, C.L. , Morgan, B.P. Membrane cofactor protein (MCP; CD46) in the rat is expressed only in male germ cells and precursors. Mol Immunol 2003; 40: 202

185. Inoue, N., Ikawa, M., Nakanishi, T., Matsumoto, M., Nomura, M., Seya, T. , Okabe, M. Disruption of mouse CD46 causes an accelerated spontaneous acrosome reaction in sperm. Mol Cell Biol 2003; 23: 2614-2622.

186. Matsumoto, A.K., Kopicky-Burd, J., Carter, R.H., Tuveson, D.A., Tedder, T.F. , Fearon, D.T. Intersection of the complement and immune systems: a signal transduction complex of the B lymphocyte-containing complement receptor type 2 and CD19. J Exp Med 1991; 173: 55-64

187. Bradbury, L.E., Kansas, G.S., Levy, S., Evans, R.L. , Tedder, T.F. The CD19/CD21 signal transducing complex of human B lymphocytes includes the target of antiproliferative antibody-1 and Leu-13 molecules. J Immunol 1992; 149: 2841-2850

188. Matsumoto, A.K., Martin, D.R., Carter, R.H., Klickstein, L.B., Ahearn, J.M. , Fearon, D.T. Functional dissection of the CD21/CD19/TAPA-1/Leu-13 complex of B lymphocytes. J Exp Med 1993; 178: 1407-1417

189. Tedder, T.F., Zhou, L.J. , Engel, P. The CD19/CD21 signal transduction complex of B lymphocytes. Immunol Today 1994; 15: 437-442

190. Carter, R.H., Spycher, M.O., Ng, Y.C., Hoffman, R. , Fearon, D.T. Synergistic interaction between complement receptor type 2 and membrane IgM on B lymphocytes. J Immunol 1988; 141: 457-463

191. Jozsi, M., Prechl, J., Bajtay, Z. , Erdei, A. Complement receptor type 1 (CD35) mediates inhibitory signals in human B lymphocytes. J Immunol 2002; 168: 2782-2788.

8

New Insights Into the Regulation of Complement Activation by Decay Accelerating Factor

Lisa Kuttner-Kondo and Edward M. Medof
Department of Pathology, Case Western Reserve University, Cleveland, Ohio 44106, USA

Abstract: Decay-accelerating factor (DAF), a ubiquitously expressed GPI-anchored protein, is an *intrinsic* regulator of complement activation that acts to dissociate autologous C3 and C5 convertases that assemble on self cells. DAF contains four ~60 amino acid long repeats termed short consensus repeats (SCRs) or complement control protein repeats (CCPs), followed by a serine/threonine (S/T)-rich region which in turn is attached to a posttranslationally-added glycosylphosphatidylinositol (GPI)-anchor. Studies with CCP deletion mutants showed that CCPs 2 and 3 are required for classical pathway (CP) function while CCP4 is additionally required for alternative pathway (AP) function. Mutagenesis studies based on a model built from the NMR structure of homologous CCPs indicated that positively charged amino acids (R^{69}, R^{96}, and R^{100} in CCP2, and K^{127} in the CCP2-CCP3 linker) and hydrophobic residues primarily in CCP3 (F^{148}, F^{169}, and L^{171}) are important for DAF's function in one or both pathways. A recent NMR solution structure of CCPs 2-3, the crystal structure of CCPs 3-4, and the crystal structure of all four CCPs have allowed mapping of the mutagenesis data on DAF's 3D structure but have raised a controversy over the flexibility of its junctions, particularly CCPs 2-3, and the roles in function of certain amino acids, particularly the positively charged residues between CCPs 2 and 3. Work on DAF's ligands indicates that DAF interacts with Y338A and Y327A residues in the von Willibrand factor type A (vWFA) domains of factor B and C2, respectively. Current work is proceeding toward understanding DAF's role as a receptor for *E. coli* expressing AFA and Dr adhesions and certain picorna viruses. The recent availability of *Daf1* knock-out mice has allowed studies of its *in vivo* function in diseases such as myasthenia gravis and autoimmune renal disease.

Key words: Decay-accelerating factor (DAF or CD55), short consensus repeats, complement control protein repeats, sushi (SCR/ CCP/ sushi), C3/C5 convertases

1.   INTRODUCTION

Decay-accelerating factor (DAF) is a cell surface regulator of complement activation whose primary role is to function *intrinsically* in the plasma membranes of self cells to dissociate any classical and alternative pathway C3 and C5 amplification convertases that assemble on their surfaces (Medof et al., 1984). In its absence, the incompletely controlled activity of the convertases on self cells would be insufficient to circumvent focused C3b and C5b deposition, local generation of C3a and C5a anaphylatoxins, and surface assembly of membranolytic C5b-9 complexes on the cells.

2.   HISTORIC BACKGROUND

The initial understanding of DAF's function grew out of the surprising observation that the purified protein, when added to cells *in vitro*, reincorporated into their plasma membranes, and once incorporated, was functionally active (Medof et al., 1984). Exploitation of this phenomenon in conjunction with the use of sequential sheep erythrocyte (E^{sh}) complement intermediates, i.e., $E^{sh}A$, $E^{sh}AC1$, $E^{sh}AC14$, and $E^{sh}AC142$, showed that the regulator had no effect on the uptake of C1 or deposition of C4b, but efficiently prevented the effective formation of functional C4b2a convertase complexes on the cell surface. The incorporation process was unaffected by trypsin- or pronase-pretreatment of the cells indicating that it did not involve a cellular receptor. It rather was inhibited by lipoproteins or serum albumin implicating a lipid interaction, a phenomenon explained two years later by the finding (Davitz et al., 1986; Medof et al., 1986) that DAF possesses a posttranslationally-added glycosylphosphatidylinositol (GPI) anchor. The (two or three) free alkyl/acyl chains contained in the inositol phospholipid (Walter et al., 1990) reintegrate with the lipid groups of other cell surface phospholipids (Walter et al., 1992). Later studies (Premkumar et al., 2001; van den Berg et al., 1995) documented that the incorporated protein, once reintegrated, fully regains its native orientation.

Mixing experiments in which incubation of $E^{sh}A$ bearing incorporated DAF protein with equal numbers of freshly prepared $E^{sh}AC142$, had no effect on C4b2a convertase activity on the untreated cells showed that DAF functions only *intrinsically*, i.e. on convertase complexes assembled on the same cells (Medof et al., 1984). This observation (Fig. 1) paved the way to the understanding that two classes of cell surface regulators exist, i.e., *extrinsic* regulators like the C3b receptor (CR1) which act on convertase complexes on other cell or substrate surfaces, and *intrinsic* regulators exemplified initially by DAF and subsequently by CD59 (Harada et al., 1990; Holguin et al., 1989; Lachmann, 1991; Meri et al., 1990) and MCP (Seya and Atkinson, 1989) which were described later.

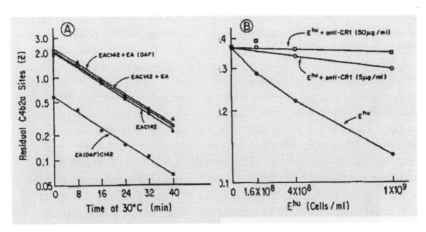

Figure 1. Inability of membrane-incorporated DAF to inhibit C3 convertase extrinsically on substrates. The effect of DAF-containing cells on the decay rate of C4b2a assembled on non-DAF-containing cells is shown in A. EACI42 (5×10^7/ml) prepared as described in the legend to Fig. 1, were mixed with an equal number of DAF-sensitized EA, which had been prepared with 14 ng/ml DAF and thoroughly washed. HDL (50 #g/ml) was added to the buffer and the mixtures placed at 30°C. The decay of C4b2a on EACI42 was then measured as a function of time as described in Materials and Methods. The decay of C4b2a on EAC 142 prepared in an identical fashion and mixed with non-treated EA was also measured in parallel as a control. As shown, the presence of DAF in the DAF-treated EA inhibited the formation of C4b2a on these cells. However, the addition of DAF-treated EA to the incubation mixture had no effect on the decay rate of C4b2a on non-DAF-treated cells. (B) The ability of monoclonal anti-CR 1 antibodies to reverse the extrinsic C3 convertase inhibition mediated by intact E h". EAC1421~m (5×10^7/ml) prepared with 300 SFU of C1, 100 SFU of C4, and ~1.5 SFU of C2 were incubated for 30 min at 30°C with increasing numbers of intact E h" in the absence or presence of pooled monoclonal anti-CR1 antibodies (57F, 44D, and 3 I D). The cells were washed and C4b2a hemolytic activity developed by addition of C3-9. Control tubes containing E ~" alone were included, and the optical density of the hemoglobin released was subtracted from the optical density in the experimental tubes. The anti-CR1 antibodies completely blocked the extrinsic inhibitory effect of the E h" on C4b2a assembled on the sheep cells. In several other experiments, we found that polyclonal mouse or rabbit anti-DAF had no effect at concentrations that reversed the DAF effect on DAF-sensitized sheep cells. Taken from (Medof, et al., 1984).

3. FUNCTION OF DAF

The initial studies of DAF (Medof et al., 1984; Nicholson-Weller et al., 1982; Pangburn et al., 1983a; Pangburn et al., 1983b) prompted questions regarding its function, i.e. 1) whether it blocks C3 and C5 convertase assembly or rather accelerates their decay following assembly, 2) its specific role in overall complement regulation, and 3) the structural features underlying its function. Data from several different types of experiments provided information concerning these issues. Using DAF incorporation assays, Fujita et al. showed that incorporated DAF in $E^{sh}AC14b2$ ($E^{sh}AC4b3bB$) cells dissociated C2a (Bb) after addition of C1 (factor D) (Fujita et al., 1987) arguing that it dissociates the C2a and Bb enzymatic components from their respective classical pathway (C4b2a) and alternative pathway (C3bBb) complexes. This finding was mirrored in a classical C3 convertase hemolytic assay where soluble urine DAF was shown to inhibit C4b2a sites if applied to $E^{sh}AC142$ but not to $E^{sh}AC14$ (Medof et al., 1987b). By means of studies of the inhibition by fluid-phase competitors of DAF-mediated Bb-decay from C3bBb complexes assembled on zymosan, Pangburn found that DAF had a higher affinity for C3bBb, C3bB, and C4b2a in the presence of Ni^+ than for uncomplexed C3b, C4b, and Bb. It differed in this regard from CR1 and factor H (Pangburn, 1986) that had higher affinity for C3b and C4b (Fearon and Collins, 1983; Seya et al., 1985). At about the same time, a crosslinking study showed that endogenous DAF both on human erythrocytes (E^{hu}) and in E^{sh} intermediates associated with C4b or C3b (Kinoshita et al., 1986). A more definitive understanding of DAF's ligand (Hourcade et al., 1999) had to await 12 years during which time structural analyses of DAF (Kuttner-Kondo et al., 1996), and the components of the convertases (Hinshelwood and Perkins, 2000a; Hinshelwood and Perkins, 2000b; Hinshelwood et al., 1999; Jing et al., 2000; Nagar et al., 1998; van den Elsen et al., 2002), as well as structure function studies of DAF (Brodbeck et al., 1996; Brodbeck et al., 2000b; Kuttner-Kondo, 2003; Kuttner-Kondo et al., 2001) were carried out.

4. MOLECULAR STRUCTURE OF DAF

4.1 Primary Structure

The cloning of DAF in 1987 (Caras et al., 1987; Medof et al., 1987a) provided an initial basis for working out its molecular mechanism of action. It showed that the regulator contains four 60-70 amino acid long consensus repeats (SCRs, CCPs, sushi's) homologous to regions in other complement as well as noncomplement proteins [reviewed in (Reid and Day, 1989)] (Fig. 2).

These CCPs are followed by a serine/threonine-rich region and finally a hydrophobic C-terminal signal that functions to direct GPI-anchoring (Caras et al., 1987; Medof et al., 1987a). This knowledge allowed dissection of DAF's sequential domains for functional mapping.

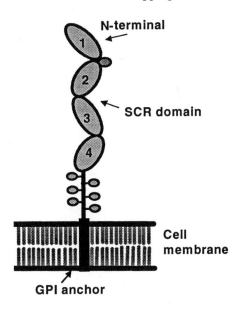

Figure 2. Diagrammatic structure of DAF. The ellipses represent the SCR domains. The spheres are O-linked or N-linked carbohydrate moieties. GPI, glycosylphosphatidylinositol. Taken from (He et al., 2002)

Using single CCP deletion mutants, functional activity was assessed in CHO cell cytotoxicity assays (Coyne et al., 1992), hemolytic assays, and C3a generation assays (Brodbeck et al., 1996). In addition, monoclonal antibodies (mAbs), some of which blocked DAF's regulatory function, could be grossly mapped (Brodbeck and Medof, 1997; Coyne et al., 1992). In cytotoxicity assays of CHO cells that had been opsonized with rabbit polyclonal antibody and human complement (Coyne et al., 1992), deletion of CCP2, CCP3, or CCP4 abrogated DAF's function. Deletion of the S/T region also abolished DAF's function, but it could be restored by addition of a spacer that projected DAF's CCPs above the membrane surface similar to the S/T region (Coyne et al., 1992). Two antibodies against CCP3, 1C6 and 1H4, abrogated DAF's function indicating that they covered an area of its regulatory site (Coyne et al., 1992).

The hemolytic and C3a generation assays showed that, while CCPs 2, 3, and 4 of DAF are required for decay acceleration of C3bBb, only CCPs 2 and 3 are required for decay acceleration of C4b2a (Brodbeck et al., 1996) demonstrating that there are structural differences underlying regulation of the classical (C4b2a) and alternative (C3bBb) pathway enzymes.

4.2   Molecular Model of 3D Structure

In the early 1990's, the NMR structures of CCP5, CCP16, and tandem CCP15-16 of factor H were determined (Barlow et al., 1992; Barlow et al., 1993; Norman et al., 1991). Building on the 3D coordinates of the CCP15-16 module, a molecular model of DAF was created with the objective of creating a framework to begin to define DAF's regulatory site(s) and clarify its mechanism of action (Kuttner-Kondo et al., 1996). CCPs are composed of five β strands allowing the ~60-70 amino acids of each CCP to take on an ellipsoid structure. Predictions made from the modeling were 1) the primary recognition site for the convertases is a positively charged surface area between CCPs 2 and 3 and an adjoining CCP2 cavity; and 2) a CCP3-4 groove and its attached cavity in CCP3 as well as a cavity in CCP4 provide additional contact points. An important aspect of this work was that since amino acids making up these sites were defined, site-directed mutagenesis could be applied to test the validity of predictions.

4.3   Lessons from Mutagenesis Studies

A preliminary experiment 1) mutated N^{61} to Q removing the N-linked glycan between CCPs 1 and 2, 2) changed $KKK^{125-127}$ to TTT in the positively charged area between CCPs 2 and 3, and 3) mutated $L^{147}F^{148}$, exposed hydrophobic residues in CCP3 that make up part of the groove between CCPs 2 and 3, to SS (Brodbeck et al., 2000a). The deletion of the N-linked glycan did not affect DAF's function. The triple substitution of T for K had a markedly negative effect in the alternative pathway, and a lesser negative effect in the classical pathway. The double S substitution completely abrogated DAF's activity in both pathways. At about the same time that these experiments on DAF were conducted, similar experiments were undertaken by others on CR1 (Krych-Goldberg et al., 1999) and C4b binding protein (C4BP) (Blom et al., 2000). Consistent with the DAF results, in CR1, F82V, the homolog of F^{148}, was shown to abrogate decay accelerating activity in both pathways. Likewise, in C4BP, K63Q, the homolog of K^{127}, caused a "medium" decrease in decay acceleration in a classical pathway C3 convertase assay. Collectively, these results indicated that F^{148} in DAF and its corresponding residue in CR1 is a critical residue in the decay acceleration process in general.

A frequently used strategy in site-directed mutagenesis is to eliminate an amino acid side chain by substituting alanine for the amino acid in question as the side chain usually provides for the residue's function. A primarily alanine-substitution mutagenesis study (Kuttner-Kondo et al., 2001) of DAF looked at residues across CCPs 2, 3, and 4, most of which had been highlighted as being potentially important by the 1996 molecular modeling study (Kuttner-Kondo et al., 1996). For analyses of each mutant's effect, a fluid-phase system was used. The mutants, consisting of the soluble modules of the functional CCPs 1-4 domains, were tested in a classical pathway C4b2a hemolytic assay and an alternative pathway C3bBb decay ELISA system. R^{69}, R^{96}, and R^{100} in CCP2 and K^{127} in the CCP2-CCP3 linker, when individually mutated to A, dramatically impaired DAF's activity in both pathways. F148A and L171A also seriously impaired DAF's function in both pathways. These findings appeared to confirm the importance of the positively charged surface area covering a portion of CCPs 2 and 3 and a binding pocket with exposed hydrophobic residues between CCPs 2 and 3. A lesser role of a potential cavity on SCR3 was indicated by mutations F154A, F163A, and S165A which had little to no negative effect on DAF's activity in either pathway. This study (Kuttner-Kondo et al., 2001) confirmed the earlier study (Brodbeck et al., 1996) that found differences in the area needed for decay acceleration of C3bBb versus C4b2a. L70A in CCP2, K126A in the linker between CCPs 2 and 3, Y160A and F169A in CCP3, and R206A and R212A in CCP4 negatively affected DAF in its ability to decay accelerate C3bBb but did not affect its ability to decay accelerate C4b2a.

Another group (Hasan et al., 2002) made several of the same mutations (Kuttner-Kondo et al., 2001) with studies of full length DAF transfected into CHO cells in which cytotoxicity of the antibody- and complement-sensitized cells was assessed after 24 hr with a Cell Titer 96 kit. This study obtained similar results on the importance of F^{148}, but diverged on the importance of L^{171} and suggested that F^{123}, F^{154}, and possibly S^{165} are additionally important for DAF's complement regulatory function. The reason for the differing results is not known. An interesting finding of this study was that mAb 1H4 which blocks DAF's activity did not recognize CHO transfectants expressing DAF mutants F148A, S155A, C156A, S165L, and L171A, while it did recognize DAF mutants F123A, F154A, G159A, Y160A, L162A, F163A, and S165A. The findings taken together with the hemolytic assay/ELISA data highlight the importance of F^{148}.

4.4   Solution and Crystal Structures of DAF

In 2003, the solution structure of CCPs 2 and 3 of DAF and the crystal structure of CCPs 3 and 4 of DAF became available (Uhrinova et al., 2003; Williams et al., 2003).   The CCP2-3 solution structure is particularly relevant since it comprises a functionally active fragment, but the orientation of CCP2 with respect to CCP3 was not well defined.   This may be influenced by the lack of CCP1 and CCP4 which might stabilize the two intervening CCP modules. Alternatively, the hinge may, in fact, be flexible. Although the NMR structure predicts few direct contacts between CCPs 2 and 3, there is evidence of a loose hydrophobic cluster on the concave side of the module. A belt of positive charge encircles the CCP2-3 junction with R^{69}, R^{96}, and K^{126} on the concave side, and R^{100} and K^{127} on the opposite side. The hydrophobic and functionally important F^{148}, F^{169}, and L^{171} align on the concave side of the molecule (Fig. 3).

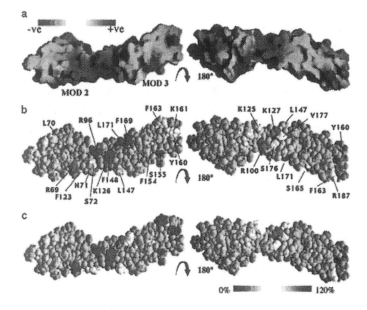

Figure 3. Electrostatic surface representation of DAF~2,3 and outcomes of mutagenesis. (a) Electrostatic surface representations: the Left view is the same as that used in Fig. 2 (but rotated ⁓90° about an axis perpendicular to the page). Red is negative and blue is positive as indicated by the upper left bar (range 1.4-128 kT). (b) Surface views as in a to illustrate outcome of mutating the labeled individual residues (20). Percentage of wild-type AP regulatory activity remaining after substitution is color coded according to the color bar (lower right). (c) As in b, but this frame summarizes the effects of the same mutations on CP regulatory activity. All mutations were to Ala except N71K and S72F. Taken from (Uhrinova et al., 2003).

The decrease in function observed from mutation, for example of K^{126} or F^{148}, could be secondary to impacting intermodular flexibility rather than eliminating a contact point between DAF and the convertases [discussed in (Uhrinova et al., 2003) and (Williams et al., 2003)]. Nevertheless, it appears that both sides of DAF near the junction of CCPs 2 and 3 interact with the convertase, perhaps occupying a groove. The determination of the crystal structure of CCPs 3 and 4 was important for several reasons. First, the CCP2-3 structure could be overlapped with the CCP3-4 structure to provide information on how the functional domains of DAF may orient themselves relative to one another. Second, it provided a scaffold for analysis of the effects of previously studied CCP3-4 site-directed mutagenesis data as well as a structure for the design of additional mutations which might shed light on DAF's interaction with the alternative pathway convertase. Finally, the functional analyses that were performed in conjunction with the CCP3-4 structure confirmed the earlier finding (Kuttner-Kondo et al., 2001) that F169A in CCP3 abrogates DAF's alternative pathway activity while not affecting its classical pathway activity.

Early in 2004, a full crystal structure of DAF's four CCPs was released (Lukacik et al., 2004). What emerged was an elongated rod shape of 160 X 50 X 30Å. Introduction of previous site-directed mutagenesis data (Kuttner-Kondo et al., 2001; Williams et al., 2003) prompted speculation that DAF's primary site of interaction with the convertases is centered in a hydrophobic patch in CCP3 (notably F169 and L171) that is part of an uncharged band circling the CCP2-3 interface. It was proposed that the positively charged residues near this junction have a predominantly structural role. A controversy currently exists as to whether the derived 3D structure is influenced by the effects of the crystallization conditions and liquor on the protein [4°C and 20% (wt/vol) monomethoxypolyethylene glycol 5000] or whether the positive surface potential at the CCP2-3 junction predicted by NMR solution structure reflects DAF's functional arrangement physiologically.

5.   DAF'S LIGANDS

For understanding DAF's function, it is necessary to include structure-function analyses of its partners (DAF ligands). The three participants in decay acceleration are the regulator, i.e. DAF, and either of the bimolecular C3 convertases, C4b2a or C3bBb. The C3 convertases are composed of two components, C4b and C2a, or C3b and Bb. Bb and C2a, themselves, are composed of two domains, a von Willibrand factor type A domain and a serine protease domain.

As indicated above, early studies provided suggestive evidence that the ligands for DAF are the bimolecular C4b2a or C3bBb complexes, but this issue remained incompletely resolved. The cloning of C2 (Bentley, 1986) and factor B (Mole et al., 1984) revealed that, like DAF, the C2b and Ba portions of these proteins are composed of CCPs, in each case 3 rather than 4 as in DAF. During C4b2a and C3bBb assembly, these 3 CCP fragments, i.e. C2b and Ba, are released into the fluid phase. Recent studies (Hourcade et al., 1999) using an ELISA with deposited C3b and factor B in the absence and presence of factor D showed that (in the absence of factor D) DAF has no effect on assembly of C3bB and cannot decay this complex. In the presence of factor D, however, following conversion to C3bBb, DAF efficiently displaces Bb. One working hypothesis (Fig. 4) is that, upon release of Ba (or C2b), the C3b (or C4b) binding sites for the 3 CCPs of the Ba fragment of factor B (or C2) are vacated and become available for binding of the functional CCPs 2-4 of DAF. This binding then displaces Bb (or C2a) and, once displaced, the affinity of DAF for the convertase decreases and it leaves C3b (or C4b).

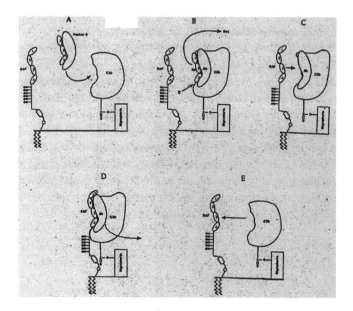

Figure 4. Proposed mechanism of action. The model proposes that DAF and the Ba fragment of factor B share common binding sites on C3b (A). Following cleavage of the Ba fragment from factor B by factor D, release of the Ba fragment from the C3bB complex, DAF binds C3bBb (B and C). The Bb fragment is destabilized (D) and displaced. Once Bb is displaced, DAF is released from the complex (E). Taken from (Kuttner-Kondo et al., 1996)

As one approach to map the residues in Bb that are important in decay acceleration by DAF (and other C3 convertase regulators), factor B was subjected to site-directed mutagenesis (primarily alanine substitutions) in its type A domain. Those mutants that were able to form viable convertase complexes with C3b were tested for their sensitivity to decay acceleration by DAF, CR1, and factor H (Hourcade et al., 2002). Two sites in the type A domain, i.e. in the α1 helix and the α4/α5 helix, were found to be essential for the decay acceleration process but apparently for different reasons. Mutations that were made in the α1 helix and adjoining loops, especially N260D, that are near a putative C3b-binding site, stabilized the C3 convertase. This made it difficult for the three regulators to accelerate the decay of C3bBb$_{mut}$. Mutations in the α4/α5 helix region, especially Y338A, negatively affected the ability of DAF and CR1, but not factor H, to accelerate the decay of C3bBb$_{mut}$. A likely explanation of these data is that DAF and CR1 interact with the alternative pathway convertase at this location, while factor H interacts at another location yet to be found (Fig. 5).

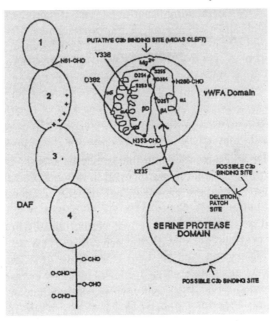

Figure 5. Proposed model of DAF's interaction with C3bBb. Locations of Y338 and D382 in the vWFA domain are approximate and based on the model of (Hinshelwood et al., 1999). The positively charged surface on DAF is schematically illustrated by "+"s. Taken from Kuttner-Kondo thesis.

A follow-up study of the interaction of DAF, CR1, and C4BP with the classical pathway convertase with mutations to C2 in its type A domain

(Kuttner-Kondo, 2003) was motivated by the knowledge that, in contrast to the alternative pathway convertase C3bBb, DAF only requires its CCPs 2 and 3 to decay accelerate the classical pathway C3 convertase C4b2a. The finding that homologous residues in the $\alpha 4/\alpha 5$ helix region of C2 are critical to DAF in its decay acceleration process would argue that CCPs 2 and/or 3, but not CCP4, are in contact with this region of C2a. Consistent with this, it was found that mutating Y327A in C2, the homologous residue to Y^{338} in factor B, abolishes DAF's ability to decay accelerate the mutant convertase supporting this proposal.

6.   DAF AS A RECEPTOR FOR BACTERIA AND VIRUSES

DAF has been shown to be a receptor for *E. coli* expressing Dr adhesins (Bernet-Camard et al., 1996; Nowicki et al., 1993; Pham et al., 1995; Pham et al., 1997). *E. coli* expressing fimbrial Dr, and afimbrial AFA-I, afimbrial AFA-III and fimbrial F1845 require CCP3 for attachment. Two dra-positive X strains (*E. coli* 8826 and *E. coli* 7372) bind CCP4 (Nowicki et al., 1990; Pham et al., 1995). DAF amino acid substitutions, S155A, C156A, and S165L (Hasan et al., 2002), completely block the binding of the Dr adhesin. Beyond DAF's CCPs, its GPI anchor appears to be involved in the Dr(+) *E. coli* internalization process (Selvarangan et al., 2000). Diseases of these bacteria include (gestational) pyelonephritis, cystitis, and diarrhea [reviewed in (Nowicki et al., 2001)]. One theory regarding the pathogenicity of *E. coli* bearing AFA/Dr adhesins in the intestine is that the adhesin-DAF interaction induces PMN transepithelial migration, and in turn the production of TNF-α and IL-1β which upregulates intestinal DAF thereby creating more receptors for the bacterial binding (Betis et al., 2003).

Accumulating evidence indicates that certain viruses in Picornaviridae bind DAF. DAF is a receptor for echovirus 7 (Ward et al., 1994), coxsackieviruses B1, B3, and B5, and enterovirus 70 (Karnauchow et al., 1996; Shafren et al., 1995). The list now includes coxsackievirus A21; echoviruses 6, 11, 12 and 30; enterovirus 68 and human rhinovirus 87 (Blomqvist et al., 2002; Shafren et al., 1997a). While members of the coxsackievirus B-like B-cluster of human enteroviruses (coxsackievirus B 1, 3, and 5; echovirus 6, 7, 11, 12, and 30) bind CCPs 2-4 of DAF, members of the poliovirus-like C-cluster of human enteroviruses (coxsackievirus A21) and members of the enterovirus 70-like D-cluster of human enteroviruses (enterovirus 70) bind CCP1 (Powell et al., 1999). However, within these clusters, the binding sites of the viruses on DAF may not be the same. Mapping echovirus 7, echovirus 11, and echovirus 12 binding data on the crystal structure of CCPs 3-4 shows that echovirus 12 binding is negatively affected by E134A while echovirus 7 binding is positively affected by F169A, an amino acid on the opposite side of DAF CCP3 (Williams et al., 2003). Often, DAF is not the sole receptor for these viruses. Coxsackievirus A21 may bind ICAM-1 as well as DAF (Shafren et al., 1997a) and coxsackievirus B3 binds the coxsackie-adenovirus receptor (CAR) (Shafren et al., 1997b). Enterovirus 70 is believed to have an additional cell surface receptor (Alexander and Dimock, 2002). Although early work indicated that ICAM-1 was required for coxsackievirus A21 to enter cells (Shafren et al., 1997a), clinical isolates have been found which appear to infect DAF expressing cells without the aid of ICAM-1 or DAF-antibody cross-linking (Newcombe et al., 2004).

7. ANIMAL MODELS OF DISEASE

Unlike humans, in the mouse there are two *Daf* genes, *Daf1* and *Daf2*. The *Daf1* gene, like the human *DAF* gene, encodes GPI-anchored DAF that is ubiquitously expressed, while the *Daf2* gene encodes transmembrane anchored DAF that is restricted in its distribution to the testes and spleen (Lin et al., 2001). Consequently for an animal model, the *Daf1* gene was targeted. *Daf1* knock-out mice (Lin et al., 2001; Miwa, 2001) provide a resource for studying several experimental animal models of disease including experimental autoimmune myasthenia gravis (EAMG), a murine model of systemic lupus erythematosus (SLE) in MRL/lpr mice, acute nephrotoxic serum (NTS)-induced nephritis, and dextran sodium sulfate (DSS)-induced colitis. In EAMG, the binding of anti-acetylcholine receptor (AChR) antibodies to the post-synaptic junction activates the classical pathway, ultimately leading to endplate damage (De Baets et al., 2003). Following anti-AChR mAb administration, as compared with $Daf1^{+/+}$ littermates which exhibited hang times of >8 min, $Daf1^{-/-}$ mice exhibited hang times <10 sec, showed greater C3b deposition, and showed larger reductions in AChR levels. These results suggest a potential therapeutic role for DAF in the treatment of myasthenia gravis (Lin et al., 2002b). In the MRL/lpr model, $Daf1^{-/-}$/MRL/lpr mice showed greater lymphadenopathy, splenomegaly, serum anti-chromatin autoantibody levels, and aggravated dermatitis indicating a protective role for DAF (Miwa et al., 2002). In the DSS-induced colitis model, $Daf1^{-/-}$ mice showed markedly greater weight loss and bloody stool and greatly retarded to completely blocked recovery from disease following discontinuation of the drug. In the NTS-induced nephritis model, $Daf1^{-/-}$ mice showed massively increased proteinuria, augmented C3b and C9 deposition in glomeruli, and massively greater podocyte destruction (Lin et al., 2002a; Lin et al., 2004). Taken together, the results of these studies and studies of other models that are underway highlight DAF's importance as a critical shield that protects self cells from direct or bystander injury during inflammation.

8.   CONCLUDING REMARKS

After many years, structural and functional studies are providing complementary information which will allow a comprehensive understanding of DAF's role as a regulator of complement activation. DAF's 3D structure and site-directed mutations will allow the mapping not only of its convertase sites but its other interactions including bacterial and viral pathogens. At the same time, studies with *Daf1* knock-out mice show that DAF is an important protein for maintaining homeostasis in a stressed system. New therapeutic approaches should become available from this expanding knowledge base.

9.   REFERENCES

1. Alexander, D. A., and Dimock, K. (2002). Sialic acid functions in enterovirus 70 binding and infection. J Virol 76, 11265-11272.
2. Barlow, P. N., Norman, D. G., Steinkasserer, A., Horne, T. J., Pearce, J., Driscoll, P. C., Sim, R. B., and Campbell, I. D. (1992). Solution structure of the fifth repeat of factor H: a second example of the complement control protein module. Biochemistry 31, 3626-3634.
3. Barlow, P. N., Steinkasserer, A., Norman, D. G., Kieffer, B., Wiles, A. P., Sim, R. B., and Campbell, I. D. (1993). Solution structure of a pair of complement modules by nuclear magnetic resonance. Journal of Molecular Biology 232, 268-284.
4. Bentley, D. R. (1986). Primary structure of human complement component C2. Homology to two unrelated protein families. Biochem J 239, 339-345.
5. Bernet-Camard, M. F., Coconnier, M. H., Hudault, S., and Servin, A. L. (1996). Pathogenicity of the diffusely adhering strain Escherichia coli C1845: F1845 adhesin-decay accelerating factor interaction, brush border microvillus injury, and actin disassembly in cultured human intestinal epithelial cells. Infect Immun 64, 1918-1928.
6. Betis, F., Brest, P., Hofman, V., Guignot, J., Kansau, I., Rossi, B., Servin, A., and Hofman, P. (2003). Afa/Dr diffusely adhering Escherichia coli infection in T84 cell monolayers induces increased neutrophil transepithelial migration, which in turn promotes cytokine-dependent upregulation of decay-accelerating factor (CD55), the receptor for Afa/Dr adhesins. Infect Immun 71, 1774-1783.
7. Blom, A. M., Zadura, A. F., Villoutreix, B. O., and Dahlback, B. (2000). Positively charged amino acids at the interface between alpha-chain CCP1 and CCP2 of C4BP are required for regulation of the classical C3-convertase. Molec Immunol 37, 445-453.

8. Blomqvist, S., Savolainen, C., Raman, L., Roivainen, M., and Hovi, T. (2002). Human rhinovirus 87 and enterovirus 68 represent a unique serotype with rhinovirus and enterovirus features. J Clin Microbiol *40*, 4218-4223.
9. Brodbeck, W. G., Kuttner-Kondo, L., Mold, C., and Medof, M. E. (2000a). Structure/function studies of human decay accelerating factor (DAF). Immunology *101*, 104-111.
10. Brodbeck, W. G., Liu, D., Sperry, J., Mold, C., and Medof, M. E. (1996). Localization of classical and alternative pathway regulatory activity within the decay-accelerating factor. J Immunol *156*, 2528-2533.
11. Brodbeck, W. G., and Medof, M. E. (1997). Use of recombinant DAF proteins to localize the epitopes recognized by monoclonal anti-CD55. Transfusion Clinique et Biologique *4*, 125-126.
12. Brodbeck, W. G., Mold, C., Atkinson, J. P., and Medof, M. E. (2000b). Cooperation between decay accelerating factor and membrane cofactor protein in protecting cells from autologous complement attack. J Immunol *165*, 3999-4006.
13. Caras, I. W., Davitz, M. A., Rhee, L., Weddell, G., Martin, D. W., Jr, and Nussenzweig, V. (1987). Cloning of decay-accelerating factor suggests novel use of splicing to generate two proteins. Nature *325*, 545-549.
14. Coyne, K. E., Hall, S. E., Thompson, E. S., Arce, M. A., Kinoshita, T., Fujita, T., Anstee, D. J., Rosse, W., and Lublin, D. M. (1992). Mapping of epitopes, glycosylation sites, and complement regulatory domains in human decay accelerating factor. J Immunol *149*, 2906-2913.
15. Davitz, M. A., Low, M. G., and Nussenzweig, V. (1986). Release of decay-accelerating factor (DAF) from the cell membrane by phosphatidylinositol-specific phospholipase C (PI-PLC). J Exp Med *163*, 1150-1161.
16. De Baets, M., Stassen, M., Losen, M., Zhang, X., and Machiels, B. (2003). Immunoregulation in experimental autoimmune myasthenia gravis--about T cells, antibodies, and endplates. Ann N Y Acad Sci *998*, 308-317.
17. Fearon, D. T., and Collins, L. A. (1983). Increased expression of C3b receptors on polymorphonuclear leukocytes induced by chemotactic factors and by purification procedures. J Immunol *130*, 370-375.
18. Fujita, T., Inoue, T., Ogawa, K., Iida, K., and Tamura, N. (1987). The mechanism of action of decay-accelerating factor (DAF). DAF inhibits the assembly of C3 convertases by dissociated C2a and Bb. J Exp Med *166*, 1221-1228.
19. Harada, R., Okada, N., Fujita, T., and Okada, H. (1990). Purification of 1F5 antigen that prevents complement attack on homologous cell membranes. J Immunol *144*, 1823-1828.
20. Hasan, R. J., Pawelczyk, E., Urvil, P. T., Venkatarajan, M. S., Goluszko, P., Kur, J., Selvarangan, R., Nowicki, S., Braun, W. A., and Nowicki, B. J. (2002). Structure-function analysis of decay-accelerating factor: identification of residues important for binding of the Escherichia coli Dr adhesin and complement regulation. Infect Immun *70*, 4485-4493.
21. Hinshelwood, J., and Perkins, S. J. (2000a). Conformational changes during the assembly of factor B from its domains by (1)H NMR spectroscopy and molecular modelling: their relevance to the regulation of factor B activity. J Mol Biol *301*, 1267-1285.
22. Hinshelwood, J., and Perkins, S. J. (2000b). Metal-dependent conformational changes in a recombinant vWF-A domain from human factor B: a solution study by circular dichroism, fourier transform infrared and (1)H NMR spectroscopy. J Mol Biol *298*, 135-147.
23. Hinshelwood, J., Spencer, D. I., Edwards, Y. J., and Perkins, S. J. (1999). Identification of the C3b binding site in a recombinant vWF-A domain of complement factor B by surface-enhanced laser desorption-ionisation affinity mass spectrometry and homology modelling: implications for the activity of factor B. J Mol Biol *294*, 587-599.

24. Holguin, M. H., Fredrick, L. R., Bernshaw, N. J., Wilcox, L. A., and Parker, C. J. (1989). Isolation and characterization of a membrane protein from normal human erythrocytes that inhibits reactive lysis of the erythrocytes of paroxysmal nocturnal hemoglobinuria. Journal of Clinical Investigation *84*, 7-17.
25. Hourcade, D. E., Mitchell, L., Kuttner-Kondo, L. A., Atkinson, J. P., and Medof, M. E. (2002). Decay-accelerating factor (DAF), complement receptor 1 (CR1), and factor H dissociate the complement AP C3 convertase (C3bBb) via sites on the type A domain of Bb. J Biol Chem *277*, 1107-1112.
26. Hourcade, D. E., Mitchell, L. M., and Medof, M. E. (1999). Decay acceleration of the complement alternative pathway C3 convertase. Immunopharmacology *42*, 167-173.
27. Jing, H., Xu, Y., Carson, M., Moore, D., Macon, K. J., Volanakis, J. E., and Narayana, S. V. (2000). New structural motifs on the chymotrypsin fold and their potential roles in complement factor B. Embo J *19*, 164-173.
28. Karnauchow, T. M., Tolson, D. L., Harrison, B. A., Altman, E., Lublin, D. M., and Dimock, K. (1996). The HeLa cell receptor for enterovirus 70 is decay-accelerating factor (CD55). J Virol *70*, 5143-5152.
29. Kinoshita, T., Medof, M. E., and Nussenzweig, V. (1986). Endogenous association of decay-accelerating factor (DAF) with C4b and C3b on cell membranes. J Immunol *136*, 3390-3395.
30. Krych-Goldberg, M., Hauhart, R. E., Subramanian, V. B., Yurcisin, B. M., II, Crimmins, D. L., Hourcade, D. E., and Atkinson, J. P. (1999). Decay accelerating activity of complement receptor type 1 (CD35). Two active sites are required for dissociating C5 convertases. J Biol Chem *274*, 31160-31168.
31. Kuttner-Kondo, L., M Dybvig, L Mitchell, N Muqim, JP Atkinson, ME Medof, D Hourcade (2003). A corresponding tyrosine residue in the C2/factor B type A domain is a hot spot in the decay acceleration of the complement C3 convertases. J Biological Chem *278*, 52386-52391.
32. Kuttner-Kondo, L., Medof, M. E., Brodbeck, W., and Shoham, M. (1996). Molecular modeling and mechanism of action of human decay-accelerating factor. Protein Engineering *9*, 1143-1149.
33. Kuttner-Kondo, L. A., Mitchell, L., Hourcade, D. E., and Medof, M. E. (2001). Characterization of the active sites in decay-accelerating factor. J Immunol *167*, 2164-2171.
34. Lachmann, P. J. (1991). The control of homologous lysis. Immunol Today *12*, 312-315.
35. Lin, F., Emancipator, S. N., Salant, D. J., and Medof, M. E. (2002a). Decay accelerating factor confers protection against complement-mediated podocyte injury in acute nephrotoxic nephritis. Lab Invest *82*, 563-569.
36. Lin, F., Fukuoka, Y., Spicer, A., Ohta, R., Okada, N., Harris, C. L., Emancipator, S. N., and Medof, M. E. (2001). Tissue distribution of products of the mouse decay-accelerating factor (DAF) genes. Exploitation of a *Daf*1 knock-out mouse and site-specific monoclonal antibodies. Immunology *104*, 215-225.
37. Lin, F., Kaminski, H. J., Conti-Fine, B. M., Wang, W., Richmonds, C., and Medof, M. E. (2002b). Markedly enhanced susceptibility to experimental autoimmune myasthenia gravis in the absence of decay-accelerating factor protection. J Clin Invest *110*, 1269-1274.
38. Lin, F., Salant, D. J., Meyerson, H., Emancipator, S., Morgan, B. P., and Medof, M. E. (2004). Respective Roles of Decay-Accelerating Factor and CD59 in Circumventing Glomerular Injury in Acute Nephrotoxic Serum Nephritis. J Immunol *172*, 2636-2642.
39. Lukacik, P., Roversi, P., White, J., Esser, D., Smith, G. P., Billington, J., Williams, P. A., Rudd, P. M., Wormald, M. R., Harvey, D. J., *et al.* (2004). Complement regulation at the

molecular level: The structure of decay-accelerating factor. Proc Natl Acad Sci U S A *101*, 1279-1284.
40. Medof, M. E., Kinoshita, T., and Nussenzweig, V. (1984). Inhibition of complement activation on the surface of cells after incorporation of decay-accelerating factor (DAF) into their membranes. J Exp Med *160*, 1558-1578.
41. Medof, M. E., Lublin, D. M., Holers, V. M., Ayers, D. J., Getty, R. R., Leykam, J. F., Atkinson, J. P., and Tykocinski, M. L. (1987a). Cloning and characterization of cDNAs encoding the complete sequence of decay-accelerating factor of human complement. Proc Natl Acad Sci U S A *84*, 2007-2011.
42. Medof, M. E., Walter, E. I., Roberts, W. L., Haas, R., and Rosenberry, T. L. (1986). Decay-accelerating factor of complement is anchored to cells by a C-terminal glycolipid. Biochemistry *25*, 6740-6747.
43. Medof, M. E., Walter, E. I., Rutgers, J. L., Knowles, D. M., and Nussenzweig, V. (1987b). Identification of the complement decay-accelerating factor (DAF) on epithelium and glandular cells and in body fluids. J Exp Med *165*, 848-864.
44. Meri, S., Morgan, B. P., Wing, M., Jones, J., Davies, A., Podack, E., and Lachmann, P. J. (1990). Human protectin (CD59), an 18-20-kD homologous complement restriction factor, does not restrict perforin-mediated lysis. J Exp Med *172*, 367-370.
45. Miwa, T., Maldonado, M. A., Zhou, L., Sun, X., Luo, H. Y., Cai, D., Werth, V. P., Madaio, M. P., Eisenberg, R. A., and Song, W. C. (2002). Deletion of decay-accelerating factor (CD55) exacerbates autoimmune disease development in MRL/lpr mice. Am J Pathol *161*, 1077-1086.
46. Miwa, T., Sun X, Ohta R, Okada N, Harris CL, Morgan BP, Song WC (2001). Characterization of glycosylphosphatidylinositol-anchored decay accelerating factor (GPI-DAF) and transmembrane DAF gene expression in wild-type and GPI-DAF gene knockout mice using polyclonal and monoclonal antibodies with dual or single specificity. Immunology *104*, 207-214.
47. Mole, J. E., Anderson, J. K., Davison, E. A., and Woods, D. E. (1984). Complete primary structure for the zymogen of human complement factor B. J Biol Chem *259*, 3407-3412.
48. Nagar, B., Jones, R. G., Diefenbach, R. J., Isenman, D. E., and Rini, J. M. (1998). X-ray crystal structure of C3d: a C3 fragment and ligand for complement receptor 2. Science *280*, 1277-1281.
49. Newcombe, N. G., Johansson, E. S., Au, G., Lindberg, A. M., Barry, R. D., and Shafren, D. R. (2004). Enterovirus capsid interactions with decay-accelerating factor mediate lytic cell infection. J Virol *78*, 1431-1439.
50. Nicholson-Weller, A., Burge, J., Fearon, D. T., Weller, P. F., and Austen, K. F. (1982). Isolation of a human erythrocyte membrane glycoprotein with decay-accelerating activity for C3 convertases of the complement system. J Immunol *129*, 184-189.
51. Norman, D. G., Barlow, P. N., Baron, M., Day, A. J., Sim, R. B., and Campbell, I. D. (1991). Three-dimensional structure of a complement control protein module in solution. Journal of Molecular Biology *219*, 717-725.
52. Nowicki, B., Hart, A., Coyne, K. E., Lublin, D. M., and Nowicki, S. (1993). Short consensus repeat-3 domain of recombinant decay-accelerating factor is recognized by *Escherichia coli* recombinant Dr adhesin in a model of a cell-cell interaction. J Exp Med *178*, 2115-2121.
53. Nowicki, B., Labigne, A., Moseley, S., Hull, R., Hull, S., and Moulds, J. (1990). The Dr hemagglutinin, afimbrial adhesins AFA-I and AFA-III, and F1845 fimbriae of uropathogenic and diarrhea-associated Escherichia coli belong to a family of hemagglutinins with Dr receptor recognition. Infect Immun *58*, 279-281.

54. Nowicki, B., Selvarangan, R., and Nowicki, S. (2001). Family of Escherichia coli Dr adhesins: decay-accelerating factor receptor recognition and invasiveness. J Infect Dis *183 Suppl 1*, S24-27.

55. Pangburn, M. K. (1986). Differences between the binding site of the complement regulatory proteins DAF, CR1 and factor H on C3 convertases. J Immunol *136*, 2216-2221.

56. Pangburn, M. K., Schreiber, R. D., and Muller-Eberhard, H. J. (1983a). Deficiency of an erythrocyte membrane protein with complement regulatory activity in paroxysmal nocturnal hemoglobinuria. Proc Natl Acad Sci U S A *80*, 5430-5434.

57. Pangburn, M. K., Schreiber, R. D., Trombold, J. S., and Muller-Eberhard, H. J. (1983b). Paroxysmal nocturnal hemoglobinuria: deficiency in factor H-like functions of the abnormal erythrocytes. J Exp Med *157*, 1971-1980.

58. Pham, T., Kaul, A., Hart, A., Golusko, P., Moulds, J., Nowicki, S., Lublin, D. M., and Nowicki, B. J. (1995). *dra*-related X adhesins of gestational pyelonephritis-associated *Escherichia coli* recognize SCR-3 and SCR-4 domains of recombinant decay - accelerating factor. Infection and Immunity *63*, 1663-1668.

59. Pham, T. Q., Goluszko, P., Popov, V., Nowicki, S., and Nowicki, B. J. (1997). Molecular cloning and characterization of Dr-II, a nonfimbrial adhesin-I-like adhesin isolated from gestational pyelonephritis-associated Escherichia coli that binds to decay-accelerating factor. Infect Immun *65*, 4309-4318.

60. Powell, R. M., Ward, T., Goodfellow, I., Almond, J. W., and Evans, D. J. (1999). Mapping the binding domains on decay accelerating factor (DAF) for haemagglutinating enteroviruses: implications for the evolution of a DAF-binding phenotype. Journal of General Virology *80*, 3145-3152.

61. Premkumar, D. R. D., Fukuoka, Y., Sevlever, D., Brunschwig, E., Rosenberry, T. R., Tykocinski, M. L., and Medof, M. E. (2001). Properties of exogenously added GPI-anchored proteins following their incorporation into cells. Journal of Cellular Biochemistry *82*, 234-245.

62. Reid, K. B., and Day, A. J. (1989). Structure-function relationships of the complement components. Immunol Today *10*, 177-180.

63. Selvarangan, R., Goluszko, P., Popov, V., Singhal, J., Pham, T., Lublin, D. M., Nowicki, S., and Nowicki, B. (2000). Role of decay-accelerating factor domains and anchorage in internalization of Dr-fimbriated Escherichia coli. Infect Immun *68*, 1391-1399.

64. Seya, T., and Atkinson, J. P. (1989). Functional properties of membrane cofactor protein of complement. Biochemical Journal *264*, 581-588.

65. Seya, T., Holers, V. M., and Atkinson, J. P. (1985). Purification and functional analysis of the polymorphic variants of the C3b/C4b receptor (CR1) and comparison with C4b-binding protein (C4bp), and decay accelerating factor (DAF). J Immunol *135*, 2661-2667.

66. Shafren, D. R., Bates, R. C., Agrez, M. V., Herd, R. L., Burns, G. F., and Barry, R. D. (1995). Coxsackieviruses B1, B3, and B5 use decay accelerating factor as a receptor for cell attachment. Journal of Virology *69*, 3873-3877.

67. Shafren, D. R., Dorahy, D. J., Ingham, R. A., Burns, G. F., and Barry, R. D. (1997a). Coxsackievirus A21 binds to decay-accelerating factor but requires intercellular adhesion molecule 1 for cell entry. J Virol *71*, 4736-4743.

68. Shafren, D. R., Williams, D. T., and Barry, R. D. (1997b). A decay-accelerating factor-binding strain of coxsackievirus B3 requires the coxsackievirus-adenovirus receptor protein to mediate lytic infection of rhabdomyosarcoma cells. J Virol *71*, 9844-9848.

69. Uhrinova, S., Lin, F., Ball, G., Bromek, K., Uhrin, D., Medof, M. E., and Barlow, P. N. (2003). Solution structure of a functionally active fragment of decay-accelerating factor. Proc Natl Acad Sci U S A *100*, 4718-4723.

70. van den Berg, C. W., Cinek, T., Hallett, M. B., Horejsi, V., and Morgan, B. P. (1995). Exogenous glycosyl phosphatidylinositol-anchored CD59 associates with kinases in membrane clusters on U937 cells and becomes Ca^{2+}-signaling competent. J Cell Biol *131*, 669-677.

71. van den Elsen, J. M., Martin, A., Wong, V., Clemenza, L., Rose, D. R., and Isenman, D. E. (2002). X-ray crystal structure of the C4d fragment of human complement component C4. J Mol Biol *322*, 1103-1115.

72. Walter, E. I., Ratnoff, W. D., Long, K. E., Kazura, J. W., and Medof, M. E. (1992). Effect of glycoinositolphospholipid anchor lipid groups on functional properties of decay-accelerating factor protein in cells. J Biol Chem *267*, 1245-1252.

73. Walter, E. I., Roberts, W. L., Rosenberry, T. L., Ratnoff, W. D., and Medof, M. E. (1990). Structural basis for variations in the sensitivity of human decay accelerating factor to phosphatidylinositol-specific phospholipase C cleavage. J Immunol *144*, 1030-1036.

74. Ward, T., Pipkin, P. A., Clarkson, N. A., Stone, D. M., Minor, P. D., and Almond, J. W. (1994). Decay-accelerating factor CD55 is identified as the receptor for echovirus 7 using CELICS, a rapid immuno-focal cloning method. Embo J *13*, 5070-5074.

75. Williams, P., Chaudhry, Y., Goodfellow, I. G., Billington, J., Powell, R., Spiller, O. B., Evans, D. J., and Lea, S. (2003). Mapping CD55 function. The structure of two pathogen-binding domains at 1.7 A. J Biol Chem *278*, 10691-10696.

9

The Role of Complement in Pregnancy and Fetal Loss

Guillermina Girardi and Jane E. Salmon
Department of Medicine, Hospital for Special Surgery-Weill Medical College of Cornell University, New York, NY 10021, USA.

Abstract: Recurrent spontaneous abortion is a significant health problem; 50 to 70% of all conceptions fail. Although in the majority of the cases the cause is unknown, an immune mechanism involving the inappropriate recognition of the embryo by the mother's immune system has been proposed. Complement activation has been proposed as a common effector in causing fetal injury initiated by different triggers. The adaptive immune system can harness innate immune mechanisms. Appropriate complement inhibition is an absolute requirement for normal pregnancy. Deficiency of complement inhibitors in mice leads to progressive embryonic lethality due to inflammation. In a murine model of antiphospholipid antibody-induced pregnancy loss we demonstrated that complement activation is required for fetal injury. Activated Th1 cells may also induce pregnancy loss through the activation of the complement cascade. Recruitment and activation of inflammatory effector cells by C3a, C5a and the C5b-9 MAC, leads to fetal injury and pregnancy loss.

Key words: Pregnancy - abortion – complement activation - fetal injury – inflammatory cells

1.   INTRODUCTION

Recurrent spontaneous abortion (RSA) is a significant health problem affecting 2 - 5% of couples worldwide (1). 78% of fertilized oocytes do not end in birth and 62% of conceptions are lost before the 12th week of pregnancy (2). RSA is generally defined as a history of three or more consecutive spontaneous abortions occurring prior to the 22nd week of gestation (3). Genetic, anatomic, hormonal and environmental factors have been implicated in the etiology of RSA, but a sizable proportion remains unexplained. It has long been suspected that approximately 80% of the unexplained RSAs are due to immunologic causes (4). Although in the majority of affected women the cause of recurrent miscarriages is unknown, an immune mechanism involving the inappropriate and subsequently injurious recognition of the embryo by the mother's immune system has been proposed.

Ever since the Nobel Prize winning immunologist Peter Medawar first likened the mammalian embryo to a tissue transplant received from a genetically different individual, immunologists have been puzzled by the basic conundrum: How do embryos survive the attack of maternal natural defenses. He noted that the embryo, being semiallogenic for the mother, was seen to survive and thrive in the face of a potentially hostile maternal immune system (5).

Studies have demonstrated that a successful pregnancy requires a state of maternal immune tolerance to accommodate the embryo (6). Failure of these mechanisms to accommodate and protect the embryo can result in pregnancy loss.

Murine models have recently been developed that are relevant to this issue. Specifically, we and others have identified a novel role for complement as an early effector in the pathway leading to pregnancy loss associated with placental inflammation. Indeed, it appears that inhibition of complement activation is an absolute requirement for normal pregnancy, and that in the antiphosphospholid syndrome, overwhelming activation of complement triggered by antibodies deposited in placenta leads to fetal injury (7).

For decades the complement system has been regarded as an effector arm of the innate immune response. The complement system acts as an effector system in host defense against invading pathogens and contributes through its activation products to the release of inflammatory mediators, promoting tissue injury at sites of inflammation. Complement has been implicated in the pathogenesis of several autoimmune, ischemic and vascular diseases (8, 9). Activation of complement promotes chemotaxis of inflammatory cells and generates proteolytic fragments that enhance phagocytosis by polymorphonuclear leukocytes (PMN) and monocytes.

2.   FETAL TOLERANCE AND COMPLEMENT

A relationship between pregnancy complications and an abnormal maternal immune response has been described in the literature (10, 11). RSA may be initiated or prevented by the maternal immune system. The fetus expresses many paternally-derived cell surface molecules foreign to the immune system of the mother. Fetal survival during pregnancy depends in significant measure on the ability of fetal tissue to avoid recognition and rejection by the maternal immune system. Evidence from murine and human pregnancy studies points to a strong association between maternal T helper 2-type (Th2-type) immunity and successful pregnancy, whereas Th1-type immune reactivity is associated with pregnancy loss (12). Fetomaternal tolerance is partially dependent on the secretion of immunoregulatory cytokines, such as TGF-β and IL-10, by the decidua and placenta (13-16). These cytokines may promote the development of Th2-type cells and regulatory T cells that provide immunosuppressive mechanisms important in fetal survival. Conditions associated with recurrent spontaneous miscarriages and preterm labor are associated with an inflammatory reaction, the production of proinflammatory cytokines such as TNF-α IL-6, IL-1, and INF-γ, and a conversion from a Th2 to a Th1 phenotype (14, 17). That autoimmune disorders, such as systemic lupus erythematosus (SLE) and the antiphospholipid syndrome are associated with poor pregnancy outcome underscores the critical role of the maternal immune response (18). Abnormalities in fetal regulation of the maternal immune response, even in the absence of autoimmunity, are a significant cause of RSA.

Whereas a clear relationship between pregnancy failure and histological evidence of inflammation has been well documented, the triggering factors involved in initiating inflammation have remained elusive in most cases of preterm labor and RSA. Recent experimental observations suggest that altered complement regulation causes and may perpetuate these complications of pregnancy (19, 20). Since fetal tissues are semi-allogeneic and alloantibodies commonly develop in the mother, the placenta is potentially subject to complement-mediated immune attack at the maternal-fetal interface (19). Although activated complement components are present in normal placentas (21, 22), it appears that uncontrolled complement activation is prevented in successful pregnancy by three regulatory proteins present on the trophoblast membrane (23, 24). Two of these membrane-bound proteins, DAF and MCP, regulate the activation of C3 and C4 on the surface of cells (25, 26). DAF inhibits the assembly and accelerates the decay of the C3 convertase enzymes that activate C3 and amplify the classical and alternative complement pathways. MCP is a cofactor for Factor I-mediated degradation and inactivation of C3b and C4b (27). The third protein, CD59, is also membrane anchored and prevents assembly of C5b-9 MAC, blocking the terminal effector functions of complement (28). Several studies have shown that the levels of activated complement components present at a given site depends on the relative effects of complement activators and their inhibitors, DAF, MCP and CD59 (25). All three proteins are expressed on the trophoblast in contact with maternal blood and tissues, providing a mechanism to protect the fetus from damage due to complement pathway activation by alloantibodies. Indeed, on the basis of their characteristic distribution patterns, it is likely that these proteins are strategically positioned for this purpose.

Little information is available about complement activation or the expression of complement regulatory proteins in normal and abnormal human pregnancy (29). During normal gestation, the levels of complement components gradually rise. Serum concentration of C3, C4, and total hemolytic complement (CH50) increase 10% to 50% (46). In some cases, modest increases in complement split products, such as C3a, occur. While levels of C3, C4, and CH50 increase in preeclampsia, marked elevation in complement split products, such as Ba, C3a, C4d, and soluble C5b-9, suggest increased complement deposition in the placenta, which has indeed been found (46,47). These findings indicate activation of both the classical and alternative pathways. However, no data are available regarding the serum levels of individual complement components or complement split products in first trimester pregnancy losses. In one small series, 3 of 10 first trimester pregnancy losses were characterized by the onset of hypocomplementemia prior to documentation by ultrasonography of the loss of embryonic viability (23). No systematic evaluation of complement deposition on the surface of the placenta and the decidua in patients with recurrent pregnancy loss has been carried out. It would be important know if a specific pattern of complement activation is predictive of impending fetal loss or fetal damage.

Recent murine studies by Molina and co-workers underscore the importance of complement regulation in fetal control of maternal processes that mediate tissue damage. In mice, Crry is a membrane-bound intrinsic complement regulatory protein whose role, like DAF and MCP, is to block C3 and C4 activation on self-membranes (13). Crry has DAF-like activity, accelerating decay of C3 convertases, and MCP-like activity, serving as a Factor I cofactor to enhance degradation of activated C3 and C4. Thus, Crry acts as an inhibitor of classical and alternative pathway C3 convertases and blocks C3, C5, and subsequent MAC activation. That appropriate complement inhibition is an absolute requirement for normal pregnancy has been demonstrated by the finding that Crry deficiency in utero leads to progressive embryonic lethality (30). Crry-/- embryos are surrounded by activated C3 fragments and PMN, primarily around the ectoplacental cone and surrounding trophoectoderm. While normal numbers of Crry-/- embryos are found on day 9, all embryos are dead by day 15 of gestation and no live births have been found in cohorts of >250 newborns. Importantly, Crry-/- embryos are completely rescued from this 100% lethality and live pups are born at a normal Mendelian frequency when Crry+/- parents are intercrossed with C3-/- mice to generate C3-/-, Crry-/- embryos (30). This outcome is genetic proof that Crry-/- embryos die *in utero* due to their inability to suppress complement activation and tissue damage mediated by C3. Lack of Crry expression on trophoblasts leads to generation of complement split products and the recruitment and activation of inflammatory cells that destroy the embryo. If this work can be extended to humans, it is possible that appropriate complement regulation may be necessary to control maternal allo-reactivity and placental inflammation and local increase in complement activation fragments may be highly deleterious to the developing fetus.

In normal pregnancy, the human placenta appears to be subjected to complement-mediated immune attack at the maternal-fetal interface (24, 31). Although there is some evidence of activated complement in the placenta, it is likely that in successful pregnancies uncontrolled complement activation is prevented by complement inhibitory proteins, such as decay-accelerating factor, membrane cofactor protein and CD59, which are present at high levels on trophoblast cells (29, 32-34). That there is hormonal regulation of the biosynthesis of several complement components and receptors expressed in the reproductive tract and that expression patterns vary during the menstrual cycle suggest that complement contributes to normal reproductive processes (35). Taken together, the murine and human findings suggest that there is recognition of fetal tissues by immune mechanisms that trigger complement fixation and that in the presence of excessive complement activation or in the absence of complement inhibitors the fetus is as risk for injury (Figure 1).

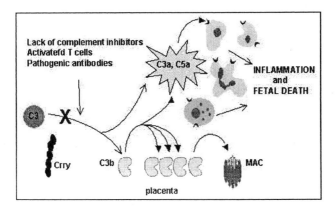

Figure 1. Complement activation leads to fetal death. Activation of the complement pathway by pathogenic antibodies (aPL-IgG) or activated T cells overwhelms the normally adequate inhibitory mechanisms and stimulates the recruitment and activation effector cells through the generation of C3a, C5a and the C5b-9 MAC. A lack of complement regulatory proteins has similar effects. The complement activation products induce inflammation and tissue injury and ultimately lead to fetal injury. In the presence of complement regulatory proteins like Crry, complement activation is blocked and normal pregnancy outcomes result

3.   **ROLE OF COMPLEMENT IN
       ANTIPHOSPHOLIPID ANTIBODY-INDUCED
       PREGNANCY LOSS**

The anti-phospholipid syndrome (APS) is characterized by recurrent fetal loss, vascular thrombosis and thrombocytopenia occurring in the presence of anti-phospholipid (aPL) antibodies. Pregnancy loss is a defining criterion for APS and occurs with particularly high frequency in systemic lupus erythematosus (SLE) patients bearing this antibody.

Over the last two decades, APS has emerged as a leading cause of pregnancy loss and pregnancy-related morbidity. It is now recognized that recurrent miscarriage occurs in 1% of couples (39-39), that up to 20% of women with recurrent miscarriage have aPL antibodies, and that in approximately 15% of otherwise apparently normal women aPL is the sole explanation for recurrent fetal loss (31, 40). The primary treatment for these patients, anticoagulation throughout pregnancy, is inconvenient, sometimes painful, expensive, and fraught with potential complications, including hemorrhage and osteoporosis. Moreover, it is often ineffective. Thus, the identification of a novel mechanism for pregnancy loss in women with aPL antibodies holds the promise of new, safer and better treatments.

The pathogenesis of fetal loss and tissue injury in APS is incompletely understood, but is thought to involve platelet and endothelial cell activation as well as the pro-coagulant effects of aPL antibodies acting directly on clotting pathway components. Recent experiments done in our laboratory are based on the hypothesis that aPL antibodies activate complement in the placenta, generating split products that mediate placental injury and lead to fetal loss and growth restriction. To test this hypothesis we used a murine model of APS in which pregnant mice were injected with human IgG containing aPL antibodies. Mice injected with aPL antibodies showed increased fetal resorption frequency. We found that inhibition of the complement cascade *in vivo*, using a soluble C3 convertase inhibitor, Crry-Ig, blocks fetal loss and growth restriction (7) (Figure 2).

Furthermore, mice deficient in complement C3 were resistant to fetal injury (pregnancy loss and fetal growth restriction) induced by aPL antibodies. To determine whether excessive complement activation occurs within the placenta in aPL-treated mice, we conducted immunohistological analyses of decidua on day 8 of pregnancy, after treatment with aPL-Ig or control IgG. In the aPL-treated mice, the decidua was abnormal morphologically, showing focal necrosis, apoptosis and PMN infiltrates. Extensive C3 deposition was noted. Treatment with Crry-Ig at the time of aPL-IgG administration completely prevented inflammation and C3 deposition. Thus, using three distinct approaches, specific complement inhibitor (Crry-Ig), genetically deficient mice (*C3-/-*), and immunohistochemical evidence that absence of C3 deposition in Crry-Ig treated mice correlates with improved outcomes, we demonstrated that complement activation is required for fetal loss and growth restriction in a murine model of APS.

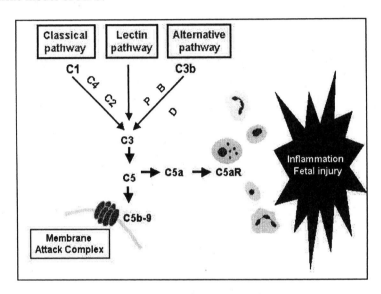

Figure 2. Effects of Crry-Ig on aPL-induced fetal resorption Representative uteri from BALB/c mice sacrificed at day 15 of pregnancy are shown. The upper panel, from a mouse treated with aPL-containing IgG, shows 1 amnion sac and 5 resorptions (arrows). The lower panel, from a mouse treated with aPL and Crry-Ig, contains 4 amnion sacs and no resorptions.

We recently demonstrated that complement C5 activation is a central mechanism of pregnancy loss in APS. We identified complement component C5, and particularly its cleavage product, C5a, as well as neutrophils as key mediators of fetal loss. We also show that treatment with antibodies or peptides that block C5a-C5a receptor interactions prevented pregnancy complications. Mice deficient in C5aR were protected from aPL-induced pregnancy complications (41).

Although the cause of tissue injury in APS is likely to prove multifactoral, our studies show that activation of complement is a critical proximal effector in aPL-induced fetal injury and that this pathway acts upstream of other important effector mechanisms.

4.   **COMPLEMENT IS AN EFFECTOR OF FETAL ALLOGRAFT REJECTION IN A MURINE MODEL**

There is a second murine model of pregnancy loss that underscores the importance of complement as a mediator of fetal injury. Indoleamine 2, 3 dioxygenase (IDO) activity during pregnancy protects developing fetuses from maternal immune responses in mice. Using IDO inhibitors, Mellor and coworkers developed a model of pregnancy loss in mice (42, 43). They showed that fetal allografts were rejected only in mating combinations where paternally inherited tissue antigens elicited potent maternal T cell responses after exposure to IDO inhibitor. IDO inhibitor treatment triggered extensive inflammation at the maternal-fetal interface, which was characterized by complement deposition and hemorrhagic necrosis. Identical inflammatory responses occurred in B cell-deficient (RAG-I-/-) mothers that carried a monoclonal cohort of CD8+ T cells specific for a single paternally inherited fetal major histocompatibility complex antigen. Thus, fetal allograft rejection was accompanied by a unique form of inflammation that was characterized by T cell-dependent, antibody-independent activation of complement. In contrast, no inflammation, complement deposition or T cell infiltration was elicited when mice carrying syngeneic fetuses were exposed to IDO inhibitor. IDO activity protects the fetus by suppressing T cell-driven local inflammatory responses to fetal alloantigens.

It appears that the inhibitory effects of Crry on complement activation are inadequate to prevent complement deposition when, under these pathological conditions, maternal T cells induce the production of large amounts of activated complement. Maternal T cells can be activated by contact with fetal cells release properdin and thereby directly provoke activation of the alternative pathway and deposition of complement at the maternal-fetal interface, causing fetal allograft rejection and death (44-45). Alternatively, maternal T cells may induce properdin release by myeloid cells. Activated T cells may thereby harness the potent inflammatory activities of complement, a constituent of the innate immune system, in a manner similar to that of antibodies. Taken together with the findings in aPL-associated pregnancy loss, these studies indicate that complement activation may be an effector in fetal damage initiated by both humoral and cellular arms of the adaptive immune system.

It is not yet known how the activation of complement is linked to the effector mechanisms associated with alterations in Th1/Th2 cytokine balance and the inflammatory reactions these cytokines provoke to induce preterm labor and spontaneous fetal loss. Interactions at many levels are likely.

Cytokines may regulate the expression of complement or its regulators (46-48). Alternatively, complement may influence local cytokine production. A major effect of C3a and C5a is to recruit inflammatory effector cells, whose many potential functions include the release of cytokines and monokines and amplification of a complement activation loop via alternative pathways. Receptors for C5a and C3a expressed on monocytes, neutrohils, mast cells, and endothelial cells initiate release of proinflammatory cytokines (Figure 3).

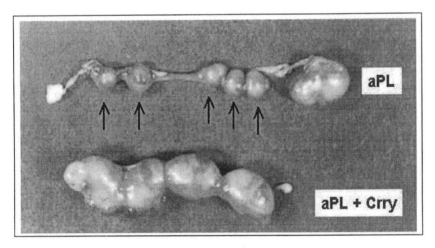

Figure 3. Uncontrolled complement activation can lead to fetal injury. The convergence of three complement activation pathways on the C3 protein results in a common pathway of effector functions. The initial step is the generation of C3a, an anaphylatoxin, and C3b. C3b attaches covalently to targets, followed by the assembly of C5 convertase with subsequent cleavage of C5 to C5a and C5b. C5a is a potent soluble inflammatory anaphylatoxic and chemotactic molecule that promotes the recruitment and activation through its receptor, C5aR. Binding of C5b to the target initiates the non-enzymatic assembly of the C5b-9 membrane attack complex (MAC). C5a is a potent anaphylotoxin , through interaction with C5a receptors on monocytes, neutrophils, mast cells and endothelial cells initiates release of cytokines, reactive oxygen species and enzymes that induce inflammation and tissue injury These and the headings shown below can be selected from the style menu. Once the subtitles written, press "enter" and the style automatically switches back to the text body style "normal".

In addition, cytokine stimulation amplifies the response of effector cells to complement activation products.

Complement activation can lead to tissue damage by binding of C5b to the target. Insertion of C5b-9 MAC can result in cell lysis through uncontrolled changes in intracellular osmolarity. However, while this mechanism operates on erythrocytes, C5b-9 MAC damages nucleated cells in disease states primarily by activating specific signaling pathways through the interaction of the membrane-associated MAC proteins with heterotrimeric G proteins (28, 49).

Thus, uncontrolled complement activation may be an initial trigger, a contributing factor that perpetuates the inflammatory response, or a final effector mechanism.

5.   CONCLUSION

Although activated complement components are present in normal placentas it appears that uncontrolled complement activation is prevented in successful pregnancy by regulatory proteins present on the trophoblast membrane. Different models of pregnancy loss in mice show that activation of complement is critical for fetal injury. In particular, a mouse model of antiphospholipid antibody-induced pregnancy loss proves that complement activation is an important effector in fetal damage initiated by both humoral and cellular arms of the adaptive immune system. Blocking complement activation prevents inflammatory response and fetal damage.

Further characterization of complement as a mediator in tissue damage and definition of the complement components necessary to trigger such injury is likely to lead to a better understanding of the pathogenesis of RSA in addition to new and improved therapies.

6.   REFERENCES

1. Hunt, J.S. (Editor) (1994). Immunobiology of Reproduction. Springer-Verlag., New York.
2. Fuzzi B, Rizzo R, Criscuoli L, Noci I, Melchorri L, Scarselli B, Bencini E, Menucucci A, Baricordi O. (2002). HLA-G expression in early embryos is a fundamental prerequisite for the obtainment of pregnancy. Eur. J. Immunol. 32:311-315.
3. Turnbull, A., and Chamberlain, G. (Editors) (1989). Obstetrics. ChurchHill Livingstone Publications., London
4. Raghupathy, R., and Tangri, S. (1996). Immunodystrophism, T Cells, Cytokines, and Pregnancy Failure. American Journal of Reproductive Immunology 35 (4) 291-296.
5. Weetman AP. (1999). The Immunology of Pregnancy. Thyroid 9(7):643-646
6. Robertson SA, Sharkey DJ. (2001). The role of semen in induction of maternal immune tolerance to pregnancy. Seminars in Immunology 13: 243-254.
7. Holers VM, Girardi G, Mo L, Guthridge JM, Molina H, Pierangeli SS, et al. Complement C3 activation is required for anti-phospholipid antibody-induced fetal loss. J Exp Med. 2002: 195:211-220.
8. Schmidt BZ, Colten HR. Complement: a critical test of its biological importance. Immunol Rev. 2000: 178:166-176.

9. Abbas AK, Lichtman AH, Pober JS. Effector mechanisms of humoral immunity. In: Fourth Ed. Cellular and molecular immunology. Philadelphia, PA: W.B. Saunders Company. 2000: 316-334.

10. Raghupathy R. Pregnancy: success and failure within the Th1/Th2/Th3 paradigm. Seminars in Immunology. 2001: 13:219-227.

11. Vince GS, Johnson PM. Materno-fetal immunobiology in normal pregnancy and its possible failure in recurrent spontaneous abortion? Human Reproduction. 1995: 10:107-113.

12. Mellor AL, Munn DH. Immunology at the maternal-fetal interface: lessons for T cell tolerance and suppression. Ann Rev Immunol. 2000: 18:367-391

13. Lu GC, Goldenberg RL. Current concepts on the pathogenesis and markers of pre-term births. Clinics in Perinatology. 2000: 27:263-283.

14. Denison FC, Kelly RW, Calder AA, Riley SC. Cytokine secretion by human fetal membranes, decidua and placenta at term. Human Reproduction. 1998: 13:3560-3565.

15. Weetman AP. The Immunology of Pregnancy. Thyroid. 1999: 9:643-646.

16. Steinborn A, Niederhut A, Solbach C, Hildenbrand R, Sohn C, Kaufmann M. Cytokine release from placental endothelial cells, a process associated with pre-term labour in the absence of intrauterine infection. Cytokine. 1999: 11:66-73.

17. Chaouat G, Menu E, Clark DA, Minkowsky M, Dy M, Wegmann TG. Control of fetal survival in CBAxDBA/2 mice by lymphokine therapy. J Reprod Fertil. 1990: 89:447-458.

18. Amigo MC, Khamashta MA. Antiphospholipid (Hughes) syndrome in Systemic Lupus Erythematosus. Rheumatic Disease Clinics of North America. 2000: 26:331-348.

19. Holmes CH, Simpson KL. Complement and pregnancy: new insights into the immunobiology of the fetomaternal relationship. Bailliere's Clinical Obstetrics and Gynecology. 1992: 6:439-459.

20. Rooney IA, Oglesby TJ, Atkinson JP. Complement in human reproduction. Activation and Control Immunol Res. 1993: 12:276-294.

21. Weir PE. Immunofluorescent studies of the uteroplacental arteries in normal pregnancy. Br J Obstet Gynaecol. 1981: 88:301-307.

22. Wells M, Bennett J, Bulmer JN, Jackson P, Holgate CS. Complement component deposition in uteroplacental (spiral) arteries in normal human pregnancy. J Reprod Immunol. 1987: 12:125-135.

23. Cunningham DS, Tichenor JR. Decay-accelerating factor protects human trophoblast from complement-mediated attack. Clin Immunol Immunopathol. 1995: 74:156-161.

24. Tedesco F, Narchi G, Radillo O, Meri S, Ferrone S, Betterle C. Susceptibility of human trophoblast to killing by human complement and the role of the complement regulatory proteins. J Immunol. 1993: 151:1562-1570.

25. Liszewski MK, Farries TC, Lublin DM, Rooney IA, Atkinson JP. Control of the complement system. Adv Immunol. 1996: 61:201-283.

26. Holers VM, Kinoshita T, Molina H. The evolution of mouse and human complement C3-binding proteins: divergence of form but conservation of function. Immunol Today. 1992: 13:231-236.

27. Oglesby TJ, Allen CJ, Liszewski MK, White DJ, Atkinson JP. Membrane cofactor protein (CD46) protects cells from complement-mediated attack by an intrinsic mechanism. J Exp Med. 1992: 175:1547-51.

28. Morgan BP, Meri S. Membrane proteins that protect against complement lysis. Springer Sem Immunopath. 1994: 15:369-396.

29. Imrie HJ, McGonigle TP, Liu DT, Jones DR. Regulation of erythrocyte complement receptor 1 (CR1) and decay accelerating factor during normal pregnancy. J Reprod Immunol. 1996: 31:221-227.
30. Xu C, Mao D, Holers VM, Palanca B, Cheng A, Molina H. A critical role for the murine complement regulator Crry in fetomaternal tolerance. Science. 2000: 287:498-501.
31. Stephenson MD. Frequency of factors associated with habitual abortion in 197 couples. Fertil Steril. 1996: 66:24-29.
32. Abramson SB, Buyon, JP. Activation of the complement pathway: Comparison of normal pregnancy, preeclampsia, and systemic lupus erythematosus during pregnancy. Am J Rep Med. 1992: 28:183-187.
33. Holmes CH, Simpson KL, Wainwright SD, Tate CG, Houliham JM, Sawyer IH. Preferential expression of complement regulatory protein decay accelerating factor at the fetomaternal interface during human pregnancy. J Immunol. 1990: 144:3099-3105.
34. Holmes CH, Simpson KL, Okada H, Okada N, Wainwright SD, Purcell DF. Complement regulatory proteins at the fetomaternal interface during human placental development distribution of CD59 by comparison with membrane cofactor protein (CD46) and decay accelerating (CD55). Eur J Immunol. 1992: 22:1579-1585.
35. Hasty LA, Lambris JD, Lessey BA, Pruksananonda K, Lyttle CR. Hormonal regulation of complement components and receptors throughout the menstrual cycle. Am J Obstet Gynecol. 1994: 170:168-175.
36. Kutteh WH. Antiphospholipid antibody-associated recurrent pregnancy loss: treatment with heparin and low-dose aspirin is superior to low-dose aspirin alone. Am J Obstet Gynecol. 1996: 174:1584-1589.
37. Rai R, Cohen H, Dave M, Regan L. Randomized controlled trial of aspirin and aspirin plus heparin in pregnant women with recurrent miscarriage associated with phospholipid antibodies. J Brit Med. 1997: 314:253-257.
38. Clifford K, Rai R, Watson H, Regan L. An informative protocol for the investigation of recurrent miscarriage: preliminary experience of 500 consecutive cases. Hum Reprod. 1994: 9:1328-1332.
39. Pattison NS, Chamley LW, Birdsall M, Zanderigo AM, Liddell HS, McDougall J. Does aspirin have a role in improving pregnancy outcome for women with the antiphospholipid syndrome? A randomized controlled trial. Am J Obstet Gynecol. 2000: 183:1008-1012.
40. Yetman DL, Kutteh WH. Antiphospholipid antibody panels and recurrent pregnancy loss: prevalence of anticardiolipin antibodies compared with other antiphospholipid antibodies. Fertil Steril. 1996: 66:540-546.
41. Girardi G, Berman J, Spruce L, Lambris JD, Holers VM and Salmon J. International Immunopharmacology 2002:2(9):1239.
42. Mellor AL, Sivakumar J, Chandler P, Smith K, Molina H, Mao D, et al. Prevention of T cell-driven complement activation and inflammation by tryptophan catabolism during pregnancy. Nature Immunol. 2002: 2:64-68.
43. Munn DH, Zhou M, Attwood JT, Bondaev I, Conway SJ, Marshall, et al. Prevention of allogenic fetal rejection by tryptophan catabolism. Science. 1998: 281:1191-1193.
44. Mellor AL, Munn DA. Tryptophan catabolism prevents maternal T cells from activation lethal anti-fetal immune responses. J Reprod Immunol. 2001: 52:5-13.
45. Schwaeble WJ, Reid KBM. Does properdin crosslink the cellular and the humoral immune response? Immunol Today. 1999: 18:17-21.
46. Sheerin NS, Zhou W, Adler S, Sacks SH. TNF-α regulation of C3 gene expression and protein biosynthesis in rat glomerular endothelial cells. Kidney Int. 1997: 51:703-710.

47. Terui T, Ishii K, Ozawa M, Tabat N, Kato T, Tagami H. C3 production of cultured human epidermal keratinocytes is enhanced by IFN-γ and TNF-α through different pathways. J Invest Derm. 1997: 108:62-67.

48. Cocuzzi ET, Bardenstein DS, Stavitsky A, Sundarraj N, Medof ME. Upregulation of DAF (CD55) on orbital fibroblasts by cytokines. Differential effects of TNF-β and TNF-α. Curr Eye Res. 2001: 23:86-89.

49. Shin ML, Rus HG, Nicolescu FI. Membrane attack by complement: assembly and biology of terminal complement complexes. Biomembranes. 1996: 4:123-149.

10

Complement Deficiencies: a 2004 Update

György Ábel[1,2] and Vincent Agnello[1,3]
[1]Department of Laboratory Medicine, Lahey Clinic, Burlington, Massachusetts, [2]Department of Pathology, Harvard Medical School, and [3]Edith Nourse Rogers Veterans Affairs Hospital, Bedford, Massachusetts, U.S.A.

Abstract: Complete hereditary deficiencies have been described for many of the complement system proteins and regulatory molecules, and a variety of disease manifestations have been associated with these deficiencies. The diseases can be grouped into two major types, autoimmune diseases and infectious diseases. The autoimmune disorders most frequently associated with complement deficiencies are SLE and SLE-like disease, and the infectious diseases are bacterial diseases, especially life-threatening infections caused by neisserial organisms. However, individuals who are completely deficient for a complement component can be free of disease, so the development of disease is undoubtedly multifactorial.

Key Words: Complement deficiency, SLE, lupus, autoimmunity

1. DEFICIENCIES OF THE COMPLEMENT SYSTEM AND DISEASE

1.1 Susceptibility to Infection

The important role the complement components play in host defenses is demonstrated by the striking association between complement deficiencies and susceptibility to infection. Deficiencies that result in significant decrease in C3 (deficiencies in C3 or factor I), the alternate pathway proteins (factor D or properdin), or in the membrane attack complex (deficiencies in C5, C6, C7, C8, or C9) are strongly associated with infections with *Neisseria* or other pyogenic bacteria. In one study of patients with *Neisseria* meningitis, 11 of the 104 patients studied were found to be completely deficient for at least one complement component (1). In a second study, of 30 patients with meningococcemia or meningitis seen in one hospital over 20 years, three patients (10%) had complement deficiencies. One of the three patients had congenital C7 deficiency and the other two patients had SLE. The prevalence of complement deficiency in the meningococcal disease was 100 times greater than the prevalence seen in the normal population (2).

Heterozygous and homozygous deficiency of MBL has been shown to be associated with several types of immunodeficiencies. A primary immunodeficiency characterized by defective yeast opsonization was described 20 years before the molecular defect that was identified as the codon 54 mutation in the MBL (3,4). Many studies have now been published, including two large studies that included 229 and 345 children with unknown primary immunodeficiencies (5,6), which have demonstrated significant associations for both homozygous and heterozygous MBL mutations with increased risk of infection. In the largest study, of the 17 homozygous MBL deficient patients identified, 13 presented with severe infections including septicemia, cellulitis and boils, severe tonsillitis, and otitis media. Homozygous MBL mutations have also been reported to be a factor in susceptibility to *Mycobacterium tuberculosis* and *avium, Trypanosoma cruzi, Klebsiella, Cryptococcus neoformans,* other fungal infections, hepatitis B virus, and influenza A.

In several published studies, MBL deficiency has been seen in increased frequency in HIV-infected men. In one study from Copenhagen (7), 96 HIV-infected men were compared to 123 healthy Danish adults and 36 Danish homosexual HIV-uninfected men. The incidence of homozygous MBL mutations was 8% in the HIV-infected men and 0% in the control groups. Infected HIV men with the most rapid progression of their disease had the lowest levels of MBL in the serum. Interpretation of these studies is controversial and work is needed to further characterize the possible role of MBL deficiency in HIV disease.

Patients deficient in CR3, the cell membrane receptor for C3, have increased susceptibility to infectious agents. In initial reported studies, about 20 patients suffering from severe recurrent infections caused by phagocyte dysfunction were identified that lacked the β chain of the CR3 molecule (8,9). These patients are missing CR3 molecules as well as the LFA-1 and CR4 membrane molecules, which share the same types of β chains. Granulocytes from these patients are defective in the ability to opsonize and adhere to foreign organisms and cell membrane. Lymphocyte function is also impaired in these individuals.

Complement receptors also may play a significant regulatory role in the activation or suppression of PMN responses to a variety of infectious agents. In recent studies (10,11), iC3b-containing immune complexes that bind to CR3 caused PMN activation and a respiratory burst in peripheral blood PMNs. This demonstrated a possible significant role for complement fragments in PMN activation during an infection. In addition, a suppressive role for CR1 was also demonstrated because the PMN respiratory burst was significantly enhanced by monoclonal antibody blockade of CR1 sites specific for C3b. The authors hypothesized that CR1 present on PMNs and RBCs in whole blood promote the degradation of immune complex bound iC3b to C3dg. This biological function would prevent binding of the complement-containing complexes to the CR3 and downregulate the PMN activation by immune complexes.

1.2 Autoimmune Manifestations of Complement Deficiencies

SLE and other rheumatic diseases have been associated for the most part with deficiencies of the early components, but there are documented rheumatic disease cases associated with virtually all complement deficiencies described. A summary of identified deficiencies and associated rheumatologic diseases found in published case reports are given in Table 1. Hereditary complement deficiencies with a complete lack of a complement protein are seen in the population at low frequencies with the exception of C1-INH, C4A, or C4B deficiencies, which are seen more frequently. Screening studies done on serum from blood donors in Osaka, Japan, found an approximate frequency of 0.003% for C5, C6, C7, and C8 deficiencies (12). In contrast, C4A and C4B deficiencies are seen much more frequently (see Chapter 4). Complement deficiencies have also been reported that are not hereditary deficiencies but rather are acquired conditions associated with the presence of anti-complement protein autoantibodies. The most frequently occurring form of acquired complement deficiency is a result of C1-INH deficiency.

1.3 Atypical Cutaneous Lupus Erythematosus: a Hallmark of Deficiencies of Early Complement Components

SLE associated with homozygous deficiency of the early components of complement was the first of the associations of early complement deficiency with lupus disease to be reported (13). A striking finding present in the first index case and subsequently confirmed was that some of the lupus disease in these patients, called *atypical cutaneous lupus erythematosus* for lack of a better term, differs from classic lupus in the following four ways: 1) increased incidence of discoid skin lesions, 2) an absence of renal disease, 3) low or absent titers of ANA and antibodies to native DNA, and 4) infrequent findings of immunoglobulin and complement in the skin lesions (see section on C2 deficiency). These features were also found in some patients with complete deficiencies of C1q, C1r-C1s, and C4 that were reported later.

Table 1. Clinical Findings in Complete* Hereditary Deficiency of Complement Components

Deficient Component	Number	% Infections	Rheumatologic Clinical Findings
C1q	42	24	MPGN, SLE, DLE, skin rash, SLE-like disease
C1r-C1s	14	22	SLE, SLE-like, glomerulonephritis
C4	25	16	SLE, SLE-like, DLE, Henoch-Schönlein and
C2	109	10	anaphylactoid purpura, cryoglobulinemia
			SLE, subacute cutaneous LE, glomerulonephritis,
			anaphylactoid purpura, vasculitis, dermatomyositis
			arthritis, arthralgias, rheumatic fever, cold
			arterioria, inflammatory bowel disease, Hodgkin's
			disease, idiopathic atrophodermia, common
			variable immunodeficiency
C3	24	60	glomerulonephritis, SLE-like
C5	27	70	SLE
C6	77	84	DLE, SLE-like, Sjögren's syndrome, arthritis
C7	73	65	SLE, CREST syndrome, pyelonephritis, hematuria
C8	73	65	SLE, hepatosplenomegaly,,
			sickle-thalassemia-hemoglobinopathy
C9	18	8	SLE
C1 INH*	hundreds	rare	Angioedema (hundreds); SLE, DLE, SLE-like (25 patients)
H	13	80	SLE, vasculitis
D	3	74	None
P	70	74	SLE, vasculitis
C4bp	3	none	Angioedema
I	23	100	SLE, vasculitis
MBL	many	60	SLE?
CR3	>20	100	None
DAF	many	none	Paroxysmal nocturnal hemoglobinuria

Data from Pickering et al. (24), Whaley and Schweble (47), and Vyse et al. (121)
  * Homozygous deficiencies, except for heterozygous C1 INH.

1.4   Hereditary C1q Deficiency

The last early complement component homozygous deficiency associated with SLE-like disease to be reported was C1q and in effect provided evidence for the hypothesis that all the early component, C1 through C4 were involved in host defenses to the development of SLE. Of the 42 patients reported 39 (93%) had a clinical syndrome similar to SLE (14-24).

Skin rash, predominantly with photosensitivity, occurred in 37 patients with negative lupus band tests in 3 of 9 cases reported. Glomerulonephritis was present in 16 patients with the membranoproliferative type present in 5 of the 8 cases characterized. Antinuclear antibodies were present in 24 of 35 patients tested but only 5 of 25 patients had antibodies to double stranded DNA. Although patients with complete C1q deficiency had some features of lupus disease, the diagnostic criteria for SLE were usually not met in most cases. The female to male ratio was 1.3:1 in the C1q deficient group compared to a ratio of 15:1 in classic SLE. Hereditary deficiencies of C1q can be subdivided into two major groups: those with normal levels of C1q and those with depressed levels of C1q protein in the blood. Only individuals with homozygous deficiency are affected.

1.5   Hereditary C1r-C1s Deficiency

There have been 14 patients with C1r-C1s patients reported in the literature (24-28). C1r and C1s deficiencies usually occur together in affected individuals, perhaps because the C1r and C1s genes are located very close to each other on chromosome 12 where simultaneous deletions of both closely linked genes may occur. Some patients have been reported to have complete absence of both C1r and C1s whereas others have complete absence of one of the molecules and significantly decreased levels of the other. Eight of the 14 (57%) had lupus disease; all had skin rash, DLE was diagnosed in two and SLE in two. Five of eight had glomerulonephritis; only one was characterized and had mesangioproliferative glomerulonephritis. The female to male ratio was 1.7:1. ANA was negative or weakly positive in 3 of 8, and DNA antibodies were negative in 3 of 5 patients studied. LE band tests were not reported.

1.6   Hereditary C4 Deficiency

C4-deficient patients of two types have been characterized: complete C4 deficiency, in which both the C4A and C4B protein products are absent, and partial C4 deficiencies, in which C4 levels are decreased and one or more of the genes for either C4A or C4B genes are missing. Complete C4 deficiency is rare; among 25 reported patients 21 (84%) had SLE or SLE-like disease (29-37). Seventeen patients had skin rash, predominately with photosensitivity; lupus band test were negative in four of the five cases studied. Nine patients had mainly mild glomerulonephritis; the mesangial type was present in all seven cases characterized. ANA was negative or weakly positive in 10 of 20 patients tested. DNA antibody tests were negative in 9 of 11 patients tested. Anti SS-A(RO) was positive in 6 of 8 patients tested. The female to male ratio of affected patients was 2:1. There were two asymptomatic patients and single case reports of Henoch-Schönlein purpura (38) and cryoglobulinemia (39) associated with complete C4 deficiency.

Partial deficiencies may exist in individuals who are missing one, two, or three of the C4 genes. See Chapter 4 for gene frequencies. Absence of both C4A genes is associated with increased susceptibility to SLE. The clinical manifestation associated with homozygous C4A deficiency has been reported in several studies. In a study from Sweden (40), homozygous C4A deficiency was found in 13 of 80 SLE patients (16%). The C4A-deficient patients had an increased incidence of photosensitivity but other clinical features were similar to the non-C4A deficient patients. No differences were seen in the percentage of anti-dsDNA, Sm, RNP, SS-A, SS-B, rheumatoid factors, or cardiolipin antibodies for these patients. In a North American study (41) that included Caucasians and Blacks, patients with homozygous C4A deficiency had less proteinuria, lower levels of anti-dsDNA, Sm, SS-A, and cardiolipin antibodies, and higher C3 levels. C4A gene deletion was found in 23.4% of 121 patients with SLE and was associated with subacute cutaneous lupus erythematosus and Sjögren's syndrome.

One large family of 35 individuals from three generations in Iceland with C4A null alleles has been reported (42). HLA typing and C4 allele typing was done by agarose–immunofixation techniques. Five of the family members had four or more criteria for SLE and an additional five members had clinical or laboratory evidence of SLE but did not fulfil four American College of Rheumatology (ACR) criteria. No other autoimmune diseases were seen in the family. The C4A null allele was highly associated with SLE in this family in that 9 of the 10 members with symptoms were C4A deficient. Interestingly, five different C4A null haplotypes were involved, including three that originated from non-consanguineous spouses.

Absence of both C4B genes is associated with increased risk of IgA nephropathy and glomerulonephritis (43). Absence of at least one C4B gene, which leads to low levels of plasma C4, has been associated with dermatological diseases, specifically discoid lupus erythematosus, angioedema, and urticaria (44). C4 deficiencies have also been shown to be associated with anti-SS-A antibodies and with anti-cardiolipin antibodies in blacks (45-46).

1.7   Hereditary C2 Deficiency

C2 deficiency is the most common homozygous complement component deficiency. The prevalence of either of C4 null genes is higher but prevalence of complete C4 deficiency, inheritance of both null genes is not (see Chapter 4). Larger numbers of patients with C1 INH deficiency than homozygous C2 patients have been reported because the inheritance of CI INH deficiency autosomal dominant (Table 1).

Homozygous C2 deficiency has an approximate prevalence of 1:20,000 in the western European Caucasian population. Over 100 patients with homozygous C2 deficiency have been reported (47). C2 deficiency was the first complement deficiency reported to be associated with SLE. This disease association has been confirmed as shown in a study of the first 52 kindred reported with homozygous C2 deficiency (48). Twenty-eight patients (34%) had lupus disease with a female to male ratio of 8:1. Eighteen patients (22%) were diagnosed as SLE but only 14 fulfilled ARA criteria for the diagnosis of SLE. The atypical aspects of the lupus disease present in the original index case (13) were also confirmed; 10 patients, a third of the patients had atypical cutaneous LE. Idiopathic glomerulonephritis was present in 9 patients and recurrent infection in 8 patients; 7 of the 9 patients with glomerulonephritis were males. The 8 patients with recurrent infections were all young children. Frequent infections have also been noted as secondary diagnosis in several of the other childhood cases of homozygous C2 deficiency. The prevalence of lupus disease in this study most likely is inflated due to a patient selection bias since the studies were mainly performed in SLE clinics. Among the non-index cases, a less biased population, only 1 of 29 (3.4%) C2 homozygotes had lupus disease; interestingly, the patient had atypical cutaneous LE. Hence, while the true prevalence of lupus disease among homozygous C2 deficient patients is not know, it most likely considerable less than 34% and much lower than the very high prevalence of lupus disease associated with C1q, C1r-C1s, and C4 complete deficiencies.

Comparison of the homozygous C2 deficient patients with SLE and atypical cutaneous lupus illustrates the four differences noted above: an increased incidence of discoid skin lesions, absence of renal disease, low or absent titers of ANA and antibodies to native DNA, and infrequent findings of immunoglobulin and complement in the skin lesions. The glomerular lesions in the patients with SLE varied in histological type and included membranoproliferative, mesangial, membranous, and focal sclerosis. Clinically and serologically these cases resemble two subgroups of classic SLE: the ANA-negative SLE with photosensitivity group and the cutaneous lesions and subcutaneous lupus erythematosus (SCLE) group 49-50).

The rash in atypical cutaneous lupus erythematosus patients bears striking resemblance to the rash in the antinuclear antibody (ANA)-negative group and to that in SCLE. The skin lesions have been described as non-scarring, papillosquamous, or annular polycyclic, with a characteristic distribution (i.e., the lesions spare the knuckles, inner aspects of the arm, axilla, lateral part of the trunk, and are rarely seen below the waist). Because the skin lesions differ from those in discoid lupus erythematosus in their clinical appearance and immunohistology, the diagnosis of the discoid type in some of these complement-deficient cases was inaccurate. The two subgroups of SLE and the complement-deficient patients with atypical cutaneous LE all share a high incidence of positivity for anti-Ro (SSA) antibody (46,49,51).

Whether there is an association of lupus disease with heterozygous C2 deficiency similar to that seen with heterozygous C4 deficiency (previous chapter) is controversial (24,52,53). There appears to be a slight increase in the prevalence of heterozygous C2 deficiency among SLE patients compared to controls. Moreover, in the study on 52 kindred with C2 deficiency cited above, the prevalence of lupus disease among the non-index heterozygous C2 deficiency cases was 0.6% compared to a prevalence of 3.4% among non-index homozygous cases suggesting that there may be an association of lupus disease with heterozygous deficiency that is 6 time less than that with homozygous C2 deficiency.

The effect of homozygous C2 deficiency on the clearance of immune complexes has been studied (54). A patient with C2 deficiency was injected with hepatitis B surface antigen–anti-HbsAg immune complexes labeled with I^{123}. The patient's uptake of complexes in the liver, spleen, and clearance of the complexes from the circulation was studied pre- and post- fresh-frozen plasma treatment. When her C2 and CH50 levels were zero, the complexes were rapidly taken up by the liver and cleared from the circulation. No binding of the complexes was seen in the spleen or on the RBCs via CR1. After treatment with fresh frozen plasma, which normalized her complement levels, the complexes cleared from the circulation more slowly and 20% of the complexes were found in the spleen. These studies suggest that uptake of immune complexes by the spleen is complement dependent and abnormal processing of immune complexes by complement-deficient patients may take place.

1.8   Hereditary C3, C5, C6, C7, and C8 Deficiencies

The major disease association with homozygous deficiencies of components C3 through C8 is infection (Table 1); few cases of SLE and SLE-like disease are associated with deficiencies of these components. The relative infrequency of these associations may indicate that no causal relationship exists, although such a relationship cannot yet be excluded because of the small numbers of cases of each deficiency studied.

Of 24 reported cases of homozygous C3 deficiency, three patients had SLE-like disease and seven had glomerulonephritis, proteinuria, or IgA nephropathy (39). The SLE-like disease patients had rash and arthralgias or arthralgias and photosensitivity (55,56). All three had negative serologic assays for ANA, LE cells, and rheumatoid factor assays.

There are two polymorphic forms of C3: S and F. The C3F form has weakly been associated with glomerulonephritis.

More typical SLE occurs among individuals with C5–C8 deficiencies. One case of homozygous C5 deficiency with SLE has been reported (57). There were no unusual features of SLE in this case. The lupus erythematosus, ANA, and dsDNA antibody tests were positive. The prominent skin lesions were typical of lupus. There were deposits of immunoglobulin and complement along the dermal–epidermal junction. There are three cases of homozygous C6 deficiency with SLE or SLE-like disease (58-60). One case had typical SLE, and one case had SLE-like disease with polyarthritis, pleurisy, and Raynaud's phenomenon. The lupus erythematosus and dsDNA tests were negative, the ANA was weakly positive, and an ssDNA test was positive. The third case had discoid lupus and Sjögren's syndrome with negative serologic test studies. Two cases of C7 deficiency have been reported with classical seropositive SLE (61). Two cases of C8 deficiencies have been reported; one had classic seropositive SLE and the other had clinical criteria for SLE with negative serologic tests for ANA and lupus erythematosus cells, and a positive rheumatoid factor (62-63).

1.9 Hereditary C9 Deficiency

Initially C9 deficiency was thought to be rare and not associated with disease. Further study of C9 deficiencies, especially in ethnic Japanese, has demonstrated that the incidence of C9 deficiency in Japan is about 0.086%, much higher than in initial studies of other populations. Three cases of SLE have been reported in association with C9 deficiencies in Japan. The first reported patient had sicca syndrome accompanied by severe Raynaud's phenomenon (64). Serologic tests for ANA and dsDNA were positive, as were assays for RNP, Sm, and SSA (Ro) antibodies and immune complexes. The other two patients (65,66) had low CH50 and absent C9 protein and function. One of the patients had recurrent urinary tract infections, pleuritis, pericarditis, proteinuria, and facial edema with a positive ANA of 1:640, and a dsDNA antibody of 28 U/ml. This patient had two other sisters with homozygous C9 deficiency with hypergammaglobulinemia and low titered ANAs (1:80). Their father was heterozygous for C9 deficiency with a positive ANA of 1:640. Four other C9-deficient patients with disease have been reported: one had sicca syndrome, and the remaining three had rheumatoid arthritis. Cases of C9 deficiency associated with neisserial meningitis have also been identified.

1.10 Hereditary MBL Deficiencies

MBL protein deficiencies, which are a result of the gene mutations of the MBL gene, have been studied in SLE. Serum levels of MBL were measured in a study with 58 SLE, 92 HIV, 30 chronic liver disease, 20 rheumatoid arthritis, and 161 healthy controls (67). Severely decreased levels of serum MBL protein were found in 12% of SLE patients, 4% of HIV patients, 3% of liver disease patients, no RA patients, and 4% of healthy controls. In one study (68), 102 Caucasian SLE patients were compared to 136 healthy controls to determine their MBL genotypes. The mutant adenine at nucleotide 230 (the codon 54 allele) was found in 41% of patients and 30% of controls, with the frequency of homozygosity for the SLE group of 10% compared to 7% for the control group. This study showed an increase but not statistically significant frequency of MBL mutation in the SLE patient group. In addition when DQA*0501/Dr3/C4A*Q0 gene studies were also done, the association with SLE for the presence of the C4 null allele and MBP genes was stronger that the association of the C4 null allele alone.

Three additional studies have been done with other racial populations. In a study of Chinese individuals in Hong Kong (69), 111 SLE patients and 123 healthy controls, 33% of patients (37) and 23% of controls (28) were positive for the codon 54 mutation. Two of the SLE patients were homozygous for the codon 54 mutation. Mean levels of MBL in the serum were about 10% of normal levels for the codon 54+ patients and controls whereas the MBL levels for SLE patients without the mutation were about 50% of the normal levels. A second study of a black cohort with SLE and matched normal controls was done to determine the gene frequency and relative risk of the codon 54, codon 57, −550, −221, HY, LY, and HX gene frequencies (70). Codon 54 mutations were found with a frequency of 0.163 in the SLE group and 0.087 in the control group; codon 57 mutations had a frequency of 0.125 in the SLE group and 0.047 in the control group. For the promoter mutations, mutations in the −550, −221, and the LX haplotype were found in increased frequency in the SLE group whereas the HY haplotype was found in increased frequency in the controls. The LY haplotype was found in equal frequency in both groups. Homozygous LX/LX haplotypes were found in 11% of the SLE group but only in 2.6% of the controls. Overall, the prevalence of any of the MBL genetic deficiencies in the SLE population was 46% compared to 23% of the control group. This study also identified an additional promoter haplotype, HX, present in three of their SLE patients. In a third study of 50 SLE patients and 49 controls in Spain (71), codon 54 mutations were found in 52% of SLE patients and 31% of controls; codon 57 mutations were found in 6% of patients and 4% of controls. Homozygosy for the codon 54 was found for two SLE patients and one control. The C4A and B genes were also determined for this group of patients. The C4B allele was at increased frequency in the SLE group (37% versus 12%) and there was a stronger association for SLE with the C4A null allele and the MBL mutant alleles than for either mutation alone.

In summary, several studies have now documented an increased frequency of MBL mutations that result in nonfunctional MBL proteins in SLE patients in a variety of racial groups. This association of MBL gene mutation with increased risk for disease appears to demonstrate a gene dosage affect associated with C4A null alleles. Additional studies are necessary to further elucidate the mechanism of this increased risk for the development of SLE.

1.11   Combined Hereditary Complement Deficiencies

Combined heterozygous C4 and C2 deficiency has been reported for 15 individuals from six families (72). About 30% of the people had SLE or another autoimmune disease. The C2 deficiencies were all due to the 28-bp deletion in the C2 gene, whereas 8 of the C4 deficiencies were all due to heterozygous C4A null alleles and five were due to C4B null alleles (the other two C4 deficiencies could not be identified as null alleles). From the frequencies of C2, C4A, and C4B deletions, the expected combined C2 and C4 deletion frequency of the population is 0.001.

A family with four children has been identified in which three of the children are homozygous deficient for factor H and two of the three children are heterozygous deficient for C2. One of the two children with both C2 and factor H deficiency had classic SLE with nephritis. Two patients have been identified with combined homozygous C7 and C4B deficiency; one of the patients was normal and one had SLE (73). The patient with SLE had a sister who was asymptomatic but was also homozygous C7 deficient. Additional patients have been identified with combined properdin and C2 deficiency, and DAF and C9 deficiency, but rheumatic disease was not reported for any of them.

2.   ACQUIRED DEFICIENCIES OF COMPLEMENT

Two forms of acquired complement deficiency states with prolonged persistent complement depression have been associated with SLE-like disease similar to that seen in hereditary complement diseases. These syndromes are early complement component depression associated with chronic hypocomplementemic cutaneous vasculitis and C3 deficiency with mesangiocapillary glomerulonephritis or SLE.

2.1   Hypocomplementemic Urticarial Vasculitis Syndrome

Hypocomplementemic cutaneous vasculitis is an acquired form of deficiency that leads to chronic decreases in complement components C1, C2, C4, and C3. The syndrome is now called hypocomplementemic urticarial vasculitis syndrome (HUVS) but in the past was identified as SLE-related syndrome, hypocomplementemic cutaneous vasculitis, chronic hypocomplementemic cutaneous vasculitis, or hypocomplementemic vasculitis urticaria syndrome. Patients with this syndrome have several distinct clinical features similar to those of SLE but do not fulfill the SLE diagnostic criteria (74-93). The typical patient is a young female with chronic rash, angioedema, and arthralgias. In clinical and serologic studie of 47 patients (37 females, 6 males, 4 sex not reported) with SLE-related syndrome, two patients developed pseudotumor cerebri (80, 89). The rash, which is the most characteristic and prominent feature of the syndrome, was initially called erythema multiforme-like because of the presence of classic target lesions (74). More recently it has been called urticaria-like but is very atypical urticaria because of the absence of itching and the persistent nature of the rash. Histologically, the skin lesions form a perivasculitis to a true leukocytoclastic vasculitis. The presence of immunoglobulins and complement in the lesions also varies, but in most cases they are absent. Renal disease, when present, is usually mild to moderate, and obstructive lung disease, which may be severe, occurs in some patients. Studies done on isolated glomeruli basement membranes demonstrated high level of antibody to C1q in the glomerular tissues (94). When pulmonary function was measured in 17 patients, 11 of them had dyspnea and severe airflow obstruction (95). Six of these patients died of respiratory failure.

The major serologic finding in the majority of patients is the presence of low-molecular-weight C1q precipitins, which have been demonstrated in most cases to be antibody to the C1q molecule (96). These antibodies can be demonstrated in this syndrome as well as in SLE, findings that are consistent with the original description of the low-molecular-weight C1q precipitin that was reported to be present not only in the first case of HUVS but in SLE patients as well (48). The majority of patients can be distinguished from those with SLE serologically because the majority of patients with the syndrome have negative ANA tests, negative assays for lupus erythematosus cells, and negative assays for dsDNA. A small number of patients identified were found to have low titered antibodies to Sm antigen. When patients with SLE were tested for anti-C1q antibodies by enzyme-linked immunosorbent assay (ELISA) 33.6% of 113 patients were positive (97). Plasma titers of anti-C1q antibodies were inversely correlated with CH50 activity. Eighty-five percent of patients with severe complement consumption had positive results for anti-C1q antibodies. Only 14% of patients with no evidence of complement consumption had positive results for anti-C1q antibodies.

The most striking serologic feature of patients with the syndrome is the marked depression of serum complement. The pattern of complement depression resembles that in SLE except that there is severe depression of C1q and associated marked depression of C2 and C4 levels. Depression of C3 tends to be moderate, and all terminal components are present at normal levels. Normal C1 esterase inhibitor levels differentiate the syndrome from the hereditary and acquired forms of angioedema.

The antibodies present in patient serums have been shown to react with a variety of epitopes on the C1q molecule. By Western blot, antibodies can be detected that react with the B and C chains in patients with HUVS. Serum from HUVS also react with the CN-CN and AN-BN dimers of the collagenous C1q fragments. Patient serums from SLE patients were negative by Western blot and thus the antibodies must be directed toward conformational epitopes of bound C1q (98).

Patients with HUVS are similar to patients with hereditary complement deficiency and SLE in that the skin rash is prominent and the ANA test is negative. However, the rash in patients with HUVS does not resemble discoid or atypical cutaneous lesions. None of the inherited forms of deficiency of C1q have similar rashes, and all are negative for antibodies to C1q. Hence, the relationship of this acquired complement deficiency to SLE appears to differ in major ways from the association of hereditary complement deficiencies and SLE.

2.2 Acquired C3 Deficiency and Systemic Lupus Erythematosus

A portion of patients with chronic mesangiocapillary glomerulonephritis will have associated depressed serum levels of C3. In a study of 21 patients with partial lipodystrophy, 17 were found to have low C3 with normal C4 and C2 concentrations (99). Seven had chronic mesangiocapillary glomerulonephritis. The patients with depressed C3 levels have been shown to have a protein in their sera capable of cleaving C3 in normal serum. This protein has been termed *C3 nephritic factor* (C3Nef) and has been shown to be an autoantibody that stabilizes the C3 convertase of the alternative pathway.

A 34-year-old Caucasian woman with partial lipodystrophy since age 5 years has been reported with classic SLE (100). The patient had pleuritis, polyarthritis, and a photosensitive rash on her arms. Lupus erythematosus cells, ANA, native DNA antibody, and rheumatoid factor tests were positive. C3 was markedly depressed, with normal levels of C1q, C2, and C4. C3Nef was demonstrated in the serum. A renal biopsy showed focal mesangial sclerosis without any electron-dense deposits on electron microscopy. This patient's lupus is classic SLE and bears little resemblance to the lupus-like syndrome seen in three of the homozygous C3-deficient cases, except that all had skin rashes and three had photosensitivity. The significance of any of these observations remains to be determined.

3. DEFICIENCIES OF REGULATORY MOLECULES

3.1 C1 Inhibitor Deficiency and Systemic Lupus Erythematosus

Genetic and acquired forms of C1-INH are associated with the syndrome of hereditary angioneurotic edema, which consists of recurrent bouts of noninflammatory swelling involving the subcutaneous tissues, intestinal walls, airways, and lungs. Twice as many males as females are affected. Two major types of the genetic deficiency exist. In approximately 85% of patients, functional and antigenic assays show low serum concentration of the inhibitor. In the variant form, which comprises approximately 15% of the cases, there is normal or elevated concentration of a functionally inactive inhibitor. Two types of acquired deficiency have been identified: type I, which is associated with B-cell lymphoproliferative disease, and type II, which is characterized by the production of anti-C1-INH antibodies. A summary of the information from 22 patients has recently been published (101). The autoantibodies are directed at epitopes at or near the reactive center of the molecule and prevent the inactivation of target proteases by the C1-INH. The levels of free antibody in the serum do not correlate with C4 levels, C1-INH functional assays, or clinical symptoms.

The clinical syndrome is very similar for the genetic and acquired forms of the disease. The severity of the clinical syndrome does not correlate directly with C1 inhibitor quantitative serum concentrations. Some affected individuals with clear depression of C1 esterase inhibitor do not have clinical manifestations of disease. During attacks patients usually develop detectable levels of free C1 esterase, which cannot be found in the circulation of normal individuals. C4 and C2, the substrates of C1 esterase, are chronically depressed in most patients. The chronic depression of C4 and C2 in these patients may be similar to levels seen in the hereditary deficiency disorders.

A number of patients with hereditary deficiencies of C1 esterase and lupus disease have been reported (44, 102-120). Of 25 affected patients 6 had SLE, 9 had discoid lupus erythematosus, and 10 had SLE-like disease. Three of the latter patients appeared to have atypical cutaneous LE; there were insufficient data on the remainder for assessment. Three of the 5 lupus bands tested performed were negative as found in the atypical cutaneous LE lesions. The female to male ratio was 7:1. As with the hereditary C2 deficiency and the C4 deficiency, the lupus disease is characterized by a high incidence of skin rash, which often has been diagnosed as discoid lupus erythematosus; some of these patients may have atypical cutaneous lupus erythematosus. most skin biopsies of the lesions showed no immunoglobulin or complement deposits. In 7 of 19 and 5 of 11 patients the ANA and 5 DNA antibody tests were negative respectively. Membranoproliferative glomerulonephritis was present in 4 of the 6 patients with SLE.

There are two published investigations of twins with hereditary C1 esterase deficiency. Identical male twins who both exhibited classic symptoms of hereditary angioedema and marked depression of C4 had discoid lupus that appeared through both clinical and immunologic studies to be typical discoid lupus erythematosus (112). In the second set of twins, identical girls with complete absence of C1 esterase inhibitor, one remains normal while the other, since age 6 years, has manifested classic symptoms of hereditary angioedema (113). At age 14 years she developed classic SLE with a positive anti-dsDNA antibody and profuse proliferative glomerulonephritis. C4 levels in the affected twin were 4% of normal, whereas the twin without clinical hereditary angioedema or SLE had C4 levels that were chronically in the range of 10–15% of normal. The findings suggest that chronic low C4 is not sufficient to predispose to lupus disease in patients with C1 esterase deficiency disease; very low levels may be required. This may be analogous to the greater association of lupus disease with homozygous C4 deficiency than with the heterozygous states. Indirect evidence for a relationship between C4 levels and lupus skin lesions has come from treatment of patients with danazol (120). Danazol, an impeded androgen, has been shown to increase C1 inhibitor levels and to control clinical symptoms in hereditary angioedema. Danazol therapy these patients resulted in complete remission of the skin rash and elimination of photosensitivity accompanied by increases in C1 esterase inhibitor and C4 levels. Discontinuation of danazol in these cases resulted in recurrence of the skin rash.

3.2   Factor I Deficiency

Twenty-three patients have been identified with homozygous factor I deficiency (121). Recurrent infections and meningitis infections with *S pneumoniae, N meningitidis, H influenzae,* and otitis media were reported in 21 of the patients (122,123). One patient was asymptomatic and one patient had a fatal systemic vasculitis following penicillin therapy. Levels of plasma and RBC associated factor I were both significantly decreased in these patients. The absence of factor I was also shown to lead to significant increases in RBC bound C3c and C3d antigens on patient red cells. In addition, there was continual formation of the alternate pathway convertase (C3bBb), which led to consumption of factor B, and C3 in the serum and to the increased formation of C3b fragments. All leukocytes from these patients are also covered with C3b fragments. When peripheral blood cells from two patients with factor I deficiency were studied, CR1 levels were significantly lower and CR2 levels were somewhat reduced on B cells; CR1 levels on monocytes and granulocytes were normal or slightly elevated.

3.3   Factor H Deficiency

Fifteen individuals from seven families have been identified with homozygous factor H deficiency (124). The disease is inherited as an autosomal-recessive trait and results in the uncontrolled cleavage of C3. This C3 cleavage depletes the factor B and properdin components of the alternative pathway and depletes C5. Patients with factor H deficiency have been associated with recurrent bacterial infections including meningococcal meningitis, glomerulonephritis, SLE, and subacute cutaneous lupus erythematosus. In 21 relatives encompassing three generations for one reported patient, 10 had low factor H levels that indicated probable heterozygous deficiencies in these relatives. Decreased factor H serum levels, C3 serum levels, C3 functional activity, factor B levels, and properdin levels were all strongly associated for these heterozygous relatives.

3.4   CR1 Deficiency

A quantitative deficiency of the number of CR1 molecules on white cells and red cells from SLE patients has been reported in many studies. Because of the possibility that the level of expression on cell membranes is related to the CR1 genotype, studies have been done to determine the frequency of CR1 alleles in SLE patients. In a group of 63 French SLE patients and 158 normal controls, a significantly higher frequency of the S (B) allele was found in patients (51%) than for controls (26%) (125). However, many other studies that have utilized the Hind III polymorphism detection method have not shown any association between SLE and the B allele (126-130). Recent studies have also shown that the CR1-C allele, smallest of the CR1 alleles, was not shown to be at increased frequency in SLE patients in either Black or Caucasian populations (131). The quantitative number of CR1 receptors on lymphocytes, granulocytes, macrophages, and RBCs has been found to be decreased in patients with a wide variety of autoimmune diseases including SLE, rheumatoid arthritis, hydralazine-induced lupus, discoid lupus erythematosus, primary phospholipid syndrome, essential mixed cryoglobulinemia, primary biliary cirrhosis, ulcerative colitis, and on cells in the MRL/lpr mouse SLE model. The decrease in receptor numbers has been correlated with disease activity and can be reversed on the red cells by the production of new red cells stimulated by erythropoietin in some patients.

3.5   CR3 Deficiency

A single reported case of the association between SLE and CR3 deficiency has been reported (132). The patient had classic SLE and an immune vasculitis. The patient had normal levels of CR3 on cell membranes but the molecule was nonfunctional. The CR3 was unable to interact with the C3bi ligand.

3.6   DAF Deficiency and Clinical Disease

Two types of deficiencies in the DAF (CD55) regulatory membrane molecule have been characterized. The acquired anemia condition of paroxysmal nocturnal hemoglobinuria (PNH) has been shown to be due to a lack of DAF and HRF20 (CD59) on red cell membranes of affected patients. The lack of CD55 and CD59 on the red cell membrane results in an increased sensitivity to complement-mediated red cell lysis because of the increased uptake of C3b and increased levels of C5-9 complexes on the cell. This is due to a lack of the regulatory functions of CD55, which disassembles the C3 convertase, and the CD59, which restricts the binding of C8 and C9 and prevents assembly of the membrane attack complex. Inherited forms of CD55 and CD59 deficiency have also been identified. Three individuals have been identified who are deficient in the Cromer red cell blood group antigens (Inab phenotype) found on the DAF molecules (133). The red cells were lacking DAF molecules. No episodes of in vivo hemolysis were reported for the patients, but the red cells were extremely sensitive to in vitro lysis. In contrast, the few patients with inherited CD59 deficiency have all been associated with hemolytic episodes. PNH associated with rheumatic disease has not been reported, but PNH and GPI-linked deficiencies have been demonstrated in aplastic anemia, hypercoagulable states, and increased susceptibility to bacterial infections.

4.   **HYPOTHESIS ON THE ROLE OF EARLY COMPLEMENT COMPONENT DEFICIENCY IN SYSTEMIC LUPUS ERYTHEMATOSUS**

There is now considerable evidence from studies on patients with hereditary deficiencies of individual complement components that complement has specific roles in host defense, independent of other systems. Specific roles have most clearly been defined for deficiencies of C3 and C5-8 that are associated with diseases caused by bacterial agents. In these instances the component is directly involved in a physiologic mechanism that eliminates the disease agent (i.e., opsonization and bacterial lysis). A hypothesis, proposed more than 25 years ago, on specific roles for early complement components in host defense was that these components protect against lupus diseases. Evidence reviewed in this chapter has confirmed that the early complement proteins, C1 through C2 are directly involved in the host defense against lupus disease. It appears from the review of the prevalence of lupus disease with other complement components that these host defenses are related to biological activities of C1, C4 and C2, and are not dependent on activation of C3 or the rest of the complement cascade.

Much of the lupus disease associated with the early complement component deficiencies lack hallmarks of classic SLE: female predominance, antibodies to dsDNA, or glomerulonephritis. The atypical cutaneous LE that lacks these features of classic SLE suggests that host defense mechanisms mediated by these components occur in the skin. For C1 and C4, these mechanisms appear to be independent of female hormones. Hence, the notion that early complement component deficiencies cause SLE is most likely incorrect. It appears more likely that these deficiencies cause specific aspects of lupus disease. Consistent with this assessment is the observation that atypical cutaneous LE constitutes 36% of the lupus disease in homozygous C2-deficient individuals but the apparent equivalent form of disease in the general populations of patients with lupus disease, subacute lupus erythematosus, affects only 9% of lupus patients. This hypothesis is similar to that proposed for murine SLE (134), i.e., multiple genetic factor predispose to lupus disease; some genes or absence or certain genes, as well as certain infectious agents, accelerate or enhance disease. The early complement component deficiency genes may be one of the accelerator or disease-enhancing groups of genes. In some deficient individuals, especially in females bearing other lupogenic genes, the result is classic SLE.

There are several other clinical observations that are relevant in considering hypotheses on the role of early complement component in the etiology of lupus disease. There is a greater prevalence of the disease in complete genetic deficiencies compared with partial ones. Similar disease associations occur in acquired deficiencies of early components as in the genetic deficiencies of these components, suggesting that the greater the deficiency of the complement protein the greater the susceptibility to disease. The initial observations that the prevalence of lupus disease with complete deficiency of C2 was lower than those of complete deficiency of C1 or C4 and a marked female predominance among affected patients with C2 but not C4 of C1 (48) have been confirmed.

At the time when the original hypothesis was formulated, the leading hypothesis on the etiology of SLE was that the disease was initiated by some yet unidentified viral agent. Hence, it was postulated that the early complement components were involved in specific host defenses to the putative viral agent. This hypothesis has not been totally excluded, but no viral etiologic agent has been identified in human SLE after 25 years of searching. A new major hypothesis on the etiology of SLE is that aberrant apoptosis leads to a breach of self-tolerance and autoimmunity. New evidence on the role of early complement components in clearance of apoptotic cells has lead to a new interesting hypothesis on how complement is involved in host defenses to lupus disease. The most widely accepted hypothesis is that these components are essential for clearance of immune complexes and since SLE disease is mediated by immune complexes, deficiencies of these components lead to disease. This hypothesis appears untenable for two reasons: 1) the existence of other complement pathways for clearing immune complexes that by pass the early components, and 2) the absence of evidence for increased immune complex disease in early component complement deficient patients.

Complement has been implicated in the apoptosis processes involved in tolerance (135) except a preliminary report that C4 participates in negative selection of autoreactive cells in mouse model studies (136). However, complement is involved in the clearance of apoptotic cell and another mechanism for breaking tolerance may be the generation of autoantigen resulting from defective clearance of apoptotic cells.

The aforementioned findings have led to the hypothesis by the Walport and Ahearn groups that C1q deficiency may predispose to autoimmune disease, that abrogation of tolerance leading to autoimmunity in SLE may be initiated in the skin lesions, and that the hierarchy of early complement component efficacy in the clearance of apoptotic cells mimics the hierarchy of prevalence of lupus disease among humans with deficiencies of these components. In the terminal phases of apoptosis the plasma membrane undergoes blebbing that results in cell surface expression of a variety of self antigens involved in autoantibody formation in lupus disease, Ro (SS-A), La (SS-B), nucleosomes, and ribosomes (137). It has been demonstrated in vitro that C1q binds independently of immunoglobulin directly to cell surface blebs on keratinocytes undergoing apoptosis following UV irradiation or viral infection (138). In addition, a C1q knockout mouse model was shown to develop a lupus-like disease characterized by antinuclear antibodies and glomerulonephritis with increased numbers of glomerular apoptotic cells (139). Further studies comparing the clearance of apoptotic cell in C1q and C4 knockout mice and glomerularnephritis in C1q and C2 knockout mice demonstrated a hierarchy in clearance with a greater deficit in C1q- than C4 deficient mice (140) and glomerulonephritis with an excess of glomerular apoptotic bodies in C1q-deficient, but not C2-deficient mice (141), respectively.

The hypotheses are appealing because they are consistent with some of the clinical findings in the hereditary C1q deficiency, i.e., UV induced lesion lacking immunoglobulins and the most severe glomerulonephritis among patients with early complement component deficiencies. The lowest prevalence and least severe glomerulonephritis occur in C2 deficient patient; the prevalence in the C4 deficient patients was similar to that among the C1q deficient patients but all were the milder mesangial lesions. Hence, the mouse C1q knockout mouse mimics the nature's C1q knockout experiment. However, there are several contrary observations. The characteristic skin lesion occurs in C4 and C2 deficient patients where C1q levels are normal. C1q deficiency alone is insufficient to cause lupus disease as illustrated by normal individuals with C1q deficiency and the requirement for an autoimmune background in mice that develop lupus disease with deletion of the C1q gene. The development of lupus disease predominantly in females, in patients with prolonged depression of C4 and C2, and with normal levels of C1q in patients with C1INH deficiency also indicates that deficiency of C4 and C2 without deficiency of C1q along with female hormones can produce susceptibility to lupus disease (134).

Thus far, studies have not been performed in human lupus to confirm the observations made on the role of apoptosis and C1q deficiency in mouse lupus models. It should also be emphasized that the etiology of SLE is unknown so that any hypothesis on the role of early complement components is purely speculative. However, studies of patients with lupus disease and complement deficiencies have lead to clues to possible etiologies and have provided a new understanding of the specific that roles complement components can play in host defense systems, as illustrated by studies on the role for C1q in the clearance of apoptotic cells.

5. REFERENCES

1. Schlessinger, M., Nave, Z., Levy, Y., et al. Prevalence of hereditary properdin. C7 and C8 deficiencies in patients with meningococcal infections. Clin Exp Immunol 1990; 81:423-7
2. Garty, B.Z., Nitzan, M., Danon, Y.L. Systemic meningococcal infections in patients with acquired complement deficiency. Pediatr Allergy Immunol 1993; 4:6-9
3. Madi, N., Steiger, G., Estreicher, J., Schifferli, J.A. Immune adherence and clearance of hepatitis B surface Ag/Ab complexes is abnormal in patients with systemic lupus erythematosus (SLE). Clin Exp Immunol 1991; 85:373-8
4. Super, M., Thiel, S., Lu, J., Levinsky, R.J., Turner, M.W. Association of low levels of mannan-binding protein with a common defect of opsonization. Lancet 1989; 2(8674)1236-9
5. Sumiya, M., Super, M., Tabona, P., et al. Molecular basis of opsonic defect in immunodeficient children. Lancet 1991; 337:1569-70
6. Garred, P., Madsen, H.O., Hofmann, B., Svejgaard, A. Increased frequency of homozygosity of abnormal mannan-binding protein alleles in patients with suspected immunodeficiency. Lancet 1995; 346:941-3
7. Summerfield, J.A., Sumiya, M., Levin, M., Turner, M.W. Association of mutations in mannose binding protein gene with childhood infection in consecutive hospital series. 1996; BMJ 314:1229-32
8. Garred, P., Madsen, H.O., Balslev, U., et al. Susceptibility to HIV infection and progression of AIDS in relation to variant alleles of mannose-binding lectin. Lancet 1997; 349:236-40
9. Anderson, D.C., Schmalstein, F.C., Finegold, M.J., et al. The severe and moderate phenotypes of heritable Mac-1 LFA-1 deficiency. Their quantitative definition and relationship to leukocyte dysfunction and clinical features. J Infect Dis 1985; 152:668-89
10. Gallin, J.I. Leukocyte adherence-related glycoproteins LFA-1, Mo-1, and pl5O,95: A new group of monoclonal antibodies, a new disease, and a possible opportunity to understand the molecular basis of leukocyte adherence. J Infect Dis 1985; 152:661-4
11. Nielsen, C.H., Antonsen, S., Matthiesen, S.H., Leslie, R.G. The roles of complement receptors type 1 (CR1, CD35) and type 3 (CR3, CD11b/CD18) in the regulation of the immune complex-elicited respiratory burst of polymorphonuclear leukocytes in whole blood. Eur J Immunol 1997; 27:2914-9
12. Inai, S., Akagaki, Y., Moriyama, T., et al. Inherited deficiencies of the late-acting complement components other than C9 found among healthy blood donors. Int Arch Allergy Appl Immunol 1989; 90:274-9
13. Agnello, V., de Bracco, M.M.E., Kunkel, H.G. Hereditary C2 deficiency with some manifestations of systemic lupus erythematosus. J Immunol 1972; 108:837-40
14. Berkel, A.L., Loos, M., Sanal, O., et al. Clinical and immunological studies in a case of selective complete C1q deficiency. Clin Exp Immunol 1979; 38:52-63
15. Leyva-Cobian, F., Mampaso, I.M.F., Sanchez-Bayle, M., et al. Familial C1q deficiency associated with renal and cutaneous disease. Clin Exp Immunol 1980; 44:173-80
16. Uenaka, A., Akimoto, T., Aoki, T., et al. A complete selective C1q deficiency in a patient with discoid lupus erythematosus (DLE). Clin Exp Immunol 1982; 48:353-8.
17. Minta, J.O., Winkler, C.J., Biggar, W.D., et al. A selective and complete absence of C1q in a patient with vasculitis and nephritis. Clin Immunol Immunopathol 22:225, 1982

18. Ziccardi, R.J., Cooper, N.R. The subunit composition and sedimentation properties of human C1. J Immunol 1977; 118:2047-52
19. Müller-Eberhard, H.J. The molecular dynamics and biochemistry of complement. p. 219. In Atkinson DE, Fox CF (eds). Modulation of Protein Function. Academic Press, San Diego, 1979
20. Muller-Eberhard, H.J. Complement. Ann Rev Biochem 1975; 44:697-724
21. Topaloglu, R., Bakkaloglu, A., Slingsby, J.H., et al: Molecular basis of hereditary C1q deficiency associated with SLE and IgA nephropathy in a Turkish family. Kidney Int 1996; 50:635-42
22. Kirschfink, M., Petry, F., Khirwadkar, K., et al. Complete functional C1q deficiency associated with systemic lupus erythematosus (SLE). Clin Exp Immunol 1993; 94:267-272
23. Bowness, P., Davies, K.A., Norsworthy, P.J., et al. Hereditary C1q deficiency and systemic lupus erythematosus. 1994; Q J Med 87:455-64
24. Pickering, M.C., Botto, M., Taylor, P.R., et al. Systemic lupus erythematosus, complement deficiency, and apoptosis. Adv Immunol 2000; 76:227-324
25. Pickering, R.J., Michael, A.F., Jr., Herdman, R.C., et al. The complement system in chronic glomerulonephritis: Three newly associated aberrations. J Pediatr 1971; 78:30-43
26. Moncada, B., Day, B., Good, R.A., et al. Lupus erythematosus-like syndrome with a familial defect of complement. N Engl J Med 1972; 286:689-93
27. Rich, K.C., Jr., Hurley, J., Gewurz, H. Inborn C1r deficiency with a mild lupus-like syndrome. Clin Immunol Immunopathol 1979; 13:77-84
28. Lee, S.L., Wallace, S.L., Barone, R., et al. Familial deficiency of two subunits of the first component of complement. Arthritis Rheum 1978; 21:958-67
29. Hauptman, G., Grosshans, E., Heid, E. Lupus erythematosus syndrome and complete deficiency of the fourth component of complement. Boll Ist Sieroter Milan 1974; 53(1):suppl:228
30. Schaller, J.G., Gilliland, B.G., Ochs, H.D., et al. Severe systemic lupus erythematosus with nephritis in a boy with deficiency of the fourth component of complement. Arthritis Rheum 1977; 20:1519-25
31. Tappeiner, G., Scholz, S., Linert, J., et al. Hereditary deficiency of the fourth component of complement (C4): Study of a family. Inserm 1978; 800:399-403
32. Ballow, M., McLean, R.H., Einarson, M., et al. Hereditary C4 deficiencyCgenetic studies and linkage to HLA. Transplant Proc 1979; 11:1710-2
33. Tappeiner, G., Hintner, H., Scholz, S., et al. Systemic lupus erythematosus in hereditary deficiency of the fourth component of complement. J Am Acad Dermatol 1982; 7:66-79
34. Tappeiner, G. Disease states in genetic complement deficiencies. Int J Dermatol 1982; 21:175-91
35. Urowitz, M.B., Gladman, D.D., Minta, J.O. Systemic lupus erythematosus in a patient with C4 deficiency. J Rheumatol 1981; 8:741-6
36. Kjellman, M., Laurell, A.B., Low, B., et al. Homozygous deficiency of C4 in a child with a lupus erythematosus syndrome. Clin Genet 1982; 22:331-9
37. Mascart-Lemone, F., Hauptmann, G., Goetz, J., et al. Genetic deficiency of the fourth component of complement presenting with recurrent infections and a SLE-like disease: Genetical and immunological studies. 1983; Am J Med 75:295-304
38. Lhotta, K., Konig, P., Hinter, H., et al. Renal disease in a patient with hereditary complement deficiency of the fourth complement component of complement. Nephron 1990; 56:206-11

39. Berliner, S., Weinberger, A., Zamir, R., et al. Familial cryoglobulinemia and C4 deficiency. Scand J Rheumatol 1984; 13:151-4
40. Sturfelt, G., Truedsson, L., Johansen, P., et al. Homozygous C4A deficiency in systemic lupus erythematosus: Analysis of patients from a defined population. Clin Genet 1990; 38:427-33
41. Petri, M., Watson, R., Winkelstein, J.A., McLean, R.H. Clinical expression of systemic lupus erythematosus in patients with C4A deficiency. Medicine (Baltimore) 1993; 72:236-44
42. Steinsson, K., Arnason, A., Erlendsson, K., et al. A study of the major histocompatibility complex in a Caucasian family with multiple cases of systemic lupus erythematosus: Association with the C4AQ0 phenotype. J. Rheumatol 1995; 22:1862-6
43. McLean, R.H., Wyatt, R.H., Julian, B.A. Complement phenotypes in glomerulonephritis, increased frequency of homozygous null C4 phenotypes in IgA nephropathy and Henoch-Schonlein purpura. Kidney Int 1984; 26:855-60
44. Gell, J., Tye, M.J., Agnello, V. Selective depression of the C4 component of complement: evidence for an association with genetic deficiency of C4 and dermatologic diseases. Diagn Immunol 1983; 1:49-55
45. Hauptmann, G. Observations presented in discussions at Symposium: Clinical Aspects of Complement Mediated Diseases, May, Bellagio, Italy, 1983
46. Provost, T.T., Arnett, F.C., Reichlin, M. Homozygous C2 deficiency, lupus erythematosus and anti-Ro (SSA) antibodies. Arthritis Rheum 1983; 26:1279-82
47. Whaley, K., Schweble, W. Complement and complement deficiencies. Semin Liver Dis 1997; 297-310
48. Agnello, V. Lupus diseases associated with hereditary and acquired deficiencies of complement. Springer Semin Immunopathol 1986; 9:161-78
49. Maddison, P.J. ANA-negative SLE. Clin Rheum Dis 1982; 8:105-19
50. Sontheimer, R.D., Thomas, J.R., Gilliam, J.N. Subacute cutaneous lupus erythematosus. Arch Dermatol 1979; 115:1409-15
51. Sontheimer, R.D., Stastny, P., Maddison, P., et al. Serologic and HLA associations in subacute cutaneous lupus erythematosus (SCLE): A clinical subset of lupus erythematosus. Ann Intern Med 1982; 97:664-71
52. Glass, D., Raum, D., Gibson, D., et al. Inherited deficiency of the second component of complement. J Clin Invest 1976; 58:853-61
53. McCarty, D.J., Tan, E.M., Zvaifler, N.J., et al. Serologic studies in a family with heterozygous C2 deficiency. Am J Med 1981; 6:945-8
54. Davies, K.A., Erlendsson, K., Beynon, H.L., et al. Splenic uptake of immune complexes in man is complement-dependent. J Immunol 1993; 151:3866-73
55. Osofsky, S.G., Thompson, B.H., Lint, L.F., et al. Hereditary deficiency of the third component of complement in a child with fever, skin rash, and arthralgias: Response to transfusion of whole blood. J Pediatr 1977; 90:180-6
56. Sano, Y., Nishimukai, H., Kitamura, H., et al. Hereditary deficiency of the third component of complement in two sisters with systemic lupus erythematosus-like symptoms. Arthritis Rheum 1981; 24:1255-60
57. Rosenfeld, S.I., Kelly, M.R., Leddy, J.P. Hereditary deficiency of the fifth component of complement in man. J Clin Invest 1976; 57:1626-34
58. Tedesco, F., Silvani, C.M., Agelli, M., et al. A lupus-like syndrome in a patient with deficiency of the sixth component of complement. Arthritis Rheum 1981; 23:1438-40
59. Trapp, R.G., Mooney, H., Coleman, T.H., et al. Hereditary complement (C6) deficiency associated with systemic lupus erythematosus, Sjögren's syndrome, and hyperthyroidism. J Rheumatol 1987; 14:1030-3

60. Mooney, E. Complement factor 6 deficiency associated with lupus. J Am Acad Dermatol 1984; 11:896-7
61. Zeitz, H.J., Miller, G.W., Lint, T.F., et al. Deficiency of C7 with systemic lupus erythematosus. Arthritis Rheum 1981; 24:87-93
62. Jasin, H.E. Absence of the eighth component of complement in association with systemic lupus erythematosus-like disease. 1977; J Clin Invest 60:709-15
63. Pickering, R.J., Rynes, R.I., LoCascio, N., et al. Identification of the subunit of the eight component of complement (C8) in a patient with systemic lupus erythematosus and absent C8 activity: Patient and family studies. Clin Immunol Immunopathol 1982; 23:323-34
64. Kawai, T., Katoh, K., Narita, M., Tani, K., Okubo, T. Deficiency of the 9th component of complement (C9) in a patient with systemic lupus erythematosus. J Rheumatol 1989; 16:5423
65. Orren, A., O'Hara, A.M., Morgan, B.P., et al. An abnormal but functionally active complement component C9 protein in an Irish family wioth subtotal C9 deficiency. Immunology 2003; 108:384-90
66. Takeda, I., Igarashi, S., Nishimaki, T., Kasukawa, R. A case of systemic lupus erythematosus in late component (C9) complement deficiency. Ryumachi 1994; 34:628-32
67. Senaldi, G., Davies, E.T., Peakman, M., et al: Frequency of mannose-binding protein deficiency in patients with systemic lupus erythematosus. Arthritis Rheum 1995; 38:1713-4
68. Davies, E.J., Snowden, N., Hillarby, M.C., et al. Mannose-binding protein gene polymorphism in systemic lupus erythematosis. Arthritis Rheum 1995; 38:110-4
69. Lau, Y.L., Lau, C.S., Chan, S.Y., Karlberg, J., Turner, M.W. Mannose-binding protein in Chinese patients with systemic lupus erythematosus. Arthritis Rheum 1996; 39:706-8
70. Sullivan, K.E., Wooten, C., Goldman, D., Petri, M. Mannose-binding protein genetic polymorphisms in black patients with systemic lupus erythematosus. Arthritis Rheum 1996; 39:2046-51
71. Davies, E.J., Teh, L-S., Ordi-Ros, J., et al. A dysfunctional allele of the mannose binding protein gene associates with systemic lupus erythematosus in a Spanish population. J Rheum 1997; 24:485-8
72. Hartmann, D., Fremeaux-Bacchi, V., Weiss, L., et al. Combined heterozygous deficiency of the classical complement pathway proteins C2 and C4. J Clin Immunol 1997; 17:176-84
73. Segurado, O.G., Arnaiz-Villena, A.A., Iglesias-Casarrubios, P., et al. Combined total deficiency of C7 and C4B with systemic lupus erythematosus (SLE). Clin Exp Immunol 1992; 87:410-4
74. Agnello, V., Koffler, D., Eisenberg, J.W., et al. C1q precipitins in the sera of patients with systemic lupus erythematosus and other hypocomplementemic states: Characterization of high and low molecular weight types. J Exp Med 1971; 134:118S,
75. Agnello, V., Winchester, R., Ruddy, S., et al. An unusual SLE related syndrome: Erythema multiforme, hypocomplementemia and circulating C1q precipitins. In Proceedings of the 13th International Congress on Rheumatology, Kyoto, Japan. Excerpta Medica, Amsterdam, International Congress Series No. 229
76. Agnello, V., Ruddy, S., Winchester, R.J. Hereditary C2 deficiency in systemic lupus erythematosus and acquired complement abnormalities in an unusual SLE-related syndrome. Birth Defects 1975; 11:312-7
77. McDuffie, F.C., Sams, W.M., Maldonado, J.E., et al. Hypocomplementemia with cutaneous vasculitis and arthritis. Mayo Clin Proc 1973; 8:340-48

78. Marder, R.J., Rent, R., Choi, E.Y., et al. C1q deficiency associated with urticarial-like lesions and cutaneous vasculitis. Am J Med 1976; 61:560-5
79. Marder, R.J., Burch, F.X., Schmid, F.R., et al. Low molecular weight C1q-precipitins in hypocomplementemic vasculitis-urticaria syndrome: Partial purification and characterization as immunoglobulin. J Immunol 1978; 121:613-8
80. Ludivico, C.I., Myers, A.R., Maurer, K. Hypocomplementemic urticarial vasculitis with glomerulonephritis and pseudotumor cerebri. Arthritis Rheum 1979; 22:1024-8
81. Zeiss, C.R., Burch, F.X., Marder, R.J., et al. A hypocomplementemic vasculitic urticarial syndrome. Am J Med 1980; 68:867-75
82. McLean, R.H., Weinstein, A., Chapitis, J., et al. Familial partial deficiency of the third component of complement (C3) and the hypocomplementemic cutaneous vasculitis syndrome. Am J Med 1980; 68:549-58
83. Schwartz, H.R., McDuffie, F.C., Black, L.F., et al. Hypocomplementemic urticarial vasculitis. Mayo Clin Proc 1982; 57:231-8
84. Sissons, J.G.P., Peters, D.K., Williams, D.G., et al. Skin lesions, angioedema, and hypocomplementemia. Lancet 1974;2:1350-2
85. Tuffanelli, D.L. Cutaneous immunopathology: Recent observations. J Invest Dermatol 1975; 65:143-53
86. Oishi, M., Takano, M., Miyachi, K., et al. A case of unusual SLE-related syndrome characterized by erythema multiforme, angioneurotic edema, marked hypocomplementemia, and C1q precipitins of the low molecular weight type. Int Arch Allergy Appl Immunol 1976; 50:463-72
87. Geha, R.S., Akl, K.F. Skin lesions, angioedema, eosinophilia, and hypocomplementemia. J Pediatr 1976; 89:724-7
88. Wara, D.W., Reiter, E.O., Doyle, N.E., et al. Persistent C1q deficiency in a patient with a systemic lupus erythematosus-like syndrome. J Pediatr 1975; 86:743-5
89. Feig, P.U., Soter, N.A., Yager, H.M., et al. Vasculitis with urticaria, hypocomplementemia, and multiple system involvement. 1976; JAMA 236:2065-8
90. Soter, N.A. Chronic urticaria as a manifestation of necrotizing vasculitis. N Engl J Med 1977; 25:1440-2
91. Mathison, D.A., Arroyave, C.M., Bhat, K.N., et al. Hypocomplementemia in chronic idiopathic urticaria. Ann Intern Med 1977; 86:534-8
92. Curd, J.G., Milgrom, H., Stevenson, D.D., et al. Potassium iodide sensitivity in four patients with hypocomplementemic vasculitis. Ann Intern Med 1979; 91:853-7
93. Gammon, W.R., Wheeler, C.E. Urticarial vasculitis. Arch Dermatol 1979; 115:76-80
94. Mannik, M., Wener, M.H. Deposition of antibodies to the collagen-like region of C1q in renal glomeruli of patients with proliferative lupus glomerulonephritis. Arthritis Rheum 1997; 40:1504-11
95. Wisnieski, J.J., Baer, A.N., Christensen, J., et al. Hypocomplementemic urticarial vasculitis syndrome. Clinical and serologic findings in 18 patients. Medicine 1995; 74:24-41
96. Wisnieski, J.J., Naff, G.B. Serum IgG antibodies to C1q in hypocomplementemic urticarial vasculitis syndrome. Arthritis Rheum 1989; 32:1119-27
97. Fremeaux-Bacchi, V.I., Weiss, L., Demouchy, C., Blouin, J., Kazatchkine, M.D. Autoantibodies to the collagen-like region of C1q are strongly associated with classical pathway-mediated hypocomplementemia in systemic lupus erythematosus. Lupus 1996; 5:216-20
98. Martensson, U., Sjoholm, A.G., Sturfelt, G., Truedsson, L., Laurell, A.B. Western blot analysis of human IgG reactive with the collagenous portion of C1q: Evidence of distinct binding specificities. Scand J Immunol 1992; 35:735-44

99.   Sissons, J.G., West, R.J., Fallows, J., et al. The complement abnormalities of lipodystrophy. N Engl J Med 1976; 294:461-5
100. Jasin, H.E. Systemic lupus erythematosus, partial lipodystrophy and hypocomplementemia. J Rheumatol 1979; 6:43-50
101. Davis, A.E., Cicardi, M. C1 Inhibitor Autoantibodies. pp. 126-131. Elsevier, 1996; New York
102. Hory, B., Panouse-Perrin, J., Suzuki, Y., et al. Immune complex nephropathy and hereditary deficiency of C1 esterase inhibitor. Nouv Presse Med 1981; 10:2193-6
103. Suzuki, Y., Nihei, H., Mimura, N., Hara, M. A case of hereditary angioneurotic edema associated with systemic lupus erythematosus. Jpn J Med 1986; 25:281-7.
104. Guillet, G., Sassolas, B., Plantin, P., et al. Anti-Ro positive lupus and hereditary angioneurotic edema. A 7-year follow-up with worsening of lupus under danazol treatment. Dermatologica 1988; 177:370-5
105. Gudat, W., Bork, K. Hereditary angioedema associated with subacute cutaneous lupus erythematosus. Dermatologica 1989; 179:211-3
106. Horiuchi, S., Baba, T., Uyeno, K., et al. A case of hereditary angioneurotic edema associated with systemic lupus erythematosus. Nippon Hifuka Gakkai Zasshi 1989; 99:921,
107. Duhra, P., Holmes, J., Porter, D.I. Discoid lupus erythematosus associated with hereditary angioneurotic edema. Br J Dermatol 1990; 123:241-4
108. Cox, N.H., West, N.C., Ive, F.A., et al. Lupus erythematosus and hereditary angio-oedema. Br J Dermatol 1991; 125:82-3
109. Perkins, W., Stables, G.I., Lever, R.S. Protein S deficiency in lupus erythematosus secondary to hereditary angio-oedema. Br J Dermatol 1994; 130:381-4
110. Donaldson, V.H., Bissler, J.J., Welch, T.R., et al. Antibody to C1-inhibitor in a patient receiving C1-inhibitor infusions for treatment of hereditary angioneurotic edema with systemic lupus srythematosus reacts with a normal allotype of residue 458 of C1-inhibitor. J Lab Clin Med 1996; 128:438-43
111. Youniou, P., Dorval, J.C., Cledes, J., et al. A study of lupus erythematosus-like disease and hereditary angio-oedema treated with danazol. Br J Dermatol 1983; 108:717-22
112. Kohler, P.F., Percy, J., Campion, W.M. Hereditary angioedema "familial" lupus erythematosus in identical twin boys. Am J Med 1974; 56:406-11
113. Rosenfeld, G.B., Partridge, R.E., Bartholomew, W., et al. Hereditary angioneurotic edema (HANE) and systemic lupus erythematosus (SLE) in one of identical twin girls. Am Acad Allergy 1974; 53:68-72
114. Donaldson, V.H., Hess, E.V., McAdams, A.J. Lupus-erythematosus-like disease in three unrelated women with hereditary angioneurotic edema. Ann Intern Med 1977; 86:312-3
115. Tuffanelli, D.L. Discoid lupus erythematosus and the variant form of hereditary angioedema. Arch Dermatol 1977; 113:374-5
116. Young, D.W., Thompson, R.A., Mackie, P.H. Plasmapheresis in hereditary angioneurotic edema and systemic lupus erythematosus. Arch Intern Med 1980 140:127-8
117. Massa, M.C., Connolly, S.M. An association between C1 esterase inhibitor deficiency and lupus erythematosus: Report of two cases and review of the literature. J Am Acad Dermatol 1982; 7:255-64
118. Jordan, R.E., Provost, T.T. The complement system and the skin. p. 7. In: Mackinson FD, Pearson RW (eds), Yearbook of Dermatology. Yearbook Medical Publishers, Chicago, 1976

119. Shiraishi, S., Watanabe, N.Y., Matsuda, K., et al. C1 inhibitor deficiency simulating systemic lupus erythematosus. Br J Dermatol 1982; 106:455-60
120. Donaldson, V.H., Hess, E.V. Effect of danazol on lupus erythematosus-like disease in hereditary, angioneurotic edema. Lancet 1980; 2:1145
121. Vyse, T.J., Spath, P.J., Davies, K.A., et al. Hereditary complement factor I deficiency. Q J Med 1994; 87:385-401
122. Moller Rasmussen, J., Jepsen, H.H., Teisner, B., et al. Quantification by ELISA of erythrocyte-bound C3 fragments expressing C3d and/or C3c epitopes in patients with factor I deficiency and with autoimmune diseases. Vox San 1989; 56:262-9
123. Marquart, H.V., Rasmussen, J.M., Leslie, R.G. Complement-activating ability of leucocytes from patients with complement factor I deficiency. Immunol 1997; 91:486-92
124. Fijen, C.A., Kuijper, E.J., Te Bulte, M., et al. Heterozygous and homozygous factor H deficiency states in a Dutch family. Clin Exp Immunol 1996; 105:511-6
125. Cornillet, P., Gredy, P., Pennaforte, J.L., et al. Increased frequency of the long (S) allotype of CR1 (the C3b/C4b receptor, CD35) in patients with systemic lupus erythematosus. Clin Exp Immunol 1992; 89:22-5
126. Van Dyne, S., Holers, V.M., Lublin, D.M., Atkinson, J.P. The polymorphism of the C3b/C4b receptor in the normal population and in patients with systemic lupus erythematosus. Clin Exp Immunol 1987; 68:570-9
127. Vik, D.P., Wong, W.W. Structure of the gene for the F allele of complement receptor type 1 and sequence of the coding region unique to the S allele. J Immunol 1993; 151:6214-24
128. Sato, H., Yokota, E., Tokiyama, K., Kawaguchi, T., Niho, Y. Distribution of the Hind III restriction fragment length polymorphism among patients with systemic lupus erythematosus with different concentrations of CR1. Ann Rheum Dis 1991; 50:765-8
129. Tebib, J.G., Martinez, O., Granados, J., Alarcon-Segovia, D., Schur, P.H. The frequency of complement receptor type 1 (CR1) gene polymorphism in nine families with multiple cases of systemic lupus erythematosus. Arthritis Rheum. 1989; 32:1465-9
130. Kumar, A., Kumar, A., Sinha, S., et al. Hind III genomic polymorphism of the C3b receptor (CR1) in patients with SLE: Low erythrocyte/CR1 expression is an acquired phenomenon. Immunol Cell Biol 1995; 73:457-62
131. Moulds, J.M., Reveille, J.D., Arnett, F.C. Structural polymorphisms of complement receptor 1 (CR1) in systemic lupus erythematosus (SLE) patients and normal controls of three ethnic groups. Clin Exp Immunol 1996; 105:302-5
132. Witte, T., Gessner, J.E., Gotze, O., Deicher, H., Schmidt, R.E. Complement receptor 3 deficiency in systemic lupus erythematosus. Immun Infekt 1992; 20:60-1
133. Merry, A.H., Rawlinson, V.I., Uchikawa, M., et al. Studies on the sensitivity to complement-mediated lysis of erythrocytes (Inab phenotype) with a deficiency of DAF (decay accelerating factor). Br J Haematol 1989; 73:248-53
134. Agnello, V., Gell, J., Tye, M. Partial genetic deficiency of the C4 component of complement in discoid lupus erythematosus and urticaria/angioedema. J Am Acad Dermatol 1983; 9:894-8
135. Fishelson, Z., Attali, G., Mevorach, D. Complement and apoptosis. Mol Immunol 2001; 38:207-19
136. Gadjeva, M., Verschoor, A., Brockman, M.A., et al. Macrophage-derived complement component C4 can restore humoral immunity in C4-deficient mice. J Immunol 2002; 169: 5489-95

137. Casciola-Rosen, L.A., Anhalt, G., Rosen, A. Autoantigens targeted in systemic lupus erythematosus are clustered in two populations of surface structures on apoptotic keratinocytes. J Exp Med 1994; 179:1317-30
138. Korb, L.C., Ahearn, J.M. C1q binds directly and specifically to surface blebs of apoptotic human keratinocytes. Complement deficiency and systemic lupus erythematosus revisited. J Immunol 1997; 158:4525-8
139. Botto, M., Dell'Agnolla, C., Bygrave, A.E., et al. Homozygous C1q deficiency causes glomerulonephritis associated with multiple apoptotic bodies. Nat Genet 1998; 19:56-9
140. Taylor, P.R., Carugati, A., Fadok, V.A., et al. A hierarchical role for classical pathway complement protein in the clearance of apoptotic cells in vivo. J Exp Med 2000; 192:359-66
141. Mitchell, D.A., Taylor, P.R., Cook, H.T., et al. C1q protects against the development of glomerulonephritis independently of C3 activation. J Immunol 1999; 162:5676-9

PART 4

EXPLOITATION OF
COMPLEMENT PROTEINS IN
INFECTION AND CANCER

11

Microbial Evasion Mechanisms Against Human Complement
Attack by Complement - Counterstrike by Micro-Organisms

Reinhard Würzner and Peter F. Zipfel*

*Institute for Hygiene and Social Medicine, Medical University of Innsbruck & Ludwig-Boltzmann-Institute for AIDS-Research, Innsbruck, Austria; and *Hans-Knöll-Institute for Natural Products Research, Jena, Germany*

Abstract: Virtually all pathogens invading the human host are attacked by the immune system directly following entry and usually also during consecutive stages of disease, especially when they are in contact with blood. In order to escape or overcome immune defence most micro-organisms have developed an effective battery of specific strategies. As the innate immune system forms an important part of the immune defence, evading the interplay between complement and the phagocytic system plays a major role for the invader in order to survive the hostile environment within the host. The measures to avoid recognition and destruction by complement via complement-mediated attraction, opsonisation and activation of phagocytic cells, and lysis involves microbial molecules which are expressed on the surface or secreted into the near vicinity and can therefore be considered as virulence factors. Of all these highly sophisticated mechanisms imitation (molecular mimicry) and employment of host complement appear to be the most evolutionary elaborated. This review concentrates on microbial evasion strategies by employing soluble host complement inhibitors, such as Factor H, FHL-1, and C4 binding protein. Acquisition of such host regulators results in downregulation of the complement attack directly at the microbial surface, inhibits formation of toxic activation products and facilitates adhesion to and invasion into host cells.

Key words: Key words: Complement – regulators – microbe host interaction – immune evasion – molecular mimicry – Factor H – FHL-1 – C4 binding protein

1. COMPLEMENT – THE ATTACK

Complement plays a major role in the innate immune system and represents an important first-line defence system of higher vertebrates against invading micro-organisms. Upon initial invasion into the human body microbes activate predominantly the alternative and lectin pathways of complement (triggered by their surface structures, such as lipopolysaccharides, sialic acids and peptidoglycans). Following induction of the adaptive immune response, antibodies bind to the surface of the intruder. C1 will bind to the Fc portion of the antibody activating the classical pathway. C1q-binding moieties on micro-organisms, however, may also directly activate the classical pathway (1-5).

Although this surveillance system has been considered primitive, as complement proteins and functions and regulatory proteins are identified early in evolution, e.g. in the teleost fish barred sand bass, which in evolution is separated from humans by 100 million years (6), four important functions can be distinguished for complement in immune defense against microorganisms. The three direct ones comprise:

i)   the attraction of phagocytic cells via newly generated anaphylatoxins to the site of infection (chemotaxis, see 1.1);

ii)   the generation of C3 fragments, mainly C3b and iC3b on the microbial surface (opsonization); these entities are recognized by complement receptors on phagocytic cells, followed by phagocytosis (see 1.2); and

iii) the lysis of the microbe by the membrane attack complex (see 1.3.).

Together with indirect actions towards the invader (see 1.4) this combination of both antibody-mediated and antibody-independent efforts lead to a limitation of the attack and a control of the infection.

1.1   Complement as Attractor

Complement activation via all three pathways eventually leads to an activation of C3 and C5 and thus to a marked release of the anaphylatoxic peptides C3a and C5a. Using their C3a- and C5a-receptors, phagocytic cells, especially polymorphonuclear phagocytes (PMNs), sense concentration gradients and migrate towards the area of highest concentration, which is the site of inflammation.

1.2   Complement as Signaller

Upon arrival at the site of infection PMNs are unable to identify the invader on its own and require complement as signaller. The deposition of complement fragments (mainly C3b and iC3b) generated on the surface of the invader (opsonisation) is a prerequisite for a sufficient engulfment and uptake via specific complement receptors (CR1 and especially CR3) displayed on the surface of the PMNs. Phagocytosis is most efficient when both C3 fragments and antibody are attached to the micro-organism, suggesting enhancement via a dual-signal-procedure.

1.3   Complement as Single Warrior

Complement, as a phylogenetically old immune defence system, is also able to act on its own as a potent first-line defence, independently of other parts of the immune system. Not only the number of C3-fragment molecules deposited on the invader but also the amount of C5b-9 inserted into the target membrane is decisive for host defence. The latter strongly correlates with bactericidal activity and inversely with complement resistance. The debate, how lysis is executed, i.e. by forming a physical hole or by generating membrane perturbations (see chapter 6), is especially interesting in the light of immune defence against *Neisseria meningitidis*. The particularly frequent occurrence of terminal complement deficiencies in patients with meningococcal infections confirms that the cytolytic activity of complement is important in resistance to gram-negative bacteria (7). It is established that the terminal pathway damages the LPS-containing cell wall (8). However, it is still unclear how the 'inner' cell membrane is destroyed: possibly via induction of injurious processes or directly by bacteria-derived lysozyme or bacterially generated ATP; alternatively, further terminal components, entering the periplasmic space via the outer membrane attack leaks, may insert into the inner membrane as MACs (9) or even as polymerized or single C9 alone (10). While lysis plays a predominant role in immune defence against *Neisseria spp.*, it appears to be less important against other micro-organisms, especially against those having a compound cell membrane or even a thick cell wall (11).

1.4   Complement as Coordinator

Complement probably represents the most important humoral part of innate immunity against micro-organisms, but, in addition, also strongly interacts with its innate cellular part, comprising macrophages, NK cells and granulocytes (1-5).

Complement thus acts at the interface between, and thus links and coordinates, innate and adaptive immunity by several ways:

(i) complement is involved in the initiation of adaptive immune responses, since antibody-independent, complement-mediated opsonization of microbes leads to an uptake and presentation of antigens via complement-receptor bearing antigen-presenting cells which then triggers the adaptive immune response (complement as initiator);

(ii) antigen-bound C3d augments antibody response by facilitating B-cell activation via crosslinking membrane IgM to the CR2/CD19/TAPA-1 complex (complement as enhancer);

(iii) non-lytic MAC induces protection to the host cell, as upon single (and erroneous) attacks it provides resistance to subsequent, otherwise lytic doses (12) (complement as protector);

(iv) non-lytic MAC activates the host cell in a procoagulant, which limits the area of attack, and proinflammatory manner, e.g. by augmenting arachidonic acid metabolism, intracellular Ca^{++} flux and protein kinase C activation (13) (complement as locally enhancing limitator); and

(v) CR1 and CR2 expressed on follicular dendritic cells are essential for the formation of memory B cells by localizing C3b- and/or C4b-bearing immune complexes in the germinal centres (complement as memorizer).

2.   MICRO-ORGANISMS – THE COUNTER STRIKE

Evolution during millions of years of both host and micro-organisms has created a commensual relationship between man and microbes, so that in many cases potentially infectious micro-organisms are not attacked and live in symbiosis with the host. Most of them only cause disease when the host defence is considerably weakened.

A different type of relationship is medically very important and scientifically most interesting: micro-organisms which are highly pathogenic but nevertheless either evade appropriate recognition or constrain suitable attack and destruction. These pathogens invading the human body are attacked by the complement system directly following entry and usually also during most stages of the disease, especially when they are in contact with human blood. However, during co-evolution alongside their obligate hosts several pathogenic micro-organisms have developed an effective battery of specific strategies to overcome the destructive human immune defence in general and complement in particular. These include both biochemical or biophysical measures to resist C3b deposition, opsonophagocytosis or complement-mediated cytolytic damage. These measures increase the likelihood of survival in a hostile environment and can be considered as virulence factors.

Micro-organisms evade complement first by avoiding appropriate recognition (see 2.1) (14) and, as this is not always efficient, by preventing eradication (see 2.2) by complement (15-19).

2.1   Avoidance of Recognition - Disguise

The easiest principle to establish survival in the host is simply the one of disguise, i.e. the host does not recognise the invasion of the pathogen. This is achieved by displaying non- or poorly-activating surface moieties. Such molecules which lead to an insufficient complement activation include sialic acids, e.g. of encapsulated bacteria or parasites as well as surface glycoproteins and lipophosphoglycans (11). Some gram-negative bacteria mask (20) or change their surface-expressed lipopolysaccharides (21) to avoid recognition. This leads to an absent or non-opsonic attachment of C3 fragments on the pathogen cell surface, resulting in an inappropriate recognition by PMNs. Likewise, this is also accomplished by displaying the complement-activating properties somewhat hidden on the surface, so that because of sterical hindrance they are inaccessible by PMNs. Not surprisingly, pathogenicity within a strain usually correlates well with its ability to prevent recognition.

2.2   Avoidance of Eradication

Once recognised by the host's complement system the invader has to introduce measures to avoid eradication by complement. This is achieved by removing (see 2.2.1), mimicking (2.2.2), or inhibiting (see 2.2.3) complement activation, or employing complement proteins via several highly sophisticated mechanisms (see 2.3.4). The principles are discussed and some representative examples are given below. A more detailed list of pathogens and their ways to avoid eradication by complement (19) and figures detailing this interaction (22) are published elsewhere. As the imitation of complement-like proteins (molecular mimicry, (19)) plays a dominant role in inhibition and employment of complement it will be presented below (see 2.2.2.) in some detail.

2.2.1   Removal of Complement

Complement can dismantled by

(i)   shedding off,
(ii)   consuming, or
(iii)   destructing complement.

2.2.1.1   Shedding off
One important way of removal of complement is by shedding off the microbial membrane

(i)   initial immune complexes, as done by *Fasciola hepatica* (23);

(ii)   C3, as executed by *Trypanosoma cruzi* (24); or

(iii)   assembling complement complexes, in particular at the membrane attack stage, as for *Naegleria fowleri* (25).

2.2.1.2   Consumption

Removal of complement is also accomplished by consumption of complement, usually following the shedding of complement activating molecules (see 2.2.1.1.) as consumption is much safer at a secure distance well away from the invader. However, this also leads to reactive lysis of bystander cells. Micro-organisms exploiting this subversive procedure, such as *Streptococcus pyogenes* (26), must have a highly sophisticated regulation to ensure that not too much detrimental activation occurs. Cleavage of C1 inhibitor by proteases is mentioned here (not under 2.2.1.3) as it resembles the destruction of an inhibitor, resulting in an uninhibited consumption of C1 (27) and consecutively of other complement proteins.

2.2.1.3   Inactivation

Proteolytic cleavage and phosphorylation of complement proteins or inactivation of anaphylatoxins by micro-organisms also represent ways to confer protection from opsonisation and lysis. Good examples are the proteinkinases of *Leishmania spp.* for phosphorilation (28), and the 56 kDa protease of *Serratia marcescens* (29) for inactivation of anaphylatoxins and the *Helicobacter pylori* urease (30) for cleavage (of C3).

2.2.2   Molecular Mimicry of Complement by Micro-Organisms

During co-evolution alongside their obligate hosts several pathogens have evolved functional or structural properties identical to those of host cells to prevent their own destruction by complement (convergent evolution). Thus, a number of distinct microbial proteins has been identified which share functional or structural similarities with complement proteins or complement receptors.

Some viruses, like Herpes virus Saimiri, share genetic similarities (antigenic cross-reactivity, sequence homology) and even functional activities (31) with complement proteins or receptors. Most likely they have, in evolutionary terms recently, incorporated complement gene segments into their genome (31).

For others a combination of convergent evolution and gene capture appears to be responsible. In the case of vaccinia virus the DNA encoding VCP, a functionally CR1-like and structurally C4bp-like complement control protein, was presumably originally acquired from the host, as it has sequence homologies to both. Over an evolutionary period the captured gene was constantly manipulated to retain only the most essential domains as any further manipulation of the small viral protein results in loss of function, indicating that the gene has achieved a maximum efficiency to encode a protein with the minimum number of amino acids (18).

Mimicry is used by pathogens both for inhibition (2.2.3) and for employment of complement (2.2.4).

2.2.3   Inhibition of Complement

A variety of mechanisms are used by pathogens to inactivate complement, such as the display of C1 binding moieties, not necessarily proteins, which directly interfere with classical pathway activation, as the *Salmonella minnesota* 39 kDa porin (32), or inhibitory molecules interfering with the potentially lytic terminal pathway, as the SIC protein of *Streptococcus pyogenes* (33).

In order to inhibit complement, some pathogens can also take advantage of their endogenously expressed complement-like molecules mimicking host complement. Well characterised examples are the parasitic (*Trypanosoma*) or viral (Vaccinia virus, Herpes simplex virus) proteins related to mammalian CR1, DAF, MCP or C4BP, which all target C4b and C3b, limiting complement attack (34-36) and confirm the importance of C3 and C4-binding molecules in host defence. The different examples of molecular mimicry of the terminal cascade inhibitory protein CD59 are also quite remarkable, comprising functional, structural and/or antigenic similarities of CD59 to Herpes virus Saimiri ORF-15 (37), the 170 kDa *Entamoeba histolytica* adhesin (38), or the 94 kDa *Schistosoma mansoni* SCIP-1 protein (39), inhibiting lysis by interacting with C8 and especially with C9.

2.2.4   Employment of Host Complement

Some micro-organisms evade complement in another very sophisticated way, namely by using host complement proteins or receptors for their own survival. Two main principles, one aggressive (see 2.2.4.1) and one defensive one (see 2.2.4.2) can be discerned: micro-organisms may employ complement to adhere to and invade into host cells or to avert their own destruction, respectively, in part by an imitation of complement components or receptors (molecular mimicry).

2.2.4.1   Adhesion and Invasion

Opsonisation of pathogens is not always harmful for the invader, and is sometimes even desired and initiated by micro-organisms, as surface-deposited complement (in particular C3b or iC3b) can act as opsonin facilitating entry of the invader into host cells via the complement receptors on the latter. This resembles a 'Trojan horse' principle as it can lead to a milder intracellular response of the phagocytes (lower respiratory burst) and thus intracellular survival and can rescue pathogens, such as *Leishmania major*, from the hostile extracellular environment (40). Opsonisation or cleavage, however, has to be very accurate so that most of the surface-deposited C3 is present in the optimum conformation (C3b or iC3b) for receptor binding. The same effect can be reached by cleaving C3, e.g. by the 56 kDa cystein protease of *Entamoeba histolytica* (41).

Even more sophisticated, molecular mimicry of complement receptor ligands also facilitates entry into host cells, employing the complement receptors on them, and does not rely on the potentially dangerous opsonisation of the pathogen. The proteins involved on the invader are antigenically and/or functionally mimicking C3, as most convincingly shown for Epstein-Barr virus gp350/220 (42). Other viruses, like measles virus or enteroviruses, are able to use complement receptors MCP or DAF, respectively, for cell entry directly (43, 44), also avoiding the potentially dangerous opsonisation procedure.

Both adhesion and possibly also inhibition can be achieved by mimicking integrins: a CR3-like molecule of the yeast *Candida albicans* facilitates not only host cell adhesion and cell invasion (45, 46), but may also bind C3 in a non-opsonising way.

2.2.4.2   Defence

Pathogens do not only employ complement for invasion but also for their own defence. Both membrane-bound (see 2.2.4.2.1) as well as fluid phase complement inhibitors (see 2.2.4.2.2) are utilized by micro-organisms.

2.2.4.2.1   Exploitation of membrane inhibitors

Intracellular pathogens, like CMV, can harness the cellular machinery for their own benefit, e.g. by inducing expression of complement regulators, such as DAF, on the surface of the infected cell, preventing its destruction by the host immune system (47).

Some virus employ complement proteins directly from the host cell membrane, e.g. upon budding HIV encoates itself with a lipid bilayer obtained from the host cell membrane and as a consequence carries, in addition to viral, also host cell membrane proteins. Of the latter especially

DAF and CD59 are of particular importance, protecting the virus from complement lysis (48).

Parasites, like *Schistosoma mansoni*, or bacteria, such as *E. coli*, can even acquire surface complement inhibitors, especially when they are glycosylphosphoinositol-linked, like DAF (49) or CD59 (50), respectively.

2.2.4.2.2. Adsorption of fluid phase inhibitors

The number of microbes that can attach host complement regulators to their surface is much higher than previously anticipated and the amount of currently identified microbial surface proteins which are involved in binding and acquisition of host complement regulators is exploding. Upon entry into an immunocompetent host microbes activate the complement system which is aimed to mark these cells as foreign and to initiate their elimination. Apparently a large number of pathogenic microbes mimic the surface structure of host cells and bind host fluid phase complement regulators. This acquisition results in a downregulation of the complement attack and in an inhibition of the generation of toxic complement activation products directly at the microbial surface. This gives a growth benefit for the microbe and allows progression in an immunocompetent host. Inhibition of complement is one of several features - other benefits for the microbe include adhesion to, as well as invasion into host cells.

Acquisition of host complement regulators has been shown for a number of microbes, including *Bordetella pertussis*, *Borrelia* species, such as *Borrelia burgdorferi* (51-57), *Escherichia coli* (58), *Neisseria meningitides* (59, 60), *N. gonorrhoeae* (60-62), *Streptococcus pyogenes* (63-68), *S. pneumoniae* (69-71), HI-Virus (72), *Candida albicans* (73), *Onchocerca volvulus* (74) and *Echinococcus granulosus* (75). These gram-positive or gram-negative bacteria, viruses, fungi and parasites acquire soluble host complement inhibitor proteins which regulate the alternative pathway, such as complement Factor H and the Factor H like protein 1 (FHL-1), and proteins which control the classical pathway of complement, i.e. the C4 binding protein (C4BP) (Table 1).

The pattern of acquired host regulators varies between strains and even further between clinical isolates of one species. Some microbes, like *Borrelia* species, bind specifically the alternative pathway regulators Factor H and FHL-1, and no *Borrelia* strain analyzed so far does bind the classical pathway regulator C4BP. In contrast, *Streptococcus pyogenes* and *Candida albicans* bind the alternative pathway regulators Factor H and FHL-1, and also the classical pathway regulator C4BP. The difference in binding suggests that at least some microbes survive by specifically inactivating the alternative pathway; others in contrast need to deal with both the alternative and the classical pathway of complement.

Table 1: Microbes and microbial proteins that are used to acquire human complement regulators

Microbe	Microbial Protein	Complement Pathway	
		Alternative	Classical
Bordetella pertussis	FHA	Factor H FHL-1	C4BP
Borrelia burgdorferi	BbCRASP-1	Factor H (19-20) FHL-1 (5-7)	
	BbCRASP-2	FHL-1 (6,7) Factor H (19,20)	
	BbCRASP-3/ErpC	Factor H (19,20)	
	BbCRASP-4	Factor H (19,20)	
	BbCRASP-5	Factor H (19,20)	
Eschericia coli	Dr-like antigen	DAF	
	OmpA		C4BP
Neisseria gonorrhoeae	Por1A	Factor H FHL-1	
	Sialic acid	Factor H	
	Por1A,Por1B		C4BP
	Type IV pilus	MCP	
Neisseria meningitis		Factor H FHL-1	C4BP
Streptococcus pyogenes	M Protein conserved	Factor H	
	Semiconserved	FHL-1 (7) FHR-3	
	Hypervariable	MCP	C4BP
	Fba	Factor H FHL-1	
Streptococcus pneumoniae	Hic/PspC	Factor H (8-11)	
	PspC	FHL-1	
HIV		Factor H	
Candida albicans		Factor H (19,20) FHL-1 (7)	C4BP (2,3)
Onchocerca volvulus		Factor H	
Echinococcus granulosis		Factor H	

When the binding domains were determined on the level of complement control protein modules, the corresponding domain is shown in parenthesis

Several of the microbial binding proteins have been characterized on a molecular level and have been shown to present important virulence factors (Table I). These include the central virulence factor of *S. pyogenes*, the M protein, which mediates antiphagocytic activity and which binds multiple host plasma proteins including immunoglobulins, fibrinogen, fibronectin and plasminogen (76).

Interestingly for the diverse variety of micro-organisms studied, rather similar or even identical patterns for binding and orientation are emerging, thus indicating a conserved mechanism for attachment of host immune regulators. Host regulators are usually attached end to end to those parts of microbial surface proteins which are located most distant from the cell so that complement activation is dealt with by the micro-organism at a safe distance. In most cases the host regulators (Factor H and FHL-1) are attached via their C-terminal ends, i.e. domain 20 of Factor H and domain 7 of FHL-1). This interaction results in a physical coat which efficiently separates the microbial cell membrane or capsule from the site of host attack and thus creates a real physical barrier which limits immune attack.

Each of the Factor H and FHL-1 attachment sites includes a heparin binding domain and consequently it has been shown for several cases that heparin affects binding. This observation suggests that the heparin binding sites of the immune regulators are involved in binding and are central for this interaction.

Factor H, FHL-1 and C4BP bound to the microbial evasion proteins maintain their complement inhibitory activities both for alternative and classical pathway regulation. Therefore acquisition of host immune regulators to a site distant form the microbial surface, inhibits the formation of complement activation products to the microbial surface, blocks the complement cascade and enhances microbial survival. With such an evasion strategy microbes subvert the host immune response.

Additional features of this interaction are summarized and characterized as follows:

- microbes utilize multiple surface proteins for binding of host proteins, e.g. *Borrelia burgdorferi* strain ZS7 uses up to five distinct surface proteins, termed BbCRASP-1 to BbCRASP-5, which acquire and bind host immune regulators and similarly *S. pyogenes* uses at least two binding proteins, i.e. the M and the Fba protein (51, 52);

- one single microbial surface protein binds multiple host regulators to distinct sites. The borrelial BbCRASP1 protein binds Factor H and FHL-1, and the streptococcal M-protein binds the two alternative pathway regulators Factor H and FHL-1 and also the classical pathway regulator C4BP (53);

- the microbial host complement inhibitor binding proteins are highly polymorphic in nature or even the binding sites of structurally conserved proteins are located in hypervariable protein domains. Binding of the host FHL-1 occurs to the hypervariable region of the streptococcal M protein and similarly the borrelial CRASP-3/Erp-3/OspE proteins represent a polymorphic protein family (76, 77).

In summary, an important way to escape the destructive action by complement is achieved by exploiting host inhibitors which are attached to the surface of the pathogen. The available data provide a common scenario which is outlined in Figure 1.

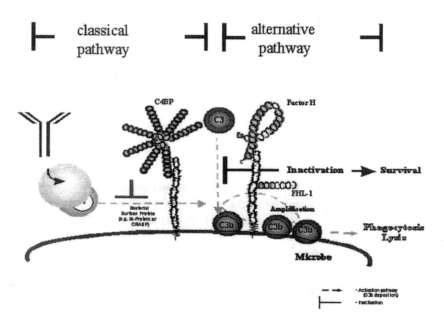

Figure 1. Immune evasion strategies of microbes: Attachment of soluble host complement regulators allows inhibition of complement attack directly at the surface of microbes.

Microbes utilize surface proteins, which attach complement inhibitors from the host to their surface, and as a consequence downregulate toxic activation products which are normally generated by complement activation in order to inactivate the invader. These inhibitory actions restrict or reduce the number of newly generated C3 convertases, leading to impaired opsonization, phagocytosis and also lysis, the latter via an insufficiently induced terminal sequence.

3.   OUTLOOK

The characterisation of molecules circumventing host defence, and complement in particular, resembles a rapid developing field. Virtually every pathogen surviving in the human blood at one stage during infection must take definite measures to avoid recognition and/or eradication – this explains why usually several defence strategies, interacting at different stages within the complement cascade, are exploited. It is important to characterise these principles in order to develop therapeutic or preventive approaches, especially as the molecules of the pathogens involved are virulence factors,

(i)   readily available on the cell surface,
(ii)   abundantly expressed, and highly conserved within each species (17).

It has been proposed that sites of molecular mimicry may represent useful targets for vaccine development (78). However, considering their multiple as yet unrevealed interactions and, more importantly, their similarity to human molecules, a detrimental effect of such a vaccine, cannot be excluded: immunisation with an microbial antigen, which mimics a host protein, may induce an antibody response against the latter (79, 80).

4.   REFERENCES

1. Morgan, B.P., Harris, C.L. eds. Complement Regulatory Proteins. London: Academic Press, 1998.
2. Rother, K., Till, G.O., Hänsch, G.M. eds. The complement system. Berlin, Heidelberg, New York: Springer, 1998.
3. Volanakis, J.E., Frank, M.M. eds. The human complement system in health and disease. New York: Marcel Dekker, 1998.
4. Walport, M. Complement. New Engl J Med 2001;344:1058-1066
5. Prodinger, W.M., Würzner, R., Stoiber, H., Dierich, M.P. Complement. In *Fundamental Immunology*, Paul, W.E. ed, Philadelphia: Lippincott-Raven, 2003.
6. Kemper, C., Gigli, I. Zipfel, P.F.. Conservation of plasma regulatory proteins of the complement system in evolution: Human and fish. Exp Clin. Immunogenetics 2000; 17: 55-62
7. Würzner, R., Orren, A., Lachmann, P.J. Inherited deficiencies of the terminal components of human complement. Immunodefic Rev 1992;3:123-147
8. O'Hara, A.M., Moran, A.P., Würzner, R., Orren, A. Complement-mediated lipopolysaccharide release and outer membrane damage in Escherichia coli J5: requirement for C9. Immunology 2001;102:365-372
9. Hänsch, G.M. Defense against bacteria. In Rother, K., Till, G.O., Hänsch, G.M. eds. The complement system. Berlin, Heidelberg, New York: Springer, 1998.
10. Taylor, P.W. Complement-mediated killing of susceptible gram-negative bacteria: an elusive mechanism. Exp Clin Immunogenet 1992;9:48-56

11. Joiner, K.A. Complement evasion by bacteria and parasites. Annu Rev Microbiol 1988;42:201-230

12. Reiter, Y., Ciobotariu, A., Fishelson, Z. Sublytic complement attack protects tumor cells from lytic doses of antibody and complement. Eur J Immunol 1992;22:1207-1213

13. Morgan, B.P. Complement membrane attack on nucleated cells: resistance, recovery and non-lethal effects. Biochem J 1989;264:1-14

14. McLaren, D.J. Disguise as an evasive strategem of parasitic organisms. Parasitology 1984;88:597-611

15. Cooper, N.R. Complement evasion strategies of microorganisms. Immunol Today 1991;12:327-331

16. Fishelson, Z. Complement-related proteins in pathogenic organisms. Springer Sem Immunopathol 1994;15:345-368

17. Jokiranta, T.S., Jokipii, L., Meri, S. Complement resistance of parasites. Scand J Immunol 1995;42:5-20

18. Kotwal, G.J. The great escape: immune evasion by pathogens. Immunologist 1997;4:157-164

19. Würzner, R. Evasion of pathogens by avoiding recognition or eradication by complement, in part via molecular mimicry. Mol Immunol 1999;36:249-260

20. Merino, S., Camprubi, S., Alberti, S., Benedi, V.J., Tomas, J.M. Mechanisms of Klebsiella pneumoniae resistance to complement-mediated killing. Infect Immun 1992;60:2529-2535

21. Liang-Takasaki, C., Saxén, H., Mäkelä, P.H., Leive, L. Complement activation by polysaccharide of lipopolysaccharide: an important virulence determinant of salmonellae. Infect Immun 1983;41:563-569

22. Würzner, R. Complement and infectious diseases. Contrib Microbiol 2003;10: 1-17

23. Duffus, W.P.H., Franks, D. In vitro effect of immune serum and bovine granulocytes on juvenile Fasciola hepatica. Clin Exp Immunol 1980;41:430-440

24. Norris, K.A. Ligand-binding renders the 160 kDa Trypanosoma cruzi complement regulatory protein susceptible to proteolytic cleavage. Microb Pathog 1996;21:235-248

25. Toney, D.M., Marciano-Cabral, F. Membrane vesiculation of naegleria fowleri amoebae as a mechnism for resisting complement damage. J Immunol 1994;152:2952-2959

26. Berge, A., Kihlberg, B.M., Sjoholm, A.G., Bjorck, L. Streptococcal protein H forms soluble complement-activating complexes with IgG, but inhibits complement activation by IgG-coated targets. J Biol Chem 1997;272:20774-20781

27. Lathem, W.W., Grys, T.E., Witowski, S.E., Torres, A.G., Kaper, J.B., Tarr, P.I., Welch, R.A. StcE, a metalloprotease secreted by Escherichia coli O157:H7, specifically cleaves C1 esterase inhibitor. Mol Microbiol 2002;45:277-288

28. Rokita, E., Makristathis, A., Presterl, E., Rotter, M.L., Hirschl, A.M. Helicobacter pylori urease significantly reduces opsonization by human complement. J Infect Dis 1998;178:1521-1525

29. Hermoso, T., Fishelson, Z., Becker, S.I., Hirschberg, K., Jaffe, C.L. Leishmanial protein kinases phosphorylate components of the complement system. EMBO J 1991;10:4061-4067

30. Oda, T., Kojima, Y., Akaike, T., Ijiri, S., Molla, A., Maeda, H. Inactivation of chemotactic activity of C5a by the serratial 56-kilodalton protease. Infect Immun 1990;58:1269-1272

31. Rother, R.P., Rollins, S.A., Fodor, W.L., Albrecht, J.C., Setter, E., Fleckenstein, B., Squinto, S.P. Inhibition of complement-mediated cytolysis by the terminal complement inhibitor of herpes virus saimiri. J Virol 1994;68:730-737

32. Stemmer, F., Loos, M. Evidence for direct binding of the first component of complement, C1, to outer membrane proteins from Salmonella minnesota. Curr Top Microbiol Immunol 1985;121:73-84

33. Fernie-King, B.A., Seilly, D., Willers, C., Würzner, R., Davies, A., Lachmann, P.J. Streptococcal inhibitor of complement inhibits the membrane attack complex by preventing uptake of C567 onto cell membranes. Immunology 2001;103:390-398

34. Norris, K.A., Bradt, B.M., Cooper, N.R., So, M. Characterization of a Trypanosoma cruzi C3 binding protein with functional and genetic similarities to the human complement regulatory protein decay accelerating factor. J Immunol 1991;147:2240-2247

35. Friedman, H.M., Cohen, G.H., Eisenberg, R.J., Seidel, C.A., Cines, D.B. Glycoprotein C of herpes simplex virus 1 acts as a receptor for the C3b complement component on infected cells. Nature 1984;309:633-635

36. Kotwal, G.J., Isaacs, S.N., McKenzie, R., Frank, M.M., Moss, B. Inhibition of the complement cascade by the major secretory protein of vaccinia virus. Science 1990;250:827-830

37. Albrecht, J.C., Nicholas, J., Camerun, K.R., Newman, C., Fleckenstein, B., Honess, R.W. Herpes virus saimiri has a gene specifying a homologue of the cellular membrane glycoprotein CD59. Virology 1992;190:527-530

38. Braga, L.L., Ninomiya, H., McCoy, J.J., Eacker, S., Wiedmer, T., Pham, C., Wood, S., Sims, P.J., Petri, W.A. Jr. Inhibition of the complement membrane attack complex by the galactose-specific adhesin of Entamoeba histolytica. J Clin Invest 1992;90:1131-1137

39. Parizade, M., Arnon, R., Lachmann, P.J., Fishelson, Z. Functional and antigenic similaries between a 94-kDa protein of schistosoma mansoni (SCIP-1) and human CD59. J Exp Med 1994;179:1625-1636

40. Da Silva, R.P., Hall, B.F., Joiner, K.A., Sacks, D.L. CR1, the C3b receptor, mediates binding of infective leishmania major metacyclic promastigotes to human macrophages. J Immunol 1989;143:617-622

41. Reed, S.L., Keene, W.E., McKerrow, J.H., Gigli, I. Cleavage of C3 by a neutral cysteine proteinase of entamoeba histolytica. J Immunol 1989;143:189-195

42. Mold, C., Bradt, B.M., Nemerow, G.R., Cooper, N.R. Epstein-Barr virus regulates activation and processing of the third component of complement. J Exp Med 1988;168:949-969

43. Dorig, R.E., Marcil, A., Chopra, A., Richardson, C.D. The human CD46 molecule is a receptor for measles virus (Edmonston Strain). Cell 1993;75:295-305

44. Bergelson, J.M., Chan, M., Solomon, K.R., Stjohn, N.F., Lin, H.M., Finberg, R.W. Decay-accelerating factor (CD55), a glycosylphosphatidyl-inositol-anchored complement regulatory protein, is a receptor for several echoviruses. Proc Natl Acad Sci USA 1994;91:6245-6248

45. Gale, C.A., Bendel, C.M., McClellan, M., Hauser, M., Becker, J.M., Berman, J., Hostetter, M.K. Linkage of adhesion, filamentous growth, and virulence in Candida albicans to a single gene, INT1. Science 1998;279:1355-1358

46. Gruber, A., Lell, C.P., Spruth, M., Lass-Flörl, C., Speth, C., Stoiber, H., Hube, B., Coleman, D., Polonelli, L., Dierich, M.P., Würzner, R. HIV-1 and its transmembrane protein gp41 bind to different *Candida* species modulating adhesion. FEMS Immunol Med Microbiol 2003;37:77-83

47. Spiller, O.B., Morgan, B.P., Tufaro, F., Devine, D.V. Altered expression of host-encoded complement regulators on human cytomegalovirus-infected cells. Eur J Immunol 1996;26:1532-1538

48. Marschang, P., Sodroski, J., Würzner, R., Dierich, M.P. Decay-accelerating factor (CD55) protects human immunodeficiency virus type I from inactivation by human complement. Eur J Immunol 1995;25:285-290

49. Pearce, E.J., Hall, B.F., Sher, A. Host-specific evasion of the alternative complement pathway by schistosomes correlates with the presence of a phospholipase C-sensitive surface molecule resembling human decay accelerating factor. J Immunol 1990;144:2751-2756

50. Rautemaa, R., Jarvis, G.A., Marnila, P., Meri, S. Acquired resistance of Escherichia coli to complement lysis by binding of glycophosphoinositol-anchored protectin (CD59). Infect Immun 1998;66:1928-1933

51. Zipfel, P.F., Skerka, C., Hellwage, J., Jokiranta, S.T., Meri, S., Brade, V., Kraiczy, P., Noris, M., Remuzzi, G. Factor H family proteins: on complement, microbes and human diseases. Biochem Soc Trans 2002;30:971-978

52. Kraiczy, P., Skerka, C., Brade, V., Zipfel, P.F. Further characterization of complement regulator-acquiring surface proteins of Borrelia burgdorferi. Infect Immun. 2001;69:7800-7809

53. Kraiczy, P., Skerka, C., Kirschfink, M., Brade, V., Zipfel, P.F. Immune evasion of Borrelia burgdorferi by acquisition of human complement regulators FHL-1/reconectin and Factor H. Eur J Immunol 2001;31:1674-1684

54. Kraiczy, P., Hellwage, J., Skerka, C., Kirschfink, M., Brade, V., Zipfel, P.F., Wallich, R. Immune evasion of Borrelia burgdorferi: mapping of a complement-inhibitor factor H-binding site of BbCRASP-3, a novel member of the Erp protein family. Eur J Immunol 2003;33:697-707

55. Alitalo, A., Meri, T., Lankinen, H., Seppala, I., Lahdenne, P., Hefty, P.S., Akins, D., Meri, S. Complement inhibitor factor H binding to Lyme disease spirochetes is mediated by inducible expression of multiple plasmid-encoded outer surface protein E paralogs. J Immunol 2002;169:3847-3853

56. Stevenson, B., El-Hage, N., Hines, M.A., Miller, J.C., Babb, K. Differential binding of host complement inhibitor factor H by Borrelia burgdorferi Erp surface proteins: a possible mechanism underlying the expansive host range of Lyme disease spirochetes. Infect Immun 2002;70:491-497

57. Alitalo, A., Meri, T., Ramo, L., Jokiranta, T.S., Heikkila, T., Seppala, I.J., Oksi, J., Viljanen, M., Meri, S. Complement evasion by Borrelia burgdorferi: serum-resistant strains promote C3b inactivation. Infect Immun. 2001;69:3685-3691

58. Prasadarao, N.V., Blom, A.M., Villoutreix, B.O., Linsangan, L.C. A novel interaction of outer membrane protein A with C4b binding protein mediates serum resistance of Escherichia coli K1. J Immunol. 2002;169:6352-6360

59. Jarva, H., Ram, S., Vogel, U., Blom, A., Meri, S. Binding of the classical pathwaxy complement inhibitor C4bp to the PorA protein of serogroup B Neisseria meningitidis. Mol. Immunol. 2003;40:175-176

60. Ram, S., Mackinnon, F.G., Gulati, S., McQuillen, D.P., Vogel, U., Frosch, M., Elkins, C., Guttormsen, H.K., Wetzler, L.M., Oppermann, M., Pangburn, M.K., Rice, P.A. The contrasting mechanisms of serum resistance of Neisseria gonorrhoeae and group B Neisseria meningitidis. Mol Immunol. 1999; 36:915-928

61. Ram, S., Cullinane, M., Blom, A.M., Gulati, S., McQuillen, D.P., Monks, B.G., O'Connell, C., Boden, R., Elkins, C., Pangburn, M.K., Dahlback, B., Rice, P.A. Binding of C4b-binding protein to porin: a molecular mechanism of serum resistance of Neisseria gonorrhoeae. J Exp Med. 2001;193:281-295

62. Ram, S., McQuillen, D.P., Gulati, S., Elkins, C., Pangburn, M.K., Rice, P.A. Binding of complement factor H to loop 5 of porin protein 1A: a molecular mechanism of serum resistance of nonsialylated Neisseria gonorrhoeae. J Exp Med. 1998;188:671-680

63. Kotarsky, H., Hellwage, J., Johnsson, E., Skerka, C., Svensson, H.G., Lindahl, G., Sjobring ,U., Zipfel, P.F. Identification of a domain in human factor H and factor H-like protein-1 required for the interaction with streptococcal M proteins. J Immunol. 1998;160:3349-3354

64. Thern, A., Stenberg, L., Dahlback, B., Lindahl, G. Ig-binding surface proteins of Streptococcus pyogenes also bind human C4b-binding protein (C4BP), a regulatory component of the complement system. J Immunol 1995;154:375-386

65. Johnsson, E., Berggard, K., Kotarsky, H., Hellwage, J., Zipfel, P.F., Sjobring, U., Lindahl, G. Role of the hypervariable region in streptococcal M proteins: Binding of a human complement inhibitor. J Immunol 1998;161:4894-490

66. Accardo, P., Sanchez-Corral, P., Criado, O., Garcia, E., Rodriguez de Cordoba, S. Binding of human complement component C4b-binding protein (C4BP) to Streptococcus pyogenes involves the C4b-binding site. J Immunol. 1996;157:4935-4939.

67. Berggard, K., Johnsson, E., Morfeldt, E., Persson, J., Stalhammar-Carlemalm, M., Lindahl, G. Binding of human C4BP to the hypervariable region of M protein: a molecular mechanism of phagocytosis resistance in Streptococcus pyogenes. Mol Microbiol. 2001;42:539-551

68. Kotarsky, H., Gustafsson, M., Svensson, H.G., Zipfel, P.F., Truedsson, L., Sjobring, U. Group A streptococcal phagocytosis resistance is independent of complement factor H and factor H-like protein 1 binding. Mol Microbiol. 2001;41:817-826

69. Neeleman, C., Geelen, S.P., Aerts, P.C., Daha, M.R., Mollnes, T.E., Roord, J.J., Posthuma, G., van Dijk, H., Fleer, A. Resistance to both complement activation and phagocytosis in type 3 pneumococci is mediated by the binding of complement regulatory protein factor H. Infect Immun. 1999;67:4517-4524

70. Jarva, H., Janulczyk, R., Hellwage, J., Zipfel, P.F., Bjorck, L., Meri, S. Streptococcus pneumoniae evades complement attack and opsonophagocytosis by expressing the pspC locus-encoded Hic protein that binds to short consensus repeats 8-11 of factor H. J Immunol. 2002;168:1886-1894

71. Lindahl, G., Sjobring, U., Johnsson, E. Human complement regulators: a major target for pathogenic microorganisms. Curr Opin Immunol. 2000;12:44-51

72. Stoiber, H., Pinter, C., Siccardi, A.G., Clivio, A., Dierich, M.P. Efficient destruction of human immunodeficiency virus in human serum by inhibiting the protective action of complement factor H. J Exp Med 1996;183:307-310

73. Meri, T., Hartmann, A., Lenk, D., Eck, R., Wurzner, R., Hellwage, J., Meri, S., Zipfel, P.F. The yeast Candida albicans binds complement regulators factor H and FHL-1.Infect Immun. 2002;70:5185-5192

74. Meri, T., Jokiranta, T.S., Hellwage, J., Bialonski, A., Zipfel, P.F., Meri, S. Onchocerca volvulus microfilariae avoid complement attack by direct binding of factor H. J Infect Dis. 2002;185:1786-1793

75. Ferreira, A.M., Irigoin, F., Breijo, M., Sim, R.B., Diaz, A. How Echinococcus granulosus deals with complement. Parasitol Today 2000;16:168-172

76. Bisno, A.L., Brito, M.O., Collins, C.M. Molecular basis of group A streptococcal virulence. Lancet Infect Dis. 2003;3:191-200

77. Blom AM. Structural and functional studies of complement inhibitor C4b-binding protein. Biochem Soc Trans. 2002;30:978-982

78. Fishelson, Z. Complement evasion by parasites: search for "Achilles' heel". Clin Exp Immunol 1991;86(Suppl.1):47-52
79. Schwimmbeck, P.L., Yu, D.T., Oldstone, M.B. Autoantibodies to HLA B27 in the sera of HLA B27 patients with ankylosing spondylitis and Reiter's syndrome. Molecular mimicry with Klebsiella pneumoniae as potential mechanism of autoimmune disease. J Exp Med 1987;166:173-181
80. Zhao, Z.S., Granucci, F., Yeh, L., Schaffer, P.A., Cantor, H. Molecular mimicry by herpes simplex virus-type 1: autoimmune disease after viral infection. Science 1998;279:1344-1347

12

Complement-Mediated Antibody-Dependent Enhancement of Viral Infections

Zoltán Prohászka[1], Ferenc D. Tóth[2†], Dénes Bánhegyi[3] and George Füst[1]

[1]*Third Department of Medicine, Faculty of Medicine, Semmelweis University, Budapest,* [2]*Institute of Medical Microbiology, Medical and Health Science Center, University of Debrecen, Debrecen,* [3]*Department of Immunology, St. László Hospital, Budapest, Hungary*

Abstract: Enhancement of in vitro infection by immune antibodies was described for several viral diseases, first for the dengue and respiratory syncytial virus infections. Immune enhancement of viral infection can be connected with vaccine failures since vaccinated individuals who develop enhancing antibodies may have an exaggerated disease upon exposure to the virus. A part of the antibody-dependent enhancement is mediated by complement activation; this enhancement is mediated by antibodies against the immunodominant part of the transmembrane protein (gp41) of HIV. Binding of the enhancing antibodies results in deposition of complement proteins (C1q) and activation products of C4 and C3 on virus particles; interaction of these proteins with the type 2 complement receptor (CR2) and the C1q receptor facilitates attachment of the HIV virions to the target cells and leads to increased virus production in vitro and probable in vivo as well. Complement mediated antibody dependent enhancement (C-ADE) was demonstrated to be clinically relevant in HIV infection by the authors of the present chapter. C-ADE was found to develop shortly after HIV-infection concomitantly with seroconversion, and strongly correlate to viral load in the course of HIV disease. C-ADE can be detected more frequently in advanced stages of HIV infection and their appearance may herald progression of disease. Combination treatment by antiviral drugs (HAART) leads to the disappearance of C-ADE; sera of the HAART-treated patients may neutralize HIV even in the presence of complement, which can be infrequently detected in untreated patients. These findings indicate that study of C-ADE may have of crucial importance at development of HIV vaccines.

Key Words: viral disease, HIV, complement, infection enhancement, enhancing antibodies

1. INTRODUCTION

Antibodies, which develop in viral infections, can be divided in three major groups according to their function. The first type of antibodies is protective, may contain infection and/or contribute to the elimination of the viral pathogen. The second type of antibodies can be designed as "antigen-reactive", their presence neither inhibits nor facilitate viral infection. Measurement of these antibodies, however, may be crucial at diagnosis of several viral diseases. The third type of antibodies, the so-called enhancing antibodies, "traitors" of the immune system, increase the growth of the viral pathogens, and facilitate progression of viral diseases. The study of enhancing antibodies is a rather neglected field of infection immunology, their presence and clinical significance was investigated only in some diseases, mainly flavivirus and HIV infections. The presence and significance of enhancing antibodies was reviewed in 1997 by one of us (1), therefore in the present review we shall mainly deal with the findings published in the last years.

There are two types of antibody-dependent infection enhancement in viral diseases: Fc receptor (FcR)-dependent, complement-independent enhancement (FcR-ADE), and complement-mediated antibody-dependent enhancement (C-ADE). It is important to note that complement may affect the course of HIV-infection and other viral diseases in several antibody-independent ways (facilitation of transport through the mucosa, trapping of viral particles on the surface of the follicular dendritic cells in the lymph nodes, HIV entry into the B cells, activation of the monocytes/macrophages through the complement-derived anaphylatoxins resulting in increased susceptibility to HIV infection, etc.) as well. These events were recently summarized in an excellent review from Manfred Dierich's group (2); therefore our review will be focused on the antibody-dependent enhancement.

2. ANTIBODY-DEPENDENT ENHANCEMENT OF VIRAL INFECTIONS

This topic was recently summarized by Sullivan (3) therefore we shall write about this topic only briefly. In vitro enhancement was observed with several viruses of the family of Flaviviridae. Later on enhancement of the in vitro growth by low titer, homotypic hyperimmune sera was described with viral strains belonging to other families like Togaviridae, Bunyviridae, etc., and recently by Retroviridae as well (reviewed in reference 3).

The possible biological significance of the ADE was raised first by the vaccine failures and other findings observed with two viruses, the respiratory syntitial virus (RSV) and the dengue virus. Sixty percent of children immunized with a formalin-inactivated RSV vaccine still became infected and the course of the disease was markedly more serious in the vaccinated than in the non-vaccinated children (4). Similar exacerbation of the disease was observed in infants with passively acquired maternal antibodies to the RSV virus (5) and to dengue virus (6).

Most studies on ADE were performed with two viruses, dengue virus and human immunodeficiency virus (HIV). Studies with ADE and HIV will be detailed in the following parts of the present chapter. Dengue virus belongs to the family of Flaviviridae. Dengue virus infections are a serious cause of morbidity and mortality in most tropical and subtropical areas in the world, mainly Southeast and South Asia. Dengue virus infection can be asymptomatic, or cause two form of illness, dengue fever and dengue haemorrhagic fever. Non-neutralizing, cross-reactive antibodies markedly augment dengue virus infection through FcR-ADE in vitro (7) and in vivo (8). C-ADE was not observed with the dengue virus infection, although according to the findings of Malasit (9) complement activation is also involved in the pathogenesis of dengue haemorrhagic fever. In addition it was recently reported by Lin et al. (10) that antibodies from dengue patient sera cross-react with endothelial cells and induce damage partly by complement-mediated cell lysis. This process may have an important role in the pathogenesis of serious dengue virus infection.

3. COMPLEMENT-MEDIATED ANTIBODY-DEPENDENT INFECTION ENHANCEMENT (C-ADE) IN HIV DISEASE

3.1 Specificity of C-ADE Initiating Antibodies, Mechanisms of C-ADE

Recent elegant studies of Mitchell et al (11) demonstrated that - in accordance with the earlier observations of Robinson at al (12,13) - the primary antigenic domains responsible for the C-ADE of HIV and SIV resides in the principal immunodominant sequence of gp41. This is a conservative sequence since according to the site-directed mutagenesis experiments of Mitchell et al. (11) it is critical for the gp120-gp41 interaction. According to their model, binding site for enhancing antibodies on the primary association site with gp41 is surrounded by amino-linked oligosaccharides, which are likely sites for the covalent attachment of the C3dg peptide of C3, the physiological ligand of the CR2 receptor. Binding site for enhancing antibodies on gp41 may be accessible after release of gp120 from gp41 or after a conformational change in gp120 upon association with CD4.

The main mechanism of the C-ADE is therefore the increased binding of C3 activation fragments to gp41 of HIV-virions and the type 2 complement receptor (CR2). By using three human anti-gp41 monoclonal antibodies we tested if there are any alternative ways of the mechanism of C-ADE (14). All monoclonals mediated increased C1q binding to solid-phase gp41. The effect of 246-D was the most pronounced. All monoclonals had a marked dose-dependent and strictly complement-dependent HIV-infection enhancing effect. Mixtures of the monoclonals with purified C1q also significantly increased HIV-1 infection. Pretreatment of the target cells with anti-CR2 antibodies only partially inhibited the enhancing effect of the monoclonals plus normal human serum. C1qD and C2D sera had a markedly lower enhancing effect than NHS (Figure 1).

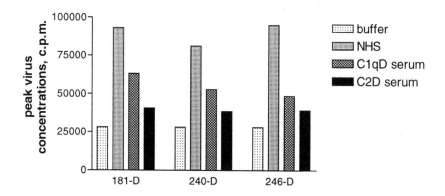

Figure 1. Enhancement of HIV-1 infection of MT-4 cells by human monoclonal anti-gp41 antibodies mixed with complement deficient sera and normal human serum (NHS) (peak virus concentrations in the MT-4 cell cultures as measured by the RT assay, c.p.m. values)

These findings indicate that besides the well-known facilitation of entry of HIV-1 by the interaction between virus-bound C3 fragments and CR2 present on the target cells, fixation of C1q to intact virions also results in an enhanced productive HIV-1 infection in the MT-4 cell cultures.

3.2   Clinical Aspects of C-ADE

In the last decade we have reported on several results supporting the role of C-ADE in the progression of HIV disease. These observations are in contrast with the findings of Montefiori et al. (15, 16) who did not observe any correlation between the extents of C-ADE in different stages of HIV disease and did not find a decreased C-ADE value in long-term non-progressors. As to be detailed below this discrepancy is most probable due to methodological differences: Montefiori's group used a procedure, which seems to be not suitable for detecting those C-ADE mediating antibodies, which are relevant in the progression of HIV infection.

3.2.1 Measurement of C-ADE by Our Group

We have applied the same method for measuring C-ADE in serum samples with only minor modifications for almost one decade (17-20). Briefly, serum or IgG samples from the patients were heat-treated (56°C, 30 min) and diluted at 1:64 in culture medium in triplicates. One hundred μl of serum or IgG dilutions were mixed with 100 μl of fresh pooled sera from HIV-seronegative healthy persons (normal human serum, NHS). HIV-1_{IIIB} (100 $TCID_{50}$) in 100 μl culture medium was added, and incubated at 37°C for 1 hour. Thus, final concentration of human complement in the samples added to target cells was 25%. In the case of each patient's serum sample mixtures without complement in which NHS was replaced by culture medium were also tested. In each series of experiments, control cultures infected with the virus alone were established, too. Then, 5×10^5 MT-4 cells in growth medium were added and incubated in this medium without change for 5 days at 37°C. Growth of HIV in the cultures was monitored on each day by the reverse transcriptase (RT) assay as outlined by Hoffman et al. (21). Peak RT values were observed almost exclusively at day 5. The results were measured as c.p.m. and expressed finally by an index (enhancement /neutralization index = E/N I) value which indicated the relationship between virus growth in serum or IgG containing samples compared to that measured in cultures infected with virus alone. Index values were calculated as follows: means of triplicate peak RT (c.p.m.) values measured in cultures infected with the mixtures of virus, patient's serum (and NHS) at day 5 were divided by the means of triplicate peak c.p.m. values measured in control cultures infected with virus alone at day 5. Samples with an E/N I less than 0.5 (two-fold decrease in virus production) were considered as neutralizing whereas samples with an E/N I exceeding 2.0 (two-fold increase in virus production) were considered as enhancing. Pooled heat-treated (56°C, 30 min) HIV-seronegative serum at the same dilution as the test samples (1:64) was used as a negative control at each measurement; it never influenced the growth of HIV-1 in the system. Variation coefficient of the method was 7.23%.

As it was pointed out above, in contrast to the results of our group Montefiori et al. (15, 16) did not find any correlation between C-ADE mediating antibodies and clinical progression. This discordance is most probably due to methodological differences: Montefiori et al. (15, 16) used much lower complement concentration, much higher input virus/cell ratio and other target cell (MT-2 vs. MT-4) for culturing the virus. To our mind, most important difference between Montefiori's group and ours is the final concentration of NHS. While we use a near-physiological (25%) NHS concentration as complement source, the other group always applied a strongly (1:20-1:27) diluted NHS. It seems reasonable to suppose that the closer the complement concentration is in the mixtures used for infecting the MT-4 cells to that in the blood, the higher the physiological relevance of the measurement. Studies of Lund et al (22) also demonstrated that the enhancing effect of complement is dose-dependent.

Paradoxically, the findings described in the studies summarized in the present chapter on the pathological role of C-ADE-mediating antibodies were obtained in a system where complement concentration is apparently non-physiological. The target cell, MT-4, is a HTLV-I infected cell-line and HIV-1$_{IIIB}$ is a laboratory, X4 strain passaged many times through T cell lines. Recent studies, however, indicate that the system is much closer to the in vivo situations than it seems to be. Nielsen et al (23) demonstrated that C-ADE occurs in vitro in peripheral blood mononuclear cells although it was not as dramatic as that detected in cell lines. The presence of complement receptor type 2 (CR2) critical for C-ADE was described in 10-50% of the circulating T cells (24, 25) indicating that the use of a CR2-carrying target cell for measuring humoral factors influencing HIV growth is reasonable.

3.2.2   Changes in C-ADE During HIV Disease

Our group demonstrated first the association between C-ADE and the clinical progression of HIV-disease (17-19). In our initial study we have found C-ADE only in 4/20 (20%) asymptomatic HIV-patients but in 12/19 (63%) patients in the symptomatic (ARC or AIDS) stage of the disease (17). This observation was supported by McDougall et al. (26) who detected C-ADE more frequently in patients with lymphocyte counts less than 400/mm^3 as compared to those in early stage of the disease. In other studies from our group (18) high titre C-ADE was found to predict rapid decline of the CD4+ cell counts and an increased probability of the AIDS development. In a five-year follow-up period AIDS developed in 33% and 83% of patients with missing or low titre C-ADE and in those with high titre C-ADE, respectively (18).

3.2.3 C-ADE Appears Concomitantly with Seroconversion

MT-4 cell cultures were infected with mixtures of the virus and heat-treated plasma samples of four different seroconversion panels (serial plasma samples of plasmapheresis donors infected by HIV during the period of sampling) diluted 1:64 with or without NHS (complement) added. HIV antibody titres were measured by the sensitive Abbott HIV ½ kit (detecting both IgG and IgM antibodies), and the amounts of HIV antigen were also measured by the Abbott kit detecting p24. The extent of the two later parameters are given as the quotient of the sample O.D. and cut-off O.D. Table 1 shows the results obtained with two seroconversion panels (J and Y) but similar results were obtained with the two other (D and P) panels (19).

Table 1. Changes in the levels of HIV p24 antigen, HIV antibodies as well as the enhancing/neutralization index measured in the presence and absence of complement in two seroconversion plasma panels

	Panel J: days after first plasmapheresis					
	0	14	26	28	32	35
Abbott antigen test, sample O.D./cut-off O.D.	0.00	5.70	0.60	0.50	0.40	0.40
Abbott IgM-IgG antibody test, sample O.D./cut-off O.D.	0.00	0.20	10.40	7.40	7.60	7.10
E/N index in the presence of complement	1.00	1.49	2.78	3.01	2.50	2.24
E/N index in the absence of complement	0.97	0.97	1.00	0.98	0.98	0.60
	Panel Y: days after first plasmapheresis					
	0	10	18	22	44	49
Abbott antigen test, sample O.D./cut-off O.D.	0.40	0.40	0.40	0.40	2.20	1.00
Abbott IgM-IgG antibody test, sample O.D./cut-off O.D.	0.00	0.20	0.10	0.20	11.80	9.90
E/N index in the presence of complement	0.98	1.01	0.98	1.49	2.72	3.55
E/N index in the absence of complement	0.95	1.01	1.03	0.98	0.97	0.50

Concomitantly with the seroconversion that is in the first sample tested positive with the Abbott antibody kit marked increase in the E/N index in the presence of complement was observed in all the 4 panels tested. In the panels J and P seroconversion was preceded by a peak p24 antigen concentration whereas in the panel Y where a long time (three weeks) passed between the collection of the last seronegative and seropositive panels a low titer p24 antigen was also found in the first seropositive plasma. In the subsequent samples E/N I measured in the cultures infected with complement-containing mixtures further increased, fluctuated or levelled off.

3.2.3.1   Close correlation between the extent of C-ADE and viral load in HIV-infected patients

HIV-1 RNA concentrations were determined by using two methods (Amplicor and NASBA) in parallel in the plasma samples of 96 patients mostly in advanced stage HIV disease. HIV infection neutralization/enhancement in the presence and absence of normal human serum (NHS) as a complement source was measured in the serum samples taken at the same time from the same patients (19). When E/N I values measured in cultures infected with virus+ heat-treated serum samples in the presence or absence of complement were plotted against HIV-1 RNA concentrations measured with the Amplicor method, a strong positive correlation was found in MT-4 cell cultures infected with complement-containing mixtures (R= 0.709 (p<0.0001). However, in cultures with no complement added a much weaker but still significant positive correlation (R=0.276 (p=0.0059) was obtained between the two parameters. Similar correlation was found between viral load measured with the NASBA method and E/N I values (R=0.627, p < 0.0001, and R=0.207, p=0.041, respectively). E/N I values measured in the presence and absence of complement strongly correlated with each other (R=0.607, p < 0.0001).

Next the E/N I values measured in sera from patients with undetectable and detectable HIV-1 RNA with the Amplicor method were compared. E/N I values measured in cultures infected in the presence of complement were significantly higher in the sera from patients with detectable than with undetectable viral load, whereas there were no significant differences between the same groups in E/N I values measured in cultures infected without complement. The patients were divided according to the E/N I values measured in cultures infected in the presence and absence of complement (Figure 2). Sera of twelve patients had an E/N I value below 0.5 implying neutralization of HIV-1 regardless of the absence or presence of complement. No HIV-1 RNA could be detected in plasma samples of either of these patients. Serum samples from 17 patients neutralized HIV-1 only in the absence of complement, while in cultures infected with complement-containing mixtures E/N I values exceeding 0.5 or even 1.0 (11/17) were measured. The median of viral load was markedly higher in this group than in the previous one, HIV-1 RNA could be detected in 10/17 plasma samples. In cultures infected with sera of 69 patients E/N I values exceeded 0.5, that is, no neutralization was found regardless of the presence or absence of complement. The median viral load was the highest in this group. According to the non-parametric ANOVA (Kruskal-Wallis test) there was a highly significant (p <0.01) difference among the three groups of the patients.

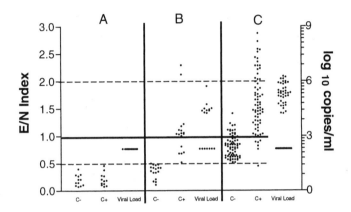

Figure 2. HIV patients were divided into three groups: A: neutralizers both in the presence and absence of complement, B: neutralizers only if complement is absent and C: non-neutralizers. The viral load in these groups is indicated on the right Y-axis. The difference of the viral load in the three groups is highly significant, as calculated by the Kruskall-Wallis test (p=0.0014)

Recently these findings were corroborated by Subbramanian et al. (27) who detected enhancement of in vitro HIV infection in the presence of complement in 72% of serum samples of HIV patients. They also concluded that the anti-HIV-1 humoral immune response consist of a mixture of antibodies that may inhibit or enhance HIV infection and whose ratios may vary in different stages of the infection.

The association between viral load and C-ADE can be explained by two different ways. It cannot be excluded that the high HIV antigen load associated with the high viral burden induce increased dose-dependent synthesis of C-ADE-mediating antibodies. However, no positive correlation between viral load and neutralizing antibodies or the total amounts of ELISA-reactive HIV antibodies has been described so far. Therefore it seems more probable that the levels of HIV-1 RNA are driven by C-ADE activity than vice versa. It is also possible that C-ADE and viral load mutually enhance each other in a vicious circle: strong C-ADE activity may increase viral load, and the resulting high viral load may further stimulate the formation of C-ADE.

3.2.3.2   Predictive value of C-ADE measurement in untreated HIV patients

E/N I values and HIV-1 RNA levels were longitudinally tested in parallel in 18 patients (19). The data obtained at the beginning and end of the 17 months (median) observation period are shown in Figure 3.

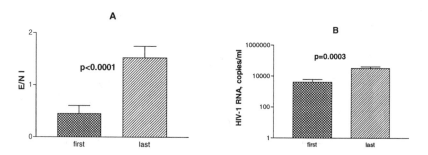

Figure 3. First and last measurements in 18 HIV patients the enhancement/neutralization index (E/N I) (A) and plasma HIV-1 RNA concentrations with the Amplicor test (B) during a 17-month observation period.

Both the E/N I values and the viral load markedly increased during the follow-up period, the differences between the initial and end values were highly significant. In line with these observations, recently it has been reported that enhancing antibodies may also contribute to the selection pressure operating on the circulating population of polymorphic HIV-1 variants (28).

3.2.3.3   Decrease of C-ADE during HAART

Recently we studied the effect of highly active antiretroviral therapy (HAART) on balance of the antibodies that enhance or neutralize growth of HIV-1$_{IIIB}$ strain in MT-4 cells in the presence or absence of human complement (20). Sequential serum samples were collected from 28 patients in advanced stage of HIV disease before and during HAART. As in our previous studies described above, the balance of the enhancing and neutralizing antibodies was expressed by an index value (E/N I). Samples with an E/N I of < 0.5 (two-fold decrease in virus production) were considered as neutralizing, whereas samples with an E/N I > 2.0 (two-fold increase in virus production) were considered as enhancing. At the beginning of HAART serum samples from 8 patients enhanced, and samples from only 2 patients neutralized the virus in the presence of complement, The median (25th-75th percentile) value of E/N I was 1.32 (0.79-2.29). In the absence of complement 10/26 samples neutralized but none enhanced HIV growth, E/N I was found to be 0.63 (0.39-0.88).

E/N I significantly (p<0.0001) dropped during the follow-up period 18.5 (10.5-23.5) of months under HAART (Table 2). No significant changes occurred during the first 8 months of treatment while a sharp decrease was registered between the 8th and 19th months of HAART. Similar changes were detected when serum samples were tested with no complement added but in these samples the decrease in E/NI I took place mainly during the first period of therapy. In the last samples neutralization (E/N index <0.5) was measured in the absence and presence of complement in 26/28 (92.9%) and 20/28 (71.4%) patients, respectively. By contrast enhancement was found with none of the samples. Viral load significantly decreased, absolute number and percentage of CD4+ T cells significantly increased, while percentage of the CD8+ cells significantly decreased during this period.

Table 2. Changes in the enhancing/neutralizing index (E/N I) values during HAART in 26 HIV-infected patients

Months of HAART, median	In the absence of complement	In the presence of complement
	Mean ± S.D.	
0	0.64 ± 0.28	1.53 ± 1.04
8	0.46 ± 0.26 **	1.22 ± 0.86
17	0.29 ± 0.19*	0.40 ± 0.23***
P values for the repeated measures ANOVA test	<0.001	<0.001

P values compared to the previous measurement, *p<0.05, **p<0.01, ***p<0.001 as calculated by the repeated measures ANOVA and Tukey post hoc tests

Our present findings indicate that HAART switches the balance of enhancement and neutralization toward neutralization. In principle our present observations can be biased by the presence of antiretroviral drugs in the test samples, which can influence the assay system we used. According to the data presented in Table 1, however, this assumption seems to be highly improbable. E/N I values were found to be markedly and significantly lower in the samples taken 19 months than in those taken 8 months after the beginning of HAART, although the patients got the same type of HAART protocols, therefore the concentration of the antiretroviral drugs in their serum samples were approximately the same at both times. Moreover, we found in control experiments that a marked drop of the E/N index values occurred when cultures inoculated with mixtures of HIV and purified IgG prepared from serum pools taken before and during HAART, respectively, were compared.

According to the findings summarized in the present chapter it seems probable that the apparent decrease in the E/N I values is due to the changes in the generation of enhancing and/or neutralizing antibodies, that is, to the drop of the production of enhancing antibodies, or an increased production of neutralizing antibodies. Changes in the titers of neutralizing antibodies in chronically infected HIV patients during HAART were studied by several groups (29-31). These studies were performed in limited numbers of patients and gave conflicting results (30, 31). It seems therefore improbable that the marked decrease observed in the E/N index values in our present study was the consequence of an increased neutralization activity -at least neutralization measured by conventional methods- during HAART.

By contrast, several observations, described above indicate that C-ADE is associated with and may potentially facilitate progression of HIV disease. Considering these observations it seems probable that drop of antigen stimulus in patients under HAART results in a markedly decreased production of the antibodies mediating C-ADE and consequently to a gradual and dramatic (more than three-fold) decrease in the E/NI index values. Most importantly, Verrier et al. (32) demonstrated that whole virus-particle-based HIV-1 vaccines in hyperimmunized rhesus macaques can play a facilitating role in the transmission of the virus and/or evolution of the disease. Therefore our present findings indicate that besides its main effect – decrease of viral load – HAART results in an additional beneficial effect: disappearance of C-ADE and shift of the balance toward dominance of the antibodies that neutralize HIV-1 *in vitro* even in the presence of complement. It was described by several groups (33, 34) that there is a drop of B cell activation and IgG levels during HAART. Our present findings indicate that the amounts of C-ADE mediating antibodies changes in parallel with the amounts of IgG-specific antibodies in the patients on HAART, similarly to the very beginning of HIV infection when the appearance of C-ADE coincides in time with the appearance of HIV-specific antibodies (see above).

3.2.4   Possible Significance of C-ADE in Vaccination

Findings summarized in the present chapter may have two implications for HIV vaccine development. First, it seems that estimation of HIV and SIV (35) neutralization and enhancement by using complement and complement-receptor carrying target cells correlates better to the natural progression of HIV infection than any other method applied for measuring HIV humoral immunity. Therefore it would be important to study if measurements by this or similar procedure can be used as correlate of HIV immune protection in animal experiments and in trials of candidate AIDS vaccines. Second, enhancing antibodies were found to develop after active and passive immunization against several virus infections including dengue haemorrhagic fever, respiratory syntitial virus and those with retroviruses such as equine infectious anaemia virus (see above). Passive immunization of rhesus macaques by serum of SIV-infected macaques led to an apparently enhanced course of the disease in association with the development of antibodies against the immunodominant region of the transmembrane glycoprotein of the virus (36, 37). Complement dependent enhancing antibodies were found in 11/19 volunteers vaccinated with high dose (640 μg) of a HIV-1 gp160 candidate vaccine (38). More recently Verrier et al. (32) demonstrated that whole virus-particle based HIV-1 vaccines in hyperimmunized rhesus macaques can play a facilitating role in the transmission of the virus and/or evolution of the disease.

4. CONCLUSIONS

In accordance with the consideration, which was raised as early as in 1988 by Robinson et al (12) and more recently by Mitchell et al. (11) and by J.P. Levy (40), the findings summarized in the present chapter indicate that it is prudent to consider the potential for development of enhancing antibodies in all vaccine preparations and trials. In principle it is possible to eliminate the gp41 epitope responsible for the development of enhancing antibodies from SIV and HIV candidate vaccines and the likely advantage of these vaccines can now be directly tested in SIV-HIV primate model systems.

5. REFERENCES

1. Füst, G. Enhancing antibodies in HIV infection. A review. Parasitology 1997; 115:S127-S140
2. Stober, H., Kacani, L., Speth, C., Würzner, R., Dierich, M.P. The supportive role of complement in HIV pathogenesis. Immunol Rev 2001;180:168-176
3. Sullivan, N.J. Antibody-mediated enhancement of viral disease. Curr Top Microbiol Immunol. 2001;260:145-169
4. Kim, H.W., Canchola, J.G., Brandt, C.D., Pyles, G., Chanock, R.M., Jensen, K., Parrott, R.H. Respiratory syncytial virus disease in infants despite prior administration of antigenic inactivated vaccine. Am J Epidemiol. 1969;89:422-434

5. Chanock, R.M., Kapikian, A.Z., Mills, J., Kim, H.W., Parrott, R.H. Influence of immunological factors in respiratory syncytial virus disease. Arch Environ Health. 1970;21:347-355
6. Halstead, S.B. Observations related to pathogensis of dengue hemorrhagic fever. VI. Hypotheses and discussion. Yale J Biol Med. 1970;42:350-362
7. Kurane, I., Innis, B.L., Nimmannitya, S., Nisalak, A., Meager, A., Janus, J., Ennis, F.A. Activation of T lymphocytes in dengue virus infections. High levels of soluble interleukin 2 receptor, soluble CD4, soluble CD8, interleukin 2, and interferon-gamma in sera of children with dengue. J Clin Invest. 1991;88:1473-1480.
8. Halstead, S.B. In vivo enhancement of dengue virus infection in rhesus monkeys by passively transferred antibody. J Infect Dis 1979;140:527-533
9. Malasit, P. Complement and dengue haemorrhagic fever/shock syndrome. Southeast Asian J Trop Med Public Health. 1987;18:316-320
10. Lin CF, Lei HY, Shiau AL, Liu CC, Liu HS, Yeh TM, Chen SH, Lin YS. Antibodies from dengue patient sera cross-react with endothelial cells and induce damage. J Med Virol. 2003;69:82-90
11. Mitchell, W.M., Ding, L., Gabriel, J. Inactivation of a common epitope responsible for the induction of antibody-dependent enhancement of HIV. AIDS, 1998;12:147-156.
12. Robinson, W.E., Montefiori, D.C., Mitchell, W.M. Antibody-dependent enhancement of human immundeficiency virus type 1 infection. Lancet 1988;1:790-794.
13. Robinson, W.E., Montefiori, D.C., Gillespie, D.H., Mitchell, W.M. Complement-mediated, antibody-dependent enhancement of HIV-1 infection in vitro is characterized by increased protein and RNA synthesis and infectious virus release. J. Acquir. Immune. Defic. Syndr. 1989; 2:33-42.
14. Prohászka, Z., Nemes, J., Hidvégi, T., Tóth, F.D., Kerekes, K., Erdei, A., Szabó, J., Thielens, N., Dierich, M.P., Spath, P., Ghebrehiwet, B., Hampl, H., Arlaud, G., Füst, G. Two parallel routes of the complement-mediated antibody-dependent enhancement of the human immunodeficiency virus type 1 infection, AIDS, 1997; 11:949-958.
15. Montefiori, D.C., Lefkowitz, L.B., Keller, R.E., Holmberg, V., Sandtstrom, E., Phairfer, J.P. and Multicenter AIDS Cohort Study: Absence of a clinical correlation for complement-mediated, infection-enhancing antibodies in plasma and sera from HIV-infected persons AIDS 1991;5:513-517.
16. Montefiori, D.C., Pantaleo, G., Fink, L.M., Zhou, J.T., Zhou, J.Y., Bilska, M., Miralles, G.D., Fauci, A.S. Neutralizing and infection-enhancing antibody responses to human immunodeficiency virus type 1 in long-term non-progressors. J. Infect. Dis.1996;173:60-67.
17. D.Tóth, F., Szabó, B., Ujhelyi, E., Pálóczi, K., Horváth, A., Füst, G., Kiss, J., Bánhegyi, D., Hollán, S.R. Neutralizing and complement-dependent enhancing antibodies in different stages of HIV infection. AIDS 1991;5:263-268.
18. Füst, G., Tóth, F.D., Kiss, J., Ujhelyi, E., Nagy, I., Bánhegyi, D. Neutralizing and enhancing antibodies measured in complement-restored serum samples from HIV-1-infected individuals correlate with immunosuppression and disease. AIDS, 1994; 8:603-609.
19. Szabó, J., Prohászka, Z., Tóth, F.D., Gyuris, Á., Segesdi, J., Bánhegyi, D., Ujhelyi, E., Minárovits, J., Füst, G. Strong correlation between the complement-mediated antibody-dependent enehancement of HIV-1 infection and plasma viral load. AIDS 1999;13:1841-1849.
20. Bánhegyi, D., Bácsi, A., Tóth, F.D., Prohászka, Z., Horváth, A., Beck, Z., Füst, G. Significant decrease of the enhancement/neutralization index in HIV patients during highly active antiretroviral therapy (HAART). Immunol Letts 2003; 89:25-30..

21. Hoffman, A.D., Banapour, B., Levy, J.A. Characterization of the AIDS-associated retrovirus reverse transcriptase and optimal conditions for its detection in virions. Virology 1985,147:326-335.
22. Lund O, Hansen J, Soorensen AM, Mosekilde E, Nielsen JO, Hansen JE. Increased adhesion as a mechanism of antibody-dependent and antibody-independent complement-mediated enhancement of human immunodeficiency virus infection. J Virol. 1995;69:2393-2400.
23. Nielsen, S.D., Moller Sorensen, A.M., Schonning, K., Lund, O., Nielsen, J.O., Hansen J-E.S. Complement-mediated enhancement of HIV-1 infection in peripheral blood mononuclear cells Scand J. Infect Dis. 1997,29: 447-452.
24. Fischer, E., Delebrias, C., Kazatchkine, M.D. Expression of CR2 (the C3dg/EBV receptor, CD21) on normal human peripheral blood lymphocytes J. Immunol. 1991, 146:865-869.
25. June, R.A., Landay, A.L., Stefanik, K., Lint, T.F., Spear, G.T. Phenotypic analysis of complement receptor 2+ T lymphocytes: reduced expression by CD4+ cells in HIV-infected persons Immunology, 1992,75: 59-65.
26. McDougall, B., Nymark, M.H., Landucci, G., Forthal, D., Robinson W.E. Jr. Predominance of detrimental humoral immune responses to HIV-1 in AIDS patients with CD4 lymphocyte counts less than 400/mm3. Scand. J. Immunol. 1997;45:103-111.
27. Subbramanian, R.A., Xu, J.M., Toma, E., Morriset, R., Cohen, E.A., Menezes, J., Ahmad, A. Comparison of human immunodeficiency virus (HIV)-specific infection-enhancing and -inhibiting antibodies in AIDS patients. J. Clin. Microbiol 2002;6:2141-2146.
28. Davis, D., Trischmann, H., Stephens, D.M., Lachmann, P.J. Antibodies raised to short synthetic peptides with sequences derived from HIV-1 SF2 gp120 can both. J Med Virol. 2001;64:207-216.
29. Binley, J.M., Trkola, A., Ketas, T., Schiller, D., Clas, B., Little, S., Richman, D., Hurley, A., Markowitz, M., Moore, J.P. The effect of highly active antiretroviral therapy on binding and neutralizing antibody responses to human immunodeficiency virus type 1 infection. J Infect Dis 2000;182:945-949.
30. Kim, J.H., Mascola, J.R., Ratto-Kim, S. VanCott, T.C., Loomis-Price, L., Cox, J.H., Michael, N,L,, Jagodzinski, L., Hawkes, C., Mayers, D., Gilliam, B.L., Birx, D.C., Robb, M.L. Selective increases in HIV-specific neutralizing antibody and partial reconstitution of cellular immune responses during prolonged, successful drug therapy of HIV infection. Selective increases in HIV-specific neutralizing antibody and partial reconstitution of cellular immune responses during prolonged, successful drug therapy of HIV infection. AIDS Res Human Retroviruses 2001;11: 2021-2034.
31. Kimura, T., Yoshimura, K., Nishihara, K., Maeda, Y., Matsumi, S., Koito, A., Matsushita, S. Reconstitution of spontaneous neutralizing antibody response against autologous human immunodeficiency virus during highly active antiretroviral therapy. J Infect Dis 2002;185:53-60.
32. Verrier, F., Moog, C., Barre-Sinoussi, F. Van der Ryst, E., Spenlehauer, C., Girard, M. Macaque immunization with virions purified from a primary isolate of the human immunodeficiency virus type 1 induced enhancement antibodies. Bull Acad Natl Med 2000;184:67-84.
33. O'Sullivan, C.E., Peng, R., Cole, K.S., Montelaro, R.C., Sturgeon, T., Jenson, H.B., Ling, P.D. Epstein-Barr virus and human immunodeficiency virus serological responses and viral burdens in HIV-infected patients treated with HAART J.Med.Virol. 2002;67:320-326.

34. Jacobson, M.A., Khayam-Bashi, H., Martin, J.N., Black, D., Ng, V. Effect of long-term highly active antiretroviral therapy in restoring HIV-induced abnormal B-lymphocyte function. J.Acquir. Immune Def. Syndr. 2002;14:472-477.
35. Montefiori, D.C., Reimann, K.A., Letvin, N,L,, Zhou, J, Hu, S,-L,: Studies of complement-activating antibodies in the SIV/macaque model of acute primary infection and vaccine protection. AIDS Res.Human Retrovir. 1995;11: 963-970.
36. Gardener, B,M,, Rosenthal, A., Jennings, M., Yee, J., Antipa, L., MacKenzie, M. Passive immunization of macaques against SIV infection J. Med .Primatol. 1994, 23:164-174.
37. Mitchell, W.M., Torres. J., Johnson, P.R., Hirsch, V., Ylma, T., Gardner, M.R., Robinson, W.E. Jr. Antibodies to the putative SIV infection-enhancing domain diminish beneficial effects of an SIV gp160 vaccine in rhesus macaques. AIDS 1995;9:27-34.
38. Keefer, M.C., Graham, B.S., Belsche, R.B., Schwartz, D., Corey, L., Bolognesi, D.P., Stablein, D.M., Montefiori, D.C., McElrath, M.J., Clenets, M.L. Studies of high doses of a human immunodeficiency virus type 1 recombinant glycoprotein 160 candidate vaccine in HIV type-1 seronegative humans. The AIDS Vaccine Clinical Trials Network. AIDS Res. Human Retrovir. 1994,10:1713-1723.
39. Lévy, J-P. AIDS Vaccine Development. Science 1998,280: 804-805.

13

Tumor Cell Resistance to Complement-Mediated Lysis

Michael Kirschfink[1] and Zvi Fishelson[2]

[1]Institute of Immunology, University of Heidelberg, Heidelberg, Germany, and [2]Department of Cell and Developmental Biology, Sackler School of Medicine, Tel Aviv University, Tel Aviv, Israel

Abstract: Complement-mediated tumor cell lysis is hampered by several protective mechanisms. Basal mechanisms of resistance are constitutively expressed in cells without a need for prior activation. These include the (over)expression of membrane-associated complement regulatory proteins, such as CD55 (DAF, Decay-Accelerating Factor), CD46 (MCP, Membrane Cofactor Protein) and CD59, on tumor cells. To generate a protective microenvironment, tumor cells secrete several soluble complement inhibitors and express on their surface ecto-proteases that degrade complement proteins or ecto-protein kinases which impair by phosphorylation the functional activity of certain complement components. Increased sialic acid expression also confers complement resistance to cancer cells and has been correlated with increased metastatic activity in certain tumors. Tumor cell protection can be also induced or augmented upon stimulation with cytokines, hormones, drugs or even with sublytic doses of complement and other pore-forming molecules. Intracellular protective pathways facilitate in cancer cells the removal of the membrane attack complexes and repair processes. Increase in cytosolic calcium ion concentration, activation of protein kinase C (PKC) and of the mitogen-activated protein kinase ERK, heat shock proteins, lipid metabolism and protein synthesis, have all been implicated in cancer cell protection from complement attack. First attempts are now being made to counteract these resistance mechanisms, including a targeted neutralisation of mCRP on tumor cells. Understanding the complex molecular mechanisms involved in basal and induced tumor cell resistance to complement is essential for development of strategies of interference with these evasion mechanisms and for effectively targeting the cytotoxic activity of the complement system to cancer cells.

Key words: cancer, complement, kinase, hsp, CD59, CD55, CD46

1.   INTRODUCTION: COMPLEMENT AND CANCER

Although complement provides a rapid and efficient mean to protect the host from invasive microorganisms (for review see: Walport, 2001a, b) its role in anti-cancer immune response remains vague and has even been questioned.

Treatment of cancer patients with microbial vaccines, dating back to the 19th century, was attempted in a hope to stimulate the immune system to arrest the malignant process. The anti-cancer effect of *Corynebacterium parvum* and *Staphylococcus aureus* protein A could be correlated with the activation of the alternative complement pathway and with macrophage infiltration (reviewed in Cooper, 1985). Although complement activation with subsequent deposition of complement components in tumor tissue has frequently been demonstrated in cancer patients (Lukas et al., 1996; Niculescu et al., 1992; Yamakawa et al., 1994; Bernet-Camard et al., 1996; Niehans et al., 1996), its role as the principal factor behind positive anti-cancer effects was not clearly shown. In clinical studies, complement levels were often found normal or even elevated in patients with various hematological neoplasia (Southam et al., 1966; Batlle Fonrodona et al., 1979; Minh et al., 1983), with neuroblastoma (Carli et al., 1979) or lung (Nishioka et al., 1976; Gminski et al., 1992), digestive tract (Maness and Orengo, 1977) and brain (Matsutani et al., 1984) tumors. Reduced CH50 and C3 (but not C4) were observed in individuals suffering from breast, gastric and colon-rectum carcinomas (Mangano et al., 1984). Classical pathway activation was assumed to be involved in the immune response against chronic lymphatic leukemia (CLL) in patients presenting low serum levels of several complement proteins and increased concentrations of circulating C1r-C1s-C1inhibitor complexes (Füst et al 1987; Hidvegi et al., 1989; Schlesinger et al., 1996). It can not be excluded that the complement system in those cancer patients was activated indirectly by immune complexes, infectious agents or substances generated within a tumor mass.

Certain tumor cell lines can activate, to some degree, complement in vitro. Oat cell carcinoma (Okada and Baba, 1974), EBV-transformed B cell lymphoma (Mc Connell et al., 1978) and Raji B lymphoblastoid cells (Budzko et al., 1976; Theofilopoulos and Perrin, 1976) are capable of activating the alternative human complement pathway in the absence of antibodies. Treatment with INFγ or TNFα led to increased C3 deposition on B lymphoblastoid cells (Yefenof et al., 1991). Pretreatment with the metabolic inhibitor puromycin accelerated Raji cell lysis (Baker et al., 1977; Schreiber et al., 1980).

Complement activation and lysis of tumor cells by homologous complement gets more effective after sensitization with potent complement-fixing antibodies and by inhibiting various metabolic processes within the tumor cells. Complement-associated anti-tumor effects of mouse monoclonal antibodies (mAb) have been observed in nude mice growing human tumors (Capone et al., 1983; Chapman et al., 1990).

As transformation to malignancy may be accompanied by an increased capacity of the cells to activate complement, it is conceivable, that cancer cells have developed means to resist complement attack in order to survive in vivo. Most of the resistant mechanisms are probably also utilized by normal tissues to resist accidental cell damage following local activation of complement.

There is a growing body of evidence indicating that resistance of tumor cells to complement-mediated lysis depends on extracellular as well as on intracellular factors (reviewed in Jurianz et al., 1999b, Fishelson et al., 2003). Extracellular protection, interfering with the cascade of complement activation at specific points or directly affecting activated complement proteins limits the quantity of components deposited on the surface of target cells. However, as we now begin to understand, resistance mechanisms also extend to intracellular pathways, which lead to the reduction of MAC-induced damage, eliminate the MAC from the cell surface and facilitate repair processes. Perhaps the best example is the elimination of the MAC from the plasma membrane by endocytosis and by vesiculation, a phenomenon which was observed in neutrophils (Campbell and Morgan, 1985), oligodendrocytes (Scolding et al., 1989) and platelets (Sims and Wiedmer, 1986), but also in Ehrlich ascites tumor cells (Carney et al., 1985), U937 and K562 cells (Morgan, 1992).

Finally, additional resistance mechanisms are induced upon stimulation of cells with cytokines, hormones, drugs, or even with sublytic doses of C5b-9 complexes and other pore-formers. As will be discussed below, blocking one or more of the protective mechanisms is required to amplify a weak spontaneous process of complement activation into an efficient lytic complement attack on homologous tumor cells.

2. EXTRACELLULAR MECHANISMS OF COMPLEMENT RESISTANCE IN TUMOR CELLS

The initial encounter of cancer cells with complement proteins occurs at their outer surface and the intensity of the attack determines its outcome. The more C3b and C5b-9 molecules are deposited at the cell surface per minute, the more severe is the damage and the lower is the capacity of the cell to survive. Nucleated cells, and particularly cancer cells, resist lysis by complement up to a threshold level of damage which is still not defined (Koski et al. 1983; Morgan, 1989). Initially, they use as shields a variety of extracellular protecting molecules that are described in this section. Once damage is inflicted to the cells, they resort to intracellular repair and support mechanisms that are described in the following section.

2.1   Utilization of Membrane Complement Regulatory Proteins (mCRP)

Like all normal cells, neoplastic cells are protected from autologous complement attack by several cell-surface complement inhibitors, such as CD35 (complement receptor type 1, CR1), CD55 (decay accelerating factor, DAF), CD46 (membrane cofactor protein, MCP) and CD59 (Protectin) (Morgan and Harris, 1999, chapters 7 and 8 in this volume).

From numerous studies which have been performed in primary tumors and in tumor cell lines it is evident that almost all cancers studied express at least one of the mCRPs and many express CD46, CD55 and CD59. Major findings are summarised in Table 1.

Table 1. Expression of CD46, CD55 and CD59 in primary tumors and tumor cell lines.

Tumor	Primary tumor	Cell line	References**
Leukemia	CD46↑/+* CD55↑/++/+ CD59↑/+/± CD55: AML ↓ ALL ↓	CD46↑/+ CD55↑/++/+ CD59↑/+/±	52, 15, 24, 25, 23, 20, 34 23
Lymphoma	CD46+, CD55+ CD59+ CD55: NHL-/±	CD46+, CD55+/± CD59+/± CD59-	15, 24, 39, 38, 53, 19, 20, 58 39, 53
Glioblastoma		CD46+ CD55+, CD59++	33
Neuroblastoma		CD46+/±, CD55+/± CD59+/± CD55-	16, 11 12, 16
Malignant glioma	CD46±, CD55± CD59++	CD46+, CD55± CD59++	42
Thyroid carcinoma	CD46++, CD55+ CD59++		61

Tumor	Primary tumor	Cell line	References**
Prostate carcinoma	CD59++/±	CD46+, CD55+ CD59++/+	31, 14
Breast carcinoma	CD46↑/+ CD55+ CD59++/± CD55-	CD46++/+/± CD55+/±, CD59++/+ CD55-	12, 27, 46, 57, 62, 14 27, 46, 57
Ovarian carcinoma	CD46++ CD55±, CD59++	CD46↑/++/+ CD55+/±, CD59++/+	5, 47, 14
Lung carcinoma	CD46↑/+ CD55↑+ CD59↑/+ CD55-	CD46↑+/+ CD55↑/+, CD59↑/+ CD55-	49, 59, 46 46, 12
Colorectal carcinoma	CD46++/+ CD55↑/± CD59↑/+/± CD46↓, CD55- CD59↓/-	CD46++/+/± CD55↑/++/+/± CD59++/±	2, 37, 38, 3 4, 29, 44, 46 32, 57, 51 28, 41, 45 1, 18 29, 46, 57, 51
Pancreatic carcinoma	CD46++ CD55± CD59↑/+	CD46++/+ CD55++/± CD59++/±	32, 51, 13
Gastric carcinoma	CD46++/+ CD55↑/+ CD59↑/++ CD55-, CD59-	CD46++/+ CD55↑/±, CD59++/±	32, 43, 51, 26, 41, 36 44, 32, 51, 30, 36
Renal carcinoma	CD46± CD55↑/+ CD59↑/± CD46↓, CD55-	CD46+, CD55+ CD59+	56, 21, 46, 6 46, 6
Oral squamous carcinoma		CD46+, CD55+ CD59++	48
Skin carcinoma	CD46+, CD55± CD59+		50
Cervical carcinoma	CD46↑, CD55± CD59±	CD46↑, CD59↑	54, 17

Tumor	Primary tumor	Cell line	References**
Hepatoma	CD46↑	CD46+, CD55+, CD59++	35, 55
Melanoma	CD46+/± CD55+/± CD59+ CD55-	CD46+, CD55+/± CD59++/+/± CD55-, CD59-	8, 9, 10, 22, 7, 60 8, 12, 60
Osteosarcoma		CD46++, CD55++ CD59++	41

*Level of mCRP expression: -, no; ±, low; +, moderate; ++, high; ↓, expression in tumor lower than in normal tissue; ↑, expression in tumor higher than in normal tissue.

** (1) Andoh et al., 2002, (2) Andrew et al., 1990, (3) Bjorge et al., 1994, (4) Bjorge et al., 1996, (5) Bjorge et al., 1997, (6) Blok et al., 2000, (7) Blom et al., 1997, (8) Brasoveanu et al., 1995, (9) Brasoveanu et al., 1996, (10) Brasoveanu et al., 1997, (11) Chen et al., 2000b, (12) Cheung et al., 1988, (13) Crnogorac-Jurcevic et al., 2002, (14) Donin et al., 2003, (15) Fukuda et al., 1991, (16) Gasque et al., 1996, (17) Gelderman et al., 2002a, (18) Gelderman et al., 2002b, (19) Golay et al., 2000, (20) Golay et al., 2001, (21) Gorter et al., 1996, (22) Goslings et al., 1996, (23) Guc et al., 2000, (24) Hara et al., 1992a, (25) Hara et al., 1995, (26) Hensel et al., 2001, (27) Hofman et al., 1994, (28) Hosch et al., 2001, (29) Inoue et al., 1994, (30) Inoue et al., 2002, (31) Jarvis et al., 1997, (32) Juhl et al., 1997 (33) Junnikkala et al., 2000, (34) Jurianz et al., 2001, (35) Kinugasa et al., 1999, (36) Kiso et al., 2002, (37) Koretz et al., 1992, (38) Koretz et al., 1993, (39) Kuraya et al., 1992, (40) Kuraya et al., 1993, (41) Li et al., 2001, (42) Maenpaa et al., 1996, (43) Mikami et al., 1998, (44) Mizuno et al., 1995, (45) Nakagawa et al., 2001, (46) Niehans et al., 1996, (47) Peng et al., 2002, (48) Ravindranath et al., 2000, (49) Sakuma et al., 1993, (50) Sayama et al., 1992, (51) Schmitt et al., 1999, (52) Seya et al., 1990, (53) Seya et al., 1994, (54) Simpson et al., 1997, (55) Spiller et al., 2000, (56) Terachi et al., 1991, (57) Thorsteinsson et al., 1998, (58) Treon et al., 2001, (59) Varsano et al., 1995, 1998, (60) Weichenthal et al., 1999, (61) Yamakawa et al., 1994, (62) Yu et al., 1999.

CD35 has only been identified on follicular dendritic cell tumors (Perez-Ordonez and Rosai, 1998), malignant endometrial tissue (Murray et al., 2000) and on leukemic blasts (Guc et al., 2000).

Immunohistochemical analysis of several human tumor tissues revealed the presence of CD59, CD55 and CD46 on uveal melanoma (Goslings et al., 1996), thyroid carcinoma (Yamakawa et al., 1994), lung and kidney cancer (Niehans et al., 1996; Terachi et al., 1991), colon adenocarcinoma (Bjørge et al., 1994) and prostate cancer (Jarvis et al., 1997). Often more detailed information has been achieved by in vitro analysis of human tumor cell lines derived from human malignant gastrointestinal tumors (Juhl et al., 1997), melanoma (Brasoveanu et al., 1995), breast cancer (Thorsteinsson et al., 1998), renal tumor (Gorter et al., 1996), Burkitt lymphoma (Kuraya et al.,

1992), neuroblastoma (Gasque et al., 1996b), ovarian (Bjørge et al., 1997; Ziegler et al., 1999) and prostate carcinoma (Donin et al., 2003). Levels of mCRP expression on malignant cells are very heterogeneous, even within the same tissues and between studies of the same tumor. A marked variation in mCRP expressions was seen among cases of breast or renal cell carcinomas (Niehans et al., 1996), which could not be correlated with complement activation and MAC deposition. In primary uterine cervix tissue the expression of CD46, but not of CD55, was found to increase during transition from normal to premalignant to malignant cells (Simpson et al., 1997). Brasoveanu et al. (1996) studied 9 melanoma cell lines with a large heterogeneity in CD59 expression where CD59 level correlated with resistance to killing by anti-ganglioside mAb and homologous complement. In samples of 16 metastatic melanoma lesions, Weichenthal et al. (1999) observed that 9 expressed both CD46 and CD59, 2 had CD59 only, 1 had CD46 only and 4 had neither CD46 nor CD59.

An increasing number of reports point, however, to an increased mCRP expression in tumors relative to the corresponding normal tissue (Bjørge et al., 1994, Hofman et al., 1994, Niehans et al., 1996, Simpson et al., 1997, Varsano et al., 1995, 1998a, Blok et al., 2000, Murray et al., 2000, Nakagawa et al., 2001, Nowicki et al., 2001). Li et al. (2001) examined colorectal and gastric carcinomas and osteosarcoma and found increased expression of CD55, whereas Kiso et al. (2002) found high levels of both CD55 and CD59 in intestinal type gastric carcinoma. Overexpression of CD59 was also identified by expression profiling for pancreatic cancer (Crnogorac-Jurcevic et al., 2002). Focal or complete loss of CD59 was recognised in malignant cells of low differentiation or on carcinomas which had already metastasised at the time of surgery (Koretz et al., 1993).

Upregulation of mCRP expression on tumor cells often correlates with increased complement resistance (Bjørge and Matre, 1995; Jurianz et al., 1999a; Kuraya et al., 1992, Gorter and Meri, 1999). In ovarian cancer, resistance to complement correlated with the level of CD55 expression (Bjørge et al., 1997). In a recent study on 136 colorectal cancer patients, 7-years survival was significantly reduced if tumors expressed high levels of CD55 (Durrant et al., 2003).

Today, we still can only speculate on mechanisms behind the variability in expression of mCRP on tumor cells. The level of expression of each mCRP may reflect a stage in differentiation of specific tumor cells. Thus, poorly differentiated colorectal carcinoma cells expressed low or no CD59, whereas differentiated carcinoma cells expressed higher CD59 levels (Koretz et al., 1993). Similarly, differentiated gastric carcinoma strongly expressed CD59 on the luminal membrane, whereas in undifferentiated tumors, CD59 was almost absent (Inoue et al., 2002). In the latter study, both differentiated and undifferentiated gastric carcinomas had higher CD55 expression than the corresponding normal cell. Loss of CD59 correlated with poor survival in 520 breast cancer patients. From this study the conclusion was drawn that reduced CD59 may offer a selective advantage for the tumor to develop into more aggressive forms (Madjd et al., 2003). Alternatively, killing or opsonization by complement could have selected for the high mCRP expressors. There is compelling underlying evidence that expression of mCRPs may be influenced by host factors, such as cytokines, growth factors or hormones which are released by neighbouring tumor or stromal cells. For example, TNFα and IL-1ß enhanced expression of CD55 and CD59 in colon adenocarcinoma cells (Bjørge et al., 1995). TNFα, IL-1α and INFγ enhanced CD55 expression on lung cancer cell lines (Varsano et al., 1998b). In hepatoma cells TNFα, IL-1ß and IL-6 have been shown to increase in vitro expression of CD55 and CD59 but to decrease CD46 expression (Spiller et al., 2000). Anoxic conditions may also affect tumor-complement interaction in situ by reducing the expression level of CD59 (Vakeva and Meri, 1998). In addition, a variety of gene or transcription abnormalities may lead to modified expression of mCRPs (Hatanaka et al., 1996).

The potency of CD59 as protector from complement-mediated killing has been convincingly demonstrated by overexpression experiments. Rat CD59 cDNA transfected into human neuroblastoma cells conferred on them resistance to killing by rat complement. Furthermore, the rat CD59 positive tumor cells grew faster in immune-deficient rats as compared to nontransfected controls (Chen et al., 2000a). Similarly, overexpression of CD59 in melanoma cells by infection with a retroviral vector carrying CD59 cDNA, conferred on them resistance to killing by anti-GD3 mAb and complement (Coral et al., 2000). There is still a great lack of knowledge on the possible impact of chemotherapeutic agents on mCRP expression. 5-azacytidine was shown to increase the levels of CD55 and CD59 on Burkitt lymphoma cell lines (Kuraya et al., 1992) but only of CD59 on melanoma cells. In contrast, levamisole reduces CD59 levels on colon adenocarcinoma cell lines (Bjørge and Matre, 1995).

Variability exists in the complement sensitivity of drug resistant tumor cells. Multiple drug resistance (MDR) of malignant cells is often mediated by the ATP-dependent efflux protein P-glycoprotein which is considered a major obstacle to successfull cancer treatment. Doxorubicin-resistant human colon carcinoma cells were more sensitive to complement than doxorubicin-sensitive cells (Gambacorti-Passerini et al., 1988). Investigations with a multidrug resistant variant of a human oral carcinoma cell line revealed a higher susceptibility to complement lysis than the corresponding parental KB-3-1 tumor cells (Bomstein and Fishelson, 1997). The increased complement sensitivity was associated with a reduced expression of CD55. Treatment of the P-glycoprotein overexpressing tumor cells with anti-P-glycoprotein mAbs reduced their sensitivity to complement. Weisburg et al. identified a P-glycoprotein overexpressing variant of the HL60 myeloid leukemia cell line which presented an increased resistance to complement-mediated cytotoxicity. Here, complement resistance could be reversed both by treatment with verapamil and with specific mAbs that bind to and block P-glycoprotein function (Weisburg et al., 1996). Analysing ovarian carcinoma cells, we also found MDR resistance to be associated with complement resistance, directly correlating with mCRP overexpression (Odening et al., 2001). Preliminary results of transfection experiments indicate that complement resistance is P-glycoprotein-independent (Odening et al., manuscript in preparation), as was also suggested by Johnstone et al. (2001). Based on a comparative analysis, it was concluded that P-glycoprotein does not affect cell lysis induced by several pore-forming molecules (Johnstone et al., 2001). At present, the data indicate that sensitivity of MDR tumor cells to complement-mediated lysis may be increased, reduced or unaffected, depending on the cell type analysed. The possible involvement of the P-glycoprotein, directly or indirectly, in the interaction of MDR tumor cells with complement requires further investigation.

2.2 Secretion of Soluble Complement Regulatory Proteins

Soluble complement inhibitors are released by hepatocytes and macrophages and also by other tissues, although in considerable smaller amounts. Secreted inhibitors may contribute to protection of tumor cell from complement attack. Indeed, a growing number of reports indicate that cancer cells of various origins secrete one or more complement inhibitor, in addition to other molecules not yet defined as conventional complement inhibitors, such as chondroitin sulfate proteoglycans.

Synthesis of C1 Inhibitor has been described for astroglioma, neuroblastoma (Gasque et al., 1995, 1996b), rhabdomyosarcoma (Gasque et al., 1996a) breast cancer cell lines, and a primary ovarian carcinoma cell line (Ziegler et al., 1999). Stimulation with IFNγ enhanced the secretion of C1 inhibitor, whereas TNFα and IL-1β had a weak or no effect on glioma cells (Gasque et al., 1993). On ovarian carcinoma cells IFNγ and TGFß augmented C1 Inhibitor secretion, whereas IL-4, IL-6 and PMA had no effect (Ziegler et al., 1999).

High pre-operative levels of C1 Inhibitor were seen in patients exhibiting early cancer recurrence (Goransson et al., 1996). In contrast, low plasma levels of functionally active C1 Inhibitor due to the presence of blocking autoantibodies are occasionally observed in patients with proliferative disorders, who eventually develop life-threatening angioedema, termed type I acquired angioedema (Alsenz et al., 1987). These autoantibodies were found to promote proteolytic cleavage of the regulator (Cicardi et al., 1996).

Factor H (fH) was coexpressed with fI by glioma and rhabdomyosarcoma cells in its plasma form (155 kDa) and in a truncated form of lower MW (Gasque et al., 1992; Legoedec et al., 1995). In glioma cells, IFNγ as well as TNFα transiently increased the secretion of fH, whereas IL-6 and IL-1β had no significant effects (Gasque et al., 1992). Similar effects were seen in neuroblastoma and myosarcoma cell lines (Legoedec et al., 1995; Gasque et al., 1996b). High levels of fH and factor H like protein-1 (fHL-1/reconectin) are secreted by certain ovarian tumor cells (Ziegler et al., 2001, Junnikkala et al., 2002) and appear to be under the regulation of IFNγ and TGFß. Various tissues, including tumor cells, exert a certain affinity to fluid phase fH which in the past had raised the question of the existance of a specific fH receptor. By secretion and binding to synovial fibroblasts, these regulators seem to confer protection against complement in rheumatoid arthritis (Friese et al. 2003). On a H2 glioblastoma line surface bound fH/fHL-1 significantly contributed to complement resistance (Junnikkala et al., 2000). For various other tumor cells in which we observed fH binding (Ziegler et al., 2001), its protective function remains to be clarified. Increased plasma levels of fH were also found in patients suffering from various urogenital tumors (Kirschfink, unpublished data). Factor H-related protein, produced by several bladder cancer cell lines has been suggested as a useful cancer marker (Kinders et al., 1998; Thomas et al., 1999).

Factor I (fI) was detected in the supernatant of ovarian carcinoma cells (Ziegler et al., 1999), as well as on myeloblasts and rhabdomyosarcoma cells (Legoedec et al., 1995).

Clusterin is expressed in various tissues and is upregulated in response to cell injury. It has been suggested that expression of clusterin may be associated with cell survival within tissues undergoing apoptosis (French et al., 1994). Clusterin and S-protein (vitronectin) were found to be also expressed in astroglioma and neuroblastoma cell lines (Gasque et al., 1995; Gasque et al., 1996b), and their secretion rate could be enhanced by IFNγ and TNFα. A possible protective effect remains to be shown.

Soluble forms of the mCRPs have been identified in most body fluids, even under normal conditions. They are either produced by alternative splicing or released from the cell surface through enzymatic cleavage. They often resemble their respective membrane forms with regard to molecular size and functional properties.

Soluble CD55 (sCD55) was found in urine (Medof et al., 1987, Nakano et al., 1991), plasma, synovial fluid, saliva and cerebrospinal fluid (Medof et al., 1987). Soluble CD59 was identified in urine (Davies et al., 1989) and amniotic fluid (Rooney and Morgan, 1992). Sera of cancer patients contain active, soluble forms of CD46 (Seya et al., 1995). Elevated CD55 concentration in stool specimens has been proposed to have a diagnostic value for patients with colorectal cancer (Mizuno et al., 1995; Iwagaki et al., 2002). Brasoveanu et al. (1997) observed the constitutive release of sCD59 from human melanoma cells which retained its activity as well as its GPI-anchor. In primary tumor sections CD55 and/or CD59 were found in the stroma of breast, colorectal, lung, renal and cervical carcinomas (Niehans et al., 1996; Li et al., 2001; Gelderman et al., 2002a,b). In vitro, endothelial cells, HeLa cells (Hindmarsh and Marks, 1998), osteosarcoma and colorectal cells (Nasu et al., 1998; Li et al., 2001) release CD55 in a soluble form or deposit it into their extracellular matrix. K562 erythroleukemia cells secrete sCD59 (Jurianz et al., 2001) as also observed for breast, ovarian and prostate carcinoma cell lines (Donin et al., 2003). Elevated plasma levels of sCR1 have been found in patients suffering from various forms of leukemia (Sadallah et al., 1999). Taken together, soluble complement regulators, secreted into the microenvironment and partly binding to the tumor cell are considered to add to the regulatory capacity of mCRP (Junnikkala et al., 2002).

In addition to well known specific complement inhibitors certain tumors may secrete molecules which protect them from complement attack. We characterized a species of chondroitin sulfate proteoglycans (CSPG) secreted by malignant human B lymphocytes which closely resembles in their structure the serum-derived C1q inhibitor (Kirschfink et al., 1997). These proteoglycans have in common a molecular mass of approx. 150 to 170 kDa with a core protein of 30 kDa released after chondroitinase ABC treatment. CSPG purified from culture supernatants of three malignant human B cell lines strongly bound to C1q. They specifically inhibited the hemolytic activity of C1q and blocked C1q receptor binding in a dose-dependent manner.

2.3   Degradation of Complement Proteins with Proteases

Cancer cells and neighbouring cells express on their surface and release into the extracellular space various proteases, including serine-, cystein- and metalloproteinases. Proteases have been shown to contribute to tumor initiation, growth, migration, extravasation, invasion, angiogenesis and to host immune evasion (reviewed in: Del Rosso et al., 2002; Krepela 2001; Lynch and Matrisian, 2002; Yoon et al., 2003). Several studies have demonstrated that such proteases can also cleave complement components and, thus, inhibit complement activation (Ollert et al., 1990; Jean et al., 1995, 1996). Best studied is the degradation of C3, a key protein in the complement cascade, by tumor proteases. Human melanoma cells contain a C3-cleaving serine protease, p65, that rapidly degrades surface deposited C3b and is mostly expressed on the surface of melanoma cell lines resistant to complement-mediated lysis (Ollert et al., 1990). Blocking studies revealed that p65 contributed to resistance of melanoma cells to human complement. A C3-cleaving cysteine protease related to procathepsin-L, p39, was also identified on the membrane and in conditioned medium of murine melanoma cells (Jean et al., 1995). Inhibition of p39 with specific antibodies caused increased susceptibility of murine melanoma cells to complement lysis. A human cystein protease, antigenically related to murine p39 and to human procathepsin-L, was purified from a highly metastatic human melanoma cell line (Jean et al., 1996). Preincubation of melanoma cells with anti-p39 not only reduced their complement resistance but also completely abolished their tumorigenicity and reduced their metastatic potential (Jean et al., 1996). In addition, transfection of procathepsin-L into non-metastatic melanoma cells, increases their tumorigenicity and makes them highly metastatic (Frade et al., 1998). Such transfectants are also highly resistant to complement-mediated lysis. Procathepsin-L was also found to be secreted by human non-small lung cancer cell lines (Heidtmann et al., 1993). Its expression directly correlated with the progression of human gliomas (Sivaparvathi et al., 1996) and colorectal carcinomas (Adenis et al., 1995). A C3-cleaving serine protease activity was also identified on the surface of U937 cells and shown to contain cathepsin-G and elastase (Maison et al., 1991). By cleaving C3 and its activated forms (C3b, iC3b, or C3d), proteases may protect tumor cells from direct complement lysis as well as from leukocyte and lymphocyte responses triggered via opsonising C3 fragments. The expression of membrane serine proteases on K562 erythroleukemia cells appears also to contribute to their complement resistance (Jurianz et al., 1999). Membrane extracts of complement resistant K562 cells express a higher proteolytic activity than those of a sensitive K562/S variant. Furthermore, treatment of K562 cells with serine protease inhibitors markedly enhances their sensitivity to complement-mediated lysis. Thus, the expression of ecto-proteases cleaving C3 and probably also other complement components could be one of the multiple mechanisms enabling tumor cells to escape immune surveillance.

2.4   Inhibition of Complement Activation by Sialic Acid

Increased expression of sialic acid on cell surface glycoconjugates, enhanced sialyl transferase activity or reduced sialidase have been reported in cancer cells and were shown to correlate with enhanced adhesion and metastasis (Yogeeswaran and Salk, 1981; Lin et al., 2002; Sawada et al., 2002; Drinnan et al., 2003). Removal of sialic acid from the cell surface with sialidase/neuraminidase (NA) has been shown to confer on certain cell types increased sensitivity to complement-mediated lysis. Thus, removal of sialic acid from red blood cells (Lauf 1975; Pangburn and Muller-Eberhard, 1978), rabbit lymph node cells (Ray and Sundaram, 1975), murine sarcoma cells (Turianskyj and Gyenes, 1976), human bladder carcinoma cells (Jacobsen, 1982), *Trypanosoma cruzi* trypomastigotes (Kipnis et al., 1981), *Neisseria meningitides* (Jarvis and Vedros, 1987) and *N. gonorrhoeae* (Ram et al., 1998), sensitized them to lysis by complement. Recently, we have revisited this issue and demonstrated that human prostate, breast and ovarian carcinoma cells also utilize sialic acid residues on their surface for protection from complement (Donin et al., 2003). Clearly, high sialic acid expression correlates with lower complement activation. Inactivation of C3b by Factors H and I occurs more efficiently on surfaces of cells that are rich in sialic acid (Pangburn and Muller-Eberhard, 1978; Kazatchkine et al., 1984; Meri and Pangburn, 1990). Therefore, following removal of sialic acid with NA, carcinoma cells probably deposit more C3b molecules and this, in turn, leads to enhanced activation of the terminal complement pathway and increased cell killing. The fact that lysis of NA-treated cells depends more on factor B than lysis of control cells (Donin et al., 2003) indicates that NA-treated cells activate better the alternative complement pathway. Involvement of the lectin complement pathway in lysis of NA-treated cells was ruled out by data showing no significant effect of 3F8 anti-MBL blocking antibodies on cell lysis (Donin et al., 2003). Interestingly, lysis of control carcinoma cells in presence of MgEGTA or of the 3F8 anti-MBL mAb was reduced by 30-40% or 12-18%, respectively (Donin et al., 2003). Hence, it appears that the alternative, lectin and classical initiation pathways cooperate in lysis of untreated carcinoma cells by antibody and complement. However, upon removal of sialic acid, the carcinoma cells appear to activate primarily the alternative and classical complement pathways (Figure 1).

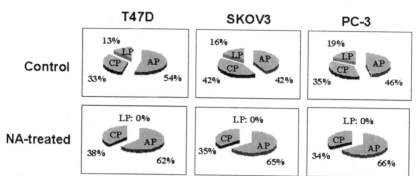

Figure 1. Pathways of complement activation by human carcinoma cell lines. Control and neuraminidase (NA)-treated cells were killed by antibody and human complement in presence of inhibitors of the classical (CP), lectin (LP) or alternative (AP) complement pathway. Data is presented in Donin et al. (2003).

It is possible that the capacity of MBL to bind to carcinoma cells or to activate the lectin pathway is controlled in a negative or positive manner by sialic acid residues.

2.5   Phosphorylation of Complement Proteins with Ecto-Protein Kinases

Ecto-protein kinases (ecto-PK) are extracellular membrane-anchored protein kinases, which have been found on the surface of many cell types. They contain an extracellular catalytic unit which utilizes extracellular ATP, present in sufficient quantities in blood plasma and probably also in other body fluids (Gordon, 1986). Ecto-PK activity is abundant on the surface of human leukemia cell lines K562, U937, HL-60 and Jurkat and carcinoma cell lines BT-474 and SKOV-3 (Paas and Fishelson, 1995; Paas et al., 1999).

Two types of ecto-PK were described, a Ser/Thr- and a Tyr-kinase. The Ser/Thr-ecto-PK has been shown to phosphorylate several exogenous substrates, including the complement C9 protein, an essential component of the terminal complement system. The C9 ecto-PK appears to be casein kinase 2 (Bohana-Kashtan et al. 1998). Phosphorylated C9 has reduced hemolytic activity and is unable to undergo Zn^{++}-induced polymerisation (Paas et al., 1999 and Bohana-Kashtan and Fishelson, unpublished). Ecto-PK is spontaneously shed from the tumor cells and can efficiently phosphorylate C9 (Paas et al., 1999). The phosphorylation site is located in the C9a fragment (Paas et al., 1999) which is involved in the interaction of the unfolded C9 with the preformed C5b-8 complex and in the formation of the MAC (Stanley et al., 1986). Based on the latter finding and the finding that unfolded C9 (by reduction/alkylation) is phosphorylated by the C9 ecto-PK much better than native C9, it was proposed (Paas et al., 1999) that phosphorylation of C9 by the ecto-PK occurs primarily during complement activation and protects tumor cells from complement, either by inhibiting MAC formation or by leading to the production of an inactive or unstable MAC. Ecto-PK of human leukemia cells (Nilsson Ekdahl and Nilsson, 1997; Paas and Fishelson, 1995) and extracellular PK released from activated platelets (Ekdahl and Nilsson, 1995) phosphorylate C3 at various sites and modulate different C3 activities. It is conceivable that phosphorylation of C3, C9 and other complement proteins by protein kinases present in the extracellular space, in a membrane-attached or soluble form, has a substantial impact on activation and regulation of complement functions. In the context of this chapter, extracellular phosphorylation may serve to assist cancer cells in complement evasion.

3. INTRACELLULAR PATHWAYS INVOLVED IN COMPLEMENT RESISTANCE

Intracellular protective mechanisms reduce the extent of damage inflicted to tumor cells by the MAC, facilitate repair processes and remove the MAC from the cell surface. These mechanisms are poorly defined, yet the following molecules appear to be involved in protection: 1. intracellular calcium ions (Morgan and Campbell, 1985), 2. cyclic AMP (Kaliner and Austen, 1974; Boyle et al., 1976) and PKA (Donin et al., 2003) 3. protein kinase C (Kraus and Fishelson, 2000), 4. mitogen-activated protein kinase ERK (Kraus et al., 2001), 5. heat-shock proteins 70 (Fishelson et al., 2001) and 90 (Sreedhar et al. 2003), and 6. Bcl-2 (Contreras et al., 2002; Attali and Fishelson, submitted for publication). In addition, active protein synthesis (Baker et al., 1977; Ohanian and Schlager, 1981) and membrane lipid metabolism (Papadimitriou et al., 1991) were shown to be required for survival under MAC attack.

In addition to their basal resistance, cancer cells can enhance their level of complement resistance in response to various stimuli. Thus, resistance to complement attack is markedly increased in cells treated for 30-50 minutes with a sublytic dose of the membrane attack complex (MAC) (Reiter et al., 1992). The insertion of a sublytic number of MAC into cell membranes causes a variety of biological responses (reviewed in Morgan, 1992), such as the release of reactive oxygen metabolites, secretion of proinflammatory mediators, such as IL-8 and MCP-1 (Kilgore et al., 1996, 1997), entry into cell cycle (Rus et al., 1996), resistance to apoptosis (Rus et al., 1996), expression of adhesion molecules (Kilgore et al., 1995; Tedesco et al., 1997) and synthesis of eicosanoides (Stahl et al., 1987; Weise et al., 1993). In addition, sublytic complement attack has been demonstrated to activate G-proteins in tumor cells (Niculescu et al., 1994) and to induce also the generation of diacylglycerol (DAG) and ceramide (Niculescu et al., 1993). The possible involvement of the latter agents in tumor cell resistance to complement still awaits clarification. The effect of sublytic MAC on increased refractoriness of the cells is transient and disappears after 8-12 hours, and is not associated with an impaired binding of antibodies or complement proteins to the cell. This phenomenon was named "complement-induced protection" and was shown to require complete MAC formation, protein and RNA synthesis and free extracellular Ca^{2+}. Tumor cells (K562) become also protected from complement lysis after treatment with the pore forming molecules perforin, mellitin and streptolysin O (Reiter et al., 1995). Sublytic complement confers on K562 cells protection also from perforin-induced lysis (Reiter et al., 1995). Transition into a stage of higher resistance requires Ca^{2+} influx, activation of cytoplasmic PKC and of MAPK as well as protein synthesis (Kraus and Fishelson, 2000; Kraus et al., 2001). Blockade of RNA and protein synthesis in tumor cells also enhances their sensitivity to complement and inhibits their capacity to undergo induced protection (Schlager et al., 1977 ; Reiter and Fishelson, 1992). This suggests that certain proteins synthesized in cells subjected to complement attack may assist in damage repair and in resistance to lysis. Cells attacked by sublytic MAC upregulate synthesis of certain proteins and downregulate synthesis of others. Which of the induced proteins contributes to cell resistance to complement is currently under investigations.

3.1   Calcium Ions in Killing and Defense

The intracellular calcium ion concentration increases dramatically within seconds after MAC formation on nucleated cells (Campbell et al., 1979). Cytosolic calcium concentrations ($[Ca^{2+}]_i$) rise due to entry of extracellular calcium as well as its release from intracellular stores (Morgan and Campbell, 1985). Whether calcium ions enter the target cell via the MAC or through another channel is still not clear. Furthermore, although it is clear that a rise in $[Ca^{2+}]_i$ induced by complement MAC (Morgan et al. 1986) or by other membrane-active toxins (Schanne et al. 1979) is toxic to cells (Trump and Berezesky, 1995), there is no strong evidence for the direct involvement of calcium ions in killing by complement, beyond the initial steps of complement activation. At high MAC doses, increasing the extracellular concentration of calcium ions increases the rate of cell lysis (Kim et al. 1987). In contrast, at low MAC doses or with relatively small lesions, excess extracellular Ca^{2+} reduces leakage through preformed complement lesions (Micklem et al. 1988). Treatment of K562 cells with a high concentration of calcium ionophores causes toxicity, whereas low concentrations are protective from death (Kraus et al. 2000). It is well accepted that an increase in $[Ca^{2+}]_i$ induced by sublytic complement is essential for its numerous stimulatory effects (reviewed in Morgan, 1992). If the rise in $[Ca^{2+}]_i$ is inhibited by removing or lowering $[Ca^{2+}]_o$, elimination of the MAC from the cell surface is slowed down (Carney et al. 1986; Morgan, 1992) and sublytic MAC is unable to induce enhanced complement resistance (Reiter et al., 1992), indicating that raised $[Ca^{2+}]_i$ is protective against complement-mediated lysis. The fact that removal of $[Ca^{2+}]_o$ and chelation of free $[Ca^{2+}]_i$ were found to reduce removal of the terminal complement complexes by vesiculation or endocytosis and to increase the susceptibility of Ehrlich ascites tumor cells to lysis by MAC (Carney et al. 1986), suggested a relationship between the $[Ca^{2+}]_i$, the elimination process and complement resistance. Calcium entry required for induction of protection by sublytic MAC occurs within 90 seconds; thereafter, its blocking has no effect on the induced protection, even though a complete protection develops only after 30-60 minutes (Fishelson and Reiter, unpublished). It is likely that at least one of the functions of $[Ca^{2+}]_i$ is to activate protein kinase C, which, as discussed below, plays a role in protection of tumor cells from lysis (Kraus et al. 2000). Another potential co-factor for PKC activation is diacylglycerol that is also produced in cells treated with sublytic MAC doses (Niculsecu et al. 1993, Cybulsky and Cyr, 1993).

3.2   Defensive Protein Kinase Cascades

The importance of protein phosphorylation cascades to rescue of cancer cells from complement-mediated lysis was suggested already in 1988 (Fishelson et al., 1988, 1989). This was based on results showing that treatment of K562 and U937 cells with PMA, a PKC activator, or cAMP, a PKA activator, conferred on them resistance to lysis, whereas treatment with a variety of protein kinase inhibitors sensitized them to lysis. A similar finding was reported for glomerular epithelial cells (Cybulsky et al., 1990). To date, the capacity of activated complement proteins to trigger protein kinase cascades within normal and cancer cells has been well documented. Nevertheless, the protective mechanisms that are induced by phosphorylation and the relevant protein substrates have not been defined yet. Rapid removal of the membrane attack complex from the target cell surface by endo- or ectocytosis has been suggested to be a protective mechanism from complement lysis (Ramm et al., 1983; Morgan et al., 1987). In support, it was shown that PKC inhibitors reduce MAC removal

(Carney et al., 1990) and increase sensitivity of tumor cells to lysis (Kraus et al., 2000). Sublytic MAC is also activating in tumor cells the mitogen activated protein kinase ERK. In JY25 B lymphoblastoid cells, MAC-induced ERK activation was shown to be dependent on G-protein activation (Niculescu et al., 1997). In K562 erythroleukemia cells, MAC-induced ERK activation was inhibited by PKC inhibitors (Kraus et al., 2001). Assuming that there is no basic difference between JY25 and K562 cells in their response to sublytic MAC, then it is possible that G-protein activation leads directly or indirectly to PKC activation or vice versa, and that both act upstream to ERK activation by sublytic MAC. Blocking of the ERK kinase MEK with PD098059 increases the sensitivity of K562 cells (Kraus et al. 2001), and of PC-3, SKOV3 and T47D carcinoma cells (Donin et al. 2003) to complement-mediated lysis. In addition, treatment of K562 cells with PD098059 and transfection of COS-7 cells with a MEK dominant-negative mutant, prevent development of complement-induced protection in these cells in response to sublytic MAC (Kraus et al., 2001). Therefore, ERK appears to be an important component of the repair or recovery machinery protecting tumor cells from the MAC. PKA, the cAMP-dependent protein kinase is yet another kinase involved in complement resistance, at least in human carcinoma cells (Donin et al., 2003). The fact that combination of a PKA inhibitor with a PKC inhibitor had no additive effects on sensitivity to complement (Donin et al., 2003), suggests that PKA and PKC act along the same protective pathway, with PKA acting either upstream or downstream of PKC.

3.3   Involvement of Heat Shock Proteins

Thermotolerance is gained by pre-exposure of cells to a sublytic heat shock (Lindquist and Craig, 1988; Li et al., 1995; Morimoto, 1998). Heat shock triggers synthesis of several transcription factors, followed by synthesis of heat shock proteins (hsp), including the hsp70 multi-gene family. Some hsps, such as hsc70 and hsp70α, are constitutively expressed and respond only poorly to heat. Under normal conditions, the hsc70 serves as a molecular chaperone, escorting proteins to their various intracellular compartments and assisting their translocation across membranes (Kang et al., 1990; Martin and Hartl, 1997; Pilon and Schekman, 1999). In addition, hsc70 plays a major role in endocytosis, uncoating clathrin-coated vesicles (de Waegh and Brady, 1989). Under stress conditions, the hsp70s participate in repair of damaged proteins and membranes and dissociation of protein aggregates. Members of the hsp70 family have been also implicated in cell protection from other toxic compounds, such as hydrogen peroxide (Bornman et al., 1998; Su et al., 1998), and from metabolic stress (Williams et al., 1993). Hsp70 can also protect cells from heat-induced apoptosis (Li et al., 1996). In contrast, hsp90 is involved in normal cellular activities such as growth and differentiation, protein transport and regulation of hormone receptors and transcription factors (Richter and Buchner, 2001).

Thermotolerance and complement-induced protection (complement-tolerance) share some resemblance. The two shock responses depend on de novo synthesis of proteins, develop within minutes and decay after several hours. Hence, the possible involvement of heat shock proteins in cell protection from complement shock was investigated. K562 cells subjected to heat shock are more resistant to complement-mediated lysis (Fishelson et al., 2001). Inhibition of hsc70 with deoxyspergualin increases the sensitivity of K562 cells to complement-mediated lysis (Fishelson et al., 2001). It is suggested that both hsc70 and hsp70 can attenuate the MAC lytic effects by a mechanism that uses their chaperone and transporter activities. MAC insertion was found to induce in K562 cells transfer of hsc70 from the cytosol to the exoplasmic side of the plasma membrane (Fishelson et al., 2000, 2001), probably as part of the L-CIP protein complex induced by sublytic MAC (Reiter et al., 1992). The relevance of this event to complement resistance is still unclear. Treatment of T lymphoma cells (Sreedhar et al., 2003) or K562 cells (Fishelson and Binyamini, unpublished) with hsp90 inhibitors, such as geldanamycin and radicicol, similarly sensitises them to lysis by MAC. Thus, the list of heat shock proteins involved in damage repair and rescue of tumor cells after complement attack has grown. Other members of the large heat shock protein family are likely to join this list.

3.4   Role for Bcl-2

Cell death induced by the complement MAC appears morphologically distinct from apoptosis, especially at the level of cytoplasmic organelles. A lytic dose of the MAC induces a loss in membrane integrity and rapid necrotic type cell death. Complement-mediated death of Ehrlich ascites tumor cells is characterized by swelling of mitochondria, dilation of the rough endoplasmic reticulum and disruption of the Golgi complex and of the plasma and nuclear membranes (Papadimitriou et al., 1994). However, there are claims that complement can also induce apoptotic cell death (reviewed in Fishelson, 2001; Nauta et al., 2002). The mitochondrion is believed to play a central role in propagation of the death signals and in determination of the type of cell death and the "point of no return". The anti-apoptotic protein Bcl-2 acts at the level of mitochondrial membranes (Vander Heiden and Thompson, 1999; Korsmeyer, 1999; Harris and Thompson, 2000). There is increasing evidence that complement may also exert anti-apoptotic effects.

Sublytic MAC induces protection in oligodendrocytes (Soane et al., 1999) and Schwann cells (Dashiell et al., 2000) from apoptosis following serum growth factor deprivation. Sublytic MAC was shown to increase synthesis of Bcl-2 (Soane et al., 1999) and to induce phosphorylation, and thus inhibition, of the pro-apoptotic protein Bad (Soane et al., 2001). These phenomena of pro-apoptotic and anti-apoptotic effects of complement have not been described yet with cancer cells, many of which are known to have enhanced Bcl-2 expression (Coultas and Strasser, 2003). The contribution of Bcl-2 to complement-mediated lysis was recently examined in Bcl-2 transfected Jurkat T lymphoma cells. Jurkat cells transfected with control vector were sensitive to lysis by antibody and complement, whereas four different transfected cell lines showed a variable resistance to lysis. Analysis by linear regression, demonstrated an inverse correlation between the degree of cell lysability and expression of Bcl-2 (Attali and Fishelson, submitted for publication). This supports the claim that Bcl-2 is not only anti-apoptotic in cancer cells, but can also protect them from complement-mediated lysis. The claim receives strong support by a report showing that gene transfer of Bcl-2 into porcine pancreatic islets confers on them resistance to killing by xenoreactive antibodies and complement (Contreras et al., 2001).

4.   INTERVENTION STRATEGIES

In recent years, new monoclonal antibodies have been designed to direct and concentrate cytotoxicity to the tumor cell (Carter, 2001). This era of targeted therapy has brought to the clinics a handful of monoclonal antibodies, including Rituxan (rituximab), designed for relapsed or refractory CD20-positive non-Hodgkin B cell lymphoma (NHL), Herceptin (trastuzumab) for breast tumors overexpressing the human epidermal growth factor receptor 2 (HER-2), Campath (alemtuzumab), binding to CD52 and administered to patients suffering from chronic lymphocytic B cell leukemia, Mylotarg (gemtuzumab ozogamicin), a chimeric antibody covalently linked to the antibiotic calicheamicin, which binds to CD33 on acute myeloid leukemia cells and Zevalin (90Y ibritumomab tiuxetan), the first radioimmuntherapeutic which, like rituximab, also targets CD20 positive NHL cells. The clinical and commercial success of such anticancer antibodies has created great interest in antibody-based therapeutics for hematopoietic malignant neoplasms and solid tumors. With the expectation of lower toxic effects on nonmalignant bystander tissues, the potential increased efficacy by conjugation to radioisotopes and other cellular toxins, and the ability to characterize the target with clinical laboratory diagnostics to improve the drug's clinical performance, current and future antibody therapeutics are likely to find substantial roles alone and in combination therapeutic strategies for treating patients with cancer. These antibodies were primarily not selected with respect to their complement-activating ability, but its analysis has been included in defining their biological functions. By introducing human IgG1 heavy and light chain domains, the antiproliferative properties of a precursor murine monoclonal anti-p185[HER] antibody to trastuzumab were extended by its capacity to induce ADCC (Carter et al. 1992) and complement activation (Jurianz et al., 1999a). The latter experiments with various HER-2 positive tumor cell lines already revealed that sensitisation with the humanized anti-p185[HER] antibody led to opsonization of the tumor cells with C3b but that complement-mediated tumor cell lysis became only possible upon neutralisation of mCRP. Part of the antitumor effect of the anti-CD20 chimeric monoclonal antibody rituximab, used in the therapy of non-Hodgkin's B cell lymphoma, has been ascribed to its capacity to bind C1q, activate complement and eventually kill the cells (Idusogie et al. 2000, 2001). The heterogeneity of the response to rituximab in different patients might have been related to mCRP expression on their tumor cells. However, as the expression level of mCRP on follicular lymphoma cells or cell susceptibility to in vitro complement-mediated lysis could not be correlated with the clinical outcome of rituximab treatment, their predictive value was questioned (Weng and Levy, 2001). As expected, the additional application of blocking anti-CD55 or anti-CD59 antibodies increased rituximab-induced complement-mediated killing in various lymphoma cell lines as well as in fresh patients-derived follicular non-Hodgkin's lymphoma and B-cell chronic leukemia samples (Golay et al. 2000, 2001; Harjunpaa et al., 2000). Studies of Treon et al. (2001) on multiple myeloma and non-Hodgkin's lymphoma cells supported these results, demonstrating that CD59 expression is associated with patients' resistance to rituximab serotherapy. By the addition of an iC3b specific antibody to rituximab-sensitised complement treated tumor cells, C3b accumulation and lysis was significantly improved (Kennedy et al., 2003). This novel treatment strategy may also promote targeted ADCC onto tumor cells. Studies of Ross et al. (1999) are of potential clinical importance. To override natural mechanisms of self-protection of iC3b-opsonised tumor cells, NK cells were primed with ß-glucan. This treatment not only led to an improvement of complement-mediated cytotoxicity but also to a tumor-localised secretion of proinflammatory cytokines.

Tumor cell directed complement activation may be improved by application of heteroconjugates composed of antitumor antibodies and cobra venom factor (CVF) (Vogel and Muller-Eberhard, 1981), C3b (Reiter and Fishelson, 1989) or iC3b (Yefenof et al., 1990). Upon conjugation of CVF or C3b to 17-1A, a mAb directed against the 17-1A antigen/epithelial cell adhesion molecule (EpCAM), Gelderman et al. (2002b) observed an up to 13-fold increase in C3 deposition which correlated with augmented complement-mediated lysis of colorectal carcinoma cells, as compared to the 17-1A mAb alone.

As demonstrated in numerous experiments, anti-mCRP blocking antibodies, which usually are poor activators of complement on their own, successfully enhance the susceptibility of tumor cells to complement-mediated lysis. For example, neutralisation of CD55 in Burkitt lymphoma cells (Kuraya et al., 1992), leukemia cells (Zhong et al., 1995; Jurianz et al., 2001; Golay et al., 2001), melanoma cells (Cheung et al., 1988) and breast cancer cells (Jurianz et al., 1999; Donin et al., 2003) increased their sensitivity to complement. In contrast, anti-CD55 mAb had no effect on killing of renal carcinoma cells (Gorter et al., 1996). Despite the expression of significant levels of CD55, blocking of this mCRP was not sufficient to sensitise prostate and ovarian carcinoma cells to complement-mediated lysis (Donin et al., 2003). The effect of blocking CD46 with neutralising mAb in augmenting cytotoxicity is often poor as shown for erythroleukemic cells (K562) and cervix carcinoma cell lines (Jurianz et al., 2001; Geldermann et al., 2002a). In contrast, neutralisation of CD59 with mAb led to efficient sensitization to complement-mediated lysis of neuroblastoma cells (Gasque et al., 1996), leukemic cells (Jurianz et al., 2001; Golay et al., 2001), breast (Jurianz et al., 1999, Donin et al., 2003), ovarian (Bjørge et al., 1997; Donin et al., 2003), renal (Gorter et al., 1996) and prostate carcinoma cells (Jarvis et al., 1997, Donin et al., 2003). CD55 and CD46 were reported to be synergistic in complement regulation by CHO cells (Brodbeck et al., 2000). This has been confirmed and extended to breast, ovarian and prostate carcinoma cell lines by using a mixture of optimal and suboptimal concentrations of neutralising mAbs directed to CD46, CD55 and CD59 (Donin et al., 2003), suggesting some type of cooperativity among CD46, CD55 and CD59.

Besides using blocking anti-mCRP mAb, attempts were made to modulate the level of expression of mCRP by treatment with cytokines or growth factors. As mentioned in section 2, most cytokines tested so far either enhanced or had no effect on mCRP expression. It is important to identify molecules that reduce mCRP expression on tumor cells. Expression of CD59 and CD46 on hepatoma cells could be decreased with INFγ (Spiller et al., 2000). Down-regulation of CD55 expression on colon cancer cells with subsequent increase of sensitivity to complement-mediated injury can be achieved in vitro by butyrate, which is normally generated in the colon by bacteria degrading dietary fibers (Andoh et al., 2002). Similarly, fludarabine treatment was shown to down-regulate the level of CD55 expression in B lymphoma cells and to increase their lysis by the anti-CD20 rituximab antibody and human complement (Di Gaetano et al., 2001).

Targeting complement regulatory proteins is a very attractive approach to tumor therapy, although great care must be taken to prevent normal tissue recognition. This could lead to uncontrolled complement deposition and extensive cell lysis. One possible approach is the construction of bispecific mAbs consisting of one F(ab) moiety directed to a tumor specific antigen and another one directed to an mCRP. However, to avoid significant binding to normal tissue, the tumor directed F(ab) moiety needs to be of high affinity (Gelderman et al., 2002a). Bispecific antibodies which recognize tumor antigens linked to an mCRP such as CD55 (Blok et al., 1998) or CD59 (Junnikkala et al., 1994; Harris et al., 1997) induced effective tumor cell killing with only marginal effects on bystander cells. Gelderman et al. (2002b) generated a bispecific mAb directed against both HLA Class I and CD55. Sensitisation of colorectal cells with an anti-HLA-anti-CD55 bispecific mAb led to increased C3 deposition as compared with anti-HLA mAb alone and with a mixture of anti-HLA and anti-CD55 mAbs.

The epithelial cell adhesion molecule (EpCAM) is a transmembrane protein associated with a variety of carcinomas. EpCAM is often strongly up-regulated or, as in the case of squamous cell carcinomas, de novo expressed. Increased C3 deposition on cervical and colorectal carcinoma cells could be achieved with a bifunctional anti-EpCAM-anti-CD55 antibody. Its opsonising capacity was as good or even better than that of an anti-EpCAM mAb conjugated with CVF or with C3b (Gelderman et al., 2002a,b). Promising results from these in vitro experiments have to be verified now in animal studies.

The introduction of anti-idiotypic antibodies mimicing mCRP are considered another interesting option in cancer immunotherapy. The human anti-idiotypic antibody 105AD7, originally isolated from a colorectal cancer patient, not only recognises the binding site of 791T/36 (an antibody directed to an osteosarcoma cell line) but also mimics CD55 (Austin et al. 1989). Immunisation of both mice and rats with 105AD7 resulted in the generation of antibodies that bind to CD55 (Austin et al., 1991). This human anti-idiotypic antibody that mimics CD55 has been used successfully in over 200 colorectal cancer and osteosarcoma patients. 70% of the patients showed CD55-specific immune responses with no associated toxicity (Durrant and Spendlove, 2001). In patients who received 105AD7 at diagnosis and prior to tumor resection, increased infiltration of CD4, CD8 and CD56 cells and increased tumor cell apoptosis was observed relative to unimmunised control patients (Spendlove at al., 2000; Amin et al., 2000). However in a following randomised double blind phase II study, 105D7 vaccination did not prolong survival in patients with advanced colorectal cancer (Maxwell-Armstrong et al. 2001).

Another future approach may be the reduction of mCRP expression by targeted RNA silencing strategies. We were recently able to show, that by the introduction of CD55 and CD46 directed antisense oligonucleotides, the expression levels of these mCRPs could be significantly reduced, thereby increasing the susceptibility of tumor cells to complement-mediated lysis (Zell et al., 2003)

5. REFERENCES

1.   Adenis A, Huet G, Zerimech F, Hecquet B, Balduyck M, Peyrat JP. Cathepsin B, L, and D activities in colorectal carcinomas: relationship with clinico-pathological parameters. Cancer Lett. 1995;96:267-275
2.   Alsenz J, Bork K, Loos M. Autoantibody-mediated acquired deficiency of C1 inhibitor. N Engl J Med. 1987;316:1360-1366
3.   Amin S, Robins RA, Maxwell-Armstrong CA, Scholefield JH, Durrant LG. Vaccine-induced apoptosis: a novel clinical trial end point? Cancer Res. 2000;60:3132-3136
4.   Andoh A, Shimada M, Araki Y, Fujiyama Y, Bamba T. Sodium butyrate enhances complement-mediated cell injury via down-regulation of decay-accelerating factor expression in colonic cancer cells. Cancer Immunol Immunother. 2002;50:663-672
5.   Andrew SM, Teh JG, Johnstone RW, Russell SM, Whitehead RH, McKenzie IF, Pietersz GA. Tumor localization by combinations of monoclonal antibodies in a new human colon carcinoma cell line (LIM1899). Cancer Res. 1990;50:5225-5230
6.   Austin EB, Robins RA, Durrant LG, Price MR, Baldwin RW. Human monoclonal anti-idiotypic antibody to the tumour-associated antibody 791T/36. Immunology. 1989;67:525-530
7.   Austin EB, Robins RA, Baldwin RW, Durrant LG. Induction of delayed hypersensitivity to human tumor cells with a human monoclonal anti-idiotypic antibody. J Natl Cancer Inst. 1991;83:1245-1248
8.   Baker PJ, Lint TF, Mortensen RF, Gewurz H. C567-initiated cytolysis of lymphoid cells: description of the phenomenon and studies on its control by C567 inhibitors. J Immunol. 1977;118:198-202
9.   Batlle Fonrodona FJ, Lopez Fernandez MF, Vicente Garcia V, Corral Alonso M, Lopez Borrasca A. Complement in hematological neoplasias. Allergol Immunopathol (Madr). 1979;7:39-46
10.   Bernet-Camard MF, Coconnier MH, Hudault S, Servin AL. Differential expression of complement proteins and regulatory decay accelerating factor in relation to differentiation of cultured human colon adenocarcinoma cell lines. Gut. 1996;38:248-253
11.   Bjorge L, Vedeler CA, Ulvestad E, Matre R. Expression and function of CD59 on colonic adenocarcinoma cells. Eur J Immunol. 1994;24:1597-1603
12.   Bjorge L, Jensen TS, Ulvestad E, Vedeler CA, Matre R. The influence of tumour necrosis factor-alpha, interleukin-1 beta and interferon-gamma on the expression and function of the complement regulatory protein CD59 on the human colonic adenocarcinoma cell line HT29. Scand J Immunol. 1995;41:350-356

13. Bjorge L, Jensen TS, Matre R. Characterisation of the complement-regulatory proteins decay-accelerating factor (DAF, CD55) and membrane cofactor protein (MCP, CD46) on a human colonic adenocarcinoma cell line. Cancer Immunol Immunother. 1996;42:185-192

14. Bjorge L, Hakulinen J, Wahlstrom T, Matre R, Meri S. Complement-regulatory proteins in ovarian malignancies. Int J Cancer. 1997;70:14-25

15. Bjorge L, Junnikkala S, Kristoffersen EK, Hakulinen J, Matre R, Meri S. Resistance of ovarian teratocarcinoma cell spheroids to complement-mediated lysis. Br J Cancer. 1997;75:1247-1255

16. Blok VT, Daha MR, Tijsma O, Harris CL, Morgan BP, Fleuren GJ, Gorter A. A bispecific monoclonal antibody directed against both the membrane-bound complement regulator CD55 and the renal tumor-associated antigen G250 enhances C3 deposition and tumor cell lysis by complement. J Immunol. 1998;160:3437-3443

17. Blok VT, Daha MR, Tijsma OM, Weissglas MG, van den Broek LJ, Gorter A. A possible role of CD46 for the protection in vivo of human renal tumor cells from complement-mediated damage. Lab Invest. 2000;80:335-344

18. Blom DJ, Goslings WR, De Waard-Siebinga I, Luyten GP, Claas FH, Gorter A, Jager MJ. Lack of effect of different cytokines on expression of membrane-bound regulators of complement activity on human uveal melanoma cells. J Interferon Cytokine Res. 1997;17:695-700

19. Bohana-Kashtan O, Paas Y, Fishelson Z. Partial characterization of the C9 ecto-protein kinase of K562 cells. Molec Immunol. 1998;35:346

20. Bomstein Y, Fishelson Z. Enhanced sensitivity of P-glycoprotein-positive multidrug resistant tumor cells to complement-mediated lysis. Eur J Immunol. 1997;27:2204-2211

21. Bornman L, Steinmann CM, Gericke GS, Polla BS. In vivo heat shock protects rat myocardial mitochondria. Biochem Biophys Res Commun. 1998;246:836-840

22. Boyle MD, Ohanian SH, Borsos T. Studies on the terminal stages of antibody-complement-mediated killing of a tumor cell. II. Inhibition of transformation of T to dead cells by 3'5' cAMP. J Immunol. 1976;116:1276-1279

23. Brasoveanu LI, Altomonte M, Gloghini A, Fonsatti E, Coral S, Gasparollo A, Montagner R, Cattarossi I, Simonelli C, Cattelan A, et al. Expression of protectin (CD59) in human melanoma and its functional role in cell- and complement-mediated cytotoxicity. Int J Cancer. 1995;61:548-556

24. Brasoveanu LI, Altomonte M, Fonsatti E, Colizzi F, Coral S, Nicotra MR, Cattarossi I, Cattelan A, Natali PG, Maio M. Levels of cell membrane CD59 regulate the extent of complement-mediated lysis of human melanoma cells. Lab Invest. 1996;74:33-42

25. Brasoveanu LI, Fonsatti E, Visintin A, Pavlovic M, Cattarossi I, Colizzi F, Gasparollo A, Coral S, Horejsi V, Altomonte M, Maio M. Melanoma cells constitutively release an anchor-positive soluble form of protectin (sCD59) that retains functional activities in homologous complement-mediated cytotoxicity. J Clin Invest. 1997;100:1248-1255

26. Brodbeck WG, Mold C, Atkinson JP, Medof ME. Cooperation between decay-accelerating factor and membrane cofactor protein in protecting cells from autologous complement attack. J Immunol. 2000;165:3999-4006

27. Budzko DB, Lachmann PJ, McConnell I. Activation of the alternative complement pathway by lymphoblastoid cell lines derived from patients with Burkitt's lymphoma and infectious mononucleosis. Cell Immunol. 1976;22:98-109

28. Campbell AK, Morgan BP. Monoclonal antibodies demonstrate protection of polymorphonuclear leukocytes against complement attack. Nature. 1985;317:164-166

29. Capone PM, Papsidero LD, Croghan GA, Chu TM. Experimental tumoricidal effects of monoclonal antibody against solid breast tumors. Proc Natl Acad Sci U S A. 1983;80:7328-7332

30. Carli M, Bucolo C, Pannunzio MT, Ongaro G, Businaro R, Revoltella R. Fluctuation of serum complement levels in children with neuroblastoma. Cancer. 1979;43:2399-2404

31. Carney DF, Koski CL, Shin ML. Elimination of terminal complement intermediates from the plasma membrane of nucleated cells: the rate of disappearance differs for cells carrying C5b-7 or C5b-8 or a mixture of C5b-8 with a limited number of C5b-9. J Immunol. 1985;134:1804-1809

32. Carney DF, Hammer CH, Shin ML. Elimination of terminal complement complexes in the plasma membrane of nucleated cells: influence of extracellular Ca2+ and association with cellular Ca2+. J Immunol. 1986;137:263-270

33. Carney DF, Lang TJ, Shin ML. Multiple signal messengers generated by terminal complement complexes and their role in terminal complement complex elimination. J Immunol. 1990;145:623-629

34. Carter P, Presta L, Gorman CM, Ridgway JB, Henner D, Wong WL, Rowland AM, Kotts C, Carver ME, Shepard HM. Humanization of an anti-p185HER2 antibody for human cancer therapy. Proc Natl Acad Sci U S A. 1992;89:4285-4289

35. Carter P. Improving the efficacy of antibody-based cancer therapies. Nat Rev Cancer. 2001;1:118-129

36. Chapman PB, Lonberg M, Houghton AN. Light chain variants of an IgG3 anti-GD3 monoclonal antibody and the relationship among avidity, effector functions, tumor targeting, and antitumor activity. Cancer Res. 1990;50:1503-1509

37. Chen S, Caragine T, Cheung NK, Tomlinson S. CD59 expressed on a tumor cell surface modulates decay-accelerating factor expression and enhances tumor growth in a rat model of human neuroblastoma. Cancer Res. 2000;60:3013-3018

38. Chen S, Caragine T, Cheung NK, Tomlinson S. Surface antigen expression and complement susceptibility of differentiated neuroblastoma clones. Am J Pathol. 2000;156:1085-1091

39. Cheung NK, Walter EI, Smith-Mensah WH, Ratnoff WD, Tykocinski ML, Medof ME. Decay-accelerating factor protects human tumor cells from complement-mediated cytotoxicity in vitro. J Clin Invest. 1988;81:1122-1128

40. Cicardi M, Beretta A, Colombo M, Gioffre D, Cugno M, Agostoni A. Relevance of lymphoproliferative disorders and of anti-C1 inhibitor autoantibodies in acquired angio-oedema. Clin Exp Immunol. 1996;106:475-480

41. Contreras JL, Bilbao G, Smyth C, Eckhoff DE, Xiang XL, Jenkins S, Cartner S, Curiel DT, Thomas FT, Thomas JM. Gene transfer of the Bcl-2 gene confers cytoprotection to isolated adult porcine pancreatic islets exposed to xenoreactive antibodies and complement. Surgery. 2001;130:166-174

42. Contreras JL, Bilbao G, Smyth CA, Eckhoff DE, Jiang XL, Jenkins S, Thomas FT, Curiel DT, Thomas JM. Cytoprotection of pancreatic islets before and early after transplantation using gene therapy. Kidney Int Suppl. 2002;61 Suppl 1:79-84

43. Cooper PD. Complement and cancer: activation of the alternative pathway as a theoretical base for immunotherapy. Adv Immun Cancer Ther. 1985;1:125-166

44. Coral S, Fonsatti E, Sigalotti L, De Nardo C, Visintin A, Nardi G, Colizzi F, Colombo MP, Romano G, Altomonte M, Maio M. Overexpression of protectin (CD59) down-modulates the susceptibility of human melanoma cells to homologous complement. J Cell Physiol. 2000;185:317-323

45. Coultas L, Strasser A. The role of the Bcl-2 protein family in cancer. Semin Cancer Biol. 2003;13:115-123

46. Crnogorac-Jurcevic T, Efthimiou E, Nielsen T, Loader J, Terris B, Stamp G, Baron A, Scarpa A, Lemoine NR. Expression profiling of microdissected pancreatic adenocarcinomas. Oncogene. 2002;21:4587-4594

47. Cybulsky AV, Salant DJ, Quigg RJ, Badalamenti J, Bonventre JV. Complement C5b-9 complex activates phospholipases in glomerular epithelial cells. Am J Physiol. 1989;257:F826-836

48. Cybulsky AV, Bonventre JV, Quigg RJ, Lieberthal W, Salant DJ. Cytosolic calcium and protein kinase C reduce complement-mediated glomerular epithelial injury. Kidney Int. 1990;38:803-811

49. Cybulsky AV, Cyr MD. Phosphatidylcholine-directed phospholipase C: activation by complement C5b-9. Am J Physiol. 1993;265:F551-560

50. Davies A, Simmons DL, Hale G, Harrison RA, Tighe H, Lachmann PJ, Waldmann H. CD59, an LY-6-like protein expressed in human lymphoid cells, regulates the action of the complement membrane attack complex on homologous cells. J Exp Med. 1989;170:637-654

51. de Waegh S, Brady ST. Axonal transport of a clathrin uncoating ATPase (HSC70): a role for HSC70 in the modulation of coated vesicle assembly in vivo. J Neurosci Res. 1989;23:433-440

52. Del Rosso M, Fibbi G, Pucci M, D'Alessio S, Del Rosso A, Magnelli L, Chiarugi V. Multiple pathways of cell invasion are regulated by multiple families of serine proteases. Clin Exp Metastasis. 2002;19:193-207

53. Di Gaetano N, Xiao Y, Erba E, Bassan R, Rambaldi A, Golay J, Introna M. Synergism between fludarabine and rituximab revealed in a follicular lymphoma cell line resistant to the cytotoxic activity of either drug alone. Br J Haematol. 2001;114:800-809

54. Donin N, Jurianz K, Ziporen L, Schultz S, Kirschfink M, Fishelson Z. Complement resistance of human carcinoma cells depends on membrane regulatory proteins, protein kinases and sialic acid. Clin Exp Immunol. 2003;131:254-263

55. Drinnan NB, Halliday J, Ramsdale T. Inhibitors of sialyltransferases: potential roles in tumor growth and metastasis. Mini Rev Med Chem. 2003;3:501-517

56. Durrant LG, Spendlove I. Immunization against tumor cell surface complement-regulatory proteins. Curr Opin Investig Drugs. 2001;2:959-966

57. Durrant LG, Chapman MA, Buckley DJ, Spendlove I, Robins RA, Armitage NC. Enhanced expression of the complement regulatory protein CD55 predicts a poor prognosis in colorectal cancer patients. Cancer Immunol Immunother. 2003;52:638-642

58. Ekdahl KN, Nilsson B. Phosphorylation of complement component C3 and C3 fragments by a human platelet protein kinase. Inhibition of factor I-mediated cleavage of C3b. J Immunol. 1995;154:6502-6510

59. Fishelson Z, Kopf E, Reiter Y. Phosphorylation, phosphatidylinositol turnover and resistance to complement damage. FASEB J. 1988;2:A872

60. Fishelson Z, Kopf E, Paas Y, Ross L, Reiter Y. Protein phosphorylation as a mechanism of resistance against complement damage. In: Melchers Fea, ed. Prog. Immunol. Vol. 7. Berlin: Springer-Verlag; 1989:205-208

61. Fishelson Z, Hochmann I, Bohana-Kashtan O. Identification of hsc70 and beta-tubulin in L-CIP, the large complement-induced protein complex. Immunopharmacol. 2000;49:97

62. Fishelson Z, Attali G, Mevorach D. Complement and apoptosis. Mol Immunol. 2001;38:207-219

63. Fishelson Z, Hochman I, Greene LE, Eisenberg E. Contribution of heat shock proteins to cell protection from complement-mediated lysis. Int Immunol. 2001;13:983-991

64. Fishelson Z, Donin N, Zell S, Schultz S, Kirschfink M. Obstacles to cancer immunotherapy: expression of membrane complement regulatory proteins (mCRPs) in tumors. Mol Immunol. 2003;40:109-123

65. Frade R, Rodrigues-Lima F, Huang S, Xie K, Guillaume N, Bar-Eli M. Procathepsin-L, a proteinase that cleaves human C3 (the third component of complement), confers high tumorigenic and metastatic properties to human melanoma cells. Cancer Res. 1998;58:2733-2736

66. French LE, Wohlwend A, Sappino AP, Tschopp J, Schifferli JA. Human clusterin gene expression is confined to surviving cells during in vitro programmed cell death. J Clin Invest. 1994;93:877-884

67. Friese MA, Manuelian T, Junnikkala S, Hellwage J, Meri S, Peter HH, Gordon DL, Eibel H, Zipfel PF. Release of endogenous anti-inflammatory complement regulators FHL-1 and factor H protects synovial fibroblasts during rheumatoid arthritis. Clin Exp Immunol. 2003;132:485-495

68. Fukuda H, Seya T, Hara T, Matsumoto M, Kinoshita T, Masaoka T. Deficiency of complement decay-accelerating factor (DAF, CD55) in non-Hodgkin's lymphoma. Immunol Lett. 1991;29:205-209

69. Fust G, Miszlay Z, Czink E, Varga L, Paloczi K, Szegedi G, Hollan SR. C1 and C4 abnormalities in chronic lymphocytic leukaemia and their significance. Immunol Lett. 1987;14:255-259

70. Gambacorti-Passerini C, Rivoltini L, Supino R, Rodolfo M, Radrizzani M, Fossati G, Parmiani G. Susceptibility of chemoresistant murine and human tumor cells to lysis by interleukin 2-activated lymphocytes. Cancer Res. 1988;48:2372-2376

71. Gasque P, Julen N, Ischenko AM, Picot C, Mauger C, Chauzy C, Ripoche J, Fontaine M. Expression of complement components of the alternative pathway by glioma cell lines. J Immunol. 1992;149:1381-1387

72. Gasque P, Ischenko A, Legoedec J, Mauger C, Schouft MT, Fontaine M. Expression of the complement classical pathway by human glioma in culture. A model for complement expression by nerve cells. J Biol Chem. 1993;268:25068-25074

73. Gasque P, Fontaine M, Morgan BP. Complement expression in human brain. Biosynthesis of terminal pathway components and regulators in human glial cells and cell lines. J Immunol. 1995;154:4726-4733

74. Gasque P, Morgan BP, Legoedec J, Chan P, Fontaine M. Human skeletal myoblasts spontaneously activate allogeneic complement but are resistant to killing. J Immunol. 1996;156:3402-3411

75. Gasque P, Thomas A, Fontaine M, Morgan BP. Complement activation on human neuroblastoma cell lines in vitro: route of activation and expression of functional complement regulatory proteins. J Neuroimmunol. 1996;66:29-40

76. Gelderman KA, Blok VT, Fleuren GJ, Gorter A. The inhibitory effect of CD46, CD55, and CD59 on complement activation after immunotherapeutic treatment of cervical carcinoma cells with monoclonal antibodies or bispecific monoclonal antibodies. Lab Invest. 2002;82:483-493

77. Gelderman KA, Kuppen PJ, Bruin W, Fleuren GJ, Gorter A. Enhancement of the complement activating capacity of 17-1A mAb to overcome the effect of membrane-bound complement regulatory proteins on colorectal carcinoma. Eur J Immunol. 2002;32:128-135

78. Gminski J, Mykala-Ciesla J, Machalski M, Drozdz M, Najda J. Immunoglobulins and complement components levels in patients with lung cancer. Rom J Intern Med. 1992;30:39-44

79. Golay J, Zaffaroni L, Vaccari T, Lazzari M, Borleri GM, Bernasconi S, Tedesco F, Rambaldi A, Introna M. Biologic response of B lymphoma cells to anti-CD20 monoclonal antibody rituximab in vitro: CD55 and CD59 regulate complement-mediated cell lysis. Blood. 2000;95:3900-3908

80. Golay J, Lazzari M, Facchinetti V, Bernasconi S, Borleri G, Barbui T, Rambaldi A, Introna M. CD20 levels determine the in vitro susceptibility to rituximab and complement of B-cell chronic lymphocytic leukemia: further regulation by CD55 and CD59. Blood. 2001;98:3383-3389

81. Goransson J, Jonsson S, Lasson A. Pre-operative plasma levels of C-reactive protein, albumin and various plasma protease inhibitors for the pre-operative assessment of operability and recurrence in cancer surgery. Eur J Surg Oncol. 1996;22:607-617

82. Gordon JL. Extracellular ATP: effects, sources and fate. Biochem J. 1986;233:309-319

83. Gorter A, Blok VT, Haasnoot WH, Ensink NG, Daha MR, Fleuren GJ. Expression of CD46, CD55, and CD59 on renal tumor cell lines and their role in preventing complement-mediated tumor cell lysis. Lab Invest. 1996;74:1039-1049

84. Gorter A, Meri S. Immune evasion of tumor cells using membrane-bound complement regulatory proteins. Immunol Today. 1999;20:576-582

85. Goslings WR, Blom DJ, de Waard-Siebinga I, van Beelen E, Claas FH, Jager MJ, Gorter A. Membrane-bound regulators of complement activation in uveal melanomas. CD46, CD55, and CD59 in uveal melanomas. Invest Ophthalmol Vis Sci. 1996;37:1884-1891

86. Guc D, Canpinar H, Kucukaksu C, Kansu E. Expression of complement regulatory proteins CR1, DAF, MCP and CD59 in haematological malignancies. Eur J Haematol. 2000;64:3-9

87. Hara T, Kojima A, Fukuda H, Masaoka T, Fukumori Y, Matsumoto M, Seya T. Levels of complement regulatory proteins, CD35 (CR1), CD46 (MCP) and CD55 (DAF) in human haematological malignancies. Br J Haematol. 1992;82:368-373

88. Hara T, Kuriyama S, Kiyohara H, Nagase Y, Matsumoto M, Seya T. Soluble forms of membrane cofactor protein (CD46, MCP) are present in plasma, tears, and seminal fluid in normal subjects. Clin Exp Immunol. 1992;89:490-494

89. Hara T, Suzuki Y, Semba T, Hatanaka M, Matsumoto M, Seya T. High expression of membrane cofactor protein of complement (CD46) in human leukaemia cell lines: implication of an alternatively spliced form containing the STA domain in CD46 up-regulation. Scand J Immunol. 1995;42:581-590

90. Harjunpaa A, Junnikkala S, Meri S. Rituximab (anti-CD20) therapy of B-cell lymphomas: direct complement killing is superior to cellular effector mechanisms. Scand J Immunol. 2000;51:634-641

91. Harris CL, Kan KS, Stevenson GT, Morgan BP. Tumour cell killing using chemically engineered antibody constructs specific for tumour cells and the complement inhibitor CD59. Clin Exp Immunol. 1997;107:364-371

92. Harris MH, Thompson CB. The role of the Bcl-2 family in the regulation of outer mitochondrial membrane permeability. Cell Death Differ. 2000;7:1182-1191

93. Hatanaka M, Seya T, Matsumoto M, Hara T, Nonaka M, Inoue N, Takeda J, Shimizu A. Mechanisms by which the surface expression of the glycosyl-phosphatidylinositol-anchored complement regulatory proteins decay-accelerating factor (CD55) and CD59 is lost in human leukaemia cell lines. Biochem J. 1996;314 (Pt 3):969-976

94. Heidtmann HH, Salge U, Havemann K, Kirschke H, Wiederanders B. Secretion of a latent, acid activatable cathepsin L precursor by human non-small cell lung cancer cell lines. Oncol Res. 1993;5:441-451

95. Hensel F, Hermann R, Brandlein S, Krenn V, Schmausser B, Geis S, Muller-Hermelink HK, Vollmers HP. Regulation of the new coexpressed CD55 (decay-accelerating factor) receptor on stomach carcinoma cells involved in antibody SC-1-induced apoptosis. Lab Invest. 2001;81:1553-1563

96. Hidvegi T, Ermolin GA, Efremov EE, Dikov MM, Kurmanova LV, Vnashenkova GV, Merkulova MV, Kokai M, Panya A, Fust G. FN-C1q and C1 INH C1r-C1s complexes as indicators of complement activation in patients with chronic lymphocytic leukaemia. Immunol Lett. 1989;22:1-6

97. Hindmarsh EJ, Marks RM. Decay-accelerating factor is a component of subendothelial extracellular matrix in vitro, and is augmented by activation of endothelial protein kinase C. Eur J Immunol. 1998;28:1052-1062

98. Hofman P, Hsi BL, Manie S, Fenichel P, Thyss A, Rossi B. High expression of the antigen recognized by the monoclonal antibody GB24 on human breast carcinomas: a preventive mechanism of malignant tumor cells against complement attack? Breast Cancer Res Treat. 1994;32:213-219

99. Hosch SB, Scheunemann P, Luth M, Inndorf S, Stoecklein NH, Erbersdobler A, Rehders A, Gundlach M, Knoefel WT, Izbicki JR. Expression of 17-1A antigen and complement resistance factors CD55 and CD59 on liver metastasis in colorectal cancer. J Gastrointest Surg. 2001;5:673-679

100. Idusogie EE, Presta LG, Gazzano-Santoro H, Totpal K, Wong PY, Ultsch M, Meng YG, Mulkerrin MG. Mapping of the C1q binding site on rituxan, a chimeric antibody with a human IgG1 Fc. J Immunol. 2000;164:4178-4184

101. Idusogie EE, Wong PY, Presta LG, Gazzano-Santoro H, Totpal K, Ultsch M, Mulkerrin MG. Engineered antibodies with increased activity to recruit complement. J Immunol. 2001;166:2571-2575

102. Inoue H, Mizuno M, Uesu T, Ueki T, Tsuji T. Distribution of complement regulatory proteins, decay-accelerating factor, CD59/homologous restriction factor 20 and membrane cofactor protein in human colorectal adenoma and cancer. Acta Med Okayama. 1994;48:271-277

103. Inoue T, Yamakawa M, Takahashi T. Expression of complement regulating factors in gastric cancer cells. Mol Pathol. 2002;55:193-199

104. Iwagaki N, Mizuno M, Nasu J, Okazaki H, Hori S, Yamamoto K, Okada H, Tsuji T, Fujita T, Shiratori Y. Advances in the development of a reliable assay for the measurement of stool decay-accelerating factor in the detection of colorectal cancer. J Immunoassay Immunochem. 2002;23:497-507

105. Jacobsen F. Increase of the in vitro complement-dependent cytotoxicity against autologous invasive human bladder tumor cells by neuraminidase treatment. Acta Pathol Microbiol Immunol Scand [C]. 1982;90:187-192

106. Jarvis GA, Vedros NA. Sialic acid of group B Neisseria meningitidis regulates alternative complement pathway activation. Infect Immun. 1987;55:174-180

107. Jarvis GA, Li J, Hakulinen J, Brady KA, Nordling S, Dahiya R, Meri S. Expression and function of the complement membrane attack complex inhibitor protectin (CD59) in human prostate cancer. Int J Cancer. 1997;71:1049-1055

108. Jean D, Hermann J, Rodrigues-Lima F, Barel M, Balbo M, Frade R. Identification on melanoma cells of p39, a cysteine proteinase that cleaves C3, the third component of complement: amino-acid-sequence identities with procathepsin L. Biochem J. 1995;312 (Pt 3):961-969

109. Jean D, Bar-Eli M, Huang S, Xie K, Rodrigues-Lima F, Hermann J, Frade R. A cysteine proteinase, which cleaves human C3, the third component of complement, is

involved in tumorigenicity and metastasis of human melanoma. Cancer Res. 1996;56:254-258

110. Johnstone RW, Tainton KM, Ruefli AA, Froelich CJ, Cerruti L, Jane SM, Smyth MJ. P-glycoprotein does not protect cells against cytolysis induced by pore-forming proteins. J Biol Chem. 2001;276:16667-16673

111. Juhl H, Helmig F, Baltzer K, Kalthoff H, Henne-Bruns D, Kremer B. Frequent expression of complement resistance factors CD46, CD55, and CD59 on gastrointestinal cancer cells limits the therapeutic potential of monoclonal antibody 17-1A. J Surg Oncol. 1997;64:222-230

112. Junnikkala S, Hakulinen J, Meri S. Targeted neutralization of the complement membrane attack complex inhibitor CD59 on the surface of human melanoma cells. Eur J Immunol. 1994;24:611-615

113. Junnikkala S, Jokiranta TS, Friese MA, Jarva H, Zipfel PF, Meri S. Exceptional resistance of human H2 glioblastoma cells to complement-mediated killing by expression and utilization of factor H and factor H-like protein 1. J Immunol. 2000;164:6075-6081

114. Junnikkala S, Hakulinen J, Jarva H, Manuelian T, Bjorge L, Butzow R, Zipfel PF, Meri S. Secretion of soluble complement inhibitors factor H and factor H-like protein (FHL-1) by ovarian tumour cells. Br J Cancer. 2002;87:1119-1127

115. Jurianz K, Maslak S, Garcia-Schuler H, Fishelson Z, Kirschfink M. Neutralization of complement regulatory proteins augments lysis of breast carcinoma cells targeted with rhumAb anti-HER2. Immunopharmacology. 1999;42:209-218

116. Jurianz K, Ziegler S, Garcia-Schuler H, Kraus S, Bohana-Kashtan O, Fishelson Z, Kirschfink M. Complement resistance of tumor cells: basal and induced mechanisms. Mol Immunol. 1999;36:929-939

117. Jurianz K, Ziegler S, Donin N, Reiter Y, Fishelson Z, Kirschfink M. K562 erythroleukemic cells are equipped with multiple mechanisms of resistance to lysis by complement. Int J Cancer. 2001;93:848-854

118. Kaliner M, Austen KF. Adenosine 3'5'-monophosphate: inhibition of complement-mediated cell lysis. Science. 1974;183:659-661

119. Kang PJ, Ostermann J, Shilling J, Neupert W, Craig EA, Pfanner N. Requirement for hsp70 in the mitochondrial matrix for translocation and folding of precursor proteins. Nature. 1990;348:137-143

120. Kazatchkine MD, Jouvin MH. Interactions between the alternative complement pathway and proteases of the coagulation system. Adv Exp Med Biol. 1984;167:235-239

121. Kennedy AD, Solga MD, Schuman TA, Chi AW, Lindorfer MA, Sutherland WM, Foley PL, Taylor RP. An anti-C3b(i) mAb enhances complement activation, C3b(i) deposition, and killing of CD20+ cells by rituximab. Blood. 2003;101:1071-1079

122. Kilgore KS, Shen JP, Miller BF, Ward PA, Warren JS. Enhancement by the complement membrane attack complex of tumor necrosis factor-alpha-induced endothelial cell expression of E-selectin and ICAM-1. J Immunol. 1995;155:1434-1441

123. Kilgore KS, Flory CM, Miller BF, Evans VM, Warren JS. The membrane attack complex of complement induces interleukin-8 and monocyte chemoattractant protein-1 secretion from human umbilical vein endothelial cells. Am J Pathol. 1996;149:953-961

124. Kilgore KS, Imlay MM, Szaflarski JP, Silverstein FS, Malani AN, Evans VM, Warren JS. Neutrophils and reactive oxygen intermediates mediate glucan-induced pulmonary granuloma formation through the local induction of monocyte chemoattractant protein-1. Lab Invest. 1997;76:191-201

125. Kim SH, Carney DF, Hammer CH, Shin ML. Nucleated cell killing by complement: effects of C5b-9 channel size and extracellular Ca2+ on the lytic process. J Immunol. 1987;138:1530-1536

126. Kinders R, Jones T, Root R, Bruce C, Murchison H, Corey M, Williams L, Enfield D, Hass GM. Complement factor H or a related protein is a marker for transitional cell cancer of the bladder. Clin Cancer Res. 1998;4:2511-2520

127. Kinugasa N, Higashi T, Nouso K, Nakatsukasa H, Kobayashi Y, Ishizaki M, Toshikuni N, Yoshida K, Uematsu S, Tsuji T. Expression of membrane cofactor protein (MCP, CD46) in human liver diseases. Br J Cancer. 1999;80:1820-1825

128. Kipnis TL, David JR, Alper CA, Sher A, da Silva WD. Enzymatic treatment transforms trypomastigotes of Trypanosoma cruzi into activators of alternative complement pathway and potentiates their uptake by macrophages. Proc Natl Acad Sci U S A. 1981;78:602-605

129. Kirschfink M, Blase L, Engelmann S, Schwartz-Albiez R. Secreted chondroitin sulfate proteoglycan of human B cell lines binds to the complement protein C1q and inhibits complex formation of C1. J Immunol. 1997;158:1324-1331

130. Kiso T, Mizuno M, Nasu J, Shimo K, Uesu T, Yamamoto K, Okada H, Fujita T, Tsuji T. Enhanced expression of decay-accelerating factor and CD59/homologous restriction factor 20 in intestinal metaplasia, gastric adenomas and intestinal-type gastric carcinomas but not in diffuse-type carcinomas. Histopathology. 2002;40:339-347

131. Koretz K, Bruderlein S, Henne C, Moller P. Decay-accelerating factor (DAF, CD55) in normal colorectal mucosa, adenomas and carcinomas. Br J Cancer. 1992;66:810-814

132. Koretz K, Bruderlein S, Henne C, Moller P. Expression of CD59, a complement regulator protein and a second ligand of the CD2 molecule, and CD46 in normal and neoplastic colorectal epithelium. Br J Cancer. 1993;68:926-931

133. Korsmeyer SJ. BCL-2 gene family and the regulation of programmed cell death. Cancer Res. 1999;59:1693s-1700s

134. Koski CL, Ramm LE, Hammer CH, Mayer MM, Shin ML. Cytolysis of nucleated cells by complement: cell death displays multi-hit characteristics. Proc Natl Acad Sci U S A. 1983;80:3816-3820

135. Kraus S, Fishelson Z. Cell desensitization by sublytic C5b-9 complexes and calcium ionophores depends on activation of protein kinase C. Eur J Immunol. 2000;30:1272-1280

136. Kraus S, Seger R, Fishelson Z. Involvement of the ERK mitogen-activated protein kinase in cell resistance to complement-mediated lysis. Clin Exp Immunol. 2001;123:366-374

137. Krepela E. Cysteine proteinases in tumor cell growth and apoptosis. Neoplasma. 2001;48:332-349

138. Kristensen T, D'Eustachio P, Ogata RT, Chung LP, Reid KB, Tack BF. The superfamily of C3b/C4b-binding proteins. Fed Proc. 1987;46:2463-2469

139. Kuraya M, Yefenof E, Klein G, Klein E. Expression of the complement regulatory proteins CD21, CD55 and CD59 on Burkitt lymphoma lines: their role in sensitivity to human serum-mediated lysis. Eur J Immunol. 1992;22:1871-1876

140. Kuraya M, Minarovits J, Okada H, Klein E. HRF20/CD59 complement regulatory protein expression is phenotype-dependent and inducible by the hypomethylating agent 5-azacytidine on Burkitt's lymphoma cell lines. Immunol Lett. 1993;37:35-39

141. Lauf PK. Immunological and physiological characteristics of the rapid immune hemolysis of neuraminidase-treated sheep red cells produced by fresh guinea pig serum. J Exp Med. 1975;142:974-988

142. Legoedec J, Gasque P, Jeanne JF, Fontaine M. Expression of the complement alternative pathway by human myoblasts in vitro: biosynthesis of C3, factor B, factor H and factor I. Eur J Immunol. 1995;25:3460-3466

143. Li GC, Mivechi NF, Weitzel G. Heat shock proteins, thermotolerance, and their relevance to clinical hyperthermia. Int J Hyperthermia. 1995;11:459-488

144. Li WX, Chen CH, Ling CC, Li GC. Apoptosis in heat-induced cell killing: the protective role of hsp-70 and the sensitization effect of the c-myc gene. Radiat Res. 1996;145:324-330

145. Li L, Spendlove I, Morgan J, Durrant LG. CD55 is over-expressed in the tumour environment. Br J Cancer. 2001;84:80-86

146. Lin S, Kemmner W, Grigull S, Schlag PM. Cell surface alpha 2,6 sialylation affects adhesion of breast carcinoma cells. Exp Cell Res. 2002;276:101-110

147. Lindquist S, Craig EA. The heat-shock proteins. Annu Rev Genet. 1988;22:631-677

148. Lucas SD, Karlsson-Parra A, Nilsson B, Grimelius L, Akerstrom G, Rastad J, Juhlin C. Tumor-specific deposition of immunoglobulin G and complement in papillary thyroid carcinoma. Hum Pathol. 1996;27:1329-1335

149. Lynch CC, Matrisian LM. Matrix metalloproteinases in tumor-host cell communication. Differentiation. 2002;70:561-573

150. Madjd Z, Pinder SE, Paish C, Ellis IO, Carmichael J, Durrant LG. Loss of CD59 expression in breast tumours correlates with poor survival. J Pathol. 2003;200:633-639

151. Maenpaa A, Junnikkala S, Hakulinen J, Timonen T, Meri S. Expression of complement membrane regulators membrane cofactor protein (CD46), decay accelerating factor (CD55), and protectin (CD59) in human malignant gliomas. Am J Pathol. 1996;148:1139-1152

152. Maison CM, Villiers CL, Colomb MG. Proteolysis of C3 on U937 cell plasma membranes. Purification of cathepsin G. J Immunol. 1991;147:921-926

153. Maness PF, Orengo A. Serum complement levels in patients with digestive tract carcinomas and other neoplastic diseases. Oncology. 1977;34:87-89

154. Mangano A, Messina L, Birgillito S, Stivala F, Bernardini A. Complement and its fractions (C3-C4) pattern in subjects with neoplasia. J Immunopharmacol. 1984;6:147-162

155. Martin J, Hartl FU. The effect of macromolecular crowding on chaperonin-mediated protein folding. Proc Natl Acad Sci U S A. 1997;94:1107-1112

156. Martin J, Hartl FU. Chaperone-assisted protein folding. Curr Opin Struct Biol. 1997;7:41-52

157. Matsutani M, Suzuki T, Hori T, Terao H, Takakura K, Nishioka K. Cellular immunity and complement levels in hosts with brain tumours. Neurosurg Rev. 1984;7:29-35

158. Maxwell-Armstrong CA, Durrant LG, Buckley TJ, Scholefield JH, Robins RA, Fielding K, Monson JR, Guillou P, Calvert H, Carmichael J, Hardcastle JD. Randomized double-blind phase II survival study comparing immunization with the anti-idiotypic monoclonal antibody 105AD7 against placebo in advanced colorectal cancer. Br J Cancer. 2001;84:1443-1446

159. McConnell I, Klein G, Lint TF, Lachmann PJ. Activation of the alternative complement pathway by human B cell lymphoma lines is associated with Epstein-Barr virus transformation of the cells. Eur J Immunol. 1978;8:453-458

160. Medof ME, Lublin DM, Holers VM, Ayers DJ, Getty RR, Leykam JF, Atkinson JP, Tykocinski ML. Cloning and characterization of cDNAs encoding the complete sequence of decay-accelerating factor of human complement. Proc Natl Acad Sci U S A. 1987;84:2007-2011

161. Medof ME, Walter EI, Rutgers JL, Knowles DM, Nussenzweig V. Identification of the complement decay-accelerating factor (DAF) on epithelium and glandular cells and in body fluids. J Exp Med. 1987;165:848-864

162. Meri S, Morgan BP, Davies A, Daniels RH, Olavesen MG, Waldmann H, Lachmann PJ. Human protectin (CD59), an 18,000-20,000 MW complement lysis restricting factor, inhibits C5b-8 catalysed insertion of C9 into lipid bilayers. Immunology. 1990;71:1-9

163. Meri S, Pangburn MK. Discrimination between activators and nonactivators of the alternative pathway of complement: regulation via a sialic acid/polyanion binding site on factor H. Proc Natl Acad Sci U S A. 1990;87:3982-3986

164. Meri S, Waldmann H, Lachmann PJ. Distribution of protectin (CD59), a complement membrane attack inhibitor, in normal human tissues. Lab Invest. 1991;65:532-537

165. Micklem KJ, Alder GM, Buckley CD, Murphy J, Pasternak CA. Protection against complement-mediated cell damage by Ca2+ and Zn2+. Complement. 1988;5:141-152

166. Mikami Y, Mikami M, Nannmoku H, Kawashima H, Sasaki T, Hada R, Inoue S. Anemia-inducing factor expressed in gastric cancer is homologous with complement regulatory factor CD59? J Exp Clin Cancer Res. 1998;17:355-360

167. Minh DQ, Czink E, Mod A, Fust G, Hollan SR. Serial complement measurements in patients with leukaemia. Clin Lab Haematol. 1983;5:23-34

168. Mizuno M, Nakagawa M, Uesu T, Inoue H, Inaba T, Ueki T, Nasu J, Okada H, Fujita T, Tsuji T. Detection of decay-accelerating factor in stool specimens of patients with colorectal cancer. Gastroenterology. 1995;109:826-831

169. Morgan BP, Campbell AK. The recovery of human polymorphonuclear leucocytes from sublytic complement attack is mediated by changes in intracellular free calcium. Biochem J. 1985;231:205-208

170. Morgan BP, Luzio JP, Campbell AK. Intracellular Ca2+ and cell injury: a paradoxical role of Ca2+ in complement membrane attack. Cell Calcium. 1986;7:399-411

171. Morgan BP, Dankert JR, Esser AF. Recovery of human neutrophils from complement attack: removal of the membrane attack complex by endocytosis and exocytosis. J Immunol. 1987;138:246-253

172. Morgan BP. Complement membrane attack on nucleated cells: resistance, recovery and non-lethal effects. Biochem J. 1989;264:1-14

173. Morgan BP, Olavesen MG, Watts MJ. Presence of a membrane attack complex inhibiting protein on the human epithelial cell line HeLa. Biochem Soc Trans. 1990;18:673-674

174. Morgan BP. Effects of the membrane attack complex of complement on nucleated cells. Curr Top Microbiol Immunol. 1992;178:115-140

175. Morgan BP, Harris, C.L. Complement Regulatory Proteins. Academic Press. San Diego; 1999

176. Morimoto RI. Regulation of the heat shock transcriptional response: cross talk between a family of heat shock factors, molecular chaperones, and negative regulators. Genes Dev. 1998;12:3788-3796

177. Morimoto RI, Santoro MG. Stress-inducible responses and heat shock proteins: new pharmacologic targets for cytoprotection. Nat Biotechnol. 1998;16:833-838

178. Murray KP, Mathure S, Kaul R, Khan S, Carson LF, Twiggs LB, Martens MG, Kaul A. Expression of complement regulatory proteins-CD 35, CD 46, CD 55, and CD 59-in benign and malignant endometrial tissue. Gynecol Oncol. 2000;76:176-182

179. Nakagawa M, Mizuno M, Kawada M, Uesu T, Nasu J, Takeuchi K, Okada H, Endo Y, Fujita T, Tsuji T. Polymorphic expression of decay-accelerating factor in human colorectal cancer. J Gastroenterol Hepatol. 2001;16:184-189

180. Nakano Y, Sugita Y, Ishikawa Y, Choi NH, Tobe T, Tomita M. Isolation of two forms of decay-accelerating factor (DAF) from human urine. Biochim Biophys Acta. 1991;1074:326-330
181. Nasu J, Mizuno M, Uesu T, Takeuchi K, Inaba T, Ohya S, Kawada M, Shimo K, Okada H, Fujita T, Tsuji T. Cytokine-stimulated release of decay-accelerating factor (DAF;CD55) from HT-29 human intestinal epithelial cells. Clin Exp Immunol. 1998;113:379-385
182. Nauta AJ, Daha MR, Tijsma O, van de Water B, Tedesco F, Roos A. The membrane attack complex of complement induces caspase activation and apoptosis. Eur J Immunol. 2002;32:783-792
183. Niculescu F, Rus HG, Retegan M, Vlaicu R. Persistent complement activation on tumor cells in breast cancer. Am J Pathol. 1992;140:1039-1043
184. Niculescu F, Rus H, Shin S, Lang T, Shin ML. Generation of diacylglycerol and ceramide during homologous complement activation. J Immunol. 1993;150:214-224
185. Niculescu F, Rus H, Shin ML. Receptor-independent activation of guanine nucleotide-binding regulatory proteins by terminal complement complexes. J Biol Chem. 1994;269:4417-4423
186. Niculescu F, Rus H, van Biesen T, Shin ML. Activation of Ras and mitogen-activated protein kinase pathway by terminal complement complexes is G protein dependent. J Immunol. 1997;158:4405-4412
187. Niehans GA, Cherwitz DL, Staley NA, Knapp DJ, Dalmasso AP. Human carcinomas variably express the complement inhibitory proteins CD46 (membrane cofactor protein), CD55 (decay-accelerating factor), and CD59 (protectin). Am J Pathol. 1996;149:129-142
188. Nilsson Ekdahl K, Nilsson B. Phosphorylation of complement component C3 after synthesis in U937 cells by a putative protein kinase, casein kinase 2, which is regulated by CD11b: evidence that membrane-bound proteases preferentially cleave phosphorylated C3. Biochem J. 1997;328 (Pt 2):625-633
189. Nishioka K, Kawamura K, Hirayama T, Kawashima T, Shimada K. The complement system in tumor immunity: significance of elevated levels of complement in tumor bearing hosts. Ann N Y Acad Sci. 1976;276:303-315
190. Nowicki S, Nowicki B, Pham T, Hasan R, Nagamani M. Expression of decay accelerating factor in endometrial adenocarcinoma is inversely related to the stage of tumor. Am J Reprod Immunol. 2001;46:144-148
191. Odening K, Jurianz K, Fishelson Z, Kirschfink M. Multi-drug resistant ovarian carcinomacells develop increased complement resistnce. Mol Immunol. 2001;38:114
192. Ohanian SH, Schlager SI. Humoral immune killing of nucleated cells: mechanisms of complement-mediated attack and target cell defense. Crit Rev Immunol. 1981;1:165-209
193. Okada H, Baba T. Rosette formation of human erythrocytes on cultured cells of tumour origin and activation of complement by cell membrane. Nature. 1974;248:521-522
194. Ollert MW, Frade R, Fiandino A, Panneerselvam M, Petrella EC, Barel M, Pangburn MK, Bredehorst R, Vogel CW. C3-cleaving membrane proteinase. A new complement regulatory protein of human melanoma cells. J Immunol. 1990;144:3862-3867
195. Paas Y, Fishelson Z. Shedding of tyrosine and serine/threonine ecto-protein kinases from human leukemic cells. Arch Biochem Biophys. 1995;316:780-788
196. Paas Y, Bohana-Kashtan O, Fishelson Z. Phosphorylation of the complement component, C9, by an ecto-protein kinase of human leukemic cells. Immunopharmacology. 1999;42:175-185

197. Pangburn MK, Muller-Eberhard HJ. Complement C3 convertase: cell surface restriction of beta1H control and generation of restriction on neuraminidase-treated cells. Proc Natl Acad Sci U S A. 1978;75:2416-2420

198. Papadimitriou JC, Carney DF, Shin ML. Inhibitors of membrane lipid metabolism enhance complement-mediated nucleated cell killing through distinct mechanisms. Mol Immunol. 1991;28:803-809

199. Papadimitriou JC, Drachenberg CB, Shin ML, Trump BF. Ultrastructural studies of complement mediated cell death: a biological reaction model to plasma membrane injury. Virchows Arch. 1994;424:677-685

200. Peng KW, TenEyck CJ, Galanis E, Kalli KR, Hartmann LC, Russell SJ. Intraperitoneal therapy of ovarian cancer using an engineered measles virus. Cancer Res. 2002;62:4656-4662

201. Perez-Ordonez B, Rosai J. Follicular dendritic cell tumor: review of the entity. Semin Diagn Pathol. 1998;15:144-154

202. Pilon M, Schekman R. Protein translocation: how Hsp70 pulls it off. Cell. 1999;97:679-682

203. Ram S, Sharma AK, Simpson SD, Gulati S, McQuillen DP, Pangburn MK, Rice PA. A novel sialic acid binding site on factor H mediates serum resistance of sialylated Neisseria gonorrhoeae. J Exp Med. 1998;187:743-752

204. Ramm LE, Whitlow MB, Koski CL, Shin ML, Mayer MM. Elimination of complement channels from the plasma membranes of U937, a nucleated mammalian cell line: temperature dependence of the elimination rate. J Immunol. 1983;131:1411-1415

205. Ravindranath NM, Nishimoto K, Chu K, Shuler C. Cell-surface expression of complement restriction factors and sialyl Lewis antigens in oral carcinoma: relevance to chemo-immunotherapy. Anticancer Res. 2000;20:21-26

206. Ray PK, Sundaram K. Cytolysis of neuraminidase-treated autochthonous lymphoid cells by autologous serum. Clin Exp Immunol. 1975;19:529-532

207. Reiter Y, Fishelson Z. Targeting of complement to tumor cells by heteroconjugates composed of antibodies and of the complement component C3b. J Immunol. 1989;142:2771-2777

208. Reiter Y, Ciobotariu A, Fishelson Z. Sublytic complement attack protects tumor cells from lytic doses of antibody and complement. Eur J Immunol. 1992;22:1207-1213.

209. Reiter Y, Fishelson Z. Complement membrane attack complexes induce in human leukemic cells rapid expression of large proteins (L-CIP). Mol Immunol. 1992;29:771-781.

210. Reiter Y, Ciobotariu A, Jones J, Morgan BP, Fishelson Z. Complement membrane attack complex, perforin, and bacterial exotoxins induce in K562 cells calcium-dependent cross-protection from lysis. J Immunol. 1995;155:2203-2210.

211. Richter K, Buchner J. Hsp90: chaperoning signal transduction. J Cell Physiol. 2001;188:281-290.

212. Rooney IA, Morgan BP. Characterization of the membrane attack complex inhibitory protein CD59 antigen on human amniotic cells and in amniotic fluid. Immunology. 1992;76:541-547

213. Ross GD, Vetvicka V, Yan J, Xia Y, Vetvickova J. Therapeutic intervention with complement and beta-glucan in cancer. Immunopharmacology. 1999;42:61-74

214. Ruefli AA, Bernhard D, Tainton KM, Kofler R, Smyth MJ, Johnstone RW. Suberoylanilide hydroxamic acid (SAHA) overcomes multidrug resistance and induces cell death in P-glycoprotein-expressing cells. Int J Cancer. 2002;99:292-298

215. Rus HG, Niculescu F, Shin ML. Sublytic complement attack induces cell cycle in oligodendrocytes. J Immunol. 1996;156:4892-4900

216. Sadallah S, Lach E, Schwarz S, Gratwohl A, Spertini O, Schifferli JA. Soluble complement receptor 1 is increased in patients with leukemia and after administration of granulocyte colony-stimulating factor. J Leukoc Biol. 1999;65:94-101

217. Sakuma T, Kodama K, Hara T, Eshita Y, Shibata N, Matsumoto M, Seya T, Mori Y. Levels of complement regulatory molecules in lung cancer: disappearance of the D17 epitope of CD55 in small-cell carcinoma. Jpn J Cancer Res. 1993;84:753-759

218. Sawada K, Morishige K, Tahara M, Ikebuchi Y, Kawagishi R, Tasaka K, Murata Y. Lysophosphatidic acid induces focal adhesion assembly through Rho/Rho-associated kinase pathway in human ovarian cancer cells. Gynecol Oncol. 2002;87:252-259

219. Sawada M, Moriya S, Saito S, Shineha R, Satomi S, Yamori T, Tsuruo T, Kannagi R, Miyagi T. Reduced sialidase expression in highly metastatic variants of mouse colon adenocarcinoma 26 and retardation of their metastatic ability by sialidase overexpression. Int J Cancer. 2002;97:180-185

220. Sayama K, Shiraishi S, Miki Y. Distribution of complement regulators (CD46, CD55 and CD59) in skin appendages, and in benign and malignant skin neoplasms. Br J Dermatol. 1992;127:1-4

221. Schanne FA, Kane AB, Young EE, Farber JL. Calcium dependence of toxic cell death: a final common pathway. Science. 1979;206:700-702

222. Schlager SI, Boyle MD, Ohanian SH, Borsos T. Effect of inhibiting DNA, RNA, and protein synthesis of tumor cells on their susceptibility to killing by antibody and complement. Cancer Res. 1977;37:1432-1437

223. Schlesinger M, Broman I, Lugassy G. The complement system is defective in chronic lymphatic leukemia patients and in their healthy relatives. Leukemia. 1996;10:1509-1513

224. Schmitt CA, Schwaeble W, Wittig BM, Meyer zum Buschenfelde KH, Dippold WG. Expression and regulation by interferon-gamma of the membrane-bound complement regulators CD46 (MCP), CD55 (DAF) and CD59 in gastrointestinal tumours. Eur J Cancer. 1999;35:117-124

225. Schreiber RD, Pangburn MK, Medicus RG, Muller-Eberhard HJ. Raji cell injury and subsequent lysis by the purified cytolytic alternative pathway of human complement. Clin Immunol Immunopathol. 1980;15:384-396

226. Scolding NJ, Houston WA, Morgan BP, Campbell AK, Compston DA. Reversible injury of cultured rat oligodendrocytes by complement. Immunology. 1989;67:441-446

227. Scolding NJ, Morgan BP, Houston WA, Linington C, Campbell AK, Compston DA. Vesicular removal by oligodendrocytes of membrane attack complexes formed by activated complement. Nature. 1989;339:620-622

228. Seya T, Hara T, Matsumoto M, Akedo H. Quantitative analysis of membrane cofactor protein (MCP) of complement. High expression of MCP on human leukemia cell lines, which is down-regulated during cell differentiation. J Immunol. 1990;145:238-245

229. Seya T, Matsumoto M, Hara T, Hatanaka M, Masaoka T, Akedo H. Distribution of C3-step regulatory proteins of the complement system, CD35 (CR1), CD46 (MCP), and CD55 (DAF), in hematological malignancies. Leuk Lymphoma. 1994;12:395-400

230. Seya T, Hara T, Iwata K, Kuriyama S, Hasegawa T, Nagase Y, Miyagawa S, Matsumoto M, Hatanaka M, Atkinson JP, et al. Purification and functional properties of soluble forms of membrane cofactor protein (CD46) of complement: identification of forms increased in cancer patients' sera. Int Immunol. 1995;7:727-736

231. Simpson KL, Jones A, Norman S, Holmes CH. Expression of the complement regulatory proteins decay accelerating factor (DAF, CD55), membrane cofactor protein (MCP, CD46) and CD59 in the normal human uterine cervix and in premalignant and malignant cervical disease. Am J Pathol. 1997;151:1455-1467

232. Sims PJ, Wiedmer T. Repolarization of the membrane potential of blood platelets after complement damage: evidence for a Ca++ -dependent exocytotic elimination of C5b-9 pores. Blood. 1986;68:556-561

233. Sivaparvathi M, Yamamoto M, Nicolson GL, Gokaslan ZL, Fuller GN, Liotta LA, Sawaya R, Rao JS. Expression and immunohistochemical localization of cathepsin L during the progression of human gliomas. Clin Exp Metastasis. 1996;14:27-34

234. Soane L, Rus H, Niculescu F, Shin ML. Inhibition of oligodendrocyte apoptosis by sublytic C5b-9 is associated with enhanced synthesis of bcl-2 and mediated by inhibition of caspase-3 activation. J Immunol. 1999;163:6132-6138

235. Soane L, Cho HJ, Niculescu F, Rus H, Shin ML. C5b-9 terminal complement complex protects oligodendrocytes from death by regulating Bad through phosphatidylinositol 3-kinase/Akt pathway. J Immunol. 2001;167:2305-2311

236. Southam CM, Siegel AH. Serum levels of second component of complement in cancer patients. J Immunol. 1966;97:331-337

237. Spendlove L, Li L, Potter V, Christiansen D, Loveland BE, Durrant LG. A therapeutic human anti-idiotypic antibody mimics CD55 in three distinct regions. Eur J Immunol. 2000;30:2944-2953

238. Spiller OB, Criado-Garcia O, Rodriguez De Cordoba S, Morgan BP. Cytokine-mediated up-regulation of CD55 and CD59 protects human hepatoma cells from complement attack. Clin Exp Immunol. 2000;121:234-241

239. Sreedhar AS, Mihaly K, Pato B, Schnaider T, Stetak A, Kis-Petik K, Fidy J, Simonics T, Maraz A, Csermely P. Hsp90 inhibition accelerates cell lysis. Anti-Hsp90 ribozyme reveals a complex mechanism of Hsp90 inhibitors involving both superoxide- and Hsp90-dependent events. J Biol Chem. 2003;278:35231-35240

240. Stanley KK, Page M, Campbell AK, Luzio JP. A mechanism for the insertion of complement component C9 into target membranes. Mol Immunol. 1986;23:451-458

241. Su CY, Chong KY, Owen OE, Dillmann WH, Chang C, Lai CC. Constitutive and inducible hsp70s are involved in oxidative resistance evoked by heat shock or ethanol. J Mol Cell Cardiol. 1998;30:587-598

242. Tedesco F, Pausa M, Nardon E, Introna M, Mantovani A, Dobrina A. The cytolytically inactive terminal complement complex activates endothelial cells to express adhesion molecules and tissue factor procoagulant activity. J Exp Med. 1997;185:1619-1627.

243. Tedesco F, Pausa M, Nardon E, Introna M, Mantovani A, Dobrina A. The cytolytically inactive terminal complement complex activates endothelial cells to express adhesion molecules and tissue factor procoagulant activity. J Exp Med. 1997;185:1619-1627

244. Terachi T, Stanescu G, Pontes JE, Medof ME, Caulfield MJ. Coexistence of autologous antibodies and decay-accelerating factor, an inhibitor of complement, on human renal tumor cells. Cancer Res. 1991;51:2521-2523

245. Theofilopoulos AN, Perrin LH. Binding of components of the properdin system to cultured human lymphoblastoid cells and B lymphocytes. J Exp Med. 1976;143:271-289

246. Thorsteinsson L, O'Dowd GM, Harrington PM, Johnson PM. The complement regulatory proteins CD46 and CD59, but not CD55, are highly expressed by glandular epithelium of human breast and colorectal tumour tissues. Apmis. 1998;106:869-878

247. Treon SP, Mitsiades C, Mitsiades N, Young G, Doss D, Schlossman R, Anderson KC. Tumor cell expression of CD59 is associated with resistance to CD20 serotherapy in patients with B-cell malignancies. J Immunother. 2001;24:263-271

248. Trump BF, Berezesky IK. Calcium-mediated cell injury and cell death. Faseb J. 1995;9:219-228

249. Turianskyj FH, Gyenes L. The effect of neuraminidase on the sensitivity of tumor cells toward lysis by antibody and complement or by sensitized lymphocytes. Transplantation. 1976;22:24-30
250. Vakeva A, Meri S. Complement activation and regulator expression after anoxic injury of human endothelial cells. Apmis. 1998;106:1149-1156
251. Vander Heiden MG, Thompson CB. Bcl-2 proteins: regulators of apoptosis or of mitochondrial homeostasis? Nat Cell Biol. 1999;1:E209-216
252. Vander Heiden MG, Thompson CB. Bcl-2 proteins: regulators of apoptosis or of mitochondrial homeostasis? Nat Cell Biol. 1999;1:E209-216
253. Varsano S, Frolkis I, Ophir D. Expression and distribution of cell-membrane complement regulatory glycoproteins along the human respiratory tract. Am J Respir Crit Care Med. 1995;152:1087-1093
254. Varsano S, Rashkovsky L, Shapiro H, Ophir D, Mark-Bentankur T. Human lung cancer cell lines express cell membrane complement inhibitory proteins and are extremely resistant to complement-mediated lysis; a comparison with normal human respiratory epithelium in vitro, and an insight into mechanism(s) of resistance. Clin Exp Immunol. 1998;113:173-182
255. Varsano S, Rashkovsky L, Shapiro H, Radnay J. Cytokines modulate expression of cell-membrane complement inhibitory proteins in human lung cancer cell lines. Am J Respir Cell Mol Biol. 1998;19:522-529
256. Vogel CW, Muller-Eberhard HJ. Induction of immune cytolysis: tumor-cell killing by complement is initiated by covalent complex of monoclonal antibody and stable C3/C5 convertase. Proc Natl Acad Sci U S A. 1981;78:7707-7711
257. Walport MJ. Complement. First of two parts. N Engl J Med. 2001;344:1058-1066
258. Walport MJ. Complement. Second of two parts. N Engl J Med. 2001;344:1140-1144
259. Weichenthal M, Siemann U, Neuber K, Breitbart EW. Expression of complement regulator proteins in primary and metastatic malignant melanoma. J Cutan Pathol. 1999;26:217-221
260. Weisburg JH, Curcio M, Caron PC, Raghu G, Mechetner EB, Roepe PD, Scheinberg DA. The multidrug resistance phenotype confers immunological resistance. J Exp Med. 1996;183:2699-2704
261. Weisburg JH, Roepe PD, Dzekunov S, Scheinberg DA. Intracellular pH and multidrug resistance regulate complement-mediated cytotoxicity of nucleated human cells. J Biol Chem. 1999;274:10877-10888
262. Weng WK, Levy R. Expression of complement inhibitors CD46, CD55, and CD59 on tumor cells does not predict clinical outcome after rituximab treatment in follicular non-Hodgkin lymphoma. Blood. 2001;98:1352-1357
263. Williams RS, Thomas JA, Fina M, German Z, Benjamin IJ. Human heat shock protein 70 (hsp70) protects murine cells from injury during metabolic stress. J Clin Invest. 1993;92:503-508
264. Yamakawa M, Yamada K, Tsuge T, Ohrui H, Ogata T, Dobashi M, Imai Y. Protection of thyroid cancer cells by complement-regulatory factors. Cancer. 1994;73:2808-2817
265. Yefenof E, Benizri R, Reiter Y, Klein E, Fishelson Z. Potentiation of NK cytotoxicity by antibody-C3b/iC3b heteroconjugates. J Immunol. 1990;144:1538-1543
266. Yefenof E, Algarra I, Ramos OF, Klein E. Activation and fixation of C3 by human B cell lines is enhanced by interferon-gamma and tumor necrosis factor alpha. Complement Inflamm. 1991;8:271-280
267. Yogeeswaran G, Salk PL. Metastatic potential is positively correlated with cell surface sialylation of cultured murine tumor cell lines. Science. 1981;212:1514-1516

268. Yoon SO, Park SJ, Yun CH, Chung AS. Roles of matrix metalloproteinases in tumor metastasis and angiogenesis. J Biochem Mol Biol. 2003;36:128-137

269. Yu J, Caragine T, Chen S, Morgan BP, Frey AB, Tomlinson S. Protection of human breast cancer cells from complement-mediated lysis by expression of heterologous CD59. Clin Exp Immunol. 1999;115:13-18

270. Zell S, Giese T, Rutz R, Schultz S, Kirschfink M. Inhibition of mCRP (C55, CD46) expression by antisense-oligonucleotides reduces complement-resistance of tumor cells. Mol Immunol. 2003;40:196

271. Zhong RK, Kozii R, Ball ED. Homologous restriction of complement-mediated cell lysis can be markedly enhanced by blocking decay-accelerating factor. Br J Haematol. 1995;91:269-274

272. Ziegler S, Jurianz K, Kirschfink M. Complement resistance of human primary ovarian carcinoma. Mol Immunol. 1999;36:317

273. Ziegler S, Jurianz K, Manuelian T, Zipfel PF, Kirschfink M. Human tumor cells secrete complement regulatory molecules Factor H and FHL-1. Mol Immunol. 2001;38:130-131

PART 5

ROLE OF COMPLEMENT IN AUTOIMMUNE DISEASES, ALLERGY AND TRANSPLANTATION

14

Complement and Autoimmunity

George C. Tsokos and Mate Tolnay
Department of Cellular Injury, Walter Reed Army Institute of Research, Silver Spring, MD 20910

Abstract: The role of complement in the regulation of the immune response has been studied extensively (1) and is reviewed elsewhere in this book. At the mature B cell level, complement 3 products bind to complement receptor 2 (CR2) expressed on the surface of B and dendritic cells and facilitate antigen localization and process, lowering the excitation threshold and deferring apoptosis. In this chapter we will discuss the impact of complement component deficiency in man and mouse on the development of autoimmunity. Differences between mice and humans will become apparent and the dual effect of complement as effector of tissue pathology and controller of the development of the immune cell repertoire will emerge.

Key words: apoptosis, B cells, complement receptors, dendritic cells, knock-out mice

1. COMPLEMENT COMPONENT DEFICIENCY AND AUTOIMMUNITY IN HUMANS

Genome wide studies of human systemic and autoimmunity have unequivocally revealed that the number of loci associated with the development of clinical disease are multiple (1-3). It can be assumed therefore, that the number of the involved genes is rather large confirming a long suspected conviction that human systemic autoimmunity is multigenic in origin. In contrast to this position have been reports of the development of systemic autoimmune disease in rare patients who miss several complement proteins. It has long been realized that deficiencies of the early components of complement pathway are associated with the autoimmune manifestations, whereas deficiency of the so-called common pathway of the complement activation is associated with infections. Almost all individuals deficient in C1q, C2 and C4 components of the complement develop either SLE or glomerulonephritis. The number of the reported cases with complement deficiency is shown in Table 1 along with the dominant autoimmune phenotype.

Table 1. Autoimmune diseases in complete complement component deficiencies (4,5)

Component	Cases	Phenotype	Frequency (%)
C1q	35	SLE	94
C1r/s	11	SLE,	55
		GN	5
C1 INH		autoantibodies	<10
		GN	<5
C4 (C4A and	24	SLE	75
C4B null)		HSP	8
		SS	4
C2	110	SLE	32
C3	21	SLE	14
		GN	23
		vasculitis	14

SLE, systemic lupus erythematosus, GN, glomerulonephritis
HSP, Henoch-Shoenlein purpura, SS, Sjogren's syndrome.

Because complement proteins and complement receptors have been considered to be important in the development of the immune response an alternative hypothesis has been adopted to understand how complement deficiency leads to the development of systemic autoimmunity. It is believed that SLE peripheral blood immune cells undergo apoptosis at increased rates. The released nuclear material enters the circulation and it binds anti-nuclear antibodies to form immune complexes. One of the main functions of the complement system is to participate in the clearance of the nuclear material and the immune complexes (5,6). If the clearance processes are defective, then an inflammatory pathology ensues which leads to tissue damage. Along these lines, C1q has been shown to bind to apoptotic cells and therefore, to participate in their clearance (7,8). Although this hypothesis has been enthusiastically adopted, it does not entertain any possible role for complement in the development and the maintenance of immune cell tolerance. Such a role is clearly implied from the data that have been generated from the study of mice in which one or two complement proteins have been deleted.

2. COMPLEMENT PROTEIN KNOCK OUT MICE

Patients with SLE have approximately 50 percent lower levels of CR1 and CR2 on the surface membrane of the B cells. It is not known (9,10) whether this decrease in receptor expression precedes the development of disease or represent an effect of disease activity. MRL/lpr mice, which develop spontaneously SLE, have decreased numbers of complement receptors prior to the initiation of the disease (11). Despite the fact that the numbers of CR2 are decreased on the surface membrane of SLE B-cells, co-engagement of surface immunoglobulin and complement receptor 2 leads to enhanced cell signalling responses (10). This is probably due to the fact that the expression of CD19 remains intact on the surface membrane of B-cells and CD19 is responsible for the transmission of the signalling message inwards (12).

The B6/lpr mouse develops minor autoimmune features. Introduction of CR1/CR2 deficiency into this mouse permits the development of intense autoimmune features (13). This observation indicates that complement receptors are important in the elimination of B-cells that display reactivity with self-antigens. This explanation assumes that self antigens initiate a strong B-cell signal which leads to cell death and the absence of the CR2-mediated enhancement of the signal permits their survival (14,15). When the complement receptor deficiency was introduced into the hen egg lysozyme (HEL) double transgenic mouse model for immune cell tolerance, the paucity of the production of anti-HEL antibodies was not reversed. It should be noted though that the numbers of the circulating B-cells increased and they responded normally to stimulation (16,17) indicating that there is some effect on B cell biology but not enough to break tolerance. These two sets of experiments suggest a relative role for CR2 in the maintenance of tolerance for self-antigens. The absence of CR2 can cause autoimmune disease only in an organism genetically predisposed to autoimmunity. Another strong piece of evidence for the involvement of CR2 in the expression of systemic autoimmunity has provided from the study of the NZM2410 mouse. A major murine SLE susceptibility locus, Sle1, which corresponds to three loci independently affecting loss of tolerance to chromatin has been identified in this congenic mouse. The congenic interval corresponding to Sle1c contains *Cr2*, which encodes CR1/CR2 (CD35/CD21). NZM2410/NZW Cr2 exhibits a single nucleotide polymorphism that introduces a novel glycosylation site, resulting in higher molecular weight proteins. This polymorphism, located in the C3d binding domain, reduces ligand binding and receptor-mediated cell signalling. Molecular modeling based on the recently solved CR2 structure in complex with C3d has revealed that this glycosylation interferes with receptor dimerization (18).

In contrast to these experiments, when Cr2-/- mice were immunized with myosin they failed to develop the expected myocarditis (19). Regardless of the claimed role of CR2 on the surface of T cells as part of an activated T cell phenotype, it is obvious that the role of complement in this inducible model of autoimmune disease is different from that in the spontaneous models of autoimmunity. This imposes distinct roles for complement as effector of tissue pathology and as regulator of positive and negative selection.

C1q deficiency alone is sufficient to cause autoimmunity in humans and it was discussed above. In contrast, in mice genetic lack of C1q is not sufficient to initiate the expression of autoimmunity. No evidence of autoimmunity was noted in C1q-deficient C57BL/6 mice, and C1q deficiency in both the C57BL/6.lpr/lpr and MRL/Mp-lpr/lpr strains did not modify the autoimmune phenotype observed in wild-type controls. However, in C1q-deficient MRL/Mp(+/+) animals an acceleration of both the onset and the severity of antinuclear antibodies and glomerulonephritis was seen. Disease was particularly pronounced in females, which developed severe crescentic glomerulonephritis accompanied by heavy proteinuria. These observations demonstrate that the expression of autoimmunity in C1q-deficient mice is strongly influenced by other background genes (20,21).

Since disruption of the C1q, C4 and CR1/CR2 lead to reduced selection against autoreactive B cells and impaired humoral responses, it was suggested that C1 and C4 act through CR1/CR2 to enhance humoral immunity and suppress autoimmunity. The Kelsoe lab (22) though has demonstrated that each complement component acts independently. High titters of spontaneous antinuclear antibody (ANA) in C4(-/)- mice and SLE-like autoimmunity developed in all C4-/- females and most male animals but not in Cr2-/- animals. The fact that the clearance of circulating ICs was impaired in pre-autoimmune C4-/-, but not Cr2-/- mice lends support to the role of nuclear antigen-anti-nuclear antibody immune complexes in the development of autoimmune disease.

Can uncontrolled activation of complement cause autoimmunity? Factor H, the main regulator of this activation, prevents formation and promotes dissociation of the C3 convertase enzyme, and, together with factor I, mediates the proteolytic inactivation of C3b. Factor H deficiency, described in 29 individuals from 12 families and in pigs, allows unhindered activation of fluid-phase C3 and severe depletion of plasma C3. Membranoproliferative glomerulonephritis (MPGN) occurs in factor H-deficient humans and pigs. Pickering et all (23) showed that that mice deficient in factor H (Cfh(-/-) mice) develop MPGN spontaneously and are hypersensitive to developing renal injury caused by immune complexes. The contribution of complement activation was confirmed because after a second mutation in the gene encoding complement factor B was introduced, which prevents C3 turnover in vivo, obviated the phenotype of Cfh(-/-) mice. Thus, uncontrolled C3 activation in vivo is essential for the development of MPGN associated with deficiency of factor H. The mechanism can include direct effect of C5b-9 on mesangial cell proliferations (24) or through the produced C5a. These data suggest that in patients with systemic autoimmunity tissue injury is not caused only by the circulating immune complexes but also through the action of complement activation products.

This concept is supported also by other data in which blockage of complement activation ameliorates glomerulonephritis. New Zealand black x New Zealand white (NZB/W) F_1 mice spontaneously develop an autoimmune syndrome with notable similarities to human systemic lupus erythematosus. Female NZB/W F_1 mice treated with a monoclonal antibody specific for the C5 component of complement that blocks the cleavage of C5 and thus prevents the generation of the potent proinflammatory factors C5a and C5b-9 developed significantly less glomerulonephritis and in markedly increased survival (25). In mice Crry, another complement activation controlling cell surface protein expressed only in mice, has been shown to control the development of glomerulonephritis either when given in a form of treatment to mice prone to develop disease (26) or when genetically expressed as a soluble form (27).

Is C3 necessary for the development of glomerulonephritis? Deposition of C3 is quite typical of glomerulonephritis in both humans and mice. Rare humans though with C3 deficiency have been described to develop glomerulonephritis. C3- and C4-deficient mice though were protected from the development of anti-glomerular basement membrane (GBM)-mediated nephritis (28). In B6/*lpr* mice that produce low titter anti-DNA antibodies but do not develop renal disease, C4 deficiency enhanced autoantibody production and the mice developed proliferate renal disease. C3 deficiency in B6/*lpr* mice had no apparent effect on antibody production and the mice did not develop renal disease (17). C3 deficiency in MRL/*lpr* mice had minimal to no effect on skin disease, spleen size, B cell or T cell number, B cell activation, pathologic renal scores, or production of autoantibodies. C3-deficient MRL/*lpr* mice did, however, manifest significantly greater albuminuria and glomerular IgG deposition compared with wild-type C3-producing littermates (29). Although, the data are not straightforward, it appears that C3 may not be needed for the development of glomerulonephritis. If it plays a role this must be protective and it may be either in the facilitation of clearance of immune complexes or in the cessation of autoreactive immune cells during the development of the immune reactivity repertoire.

The above-discussed experiments point out to a dichotomous effect of complement in the immune response in pathology. A role in the negative and positive selection of the immune cell repertoire and a second in the effector part. It also seems that unlike in humans, in mice complement deficiency adds to an autoimmunity-predisposing environment. Treatment of established disease with complement activation inhibitors should prove rewarding, unless complement proteins and or complement activation products control the maintenance of the peripheral immune cell repertoire. We do not know anything about the latter.

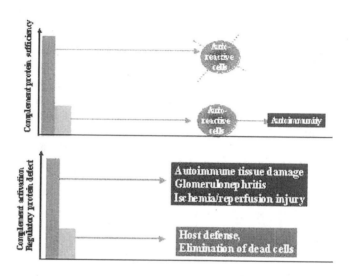

Figure 1. Diagrammatic depiction of discussed concepts. Upper level: Sufficient levels of complement proteins, such as C4 and of the receptors where main breakdown products bind to, such as CR2 are necessary for the deletion of autoreactive lymphocytes during ontogeny. When complement proteins are not expressed at sufficient levels, autoreactive cells survive and in the proper genetic background and environment lead to the expression of autoimmune manifestations. Lower level: Sufficient ongoing and induced (under controlled conditions) complement activation is needed for the performance of house-keeping complement functions, such as host defense and elimination of dead cells. Excessive and inappropriate activation of complement may lead to autoimmune pathology and tissue damage.

The opinions contained herein are the private ones of the authors and are not to be construed as official policy or reflecting the views of the Department of Defence. Work in the authors Laboratory was supported by MRMC STO R and PHS RO1 AI 42782.

3.   REFERENCES

1.   Tolnay, M. and G. C. Tsokos. 1998. Complement receptor 2 in the regulation of the immune response. Clin. Immunol. Immunopathol. 88:123-132.

2. Harley, J. B., K. L. Moser, P. M. Gaffney, and T. W. Behrens. 1998. The genetics of human systemic lupus erythematosus. Curr. Opin. Immunol. 10:690-696.

3. Shirai, T., H. Nishimura, Y. Jiang, and S. Hirose. 2002. Genome screening for susceptibility loci in systemic lupus erythematosus. Am. J. Pharmacogenomics. 2:1-12.

4. Atkinson, J. P. and P. M. Schneider. 1999. Genetic susceptibility and class III complement genes. In Systemic Lupus Erythematosus. R. G. Lahita, ed. Academic Press., New York, pp. 87-102.

5. Barilla-LaBarca, M. L. and J. P. Atkinson. 2003. Rheumatic syndromes associated with complement deficiency. Curr. Opin. Rheumatol. 15:55-60.

6. Vaishnaw, A. K., J. D. McNally, and K. B. Elkon. 1997. Apoptosis in the rheumatic diseases. Arthritis Rheum. 40:1917-1927.

7. Navratil, J. S. and J. M. Ahearn. 2001. Apoptosis, clearance mechanisms, and the development of systemic lupus erythematosus. Curr. Rheumatol. Rep. 3:191-198.

8. Navratil, J. S., S. C. Watkins, J. J. Wisnieski, and J. M. Ahearn. 2001. The globular heads of C1q specifically recognize surface blebs of apoptotic vascular endothelial cells. J. Immunol. 166:3231-3239.

9. Wilson, J. G., W. D. Ratnoff, P. H. Schur, and D. T. Fearon. 1986. Decreased expression of the C3b/C4b receptor (CR1) and the C3d receptor (CR2) on B lymphocytes and of CR1 on neutrophils of patients with systemic lupus erythematosus. Arthritis. Rheum. 29:739-747.

10. Mitchell, J. P., E. J. Enyedy, M. P. Nambiar, A. Lees, and G. C. Tsokos. 2002. Engagement of complement receptor 2 on the surface of B cells from patients with systemic lupus erythematosus contributes to the increased responsiveness to antigen stimulation. Lupus 11:299-303.

11. Theofilopoulos, A. N., R. A. Eisenberg, M. Bourdon, J. S. Crowell, Jr., and F. J. Dixon. 1979. Distribution of lymphocytes identified by surface markers in murine strains with systemic lupus erythematosus-like syndromes. J. Exp. Med. 149:516-534.

12. Smith, K. G. and D. T. Fearon. 2000. Receptor modulators of B-cell receptor signalling-- CD19/CD22. Curr. Top. Microbiol. Immunol 245:195-212.

13. Boackle, S. A. and V. M. Holers. 2003. Role of complement in the development of autoimmunity. Curr. Dir. Autoimmun. 6:154-168.

14. Dempsey, P. W., M. E. Allison, S. Akkaraju, C. C. Goodnow, and D. T. Fearon. 1996. C3d of complement as a molecular adjuvant: bridging innate and acquired immunity. Science 271:348-350.

15. Tsokos, G. C., J. D. Lambris, F. D. Finkelman, E. D. Anastassiou, and C. H. June. 1990. Monovalent ligands of complement receptor 2 inhibit whereas polyvalent ligands enhance anti-Ig-induced human B cell intracytoplasmic free calcium concentration. J. Immunol. 144:1640-1645.

16. Fischer, M. B., S. Goerg, L. Shen, A. P. Prodeus, C. C. Goodnow, G. Kelsoe, and M. C. Carroll. 1998. Dependence of germinal center B cells on expression of CD21/CD35 for survival. Science 280:582-585.

17. Prodeus, A. P., S. Goerg, L. M. Shen, O. O. Pozdnyakova, L. Chu, E. M. Alicot, C. C. Goodnow, and M. C. Carroll. 1998. A critical role for complement in maintenance of self-tolerance. Immunity. 9:721-731.

18. Boackle, S. A., V. M. Holers, X. Chen, G. Szakonyi, D. R. Karp, E. K. Wakeland, and L. Morel. 2001. Cr2, a candidate gene in the murine Sle1c lupus susceptibility locus, encodes a dysfunctional protein. Immunity 15:775-785.

19. Kaya, Z., M. Afanasyeva, Y. Wang, K. M. Dohmen, J. Schlichting, T. Tretter, D. Fairweather, V. M. Holers, and N. R. Rose. 2001. Contribution of the innate immune system to autoimmune myocarditis: a role for complement. Nat. Immunol. 2:739-745.

20. Botto, M. and M. J. Walport. 2002. C1q, autoimmunity and apoptosis. Immunobiology 205:395-406.

21. Moldenhauer, F., J. David, A. H. Fielder, P. J. Lachmann, and M. J. Walport. 1987. Inherited deficiency of erythrocyte complement receptor type 1 does not cause susceptibility to systemic lupus erythematosus. Arthritis Rheum. 30:961-966.

22. Chen, Z., S. B. Koralov, and G. Kelsoe. 2000. Complement C4 inhibits systemic autoimmunity through a mechanism independent of complement receptors CR1 and CR2. J. Exp. Med. 192:1339-1352.

23. Pickering, M. C., H. T. Cook, J. Warren, A. E. Bygrave, J. Moss, M. J. Walport, and M. Botto. 2002. Uncontrolled C3 activation causes membranoproliferative glomerulonephritis in mice deficient in complement factor H. Nat. Genet. 31:424-428.

24. Niculescu, F., H. Rus, T. van Biesen, and M. L. Shin. 1997. Activation of Ras and mitogen-activated protein kinase pathway by terminal complement complexes is G protein dependent. J Immunol 158:4405-4412.

25. Wang, Y., Q. Hu, J. A. Madri, S. A. Rollins, A. Chodera, and L. A. Matis. 1996. Amelioration of lupus-like autoimmune disease in NZB/WF1 mice after treatment with a blocking monoclonal antibody specific for complement component C5. Proc. Natl. Acad. Sci. U. S. A 93:8563-8568.

26. Quigg, R. J., Y. Kozono, D. Berthiaume, A. Lim, D. J. Salant, A. Weinfeld, P. Griffin, E. Kremmer, and V. M. Holers. 1998. Blockade of antibody-induced glomerulonephritis with Crry-Ig, a soluble murine complement inhibitor. J. Immunol. 160:4553-4560.

27. Quigg, R. J., C. He, A. Lim, D. Berthiaume, J. J. Alexander, D. Kraus, and V. M. Holers. 1998. Transgenic mice overexpressing the complement inhibitor crry as a soluble protein are protected from antibody-induced glomerular injury. J. Exp. Med. 188:1321-1331.

28. Sheerin, N. S., T. Springall, M. C. Carroll, B. Hartley, and S. H. Sacks. 1997. Protection against anti-glomerular basement membrane (GBM)-mediated nephritis in C3- and C4-deficient mice. Clin. Exp. Immunol. 110:403-409.

29. Sekine, H., C. M. Reilly, I. D. Molano, G. Garnier, A. Circolo, P. Ruiz, V. M. Holers, S. A. Boackle, and G. S. Gilkeson. 2001. Complement component C3 is not required for full expression of immune complex glomerulonephritis in MRL/lpr mice. J. Immunol. 166:6444-6451.

15

The Complex Roles of Anaphylatoxins in Allergic Asthma and Autoimmune Diseases

Heiko Hawlisch[1], Marsha Wills-Karp[2], Christopher L. Karp[1], and Jörg Köhl[1]

[1] *Division of Molecular Immunology and* [2] *Division of Immunobiology, Cincinnati Children's Hospital Medical Center and University of Cincinnati College of Medicine, Cincinnati, Ohio, USA*

Abstract: Complement has a long-recognized role as a lytic effector system that protects against microbial pathogens as well as a mediator of acute and chronic inflammatory responses. Many of the inflammatory properties related to complement activation can be related to the complement cleavage fragments C3a and C5a, the so-called anaphylatoxins. Cloning and subsequent gene targeting of their corresponding receptors, as well as generation of specific C3a and C5a inhibitors, have fueled new interest in studies aimed at defining the roles of the anaphylatoxins in inflammatory diseases. Traditionally, the anaphylatoxins have been considered mediators of end-stage effector mechanisms. However, recent data from animal models of allergic asthma suggest that C3a and C5a provide a critical link between innate and adaptive immunity. Further, the anaphylatoxins appear to form a sophisticated regulatory network together with immunoglobulin G Fc receptors that links regulatory events with effector activities in autoimmune disease. In this review, we will focus exclusively on the role of C3a and C5a in allergic asthma and autoimmune disease.

Key words: allergy, anaphylatoxins, asthma, autoimmune disease, interleukins, B cells, complement receptors, intracellular signaling

1. ALLERGIC ASTHMA

1.1 Epidemiology and Pathogenesis

The worldwide prevalence and severity of allergic asthma have increased dramatically in recent decades. In the U.S. alone, 15 million people suffer from asthma (1). The mechanisms underlying these epidemiological shifts remain obscure (2). Further, the development of effective therapies has lagged behind the growing prominence of the disease, and asthma morbidity and mortality continue to rise. Both epidemiologic and therapeutic investigation has been hindered by the lack of a detailed understanding of asthma pathogenesis. Recent advances have been driven by the insight that asthma is, in essence, an inflammatory disorder. The cardinal features of allergic asthma include airway hyperresponsiveness (AHR) to a variety of specific and nonspecific stimuli, excessive airway mucus production, pulmonary eosinophilia, and elevated concentrations of serum IgE. Although asthma is multifactorial in origin, it is generally accepted that it arises as a result of inappropriate immunological responses to common environmental antigens in genetically susceptible individuals. Specifically, a multitude of evidence suggests that CD4+ T cells producing Th2 cytokines (IL-4, IL-5, IL-13) play a pivotal role in disease pathogenesis (3). Although extensive research is ongoing into the processes underlying the development of deleterious immune responses to the ubiquitous, otherwise harmless, antigens that drive the expression of allergic asthma, these mechanisms remain a mystery. Recent data from animal models and humans provide evidence that the complement system is strongly activated during the disease and that bioactive complement cleavage fragments are important in disease pathogenesis and expression (4-10).

1.2 Complement Activation, Regulation and Effector Functions

Recent years have brought growing mechanistic awareness of the profound influence of the innate immune system on adaptive immune responses. The complement system, a phylogenetically ancient part of the innate immune system, is no exception. In addition to its long-recognized role as a lytic effector system that protects against microbial pathogens, it is clear that the complement system regulates adaptive immunity at many levels. First, the complement system is an important regulator of B cell activation, providing an important mechanism for pathogen (or "danger") recognition by B lymphocytes (11). Second, the engagement of complement receptors on antigen-presenting cells (APC) leads to potent effects on the production of immunoregulatory cytokines such as IL-12 (12,13). Third, while the anaphylatoxins (the complement activation products C3a, C5a and C5adesArg) have long been appreciated for their effects on myeloid cell migration, activation, and effector functions, it has recently become clear these molecules can also regulate the functions of APC, and lymphocytes (4, 14-17).

Activation of the complement system occurs by 3 different pathways: the classical pathway, the lectin pathway and the alternative pathway (for review see (18,19). All 3 pathways lead to C3 activation, with liberation of the anaphylatoxin C3a, and generation of C3b. Downstream cleavage of C5 leads to liberation of the anaphylatoxin C5a, and generation of C5b. In turn, C5b nucleates formation of the membrane attack complex (MAC). A variety of biological outcomes are downstream of C3 and C5 activation. In addition to microbial lysis, these include: (a) activation of granulocytes and endothelia by sublytic quantities of MAC; (b) deposition of C3 fragments (e.g. C3b, iC3b) on membranes and/or particles (e.g. Ag-Ab complexes, microbes) leading to phagocytosis; immune complex clearance; clearance of apoptotic bodies; B-cell activation; and alterations in immune cell signal transduction, adhesion, activation, and cytokine production; and (c) anaphylatoxin-mediated effects. Most such activities depend upon the engagement of specific complement receptors. These include some regulator of complement activation (RCA) family members (CR1, CR2, MCP, DAF), the ß-integrins CR3 and CR4, and the anaphylatoxin receptors C3a receptor (C3aR) and C5a receptor (C5aR), among others.

1.3 Anaphylatoxins: Mode of Generation and Effector Functions

How complement is activated in asthma, whether during antigen priming or during the effector phase of the response, remains unclear. Anaphylatoxins may be generated by several different pathways, including: (a) activation through the classical pathway as a result of allergen-antibody complex formation (necessarily an event downstream of Ag presentation unless due to natural antibodies); (b) activation of the lectin pathway through engagement of carbohydrate structures on allergens; (c) alternative pathway activation on allergen surfaces; (d) cleavage of C5 and C3 by proteases released from inflammatory cells; and, most interestingly (e) direct cleavage of C3 and C5 by allergen proteases (20-22).

Complement activation by any pathway results in formation of the anaphylatoxins, which were initially defined functionally by their activities on small blood vessels, smooth muscle, mast cells, and peripheral blood leukocytes. The anaphylatoxins have a plethora of proinflammatory actions, including: (a) promotion of leukocyte chemotaxis; (b) enhancement of neutrophil-endothelial cell adhesion; (c) upregulation of vascular permeability; (d) induction of granule secretion by phagocytes; and (d) induction of the production and release of a variety of proinflammatory cytokines (e.g. IL-1, IL-6, and IL-8) (23). The potent effects of the anaphylatoxins on the trafficking and activation of effector cells of the allergic response is likely to be of particular relevance to asthma. Notably,

C5a is chemotactic for macrophages, activated B and T lymphocytes (17,24), and both anaphylatoxins are chemotactic for eosinophils and mast cells (23,25). In addition to recruiting leukocytes into the airways, the anaphylatoxins also stimulate their effector mechanisms, leading to rapid release of histamine from basophils and mast cells (26), and to upregulation of eosinophil cationic protein synthesis (27,28). The anaphylatoxins can also induce smooth muscle contraction (see 1.6).

All of the effector functions are mediated through specific receptors, C3aR or C5aR (CD88), both belonging to the group of G-protein-coupled receptors (GPCR) (29-32). In leukocytes, C3aR and C5aR mediate their effects via coupling to pertussis-sensitive and -insensitive G-proteins ($G_{\alpha i}$ and $G_{\alpha 16}$, respectively; see 2.3.1, Fig. 2) (33-36). C3aR also couples to $G_{\alpha 12}$ and $G_{\alpha 13}$ in endothelial cells (37). Recently, the orphan receptor C5L2 (human and murine) has been described as a second receptor for C5a (38,39). Interestingly, C5L2 binds C5adesArg with a ten-fold higher affinity than CD88 does. In contrast to CD88, engagement of C5L2 on C5L2 transfected rat basophilic Leukemia (RBL)-2H3 cells does not induce degranulation, nor does it increase intracellular Ca^{2+} or receptor internalization. C5L2 does not couple to heterotrimeric G proteins mainly because of an amino acid replacement in the DRY motif at the end of the third transmembrane segment (39). However, several reports have revealed that GPCR can use other intracellular signaling molecules as well (40), suggesting that C5L2 may induce effector functions independent of G proteins. In support of this view, recent data suggest that signaling through C5L2 induces triglyceride synthesis in adipose tissue (41). Human and murine C5L2 show an almost identical mRNA expression pattern in multiple tissues (39).

1.4 Experimental Models

The role of complement in the pathogenesis of allergic asthma has not been studied in detail yet, despite knowledge of the fact that several pathophysiologic features of allergic asthma (e.g. smooth muscle contraction, increased vascular permeability, mucus secretion and recruitment of inflammatory cells) have long been known to be consonant with well-defined effects of the anaphylatoxins (23,42,43). Indeed, the fact that the complement system is highly activated at sites of disease (i.e. in the human asthmatic lung) is well-documented (6,10,44). However, recent awareness of the key immunoregulatory role of complement in other infectious and inflammatory disease models has fueled a new interest in its role in asthma and allergic disease.

1.4.1 C5 and C5a

A recent study by Karp et al. pursued genetic susceptibility loci in a murine model that mimics the pathophysiology of human asthma (4). In this antigen-driven model of asthma, A/J mice are susceptible, exhibiting AHR along with mucus metaplasia and an inflammatory response characterized by marked pulmonary eosinophilia and elevated IgE levels after antigen challenge. C3H/HeJ mice are resistant, do not develop AHR or elevations in IgE production, and exhibit a reduced eosinophilic inflammatory response. Notably, A/J mice are deficient in C5 whereas C3H/HeJ mice are C5 sufficient (45). Susceptibility to the development of allergen-induced AHR in this model is associated with a Th2 dominant cytokine pattern, whereas resistance is associated with Th1 cytokine production. IL-12 is a cytokine that is critical for the development of Th1 responses in most systems (46). As might therefore be expected, allergen-induced AHR is prevented or ablated by exogenous IL-12 in susceptible strains (47), whereas neutralization of IL-12 renders resistant strains susceptible (48).

Microarray analysis of pulmonary gene expression and single nucleotide polymorphism-based genotyping, combined with quantitative trait locus analysis, identified C5 as a susceptibility locus for allergen-induced AHR (4). Given the facts that (i) C3 fragments (C3b, iC3b) inhibit production of IL-12 by APCs (12,13,49), and (ii) C5a promotes monocyte/macrophage production of TNF-α, IL-1β, and IL-6, the effects of ablating C5a-mediated signaling was investigated in monocytic cells in a mechanistic search for the link between C5 and susceptibility to allergen-induced AHR. To model the in vivo lack of access to C5a in the macrophages of susceptible mice, ablation of C5a-mediated signaling was studied in human monocyte/macrophages cultured in the absence of serum. C5aR signaling was blocked with a C5aR antagonist (C5aRA) (50). Of note, blockade of the C5aR caused marked, dose dependent inhibition of IL-12 production from primary human monocytes. Such blockade also inhibited the secretion of TNF-α, albeit less potently. Interestingly, while inhibition of C5aR signaling had no overall effect on bacterially-driven IL-10 production, IFN-γ–mediated suppression of IL-10 production was reversed (4). The suppression of IL-12 production seen in vitro in human monocytes, was found to be recapitulated ex vivo in murine macrophages from sensitive and resistant strains. Peritoneal (PE) macrophages from C5-/- A/J mice produce significantly less IL-12 than those obtained from C5+/+ C3H/HeJ mice.

This finding appeared, superficially, to be in conflict with other data demonstrating that high concentrations of C5a can itself lead to IL-12 inhibition (14,15). However, suppression of IL-12 production induced by C5a is mechanistically separable from that resulting from ablation of C5aR signaling. Suppression of IL-12 production by both a C5aRA and C5a suggests a model in which some C5aR signaling is needed to render monocyte/macrophages competent for IL-12 production, while further exposure to C5a leads to inhibition of the production of this potentially toxic cytokine (Fig. 1).

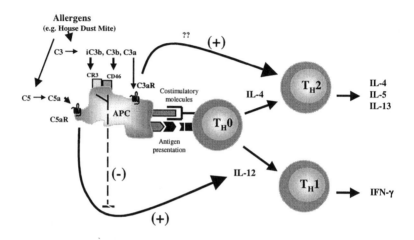

Figure 1. Proposed effects of C3 cleavage products and C5a on T cell polarization in allergic asthma. C3 and C5 may be secreted from pulmonary resident cells (e.g. epithelial cells, macrophages) and/or may be derived from plasma leakage. Proteases derived from allergens (e.g. house dust mite, *Aspergillus fumigatus*) or released from activated macrophages/mast cells are able to cleave C3/C5. Once generated, C3a, C5a, C3b and iC3b cleavage products bind to their corresponding receptors on APC. Some C5aR signaling appears to be needed to render APC competent for IL-12 production and to drive a Th1 response. Conversely, the C3 cleavage products C3b and iC3b can suppress IL-12 production by APC, and favor the development of a Th2 response. Further, C3a appears to promote a Th2 response, the mechanisms of which are yet unknown. C3a may induce or modulate Th2 cytokine release from basophils/mast cells or Th2 polarization during allergen sensitization (on APC), and/or may interact with activated T-cells to promote the maintenance of a Th2 response. Through these opposing actions, C3a (and C3b/iC3b) and C5a play a major role in skewing the T-cell response towards a Th2 phenotype and, consequently, play a major role in the development of allergic airway response.

These results may provide insight into other models of genetic deletion or Ab-mediated inhibition of C5, C5a, or the C5aR. Notably, such models have suggested a central role for C5 in the pathogenesis of collagen-induced arthritis, DTH responses, and endotoxic shock, as well as in resistance to *Listeria monocytogenes* and to blood-stage malaria infection (16,51-54). While C5a has pleiotropic effects, all of these models depend on, or are exacerbated by IL-12, and downmodulated by IL-10 (36). Likewise in vivo deficiencies of C5 and the C5aR are associated with blunted production of TNF-α (37).

Taken together these studies suggest that C5a normally serves to facilitate IL-12 production by APC, and that C5a deficiency leads to skewing towards Th2 immune responses due to deficient IL-12 production by such cells. The exact mechanisms by which C5a leads to polarization of the T-cell response remain to be defined.

1.4.2 C3 and C3a

Humbles et al. (6) have shown that C3aR$^{-/-}$ mice (Balb/c x 129) are protected from ovalbumin- (OVA-) driven AHR. Of note, the pattern and magnitude of inflammatory cell infiltration was similar in the lungs of allergen-exposed C3aR wildtype and knockout mice, suggesting that, in contrast to current dogma, C3 plays a major role in the allergic response that is independent of its chemoattractant properties (on eosinophils). Similarly, Bautsch et al. have shown that the allergen-induced, early-phase bronchoconstriction depends on C3aR pathway activation as well. Guinea pigs with a naturally occurring deficiency in the C3aR exhibit a significant decrease in bronchoconstriction compared with wild-type controls (6). As in the mouse model, no change was evident in the cellular inflammatory response. Further, AHR induced by airway exposure to a non-antigenic environmental stimulus (urban ambient air-derived particulate matter) is also dependent on C3; C3$^{-/-}$ mice (C57BL/6 background) fail to develop AHR (55). The particulate matter-induced inflammatory response was unchanged in the knockouts in this model as well. Airway challenge with particulate matter was associated with marked deposition of C3 along the airway epithelium and subepithelial smooth muscle in wildtype mice. Finally, a similar dependence on C3 for the elevation in AHR was recently found to be associated with atypical RSV in murine models (56). The fact that the effects of C3/C3a on the local inflammatory process can clearly be separated from its effects on the degree of Th2 polarization and AHR in these models (something well-described in murine models of asthma (57), indicates that C3/C3a can impact both immunoregulation and inflammation.

However, not all studies have been able to separate the chemotactic from immunoregulatory effects of C3. Both, suppressed pulmonary Th2 responses and reduced eosinophil and neutrophil infiltrates were described in C3$^{-/-}$ (compared with C3$^{+/+}$) mice challenged with *Aspergillus fumigatus* and OVA (8). Similar results were found using a C3aR$^{-/-}$ strain by the same authors (7). The differences in the linkage between inflammation and Th2 polarization seen in different C3aR$^{-/-}$ models may be explained by (a) the different antigens used; and/or (b) the different backgrounds to which these C3aR$^{-/-}$

mice were back-crossed (BALB/c vs. C57BL/6), given the multigenic nature of allergic asthma.

Taken together, these studies suggest that C3, in particular C3a, is important for the development of pulmonary Th2 responses and AHR. The data are consistent with an upstream immunoregulatory role for C3a, i.e. the promotion of T cell polarization towards a Th2 phenotype, in addition to a role as a chemoattractant and a mediator of inflammation (Fig. 1).

1.4.3 Summary

Altogether, these data strongly support a role for anaphylatoxins in the pathogenesis of allergic asthma. While C3a and C5a have similar functions as chemoattractants (for mast cells and eosinophils), these studies highlight a likely divergent role in their immunoregulatory effects. Specifically, these data suggest that C3a and C5a have directly opposing immunoregulatory effects, with C3a production driving Th2 immune responses and C5a inhibiting the development of such responses (Fig. 1). The effects of the complement system on asthma pathogenesis are thus likely to be quite complex, with different complement activation products having similar or opposing actions depending on where and when they impact upon the immunopathogenetic process. It is tempting to hypothesize that anaphylatoxins regulate the immunopathogenesis of allergic asthma at two levels, at least: (1) modulation of Th1/Th2 polarization at the time and place of antigen presentation, and/or maintenance of such polarization at sites of disease (i.e. the lung); and (2) regulation of allergic effector mechanisms (smooth muscle contraction, airway inflammation, mucus secretion) in the lung.

1.5   Modulation of Th1/Th2 Polarization by Anaphylatoxins: Potential Mechanisms

The molecular mechanisms underlying the Th1/Th2 polarization of CD4+ T cells have been reviewed recently (46,58). A critical upstream event in this process is the cytokine milieu present during the priming of naive T cells. Dendritic cells (DC) represent the principal APC for naive T cells. Immature DC (iDC) reside in tissues, where they actively survey their environment. In order to process and present a given antigen, DC need to undergo activation and maturation (a processes induced by multiple stimuli, including microbial products and ligands on activated T cells). With maturation, DCs migrate to secondary lymphoid organs where they are able to activate Ag-specific naive T cells. While Ag dose, costimulation, and genetic modifiers can all alter the path of differentiation of activated, naïve T cells, the cytokines IL-12 and IL-4 have clearly been shown to be critical determinants of the polarization of Th1 and Th2 cells, respectively. IL-12 is made by DCs and other APC. The relevant source of IL-4 remains unclear.

IL-12 production by APCs is modulated by anaphylatoxins (4,14,15), both in vitro and ex vivo. Recently, a further member of the IL-12 family was described and termed IL-27 (59). IL-27 appears to be produced early by activated APC. It is able to induce clonal proliferation of naïve but not memory CD4+ T cells and synergizes with IL-12 in IFN-γ production by naïve CD4+ T cells. It is likely that IL-27 and IL-12 function sequentially in initiating and maintaining Th1 responses, respectively (59,60) (with IL-27 acting before IL-12). Differentiated effector T cells traffic to nonlymphoid organs and tissue. There, functional Th1 polarization appears to be maintained by local production of IL-12 and IL-18 (58). Activation of Th1 memory cells appears to be restricted to the new IL-12 family member IL-23 (58).

It will be of major interest to determine whether the anaphylatoxins modulate the expression of other members of the IL-12 family (and of IL-18) to obtain a more comprehensive understanding of CD4+ T-cell polarization and/or maintenance by C3a and C5a.

Anaphylatoxin receptors are expressed on DC and have been found to induce several effector functions: (a) DCs isolated from rat respiratory tract tissue, or generated in vitro from human peripheral blood monocytes, migrate in response to C5a (61); (b) human Langerhans cells (a type of dermal iDC) express C5aR and respond chemotactically to C5a (62); (c) Langerhans cell C5aR expression increases during maturation and tissue trafficking (63); (d) freshly isolated, cultured human dermal DCs, and monocyte derived iDCs, express C5aR and C3aR (64); (e) C5a induces calcium fluxes in such dermal DCs, whereas C3a does not; (f) expression of both anaphylatoxin receptors is downregulated on such dermal DC by TNF-α (65); and (g) both human and murine monocyte-derived iDCs and mature DCs (mDCs) respond to C5a as determined by chemotaxis and Ca^{2+} mobilization (65). Thus, interactions with C5a have potent functional effects on both mDCs and iDCs.

Low basal expression of C5aR has been reported on primary, unstimulated T cells, with striking upregulation upon mitogen stimulation (24). T cells have also been shown to express C5aR mRNA, and to migrate in response to nanomolar concentrations of C5a (66). Further, Werfel et al.(66) showed expression of C3aR on blood- or skin-derived CD4+ and CD8+ T cell clones derived from birch pollen-sensitized patients with atopic dermatitis but not on unstimulated T cells. By contrast, these authors did not find C5aR expression in either of their experimental settings.

The fact that functional anaphylatoxin receptors are expressed on DCs and on activated T cells, as well as tissue macrophages, suggests a variety of direct ways by which anaphylatoxins may modulate Th1/Th2 differentiation, as well as maintain the Th1/Th2 phenotype of effector T cells (Fig.1).

1.6 Modulation of Airway Smooth Muscle Contraction by Anaphylatoxins: Potential Mechanisms

Among the various effector pathways of the asthmatic response, anaphylatoxins have long been recognized as potent contractile agonists for smooth muscle. Controversy exists, however, as to whether these effects are direct or secondary to the release of histamine and/or products of arachidonic acid metabolism. Most data were obtained in guinea pig systems 20 years ago. Such data support a model in which C5a-stimulated contraction of isolated tracheal strips was due, in part, to histamine release and production of cysteinyl leukotrienes (67). C3a is considerably less potent than C5a in inducing the contraction of lung tissues, and appears to act primarily by causing the release of prostaglandins (68). Anaphylatoxins thus stimulate release of many of the same mediators from lung tissues that are released by antigen challenge during asthma, and may therefore play an important, if indirect, role in the pathogenesis of allergic bronchospasm. However, both C5a and C3a appear to have direct effects on contractile cells within the lung as well (69,70).

The exact contribution of direct and/or indirect effects of anaphylatoxins on airway smooth muscle cells remains to be elucidated. C3aR is expressed on bronchial smooth muscle cells in normal human and mouse lung. Interestingly, C3aR expression is upregulated on murine bronchial smooth muscle cells after allergen and endotoxin challenge (71). These authors found C5aR expression in naïve human (but not mouse) lung (71). The functional consequences of triggering either C3aR or C5aR signaling pathways in airway smooth muscle cells are currently unknown.

1.7 Conclusion

Taken together the accumulated data support the hypothesis that the skewed T-cell responses and allergen-induced AHR arise either as a result of impaired generation of C5a (or C5aR activation) and/or as a result of enhanced C3a generation (or C3aR activation), or both. This imbalance in triggering the C3aR/C5aR pathways may predispose to deleterious Th2 immune response and disturbance of the local environment of the lung following allergen exposure resulting in the known pathologic feature of the asthmatic response. Clearly, further studies are needed to address more precisely the role of C3a and C5a in the pathogenesis of asthma.

2.   AUTOIMMUNE DISEASES

2.1   Epidemiology and Pathogenesis

Autoimmune diseases are chronic disabling disorders in which immune dysregulation leads the body to attack its own organs and tissues. More than 80 autoimmune diseases have been identified. The most common of these diseases include systemic lupus erythematosus (SLE), multiple sclerosis, type 1 diabetes, autoimmune thyroid diseases, myasthenia gravis, and rheumatoid arthritis (RA). Collectively, autoimmune diseases are thought to affect approximately 14–22 million people in the U.S. and represent a significant physical, emotional, social, and fiscal burden to the country's health care system. For reasons that are not clear, the prevalence of autoimmune diseases appears to be rising. Further, the development of effective therapies has lagged behind the growing prominence of these diseases.

Immune complexes (IC) are integral to the pathogenesis of several autoimmune diseases, including SLE and RA. The prototypic experimental model of soluble IC disease, the Arthus reaction, has served as the basis for dissecting the cellular and molecular events triggered by IC deposition and serves as the basis for our understanding of the pathophysiology of IC–mediated diseases. Recent data obtained in this model suggest that both FcγR and complement receptors are integral to the regulation of IC–driven inflammatory processes.

2.2   Complement Pathways

The inflammatory process in IC disease appears to be regulated by two different arms of the complement system: (1) cleavage products of C3, (C3b and iC3b) that opsonize IC and target them to CR1 (C3b) and CR3 (iC3b); and (2) anaphylatoxins, which recruit and activate polymorphonuclear granulocytes (PMN), tissue macrophages and mast cells.

IC can activate the complement cascade by the classical and the alternative pathway and become the nucleus of opsonization by different C3 cleavage products. Upon binding of C3 to IC IgG, C3 is cleaved into C3b and C3a. In the fluid phase, C3b is rapidly degraded to iC3b by factors H and I. iC3b opsonized IC are target for CR3, the interaction of which results in IC phagocytosis and, consequently, IC clearance. Ongoing release of antigens in case of persistent infection and/or the failure of apoptotic clearance of autoantibody-producing lymphocytes may overwhelm clearance mechanisms and result in a persistent inflammatory response: IC disease.

Complement activation by any pathway results in formation of the anaphylatoxins, the cellular effector functions of which are mediated by specific GPCR. Cellular responses to C5a reflect the prominent proinflammatory character of the molecule. Potent chemotactic activity for PMN is paradigmatic. Consistent with this direct chemotactic property, C5a has been shown to act as a proadhesive stimulus for PMN by increasing the expression of P-selectin (72) and the β2 integrin CD11b/CD18 (MAC-1, or CR3) (73). C5a is also a potent activator of PMN and induces release of all known classes of secretory granules. In addition, C5a activates the NADPH-oxidase pathway in PMN, leading to the oxidative burst (74). C5a also triggers mast cell activation and chemotaxis (75,76). In murine and rat peritoneal mast cells, and the human mast cell line HMC-1, degranulation occurs, resulting in liberation of potent vasoactive mediators such as histamine and serotonin (77-79). Further, C5a induces the production of eicosanoid products such as thromboxane A2, and cysteinyl-leukotrienes (80). In monocytes and macrophages, C5a is capable of either directly inducing or synergistically enhancing LPS-induced production of inflammatory cytokines and chemokines, including IL-1 (81), IL-6 (82) and IL-8 (83). Further, C5a is chemotactic for human monocytes (84,85) and upregulates the expression of CR3 (86).

In contrast to the broad pro-inflammatory functions of C5a, the effects of C3a appear to be much more selective in terms of cellular responsiveness, and less specifically proinflammatory. Although a specific C3a receptor has been demonstrated on PMN (87,88), C3a is neither chemotactic for PMN nor does it induce any of above-noted effector functions exerted by C5a. In monocytes and macrophages, C3a acts as an anti-inflammatory molecule, suppressing the release of pro-inflammatory cytokines (89). The pro-inflammatory properties of C3a appear to be restricted to eosinophils and MC in which the effector functions are almost identical to those of C5a (23).

2.3 Complement Receptors

2.3.1 The C5a Receptor (C5aR)

C5a exerts its effector functions by ligating a specific GPCR (CD88). G-proteins consist of three subunits, α, β, and γ. When signaling, they function in essence as dimers, as the signal is communicated either by the Gα subunit or the Gβγ complex (Fig.2).

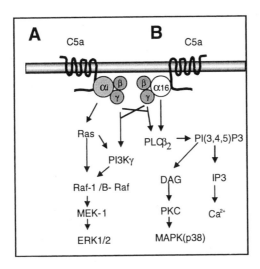

Figure 2. C5aR signaling pathways. (A) coupling to Gα$_i$ (light gray, PTX sensitive); (B) coupling to Gα$_{16}$ (white, PTX insensitive).

C5aR coupling to two distinct Gα-subunits has been demonstrated: Gα$_i$ (pertussis toxin [PTX] sensitive) and Gα$_{16}$ (Gα$_{15}$ in mice; PTX insensitive). Many of the effector functions of C5a (e.g. superoxide generation, chemotaxis) are entirely PTX sensitive, however, certain functions, such as IL-8 release or modulation of IL-12 are only partially blocked by this treatment. The downstream pathways have been intensively studied in human PMN (90,91). In such cells, C5aR signals through Gα$_i$ and activates class IB phophoinositide-3-kinase γ (PI3Kγ, Fig. 2A). PI3Kγ belongs to a family of lipid kinases involved in generating distinct phosphoinositides, that are important second messengers for intracellular signalling (92). C5a appears to activate PI3Kγ by two distinct pathways signaling through: (1) Gα$_i$, which activates the small GTPase Ras; and (2) Gβγ. In turn, PI3Kγ activates the Raf/MEK/ERK pathway. In monocytes and macrophages, coupling to both Gα$_i$ and Gα$_{16}$ has been described (93). The Gα$_{16}$ subunit (Fig. 2B) signals through activation of phosphoinositide-specific phospholipase C (PLC) subtype β, which is a multidomain phosphodiesterase that generates the second messenger inositol 1,4,5-trisphosphate (IP3) and diacylglycerol (DAG). These latter molecules mediate Ca^{2+} mobilization and the activation of protein kinase C (PKC).

Ligation of C5aR has been found to activate only the β2 subunit of PLC (PLC β2) (94).

2.3.2 Complement Receptor 3 (CR3)

CR3 is a remarkably versatile adhesion and recognition receptor, binding both endogenous ligands (including iC3b) as well as an array of microbial molecules. CR3 is a primary phagocytic receptor on macrophages and PMN, mediates phagocyte migration, and has prodigious signaling capabilities via pathways that include PI3K cascades and cytoskeletal rearrangement (95). A complex issue that has yet to be completely resolved, concerns the two-way activation signals that, on the one hand, are required for generation of the high-affinity ligand-binding state of CR3 (inside-out signaling) and, on the other, for CR3-mediated phagocyte activation (outside-in signaling). Full activation of PMN and monocytes, including the capacities for phagocytosis, adhesion, migration, and degranulation, are critically dependent on CR3-mediated activation (96). Paradoxically, such activation of leukocyte effector functions is dependent, in turn, on prior activation of the CR3 integrin itself. This is accomplished by one of two mechanisms. The first involves receptor clustering, depends on ligation of co-receptors such as FcγR or selectins, and requires rearrangement of the actin cytoskeleton. The second is induced by ligation of chemoattractant GPCR (e.g. C5aR, CXCR2) and is independent of actin reorganization. Recently, the receptor-clustering pathway has been shown to signal via class IA PI3K, whereas the G protein pathway is PI3K-independent (97).

In contrast to FcγR, phagocytosis by CR3 is characterized by an absent respiratory burst and the failure to elicit proinflammatory signals. In fact, CR3 by itself is not an activating receptor on phagocytes despite its role as an important component of innate immune responses. This paradox resolves when CR3 is considered in relation to other leukocyte receptors such as FcγR. It has been shown in human PMN that CR3 clusters with FcγRIIA or FcγRIIIA to stimulate a respiratory burst and to facilitate IC dependent phagocytosis (98). Although such cooperation between activating FcγR and CR3 is desirable during an infection, it is a double edged-sword in that it amplifies IC-mediated inflammatory responses. In fact, PMN trafficking into the peritoneal cavity during IC peritonitis is abolished by i.p. administration of a CR3 neutralizing mAb (our unpublished results). This result underscores the importance of CR3 signaling in initiating inflammatory responses. On the other hand, CR3 may also play an important role in regulating C5aR and activating FcγR signaling. It has recently been demonstrated that stimuli that activate the NADPH-oxidase system in PMN (such as C5a) induce the association of the SH2-domain-containing 5'-

inositol phosphatase (SHIP) with CR3. As will be discussed below (2.5) SHIP has the capacity to downregulate the signaling pathways of chemoattractant GPCR (C5aR, CXCR2) and of activating FcγR (Fig. 3).

2.4 The Receptors for CXC Chemokines with an ELR Motif

Ligation of C5aR and of activating FcγR mediates the release of CXC chemokines which contribute significantly to inflammation in IC disease. To date, there are over 15 known CXC chemokines and five CXC chemokine receptors (CXCR). Of these, CXCR1 and CXCR2 appear the most relevant to IC disease. CXCR1 and 2 couple to PTX sensitive G-proteins and their signaling pathways resemble that of the C5aR in many steps (91). In addition to IL-8, both receptors bind CXC chemokines with a glutamic acid-leucine-arginine motif (ELR). These include ENA-78, GCP-2, NAP-2, GRO-α, GRO-β and GRO-γ. IL-8 is highly selective for CXCR1. However, no rodent counterpart of human IL-8 is present and mice lack CXCR1. Mice express CXCR2 as an exclusive receptor for ELR CXC chemokines. Three different ligands for CXCR2 have been described in mice: (1) cytokine-induced neutrophil chemoattractant (KC [CXCL1]; homolog to hGRO-α), macrophage inflammatory protein-2 (MIP-2 [CXCL2]; homolog to hGRO-β) and LPS-induced CXC chemokine (LIX (CXCL5]; homolog to two human chemokines, ENA-78 and GCP-2). CXCR2 is highly expressed on murine PMN and macrophages (99), the human mast cell line HMC-1, and blood-derived cultured human mast cells (100,101). Ligation of CXCR2 on PMN results in chemotaxis, Ca^{2+} mobilization and degranulation (102). Recently, it has also been demonstrated that CXCR2 signaling induces upregulation of IL-1β and TNF-α(103) mRNA. Further, CXCR2 stimulates the activation of CR3 in PMN.

2.5 Fc Receptors for Immunoglobulin G (FcγR)

FcγR provide a critical link between the humoral and cellular arms of the immune system. Recognition of IgG by FcγR results in receptor cross-linking, cellular activation, and the induction of effector functions, including: (a) IC-clearance; (b) phagocytosis; (c) release of toxic oxygen metabolites; (d) production and secretion of cytokines and chemokines and; (e) modulation of cell proliferation and differentiation. Three distinct classes of FcγR, differing in molecular size, cellular distribution, functions and affinity for IgG isotypes, have been defined on leukocytes in humans and mice: FcγRI (CD64), FcγRII (CD32), and FcγRIII (CD16). In mice, FcγRI and FcγRIII function as activating receptors, forming multimeric complexes together with their signal transduction subunit, the FcR γ-chain, characterized by the presence of an immunoreceptor tyrosine-based activation motif (ITAM) in its cytoplasmic domain (Fig. 3A).

FcγRI is mainly expressed on macrophages and dendritic cells and binds IgG (IgG2a and IgG2b, but not IgG1) with high affinity. FcγRIIB and FcγRIII (the murine homolog of human FcγRIIIA) are low affinity receptors for complexed IgG1, IgG2a and IgG2b but not IgG3. The inhibitory FcγRIIB is a monomeric receptor containing an immunoreceptor tyrosine-based inhibition motif (ITIM) in its cytoplasmic domain. FcγRIIB and FcγRIII are co-expressed on myeloid cells including PMN, mast cells, and macrophages. Among lymphocytes, FcγRIIB is present on B cells, while NK cells express FcγRIII. FcγRIIB does not trigger cellular activation to aggregated IgG, unless the ligand coengages FcγRIIB and an ITAM containing activation receptor such as the BCR on B cells, FcγRIII and FcεRI on mast cells, and FcγRI and/or FcγRIII on phagocytes (Fig. 3B).

The activating FcγRIII and the inhibitory FcγRIIB bind IC with comparable affinity and specificity. These two opposing signaling pathways appear to act in concert, determining the magnitude of effector cell responses in IC-mediated inflammation in vivo 104. In fact, in non-inflamed tissues, the ratio of activating to inhibitory FcγR is low. It increases substantially in an inflamed environment. Several cytokines modulate this ratio: IFN-γ increases it through upregulation of activating FcγR and downregulation of inhibitory FcγR 9105); IL-4 and TGF-β decrease the ratio through upregulation of inhibitory FcγRIIB (106) (IL-4) or downregulation of the γ-chain (107) (TGF-β). Of note, administration of IL-4 protects against lung injury following intrapulmonary IC challenge in rats (108).

The initial event in inhibitory signaling by FcγRIIB is phosphorylation of the ITIM motif by the SRC-family kinase Lyn. This results in the recruitment of SH2-domain-containing phosphatases (SHP), predominantly SHIP, which is the primary signaling effector of FcγRIIB mediated inhibition. The main substrate of SHIP is phosphatidylinositol-3,4,5-trisphospshate (PI[3,4,5]P3), which is formed by the action of PI3K. Thus, SHIP inhibits the generation of the second messengers IP3 and DAG, which are important to C5aR and CXCR2 signaling (Fig.2). Further, phosphorylated SHIP is a docking site for DOK, which recruits Ras-GAP and catalyzes the conversion of Ras-GTP to Ras–GDP, leading to inhibition of the ERK pathway (109). ERK is a critical second messenger of the $G\alpha_i$ pathway that is activated by ligation of the C5aR and CXCR2 (Fig. 2).

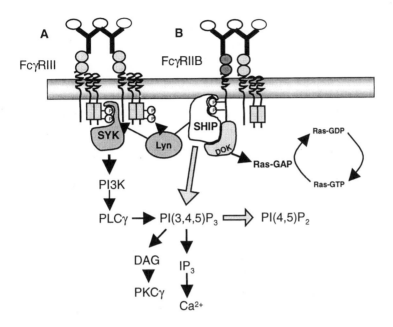

Figure 3. Signaling mechanisms of activating and inhibitory FcγR. (A) IC-mediated aggregation of activating FcγRIII (and FcγRI) results in the phosphorylation of the ITAM motif in its associated cytoplasmic γ-chain (both in light gray). Phosphorylated ITAM is a docking site for the syk kinase, which activates class IA PI3K. Various target proteins function downstream of PI3K; (B) Co-aggregation of FcγRIII and FcγRIIB (dark gray) results in phosphorylation of the ITIM motif and recruitment of SHIP.

2.6 Complement and FcγR in experimental models of IC-mediated disease

2.6.1 The Arthus Reaction

The Arthus reaction was first described almost 100 years ago by Maurice Arthus, who observed perivascular edema, infiltration of PMN and tissue damage following repeated injection of antigen intradermally (110). Today, the most commonly used experimental model is the reverse passive Arthus reaction. Preformed IgG antibodies are deposited in a desired tissue, followed by systemic application of the related antigen. Based on work in the 1960's and 1970's, it was understood that such induced IC-formation propagates tissue injury entirely by complement activation via the classical pathway. As outlined below, however, recent studies in gene-targeted mice established critical roles for FcγR as well as for the involvement of C5a generated by the alternative pathway of complement activation. Moreover, these effector systems appear to be connected by bidirectional interactions between C5aR and the different FcγR at the site of inflammation.

2.6.1.1 The cutaneous Arthus reaction

FcR γ-chain$^{-/-}$mice, deficient in signaling through activating FcγRI and FcγRIII, exhibit a strongly attenuated cutaneous Arthus reaction despite the presence of a functional complement system (111). Further characterization showed that the Arthus reactions are attenuated in mast cell deficient mice, and that the inflammatory response can be reconstituted with MC from control mice but not with mast cells from FcR γ-chain mutant mice (112). FcR γ-chain$^{-/-}$ and FcγRIII$^{-/-}$ mice share similar phenotypes, and it has thus been concluded that FcγRIII expressing MC are mainly responsible for triggering IgG-dependent inflammation (113). However, this leaves the specific contribution of complement unclear. The finding that genetic deletion of C3 and C4 does not cause an impaired Arthus reaction has been taken as evidence for the concept that complement plays no role, or participates only secondarily (111,114). This view does not encompass recognition of the fact that C3 deficiency does not disrupt the inflammatory properties of the complement system in general. For example, C3b-independent activation of C5 in the generation of C5a has been shown to account for an efficient Arthus reaction in C3$^{-/-}$ mice, which thus represents a potential bypass to the classical complement cascade (115). Moreover, pharmacological inhibition or genetic inactivation of C5aR is effective in preventing IC-mediated inflammation (50,116-118). Comparative studies of complement and FcγR under the same experimental conditions has revealed a co-dominant role for FcγR and complement, with FcγRIII and C5aR being the most relevant molecules (119,120). These results argue for a model of the Arthus reaction in which FcγR-mediated effector responses are integrated through C5aR activation (120-121) (Fig. 4).

2.6.1.2 The pulmonary Arthus reaction

The anatomy of the lung has allowed a more detailed analysis of the involved chemotactic cytokines, due to the possibility of obtaining bronchoalveolar lavage (BAL) specimens. Large amounts of TNF-α and IL-1β, as well as of MIP-2 and KC, are found in BAL during IC alveolitis. Such cytokine production depends critically on signaling through FcγRIII (122). In contrast to the skin, C3 deficiency decreases PMN trafficking into the lung and lowers cytokine production (115). TNF-α is strictly required for alveolar PMN infiltration and IL-1β synthesis, but not for MIP-2 and KC secretion. Importantly, FcγRIII-mediated chemokine production by alveolar macrophages is dependent on the presence of C5a (123,124). Co-stimulation of IC with C5a results in strong enhancement of FcγRIII-triggered cellular activation in vitro and in vivo (124). Further, C5aR ligation upregulates activating FcγRIII and downregulates inhibitory FcγRIIB on alveolar macrophages, something that appears crucial for efficient cytokine production (124). Thus C5a functions as a critical regulator of the FcγIIB/III ratio, connecting complement and FcγR effector pathways in IC-mediated inflammation.

2.6.1.3 The Peritoneal Arthus reaction

In the peritoneum, PMN trafficking is also dependent on the presence of C5aR ligation - as demonstrated by pharmacological blockade (50,118) or deletion of the C5aR (117). Surprisingly, PMN recruitment is unaffected in FcγRIII$^{-/-}$ (125) mice and is only slightly (although significantly) reduced in FcγRI$^{-/-}$ mice (our unpublished results). By contrast, PMN migration is abolished in FcR γ-chain$^{-/-}$ mice, suggesting that either FcγRI or FcγRIII signaling is sufficient to mediate peritoneal trafficking of PMN. As FcγRI expression is restricted to macrophages and dendritic cells, these data suggest an important role for FcγRI signaling in macrophage-mediated PMN trafficking. In support of this view, depletion of macrophages impairs PMN recruitment (our unpublished results).

As in IC alveolitis, TNF-α is also released in large amounts into the peritoneum in IC-mediated peritonitis. This is critically dependent on ligation of FcγRIII (125). However, as deletion of FcγRIII does not alter PMN recruitment, the role of TNF-α in peritoneal PMN recruitment is at most redundant. This view is further supported by data showing that functional inhibition of TNF-α has no effect on PMN infiltration (125), although a protective effect was demonstrated in a single study (126). In addition, substantial amounts of KC and MIP-2 are found in peritoneal lavage fluid during IC peritonitis, the release of which critically depends on FcγR- and on C5aR ligation on resident peritoneal cells (our unpublished results). Blockade of KC and MIP-2, but not of MIP-2 alone, reduces PMN recruitment by 50% suggesting that KC and MIP-2 act together as important downstream mediators of PMN recruitment.

C5aR ligation in peritoneal macrophages upregulates FcγRIII expression and downregulates expression of FcγRIIB (similar to alveolar macrophages (124). In turn, ligation of FcγR modulates signaling pathway(s) downstream of the C5aR. In fact, PMN migration towards C5a is substantially reduced by ligation of inhibitory FcγRIIB. Moreover, migration towards KC is impaired as well, suggesting an even broader downregulation of chemoattractant GPCR functions by FcγRIIB (our unpublished results).

2.6.2 Other IC Disease Models

Although the Arthus reaction has long been used to model human IC-mediated autoimmune disease, the question arises as to whether the immune mechanisms mediating inflammation in the Arthus reaction mirror the mechanisms important in human disease. As shown in two models of RA and SLE nephritis that comprise many clinical features of the human diseases, this is likely the case.

2.6.2.1 Rheumatoid arthritis

Many pathological features of rheumatoid arthritis are found in the K/BxN T cell transgenic mouse model. Disease in such animals occurs specifically in the joints but is caused by autoreactivity against the widely expressed antigen, glucose-6-phosphate isomerase (GPI) (127). T and B cells are both required for disease initiation, but anti-GPI IgGs alone can induce arthritis in lymphocyte deficient recipient mice (128). The GPI autoantibody-induced joint disease requires both FcγR and the alternative pathway of complement (52). Deposition of GPI:anti-GPI complexes on articular surfaces initiate the inflammatory cascade and full or virtually full protection against arthritis is observed in FcR γ-chain$^{-/-}$ or FcγRIII$^{-/-}$ mice, respectively, while FcγRI appears to play a minor, if any role. Complete prevention is also achieved by deficiency of C5 or C5aR, or by anti-C5 antibody treatment. This illustrates that adaptive autoimmunity can induce inflammation that, in the effector phase, uses similar mechanisms to that identified by passive Arthus reaction models.

2.6.2.2 Lupus nephritis

Lupus nephritis is another example in which C5a/C5aR together with activating FcγR, especially FcγRIII, can initiate inflammation and tissue damage. Defective FcγR-mediated IC clearance, and correlation with FcγR polymorphism have been described in patients suffering from SLE and severe glomerulonephritis (129). Experimental induction of glomerular injury in the mouse reveals the critical involvement of complement (C1q, C3 and C5), as well as FcγR. In a passive model of acute anti-glomerular basement membrane (GBM) nephritis, PMN recruitment is abrogated in both FcR γ-chain$^{-/-}$ and FcγRIII$^{-/-}$ mice, indicating an essential contribution of the activating FcγRIII (130). Importantly, early renal production of CC and CXC chemokines (MCP-1, MIP-2 and KC) and cellular infiltration is dependent on downregulation of the constitutively expressed FcγRIIB on glomerular mesangial cells. FcγRIIB deficiency can exacerbate kidney injury. The importance of the inhibitory FcγRIIB to limit the FcγRIII-mediated inflammatory response is well established and is consistently seen in FcγRIIB$^{-/-}$ mice that display enhanced susceptibility in the Arthus reaction (131), collagen-induced arthritis (132) and Goodpasture's syndrome (133). The observation that ligation of FcγRIIB impairs signal transduction by chemoattractant GPCR (C5aR, CXCR2) provides a regulatory link between cellular (FcγR) and humoral (complement) immunity and adds a novel function to the complex regulatory role of FcγRIIB in autoimmune disease (Fig.4).

2.7 Conclusion

Taken together, it is now clear that both complement receptors and FcγR regulate IC-mediated autoimmunity. C5aR plays a role similar in importance to that played by activating FcγR. Ablation of either FcγR or C5aR signaling almost completely blocks inflammation in the Arthus models in skin, lung, peritoneum, as well as in acute arthritis. C5aR acts upstream of FcγR through modifying the balance of activating FcγRIII and inhibitory FcγRIIB. Moreover, C5aR ligation defines the threshold of FcγR-dependent effector responses in IC-peritonitis. In turn, FcγR signaling can modulate C5aR-driven effector functions and, even more generally, those of a variety of chemoattractant GPCR (Fig. 4).

Thus, the available data support a model of bidirectional interaction, in which complement activation at the site of inflammation initiates inflammation by controlling the ratio of activating to inhibitory FcγR (Fig. 4B). Under conditions that favor a low ratio of activating to inhibitory receptors (e.g. by IL-4, Fig. 4C), FcγRIIB downregulates C5aR mediated effector functions, most likely by modulation of intracellular signaling pathways (Fig. 4D).

Clearly further studies are needed to define the molecular mechanisms underlying the bidirectional regulation of chemoattractant GPCR and FcγR.

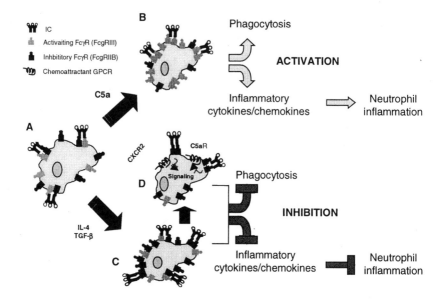

Figure 4. Model of bidirectional regulation of C5aR and FcγR that controls the inflammatory response in IC-mediated disease. (A) In a non-inflamed environment, activating and inhibitory FcγR are expressed at a low level with a preponderance of inhibitory FcγRIIB (here shown on a tissue MØ). (B) IC-induced generation of C5a upregulates FcγRIII and downregulates FcγRIIB, resulting in a lowered threshold for IC stimulation and, consequently, an enhanced inflammatory response; (C) Conversely, upregulation of the FcγRIIB (by IL-4) or downregulation of the common γ-chain (by TGF-β) raises the threshold for IC stimulation and suppresses the inflammatory response; (D) Further, ligation of FcγRIIB leads to inhibition of chemoattractant GPCR (C5aR, CXCR2) signaling as a novel means to suppress inflammation.

3.   REFERENCES

1. Anonymous. Surveillance for asthma - United States, 1960-1995. 47, 1-28. 1-1-1998. Morb. Mort. Wkly Rep.
2. Wills-Karp, M., J. Santeliz, and C. L. Karp. 2001. The germless theory of allergic disease: revisiting the hygiene hypothesis. *Nat.Rev.Immunol.* 1:69-75.
3. Wills-Karp, M. 1999. Immunologic basis of antigen-induced airway hyperresponsiveness. *Annu.Rev.Immunol.* 17:255-281.
4. Karp, C. L., A. Grupe, E. Schadt, S. L. Ewart, M. Keane-Moore, P. J. Cuomo, J. Kohl, L. Wahl, D. Kuperman, S. Germer, D. Aud, G. Peltz, and M. Wills-Karp. 2000. Identification of complement factor 5 as a susceptibility locus for experimental allergic asthma. *Nat.Immunol.* 1:221-226.

5.   Bautsch, W., H. G. Hoymann, Q. Zhang, I. Meier-Wiedenbach, U. Raschke, R. S. Ames, B. Sohns, N. Flemme, z. Meyer, V, M. Grove, A. Klos, and J. Kohl. 2000. Cutting edge: guinea pigs with a natural C3a-receptor defect exhibit decreased bronchoconstriction in allergic airway disease: evidence for an involvement of the C3a anaphylatoxin in the pathogenesis of asthma. *J.Immunol.* 165:5401-5405.
6.   Humbles, A. A., B. Lu, C. A. Nilsson, C. Lilly, E. Israel, Y. Fujiwara, N. P. Gerard, and C. Gerard. 2000. A role for the C3a anaphylatoxin receptor in the effector phase of asthma. *Nature* 406:998-1001.
7.   Drouin, S. M., D. B. Corry, T. J. Hollman, J. Kildsgaard, and R. A. Wetsel. 2002. Absence of the Complement Anaphylatoxin C3a Receptor Suppresses Th2 Effector Functions in a Murine Model of Pulmonary Allergy. *J.Immunol.* 169:5926-5933.
8.   Drouin, S. M., D. B. Corry, J. Kildsgaard, and R. A. Wetsel. 2001. Cutting edge: the absence of C3 demonstrates a role for complement in Th2 effector functions in a murine model of pulmonary allergy. *J.Immunol.* 167:4141-4145.
9.   Walters, D. M., P. N. Breysse, B. Schofield, and M. Wills-Karp. 2002. Complement factor 3 mediates particulate matter-induced airway hyperresponsiveness. *Am.J.Respir.Cell Mol.Biol.* 27:413-418.
10. Krug, N., T. Tschernig, V. J. Erpenbeck, J. M. Hohlfeld, and J. Kohl. 2001. Complement factors c3a and c5a are increased in bronchoalveolar lavage fluid after segmental allergen provocation in subjects with asthma. *Am.J.Respir.Crit Care Med.* 164:1841-1843.
11. Fearon, D. T. and M. C. Carroll. 2000. Regulation of B lymphocyte responses to foreign and self-antigens by the CD19/CD21 complex. *Annu.Rev.Immunol.* 18:393-422.
12. Karp, C. L., M. Wysocka, L. M. Wahl, J. M. Ahearn, P. J. Cuomo, B. Sherry, G. Trinchieri, and D. E. Griffin. 1996. Mechanism of suppression of cell-mediated immunity by measles virus. *Science* 273:228-231.
13. Marth, T. and B. L. Kelsall. 1997. Regulation of interleukin-12 by complement receptor 3 signaling. *J.Exp.Med.* 185:1987-1995.
14. Wittmann, M., J. Zwirner, V. A. Larsson, K. Kirchhoff, G. Begemann, A. Kapp, O. Gotze, and T. Werfel. 1999. C5a suppresses the production of IL-12 by IFN-gamma-primed and lipopolysaccharide-challenged human monocytes. *J.Immunol.* 162:6763-6769.
15. Braun, M. C., E. Lahey, and B. L. Kelsall. 2000. Selective suppression of IL-12 production by chemoattractants. *J.Immunol.* 164:3009-3017.
16. Tsuji, R. F., I. Kawikova, R. Ramabhadran, M. Akahira-Azuma, D. Taub, T. E. Hugli, C. Gerard, and P. W. Askenase. 2000. Early local generation of C5a initiates the elicitation of contact sensitivity by leading to early T cell recruitment. *J.Immunol.* 165:1588-1598.
17. Ottonello, L., A. Corcione, G. Tortolina, I. Airoldi, E. Albesiano, A. Favre, R. D'Agostino, F. Malavasi, V. Pistoia, and F. Dallegri. 1999. rC5a directs the in vitro migration of human memory and naive tonsillar B lymphocytes: implications for B cell trafficking in secondary lymphoid tissues. *J.Immunol.* 162:6510-6517.
18. Walport, M. J. 2001. Review Articles: Advances in Immunology: Complement (First of Two Parts). *N.Engl.J.Med.* 344:1058-1066.
19. Walport, M. J. 2001. Complement. Second of two parts. *N.Engl.J.Med.* 344:1140-1144.
20. Nagata, S. and M. M. Glovsky. 1987. Activation of human serum complement with allergens. I. Generation of C3a, C4a, and C5a and induction of human neutrophil aggregation. *J.Allergy Clin.Immunol.* 80:24-32.

21. Castro, F. F., M. Schmitz Schumann, U. Rother, and M. Kirschfink. 1991. Complement activation by house dust: reduced reactivity of serum complement in patients with bronchial asthma. *Int.Arch.Allergy Appl.Immunol.* 96:305-310.
22. Maruo, K., T. Akaike, T. Ono, T. Okamoto, and H. Maeda. 1997. Generation of anaphylatoxins through proteolytic processing of C3 and C5 by house dust mite protease. *J.Allergy Clin.Immunol.* 100:253-260.
23. Ember, J. A., M. A. Jagels, and T. E. Hugli. 1998. Characterization of complement anaphylatoxins and their biological responses. In *The human complement system in health and disease*. J. E. Volanakis and M. M. Frank, eds. Marcel Dekker Inc., New York, pp. 241-284.
24. Nataf, S., N. Davoust, R. S. Ames, and S. R. Barnum. 1999. Human T cells express the C5a receptor and are chemoattracted to C5a. *J.Immunol.* 162:4018-4023.
25. Schulman, E. S., T. J. Post, P. M. Henson, and P. C. Giclas. 1988. Differential effects of the complement peptides, C5a and C5a des Arg on human basophil and lung mast cell histamine release. *J Clin.Invest.* 81:918-923.
26. Eglite, S., K. Pluss, and C. A. Dahinden. 2000. Requirements for C5a receptor-mediated IL-4 and IL-13 production and leukotriene C4 generation in human basophils. *J.Immunol.* 165:2183-2189.
27. Takafuji, S., K. Tadokoro, K. Ito, and C. A. Dahinden. 1994. Degranulation from human eosinophils stimulated with C3a and C5a. *Int.Arch.Allergy Immunol.* 104:27-29.
28. Takafuji, S., K. Tadokoro, and K. Ito. 1996. Effects of interleukin (IL)-3 and IL-5 on human eosinophil degranulation induced by complement components C3a and C5a. *Allergy* 51:563-568.
29. Crass, T., U. Raffetseder, U. Martin, M. Grove, A. Klos, J. Kohl, and W. Bautsch. 1996. Expression cloning of the human C3a anaphylatoxin receptor (C3aR) from differentiated U-937 cells. *Eur.J.Immunol.* 26:1944-1950.
30. Ames, R. S., Y. Li, H. M. Sarau, P. Nuthulaganti, J. J. Foley, C. Ellis, Z. Zeng, K. Su, A. J. Jurewicz, R. P. Hertzberg, D. J. Bergsma, and C. Kumar. 1996. Molecular cloning and characterization of the human anaphylatoxin C3a receptor. *J Biol.Chem.* 271:20231-20234.
31. Gerard, N. P. and C. Gerard. 1991. The chemotactic receptor for human C5a anaphylatoxin. *Nature* 349:614-617.
32. Boulay, F., L. Mery, M. Tardif, L. Brouchon, and P. Vignais. 1991. Expression cloning of a receptor for C5a anaphylatoxin on differentiated HL-60 cells. *Biochemistry* 30:2993-2999.
33. Norgauer, J., G. Dobos, E. Kownatzki, C. Dahinden, R. Burger, R. Kupper, and P. Gierschik. 1993. Complement fragment C3a stimulates Ca2+ influx in neutrophils via a pertussis-toxin-sensitive G protein. *Eur.J.Biochem.* 217:289-294.
34. Zwirner, J., O. Gotze, A. Moser, A. Sieber, G. Begemann, A. Kapp, J. Elsner, and T. Werfel. 1997. Blood- and skin-derived monocytes/macrophages respond to C3a but not to C3a(desArg) with a transient release of calcium via a pertussis toxin-sensitive signal transduction pathway. *Eur.J.Immunol.* 27:2317-2322.
35. Buhl, A. M., S. Osawa, and G. L. Johnson. 1995. Mitogen-activated protein kinase activation requires two signal inputs from the human anaphylatoxin C5a receptor. *J.Biol.Chem.* 270:19828-19832.
36. Vanek, M., L. D. Hawkins, and F. Gusovsky. 1994. Coupling of the C5a receptor to Gi in U-937 cells and in cells transfected with C5a receptor cDNA. *Mol.Pharmacol.* 46:832-839.

37. Schraufstatter, I. U., K. Trieu, L. Sikora, P. Sriramarao, and R. DiScipio. 2002. Complement c3a and c5a induce different signal transduction cascades in endothelial cells. *J.Immunol.* 169:2102-2110.

38. Cain, S. A. and P. N. Monk. 2002. The orphan receptor C5L2 has high affinity binding sites for complement fragments C5a and C5a des-Arg(74). *J.Biol.Chem.* 277:7165-7169.

39. Okinaga, S., D. Slattery, A. Humbles, Z. Zsengeller, O. Morteau, M. B. Kinrade, R. M. Brodbeck, J. E. Krause, H. R. Choe, N. P. Gerard, and C. Gerard. 2003. C5L2, a Nonsignaling C5A Binding Protein. *Biochemistry* 42:9406-9415.

40. Marinissen, M. J. and J. S. Gutkind. 2001. G-protein-coupled receptors and signaling networks: emerging paradigms. *Trends Pharmacol.Sci.* 22:368-376.

41. Kalant, D., S. A. Cain, M. Maslowska, A. D. Sniderman, K. Cianflone, and P. N. Monk. 2003. The chemoattractant receptor-like protein C5L2 binds the C3a des-Arg77/acylation-stimulating protein. *J.Biol.Chem.* 278:11123-11129.

42. Kohl, J. and D. Bitter-Suermann. 1993. Anaphylatoxins. In *Complement in Health and Disease.* K. Whaley, M. Loos, and J. M. Weiler, eds. Kluwer Academic Publishers, Dordrecht, pp. 295-320.

43. Gerard, C. and N. P. Gerard. 1994. C5A anaphylatoxin and its seven transmembrane-segment receptor. *Annu.Rev.Immunol.* 12:775-808.

44. van de Graaf, E. A., H. M. Jansen, M. M. Bakker, C. Alberts, J. K. Eeftinck Schattenkerk, and T. A. Out. 1992. ELISA of complement C3a in bronchoalveolar lavage fluid. *J.Immunol.Methods* 147:241-250.

45. Wetsel, R. A., D. T. Fleischer, and D. L. Haviland. 1990. Deficiency of the murine fifth complement component (C5). A 2-base pair gene deletion in a 5'-exon. *J.Biol.Chem.* 265:2435-2440.

46. Murphy, K. M. and S. L. Reiner. 2002. The lineage decisions of helper T cells. *Nat.Rev.Immunol.* 2:933-944.

47. Gavett, S. H., D. J. O'Hearn, X. Li, S. K. Huang, F. D. Finkelman, and M. Wills-Karp. 1995. Interleukin 12 inhibits antigen-induced airway hyperresponsiveness, inflammation, and Th2 cytokine expression in mice. *J.Exp.Med.* 182:1527-1536.

48. Keane-Myers, A., M. Wysocka, G. Trinchieri, and M. Wills-Karp. 1998. Resistance to antigen-induced airway hyperresponsiveness requires endogenous production of IL-12. *J.Immunol.* 161:919-926.

49. Sutterwala, F. S., G. J. Noel, R. Clynes, and D. M. Mosser. 1997. Selective suppression of interleukin-12 induction after macrophage receptor ligation. *J.Exp.Med.* 185:1977-1985.

50. Heller, T., M. Hennecke, U. Baumann, J. E. Gessner, A. M. zu Vilsendorf, M. Baensch, F. Boulay, A. Kola, A. Klos, W. Bautsch, and J. Kohl. 1999. Selection of a C5a receptor antagonist from phage libraries attenuating the inflammatory response in immune complex disease and ischemia/reperfusion injury. *J.Immunol.* 163:985-994.

51. Czermak, B. J., V. Sarma, C. L. Pierson, R. L. Warner, M. Huber-Lang, N. M. Bless, H. Schmal, H. P. Friedl, and P. A. Ward. 1999. Protective effects of C5a blockade in sepsis. *Nat.Med.* 5:788-792.

52. Ji, H., K. Ohmura, U. Mahmood, D. M. Lee, F. M. Hofhuis, S. A. Boackle, K. Takahashi, V. M. Holers, M. Walport, C. Gerard, A. Ezekowitz, M. C. Carroll, M. Brenner, R. Weissleder, J. S. Verbeek, V. Duchatelle, C. Degott, C. Benoist, and D. Mathis. 2002. Arthritis critically dependent on innate immune system players. *Immunity.* 16:157-168.

53. Sam, H. and M. M. Stevenson. 1999. Early IL-12 p70, but not p40, production by splenic macrophages correlates with host resistance to blood-stage Plasmodium chabaudi AS malaria. *Clin.Exp.Immunol.* 117:343-349.

54. Gervais, F., C. Desforges, and E. Skamene. 1989. The C5-sufficient A/J congenic mouse strain. Inflammatory response and resistance to Listeria monocytogenes. *J.Immunol.* 142:2057-2060.

55. Walters, D. M., P. N. Breysse, B. Schofield, and M. Wills-Karp. 2002. Complement factor 3 mediates particulate matter-induced airway hyperresponsiveness. *Am.J.Respir.Cell Mol.Biol.* 27:413-418.

56. Polack, F. P., M. N. Teng, P. L. Collins, G. A. Prince, M. Exner, H. Regele, D. D. Lirman, R. Rabold, S. J. Hoffman, C. L. Karp, S. R. Kleeberger, M. Wills-Karp, and R. A. Karron. 2002. A role for immune complexes in enhanced respiratory syncytial virus disease. *J.Exp.Med.* 196:859-865.

57. Wills-Karp, M. 2000. Murine models of asthma in understanding immune dysregulation in human asthma. *Immunopharmacology* 48:263-268.

58. Brombacher, F., R. A. Kastelein, and G. Alber. 2003. Novel IL-12 family members shed light on the orchestration of Th1 responses. *Trends Immunol.* 24:207-212.

59. Pflanz, S., J. C. Timans, J. Cheung, R. Rosales, H. Kanzler, J. Gilbert, L. Hibbert, T. Churakova, M. Travis, E. Vaisberg, W. M. Blumenschein, J. D. Mattson, J. L. Wagner, W. To, S. Zurawski, T. K. McClanahan, D. M. Gorman, J. F. Bazan, M. R. de Waal, D. Rennick, and R. A. Kastelein. 2002. IL-27, a heterodimeric cytokine composed of EBI3 and p28 protein, induces proliferation of naive CD4(+) T cells. *Immunity.* 16:779-790.

60. Yoshida, H., S. Hamano, G. Senaldi, T. Covey, R. Faggioni, S. Mu, M. Xia, A. C. Wakeham, H. Nishina, J. Potter, C. J. Saris, and T. W. Mak. 2001. WSX-1 is required for the initiation of Th1 responses and resistance to L. major infection. *Immunity.* 15:569-578.

61. McWilliam, A. S., S. Napoli, A. M. Marsh, F. L. Pemper, D. J. Nelson, C. L. Pimm, P. A. Stumbles, T. N. Wells, and P. G. Holt. 1996. Dendritic cells are recruited into the airway epithelium during the inflammatory response to a broad spectrum of stimuli. *J.Exp.Med.* 184:2429-2432.

62. Morelli, A., A. Larregina, E. Chuluyan, E. Kolkowski, and L. Fainboim. 1997. Functional expression and modulation of C5a receptor (CD88) on skin dendritic cells. *Adv.Exp.Med.Biol.* 417:133-138.

63. Morelli, A., A. Larregina, I. Chuluyan, E. Kolkowski, and L. Fainboim. 1996. Expression and modulation of C5a receptor (CD88) on skin dendritic cells. Chemotactic effect of C5a on skin migratory dendritic cells. *Immunology* 89:126-134.

64. Kirchhoff, K., O. Weinmann, J. Zwirner, G. Begemann, O. Gotze, A. Kapp, and T. Werfel. 2001. Detection of anaphylatoxin receptors on CD83+ dendritic cells derived from human skin. *Immunology* 103:210-217.

65. Yang, D., Q. Chen, S. Stoll, X. Chen, O. M. Howard, and J. J. Oppenheim. 2000. Differential regulation of responsiveness to fMLP and C5a upon dendritic cell maturation: correlation with receptor expression. *J.Immunol.* 165:2694-2702.

66. Werfel, T., K. Kirchhoff, M. Wittmann, G. Begemann, A. Kapp, F. Heidenreich, O. Gotze, and J. Zwirner. 2000. Activated human T lymphocytes express a functional C3a receptor. *J.Immunol.* 165:6599-6605.

67. Stimler, N. P., M. K. Bach, C. M. Bloor, and T. E. Hugli. 1982. Release of leukotrienes from guinea pig lung stimulated by C5ades Arg anaphylatoxin. *J Immunol* 128:2247-2252.

68. Stimler, N. P., C. M. Bloor, and T. E. Hugli. 1983. C3a-induced contraction of guinea pig lung parenchyma: role of cyclooxygenase metabolites. *Immunopharmacology* 5:251-257.

69. Scheid, C. R., R. O. Webster, P. M. Henson, and S. R. Findlay. 1983. Direct effect of complement factor C5a on the contractile state of isolated smooth muscle cells. *J Immunol* 130:1997-1999.

70. Stimler-Gerard, N. P. 1986. Immunopharmacology of anaphylatoxin-induced bronchoconstrictor responses. *Complement* 3:137-151.

71. Drouin, S. M., J. Kildsgaard, J. Haviland, J. Zabner, H. P. Jia, P. B. McCray, B. F. Tack, and R. A. Wetsel. 2001. Expression of the complement anaphylatoxin C3a and C5a receptors on bronchial epithelial and smooth muscle cells in models of sepsis and asthma. *J.Immunol.* 166:2025-2032.

72. Mulligan, M. S., E. Schmid, G. O. Till, T. E. Hugli, H. P. Friedl, R. A. Roth, and P. A. Ward. 1997. C5a-dependent up-regulation in vivo of lung vascular P-selectin. *J.Immunol.* 158:1857-1861.

73. Kishimoto, T. K., M. A. Jutila, E. L. Berg, and E. C. Butcher. 1989. Neutrophil Mac-1 and MEL-14 adhesion proteins inversely regulated by chemotactic factors. *Science* 245:1238-1241.

74. Huber-Lang, M. S., N. C. Riedeman, J. V. Sarma, E. M. Younkin, S. R. McGuire, I. J. Laudes, K. T. Lu, R. F. Guo, T. A. Neff, V. A. Padgaonkar, J. D. Lambris, L. Spruce, D. Mastellos, F. S. Zetoune, and P. A. Ward. 2002. Protection of innate immunity by C5aR antagonist in septic mice. *FASEB J.* 16:1567-1574.

75. Hartmann, K., B. M. Henz, S. Kruger-Krasagakes, J. Kohl, R. Burger, S. Guhl, I. Haase, U. Lippert, and T. Zuberbier. 1997. C3a and C5a stimulate chemotaxis of human mast cells. *Blood* 89:2863-2870.

76. Nilsson, G., M. Johnell, C. H. Hammer, H. L. Tiffany, K. Nilsson, D. D. Metcalfe, A. Siegbahn, and P. M. Murphy. 1996. C3a and C5a are chemotaxins for human mast cells and act through distinct receptors via a pertussis toxin-sensitive signal transduction pathway. *J.Immunol.* 157:1693-1698.

77. Cochrane, C. G. and H. J. Müller-Eberhard. 1968. The derivation of two distinct anaphylatoxin activities from the third and fifth components of human complement. *J.Exp.Med.* 127:371-386.

78. Basta, M., F. Van Goor, S. Luccioli, E. M. Billings, A. O. Vortmeyer, L. Baranyi, J. Szebeni, C. R. Alving, M. C. Carroll, I. Berkower, S. S. Stojilkovic, and D. D. Metcalfe. 2003. F(ab)(2)-mediated neutralization of C3a and C5a anaphylatoxins: a novel effector function of immunoglobulins. *Nat.Med.* 9:431-438.

79. Ramos, B. F., Y. Zhang, and B. A. Jakshik. 1994. Neutrophil elicitation in the reverse passive Arthus reaction. Complement-dependent and -independent mast cell involvement. *J Immunol.* 152:1380-1384.

80. Clancy, R. M., C. A. Dahinden, and T. E. Hugli. 1985. Complement-mediated arachidonate metabolism. *Prog.Biochem.Pharmacol.* 20:120-131.

81. Okusawa, S., C. A. Dinarello, K. B. Yancey, S. Endres, T. J. Lawley, M. M. Frank, J. F. Burke, and J. A. Gelfand. 1987. C5a induction of human interleukin 1. Synergistic effect with endotoxin or interferon-gamma. *J Immunol* 139:2635-2640.

82. Scholz, W., M. R. McClurg, G. J. Cardenas, M. Smith, D. J. Noonan, T. E. Hugli, and E. L. Morgan. 1990. C5a-mediated release of interleukin 6 by human monocytes. *Clin.Immunol.Immunopathol.* 57:297-307.

83. Ember, J. A., S. D. Sanderson, T. E. Hugli, and E. L. Morgan. 1994. Induction of interleukin-8 synthesis from monocytes by human C5a anaphylatoxin. *Am.J.Pathol.* 144:393-403.

84. Pieters, W. R., L. A. Houben, L. Koenderman, and J. A. Raaijmakers. 1995. C5a-induced migration of human monocytes is primed by dexamethasone. *Am.J.Respir.Cell Mol.Biol.* 12:691-696.

85. Soruri, A., Z. Kiafard, C. Dettmer, J. Riggert, J. Kohl, and J. Zwirner. 2003. IL-4 Down-Regulates Anaphylatoxin Receptors in Monocytes and Dendritic Cells and Impairs Anaphylatoxin-Induced Migration In Vivo. *J.Immunol.* 170:3306-3314.

86. Monk, P. N., M. D. Barker, and L. J. Partridge. 1994. Multiple signalling pathways in the C5a-induced expression of adhesion receptor Mac-1. *Biochim.Biophys.Acta* 1221:323-329.

87. Martin, U., D. Bock, L. Arseniev, M. A. Tornetta, R. S. Ames, W. Bautsch, J. Kohl, A. Ganser, and A. Klos. 1997. The human C3a receptor is expressed on neutrophils and monocytes, but not on B or T lymphocytes. *J.Exp.Med.* 186:199-207.

88. Hawlisch, H., R. Frank, M. Hennecke, M. Baensch, B. Sohns, L. Arseniev, W. Bautsch, A. Kola, A. Klos, and J. Kohl. 1998. Site-directed C3a receptor antibodies from phage display libraries. *J.Immunol.* 160:2947-2958.

89. Takabayashi, T., E. Vannier, B. D. Clark, N. H. Margolis, C. A. Dinarello, J. F. Burke, and J. A. Gelfand. 1996. A new biologic role for C3a and C3a desArg: regulation of TNF- alpha and IL-1 beta synthesis. *J.Immunol.* 156:3455-3460.

90. Buhl, A. M., N. Avdi, G. S. Worthen, and G. L. Johnson. 1994. Mapping of the C5a receptor signal transduction network in human neutrophils. *Proc.Natl.Acad.Sci.U.S.A* 91:9190-9194.

91. Knall, C., S. Young, J. A. Nick, A. M. Buhl, G. S. Worthen, and G. L. Johnson. 1996. Interleukin-8 regulation of the Ras/Raf/mitogen-activated protein kinase pathway in human neutrophils. *J.Biol.Chem.* 271:2832-2838.

92. Koyasu, S. 2003. The role of PI3K in immune cells. *Nat.Immunol.* 4:313-319.

93. Davignon, I., M. D. Catalina, D. Smith, J. Montgomery, J. Swantek, J. Croy, M. Siegelman, and T. M. Wilkie. 2000. Normal hematopoiesis and inflammatory responses despite discrete signaling defects in Galpha15 knockout mice. *Mol.Cell Biol.* 20:797-804.

94. Jiang, H., Y. Kuang, Y. Wu, A. Smrcka, M. I. Simon, and D. Wu. 1996. Pertussis toxin-sensitive activation of phospholipase C by the C5a and fMet-Leu-Phe receptors. *J.Biol.Chem.* 271:13430-13434.

95. Giancotti, F. G. and E. Ruoslahti. 1999. Integrin signaling. *Science* 285:1028-1032.

96. Plow, E. F. and L. Zhang. 1997. A MAC-1 attack: integrin functions directly challenged in knockout mice. *J.Clin.Invest* 99:1145-1146.

97. Jones, S. L., U. G. Knaus, G. M. Bokoch, and E. J. Brown. 1998. Two signaling mechanisms for activation of alphaM beta2 avidity in polymorphonuclear neutrophils. *J.Biol.Chem.* 273:10556-10566.

98. Zhou, M. J. and E. J. Brown. 1994. CR3 (Mac-1, alpha M beta 2, CD11b/CD18) and Fc gamma RIII cooperate in generation of a neutrophil respiratory burst: requirement for Fc gamma RIII and tyrosine phosphorylation. *J.Cell Biol.* 125:1407-1416.

99. Boisvert, W. A., R. Santiago, L. K. Curtiss, and R. A. Terkeltaub. 1998. A leukocyte homologue of the IL-8 receptor CXCR-2 mediates the accumulation of macrophages in atherosclerotic lesions of LDL receptor-deficient mice. *J.Clin.Invest* 101:353-363.

100. Nilsson, G., J. A. Mikovits, D. D. Metcalfe, and D. D. Taub. 1999. Mast cell migratory response to interleukin-8 is mediated through interaction with chemokine receptor CXCR2/Interleukin-8RB. *Blood* 93:2791-2797.

101. Inamura, H., M. Kurosawa, A. Okano, H. Kayaba, and M. Majima. 2002. Expression of the interleukin-8 receptors CXCR1 and CXCR2 on cord-blood-derived cultured human mast cells. *Int.Arch.Allergy Immunol.* 128:142-150.

102. Baggiolini, M., B. Dewald, and B. Moser. 1997. Human chemokines: an update. *Annu.Rev.Immunol.* 15:675-705.
103. Chandrasekar, B., P. C. Melby, H. M. Sarau, M. Raveendran, R. P. Perla, F. M. Marelli-Berg, N. O. Dulin, and I. S. Singh. 2003. Chemokine-cytokine cross-talk. The ELR+ CXC chemokine LIX (CXCL5) amplifies a proinflammatory cytokine response via a phosphatidylinositol 3-kinase-NF-kappa B pathway. *J.Biol.Chem.* 278:4675-4686.
104. Ravetch, J. V. and S. Bolland. 2001. IgG Fc receptors. *Annu.Rev.Immunol.* 19:275-90.:275-290.
105. Weinshank, R. L., A. D. Luster, and J. V. Ravetch. 1988. Function and regulation of a murine macrophage-specific IgG Fc receptor, Fc gamma R-alpha. *J.Exp.Med.* 167:1909-1925.
106. Tridandapani, S., K. Siefker, J. L. Teillaud, J. E. Carter, M. D. Wewers, and C. L. Anderson. 2002. Regulated expression and inhibitory function of Fcgamma RIIb in human monocytic cells. *J.Biol.Chem.* 277:5082-5089.
107. Tridandapani, S., R. Wardrop, C. P. Baran, Y. Wang, J. M. Opalek, M. A. Caligiuri, and C. B. Marsh. 2003. TGF-beta1 Supresses Myeloid Fcgamma Receptor Function by Regulating the Expression and Function of the Common gamma-Subunit. *J.Immunol.* 170:4572-4577.
108. Mulligan, M. S., R. L. Warner, J. L. Foreback, T. P. Shanley, and P. A. Ward. 1997. Protective effects of IL-4, IL-10, IL-12, and IL-13 in IgG immune complex-induced lung injury: role of endogenous IL-12. *J.Immunol.* 159:3483-3489.
109. Takai, T. 2002. Roles of Fc receptors in autoimmunity. *Nat.Rev.Immunol.* 2:580-592.
110. Arthus, M. 1903. Inections repetees de serum de cheval chez le lapin. *C.R.Soc.Biol.* 55:817.
111. Sylvestre, D., R. Clynes, M. Ma, H. Warren, M. C. Carroll, and J. V. Ravetch. 1996. Immunoglobulin G-mediated inflammatory responses develop normally in complement-deficient mice. *J Exp.Med.* 184:2385-2392.
112. Sylvestre, D. L. and J. V. Ravetch. 1996. A dominant role for mast cell Fc receptors in the Arthus reaction. *Immunity.* 5:387-390.
113. Sylvestre, D. L. and J. V. Ravetch. 1994. Fc receptors initiate the Arthus reaction: redefining the inflammatory cascade. *Science* 265:1095-1098.
114. Ravetch, J. V. and R. A. Clynes. 1998. Divergent roles for Fc receptors and complement in vivo. *Annu.Rev.Immunol.* 16:421-32.:421-432.
115. Baumann, U., N. Chouchakova, B. Gewecke, J. Kohl, M. C. Carroll, R. E. Schmidt, and J. E. Gessner. 2001. Distinct tissue site-specific requirements of mast cells and complement components C3/C5a receptor in IgG immune complex-induced injury of skin and lung. *J.Immunol.* 167:1022-1027.
116. Bozic, C. R., B. Lu, U. E. Hopken, C. Gerard, and N. P. Gerard. 1996. Neurogenic amplification of immune complex inflammation. *Science* 273:1722-1725.
117. Hopken, U. E., B. Lu, N. P. Gerard, and C. Gerard. 1997. Impaired inflammatory responses in the reverse arthus reaction through genetic deletion of the C5a receptor. *J.Exp.Med.* 186:749-756.
118. Strachan, A. J., T. M. Woodruff, G. Haaima, D. P. Fairlie, and S. M. Taylor. 2000. A new small molecule C5a receptor antagonist inhibits the reverse-passive Arthus reaction and endotoxic shock in rats. *J.Immunol.* 164:6560-6565.
119. Baumann, U., J. Kohl, T. Tschernig, K. Schwerter-Strumpf, J. S. Verbeek, R. E. Schmidt, and J. E. Gessner. 2000. A codominant role of Fc gamma RI/III and C5aR in the reverse Arthus reaction. *J.Immunol.* 164:1065-1070.
120. Kohl, J. and J. E. Gessner. 1999. On the role of complement and Fc gamma-receptors in the Arthus reaction. *Mol.Immunol.* 36:893-903.

121. Kohl, J. 2001. Anaphylatoxins and infectious and non-infectious inflammatory diseases. *Mol.Immunol.* 38:175-187.
122. Chouchakova, N., J. Skokowa, U. Baumann, T. Tschernig, K. M. Philippens, B. Nieswandt, R. E. Schmidt, and J. E. Gessner. 2001. Fc gamma RIII-mediated production of TNF-alpha induces immune complex alveolitis independently of CXC chemokine generation. *J.Immunol.* 166:5193-5200.
123. Czermak, B. J., V. Sarma, N. M. Bless, H. Schmal, H. P. Friedl, and P. A. Ward. 1999. In vitro and in vivo dependency of chemokine generation on C5a and TNF-alpha. *J.Immunol.* 162:2321-2325.
124. Shushakova, N., J. Skokowa, J. Schulman, U. Baumann, J. Zwirner, R. E. Schmidt, and J. E. Gessner. 2002. C5a anaphylatoxin is a major regulator of activating versus inhibitory FcgammaRs in immune complex-induced lung disease. *J.Clin.Invest* 110:1823-1830.
125. Heller, T., J. E. Gessner, R. E. Schmidt, A. Klos, W. Bautsch, and J. Kohl. 1999. Cutting edge: Fc receptor type I for IgG on macrophages and complement mediate the inflammatory response in immune complex peritonitis. *J.Immunol.* 162:5657-5661.
126. Zhang, Y., B. F. Ramos, and B. A. Jakschik. 1992. Neutrophil recruitment by tumor necrosis factor from mast cells in immune complex peritonitis. *Science* 258:1957-1959.
127. Matsumoto, I., A. Staub, C. Benoist, and D. Mathis. 1999. Arthritis provoked by linked T and B cell recognition of a glycolytic enzyme. *Science* 286:1732-1735.
128. Kouskoff, V., A. S. Korganow, V. Duchatelle, C. Degott, C. Benoist, and D. Mathis. 1996. Organ-specific disease provoked by systemic autoimmunity. *Cell* 87:811-822.
129. Kyogoku, C., H. M. Dijstelbloem, N. Tsuchiya, Y. Hatta, H. Kato, A. Yamaguchi, T. Fukazawa, M. D. Jansen, H. Hashimoto, J. G. van de Winkel, C. G. Kallenberg, and K. Tokunaga. 2002. Fcgamma receptor gene polymorphisms in Japanese patients with systemic lupus erythematosus: contribution of FCGR2B to genetic susceptibility. *Arthritis Rheum.* 46:1242-1254.
130. Radeke, H. H., I. Janssen-Graalfs, E. N. Sowa, N. Chouchakova, J. Skokowa, F. Loscher, R. E. Schmidt, P. Heeringa, and J. E. Gessner. 2002. Opposite regulation of type II and III receptors for immunoglobulin G in mouse glomerular mesangial cells and in the induction of anti-glomerular basement membrane (GBM) nephritis. *J.Biol.Chem.* 277:27535-27544.
131. Clynes, R., J. S. Maizes, R. Guinamard, M. Ono, T. Takai, and J. V. Ravetch. 1999. Modulation of immune complex-induced inflammation in vivo by the coordinate expression of activation and inhibitory Fc receptors. *J.Exp.Med.* 189:179-185.
132. Yuasa, T., S. Kubo, T. Yoshino, A. Ujike, K. Matsumura, M. Ono, J. V. Ravetch, and T. Takai. 1999. Deletion of fcgamma receptor IIB renders H-2(b) mice susceptible to collagen-induced arthritis. *J.Exp.Med.* 189:187-194.
133. Nakamura, A., T. Yuasa, A. Ujike, M. Ono, T. Nukiwa, J. V. Ravetch, and T. Takai. 2000. Fcgamma receptor IIB-deficient mice develop Goodpasture's syndrome upon immunization with type IV collagen: a novel murine model for autoimmune glomerular basement membrane disease. *J.Exp.Med.* 191:899-906.

16

Role of Complement in Allergy

Lilian Varga, Henriette Farkas and George Füst
Third Department of Internal Medicine and Angoedema and Allergy Center, Semmelweis University, Budapest, Hungary

Abstract: For several decades the role for complement as a mediator of type I hypersensitivity reaction was not considered important. In the last ten years, however, the role of complement in allergy and asthma has been revisited and revised. This chapter summarizes the recent results on this topic. In *in vitro* and animal experiments several findings on the role of complement activation in both the sensitization and effector phases of allergic reactions have been published. Association between allergy-induced provocation of airway symptoms and generation of complement activation products was demonstrated in patients as well. Our group studied the mechanism of complement activation by allergens, and revealed a strong correlation between the extent of in vitro activation by ragweed allergen and the severity of clinical symptoms in the ragweed season in the same allergic patients. The results of most experiments described in the chapter have therapeutic relevance; clinical trials are expected to be started in the near future.

Key words: complement, allergy, type I hypersensitivity reactions, ragweed, C3bBbP, C3a, C5a, symptoms of allergy

1.   INTRODUCTION

Several decades ago it was shown that crude allergen extracts may activate the complement system *in vitro* (1,2,3). For several decades, however, except for the works from the group of Lubertus Berrens (4,5), no studies on the interaction between allergens and the complement system were published. Traditionally, complement activation was not considered important in the pathogenesis of type I hypersensitivity reactions. Berrens' group has studied the role of complement in both the induction and effector phases of allergy but their work has been rather neglected by mainstream allergology researchers.

The situation, however, has considerably changed in the last years. Several experimental and clinical works were published which demonstrated that complement activation not only takes place during the exposition of sensitized individuals to specific allergens but it modifies its pathogenesis as well. Our group was involved in the description of the mechanism of allergen-induced complement activation, and demonstrated a strong correlation between the extent of complement activation in the sera of the ragweed-allergic patients (most common pollen allergy in Hungary) and the number and severity of the symptoms in the same patients. In this chapter we summarize the most important findings reported in the last decade on the role of complement in allergy.

2.   MECHANISM OF COMPLEMENT ACTIVATION BY ALLERGEN EXTRACTS

For a long time it has been well known that some allergens are as potent activators of complement, as aggregated IgG or endotoxins (4, 6). These and more recent studies (7) strongly suggest that initial complement activation by some allergens is triggered mainly via the classical pathway, although help of the alternative pathway may occur.

Experiments from our group (8) also supported the involvement of the classical pathway in the initiation of allergen-induced complement activation. Serum samples from 3 non-allergic normocomplementaemic individuals, as well as from three C2-deficient patients and a C2-depleted serum preparation were incubated with 100 AU/ml RWA and as control with veronal-buffered saline (VBS). Formation of two complement activation products, C3bBbP and C3a were measured. In the complement-sufficient sera RWA induced a strong C3bBbP formation (332 %, p<0.001) and a significant C3a generation (135 %, p<0.05) as compared to VBS. By contrast, significant C3BbP and/or C3a generation were not observed in any of the three homozygous C2 deficient patients tested. Similar absence of complement activation was found in the C2-depleted human serum preparation.

The precise mechanism of classical pathway activation by allergen extracts, however, has remained obscure until now. Two explanations were offered on the basis of the experimental data available at that time. According to Berrens et al. (4) C1 activation is immunoglobulin-independent, and is largely mediated by interactions between unknown serum factors and soluble degradation products in allergen extracts. In contrast, on the basis of studies performed with unrefined house dust extracts (7) it was concluded that activation of the classical pathway by allergens is mediated by natural IgM antibodies directed to polysaccharide antigens in the extracts.

Recently, as part of an international collaborative study, we have examined the mechanism of the early steps of allergen-induced activation of complement in detail (9). Two allergen preparations, house dust (HD) and *Parietaria judaica* (PA) were found to be strong activators of complement in preliminary experiments.

In the first series of these experiments we demonstrated significant increase in the formation of C4d, an activation product of the early steps of complement activation, in human serum following incubation with HD and PA allergen extracts in the 0.05-1 mg/ml dose range. Complement activation by allergen extracts at a final concentration of 0.05-1 mg/ml was seen in serum from both allergic and non-allergic individuals. As a control heat-aggregated human IgG was used at a final concentration of 0.05-1 mg/ml. HD and PA extracts generated C4d in amounts comparable to that formed with aggregated IgG in the same sera.

In subsequent experiments the allergens were mixed with sera from three hypogammaglobulinaemic subjects, and, as positive control, with sera from three non-allergic normogammaglobulinaemic individuals. Figure 1 shows the results obtained with 1-1 serum samples.

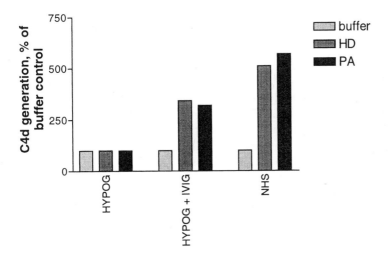

Figure 1. Generation of C4d in serum samples from a healthy, non-allergic individual (NHS), as well as a patient with severe hypogammaglobulinaemia (HYPOG) with or without a purified immunogloblin preparation (IVIG)

In all hypogammaglobulinaemic sera the HD and PA extracts did not generate C4d above the buffer control level. In normal sera the same doses of the allergens led to formation of C4d, approximately three-fold above the buffer control. When IgG in hypogammaglobulinaemic sera was reconstituted to about 5 g/l, the ability to generate C4d of both allergen extracts has significantly improved (Figure 1).

Second, interaction of allergens with C1q, MBL and their ability to activate C1 were investigated by using purified complement proteins. The allergen extracts bound to the globular head of C1q and interacted with purified mannan-binding lectin, MBL, as measured by solid phase ELISA. HD-induced C4d generation was about the same in MBL-depleted serum and in normal sera. In contrast PA induced no C4d formation in the MBL-depleted serum, whereas reconstitution with purified MBL restored C4d generation.

The HD extract and, as a control, heat-aggregated IgG (HAIgG), were added to a C1 preparation which was reconstituted from purified C1q and recombinant proenzymes C1r and C1s. Activation of C1 was monitored by Western blot analysis which detects C1s cleavage as a marker of C1 activation. Allergens were used at concentrations that were shown to generate high proportions of C4d in normal serum. Almost complete cleavage of C1s occurred when reconstituted C1 was incubated with different doses of HAIgG whereas no C1s cleavage could be detected in presence of HD extract.

These *in vitro* findings indicate that although the allergen extracts can bind purified C1q and MBL, they require IgG for efficient complement activation. Depending on the allergens, this activation may be initiated through C1, MBL, or both. It can be definitely excluded that antibodies, specific for different allergen epitopes, are involved in the allergen induced complement activation. Firstly, allergen extracts may induce marked classical pathway activation in the sera of individuals non-allergic to these extracts (5,7,8,10). Moreover, several lines of evidence published by Berrens (11), Berrens and de la Cuedra, (12) and Berrens et. al., (13) indicate that there is a constant quantitative relationship between the complement activating potentials of distinct allergen extracts, which is independent of the serum samples used. Accordingly, very strong correlation was observed in the extent of complement activation induced by several allergens in different sera from either allergic or non-allergic individuals. Thus, complement activation can possibly be explained by immune complex formation between ubiquitous polysaccharide epitope(s) present in different densities in various allergen extracts with cross-reacting naturally occurring antibodies present in sera of various individuals (7).

Concerning the nature of the allergen antigen epitopes, Berrens and coworkers (12,13) identified polyphenilic (flavonoid) structures complexed with or chemically conjugated to the pollen proteins that were able to activate the complement system. This type of structure(s), may represent the common epitope for cross-reacting, naturally occurring IgG antibodies, although direct proof of this structure remains to be obtained.

3.   ROLE OF COMPLEMENT ACTIVATION PRODUCTS IN THE INDUCTION PHASE OF TYPE 1 HYPERSENSITIVITY REACTIONS

Recent experiments performed with up-to-date molecular biological techniques indicate that complement has a major role in the sensitization of patients to different allergens. Karp et al. (14) compared two groups of inbred mouse strains that exhibited low and high responsiveness to metacholine challenge. They have demonstrated that the C5 gene conferred decreased bronchial responsiveness following allergen challenge: responsiveness of the genetically C5-deficient strains was significantly higher than that in the C5 sufficient animals. Authors explained their finding with the ability of C5a to inhibit IL-12 release from monocytes and macrophages and the consequent Th1 response. When C5 is absent, that is, no C5a can be generated, the balance of immune response switches toward the Th2 type response that is characteristic of allergy. In accordance with this observation, at genome-wide scanning of asthma susceptibility loci it was found that among the asthma-associated genetic regions the C5 gene in chromosome 9 and that for the C5a receptor in chromosome 19 (15,16,17) are present.

In contrast to the results obtained with C5, Drouin et al. demonstrated that C3 (18) and the C3a receptors (C3aR) (19) are necessary for an effective Th2 type response to occur after allergen challenge. Mice deficient in C3a exhibited not only a diminished airway hyperresponsiveness and lung eosonophilia after intranasal challenge with *Aspergillus fumigatus* + BSA allergen (see below), but they had a dramatically reduced numbers of IL-4 producing cells and attenuated IgE and IgG1 responses (18). Similarly, C3aR knock out mice had an 59% reduction of IL-4 producing cells, diminished levels of Th2 type cytokines IL-5 and IL-13 in bronchoalveolar lavage fluid, decreased IgE titers and reduced mucus production (19). These data implicate C3a and its receptor in the Th2 response development in this model and indicate a role of the complement system in sensitization stage by promoting Th2 effector functions in asthma and other types of allergic diseases.

4.   ROLE OF COMPLEMENT ACTIVATION
PRODUCTS IN THE EFFECTOR PHASE OF
TYPE 1 HYPERSENSITIVITY REACTIONS

4.1   Formation of Complement Activation Products in
Experimental Allergy Models

Several findings indicate that complement activation takes places on the allergen-exposed mucosa of allergic individuals. C3a generated during complement activation can lead to increased vascular permeability it markedly facilitates mucus formation in the lower parts of respiratory tract (20) and induces production and release of interleukin 1 by cultured human monocytes (21). Fraser et al. (22) in a guinea pig model, using trimellitic anhydride (TMA), (a small molecular weight industrial compound that can cause asthma-like symptoms in humans), could directly prove the role of complement in the allergic response of the lung. Depletion of complement by cobra venom factor in the animals prior to their exposition to TMA prevented inflammatory cell infiltration in TMA-induced asthma.

Recently several new findings obtained in different animal allergy models support the role of the complement activation in the effector phase of type 1 hypersensitivity reactions (reviewed by Gerard and Gerard (23)). Abe et al. (24) examined rats sensitized to ovalbumin (OVA). The animals were repeatedly exposed intranasally to OVA and the pulmonary resistance was determined. Before exposure the rats were treated with two types of complement inhibitor, soluble complement receptor type 1 (sCR1) and futan (nafomostate mesylate). Pretreatment with both substances inhibited immediate airway response. Pretreatment with sCR1 and a C5aR antagonist blocked the development of the late airway responsiveness (LAR), as well as esosinophil and neutrophil infiltration of the submucosa. The preventive effect of sCR1 could be reversed by addition of rat C5a-des-arg, further indicating the complement dependence of LAR.

Several recent data obtained in C3 or C3aR deficient animals support the role of C3a in the allergy models. Drouin et al. (18) used OVA mixed with *Aspergillus fumigatus* filtrate for sensitization and challenge of C3-deficient mice. When challenged with allergen mice deficient in C3 exhibited diminished airway hyperresponsiveness and lung eosinophilia. Humbles et al. (25) observed near complete protection from the development of airway hyperresponsiveness to aerosolized metacholine in OVA-sensitized C3aR KO mice. Similar results were obtained by Bautsch et al. (26) in guinea pig with a natural deletion of C3aR and by Drouin et al. (19) in C3aR KO mice. A significant protection from airway bronchoconstriction following allergen challenge was observed in OVA-sensitized animals by both groups. Drouin et al. (19) used the OVA+*Aspergillus fumigatus* model in C3aR KO mice. In addition to an airway responsiveness after challenge the C3aR deficient animals also had an 88% decrease in airway eosinophils and diminished levels od Th2 cytokines, IL-5 and IL-13 in bronchoalveolar lavage fluids.

4.2 Detection of Complement Activation Products in the Blood or Lavage Fluids After Allergen-Provocation in Allergic Patients

Several years ago we tested the complement-activation dependent granulocyte aggregating activity in sera of workers exposed to textile dust inhalation. (27). Granulocyte aggregation is a sensitive method suitable for detection of C5a formation due to even a minimal extent of systemic complement activation. Using this procedure we were able to demonstrate a significant increase (from 10 ± 4 to 29 ± 4 zymosan-equivalent units) in the aggregation of the granulocytes exposed to serum samples from 12 textile workers taken immediately after inhalative exposition to textile dust as compared to the samples taken before exposition. By contrast, no increase in granulocyte aggregation activity was found in 5 controls after the same exposition. It seems that in these patients massive complement activation took place, since later on any attempts to detect systemic complement activation in patients with allergic asthma remained unsuccessful (Durham et al, 1984 (24, 28).

Therefore more recently the levels of complement activation products were measured in nasal of bronchial lavage fluids. Ballow et al. (29) detected C3a anaphylatoxin in the tears of patients with allergic conjunctivitis. Andersson et al. (30) reported a generation of two complement activation products (C3a-des-arg and C5a-des-arg) in some minutes after nasal allergen with birch and timothy grass-pollen concomitantly with the development of nasal symptoms in patients with seasonal allergic rhinitis allergic to these pollens. Recently we could reproduce this observation in ragweed-allergic patients (31). The study was performed in 15 adolescents allergic to ragweed and in 6 non-allergic healthy volunteers. Following baseline measurements subjects were challenged with increasing doses of ragweed allergen after which symptoms, nasal inspiratory peak flow and nasal temperature were registered. Lavage fluid were collected and tested for complement activation product (C3bBbP). The allergic patients responded to allergen provocation with a significant ($p<0.001$) more than four-fold (from 2.23 to 9.73 U/ml) increase in C3bBbP formation compared to the initial lavage. In non-allergic volunteers C3bBbP remained low in the lavage fluids after challenge. We found a strong correlation between the threshold dose inducing symptoms and the dose where the maximum complement activation was detected ($r=0.78$, $p<0.001$).

Similar studies were reported on the generation of complement activation products in bronchoalveolar lavage fluid (BAL) of patients with asthma. C3a was higher in the BAL of patients with stable asthma compared healthy control subjects (32). Humbles et al. (25) found C3a to be elevated 4-6 hours after segmental allergen challenge compared with shame challenge in patients with mild asthma. Krug et al. (33) measured C3a/C3a-des-arg and C5a/C5a-des-arg concentrations in BAL in a group of 15 patients with mild asthma after challenge with allergens to which they were allergic according to skin prick test and IgE antibody determinations. Both C3a and C5a levels in BAL were significantly increased 24 hours after allergen challenge compared with baseline results. In the group of healthy volunteers the concentrations of both complement activation products remained unchanged. Importantly, the authors found significant correlation between C3a and C5a concentration and the number of eosinophils ($p<0.01$) and neutrophils ($p<0.05$) in BAL.

These data suggest the contribution of complement activation products in the pathogenesis of allergic rhinitis and asthma.

5.   RELATIONSHIP BETWEEN COMPLEMENT ACTIVATION AND THE SEVERITY OF ALLERGIC SYMPTOMS.

5.1   Correlation Between the Extent of In Vitro Complement Activation by Allergens and the Clinical Symptoms in the Same Patients

Recently we published several findings indicating that complement activation occurs on the allergen-exposed mucosa of the sensitized patients, contribute to the development of allergic inflammation and may determine the severity of symptoms. Ragweed (RW) allergy was selected as a model of pollen allergy since it is the most common inhalation allergen in Hungary and in the United States, too.

In early August 1992 (that is during the RW blooming season) blood samples were taken from 40 RW allergic patients (8). These sera were incubated with ragweed allergen extract (RWA) (20 AU/ml) and the formation of complement activation products was determined. After taking blood samples the allergic patients were asked to fill diaries about their symptoms during the subsequent 4 weeks. This diary included subjective scores to be given to nasal-, eye-, throat-, pulmonary-, and ear symptoms (0 = no symptom, 1 = mild symptom, 2 = medium symptom, 3 = severe symptom, disturbing daily life). Symptoms' scores were summed. 26 of the diaries could be evaluated, and compared to RWA induced AP activation (C3bBbP formation). We found a significant positive correlation between eye-, and throat symptoms and the activation of the AP ($p=0.03$) and $p=0.006$, respectively). The correlation between nasal symptoms and C3bBbP formation was of marginal significance ($p=0.07$).

When the 26 allergic subjects were divided into two groups according to the extent of C3bBbP formation (>120 %, n=15 or ≤120 %, n=11 compared to buffer control) upon incubation with 20 AU/ml RWA, we found that the sum of eye and nasal symptoms' scores that developed in a 4-week period subsequent to blood sampling obtained in different patients were significantly higher in patients with more pronounced allergen-induced AP activation (128 ± 22 vs. 28 ± 6, $p=0.0009$, and 149 ± 22 vs. 57 ± 13, $p=0.0032$, respectively)

An other study was performed in twenty-two 15-17 year old RW allergic adolescents (34). Serum samples taken during the RW blooming season were incubated with 100 µg/ml RWA and the generation of different complement activation products were measured by ELISA or RIA tests. Symptom scores were registered for 4 weeks during the RW blooming season. The patients were divided according to the extent (low or high) of generation of the complement activation products and symptom scores registered in the two groups were compared by using the two-way ANOVA method. Significantly higher symptom scores were obtained in the high than in the low complement activation group (p values: 0.049 for C1rC1sC1inh, 0.022 for C3bBbP, 0.015 for C5b-9, 0.0001 for C3a, 0.0008 for C5a). Similar results were obtained at the measurement performed in the sera obtained from the same patients half a year before the season (p values: 0.022 for C3bBbP, 0.005 for C5b-9) (Figure 2).

Next, we analyzed the relationship between the results of the usual allergologic tests (IgE estimation, titration skin prick test) and the extent of in vitro ragweed allergen extract (RWA)-induced complement activation in the sera of the same 48 patients suffering from late-summer allergy (35). For obtaining estimation about skin reactivity to RWA of a patient, skin prick testing was performed by titration. The aqueous extract of RWA was applied in three different concentrations (10^3, 10^4, and 10^5 biological units [BU]/ml). The results were evaluated after 15 minutes. The lowest concentration which gave rise to a histamine-equivalent positive reaction was considered as the measure of skin reactivity and was expressed in arbitrary units. Skin reactivity was designated as one arbitrary skin reactivity unit (SRU) if 10^5 BU/ml RWA produced a wheal with a diameter equal to the histamine control at a given patient, while 10^3 and 10^4 BU/ml RWA induced less or no reaction.

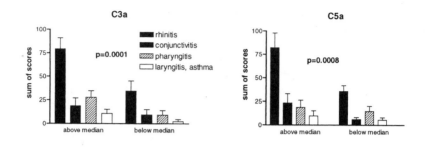

Figure 2. Symptoms scores registered during the ragweed blooming seasons in 22 ragweed allergic adolescents with high (above median of the whole group) and low (below median) C3a and C5a generation in their serum samples incubated with 100 µg/ml RWA

Skin reactivity was designated as 10 or 100 SRU if histamine-equivalent positive reaction was obtained already with 10^4 and 10^3 BU/ml RWA, respectively. Sera of these patients were incubated with 20, 100, and 400 U/ml RWA and generation of two complement activation products, alternative pathway C3-convertase (C3bBbP) and terminal pathway activation complex (C5b-9) was measured by ELISA methods. A strong positive correlation (Spearman correlation coefficient r = 0.495, p=0.0004, and r = 0.454, p=0.0012, respectively) was found between individual skin reactivity to RWA and C3bBbP generation induced by 20 and 100 allergological units/ml (U/ml) RWA (Figure 3).

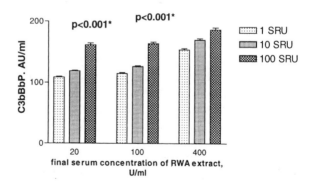

Figure 3. Correlation between the skin reactivity to ragweed as determined by a dilution prick test and the extent of C3bBbP formation in the sera of ragweed allergic patients incubated with different amounts of ragweed allergen extract. *Compared to 1SRU, Mann-Whitney test

6. RELATIONSHIP BETWEEN THE IGE-MEDIATED AND COMPLEMENT-MEDIATED PROCESSES IN THE MEDIATION OF THE ALLERGIC REACTION

6.1 Differences in the Complement Activating and IgE-Binding Structures of the Allergens

We compared the effect on the complement activating and IgE-binding capacity of the RWA by using two types of treatment (36). Elimination of the physically adsorbed (flavonoid) pigments from the allergenic proteins had no significant effect in their complement activating capacity. By contrast the same treatment led to an about 100-fold decrease in the IgE binding capacity of the RWA extract. Removal of trypsin inhibitor present in various allergenic pollen including ragweed (37) resulted in a significant increase in the complement activation by RWA whereas in did not affect IgE-binding.

These findings indicate that complement activation and IgE binding are distinct molecular properties of the RWA extract.

6.2 A Hypothesis on the Role of Complement Activation in type I Allergy Reactions

Results summarized in the chapter clearly indicate that allergens can activate the complement system both in RW-allergic and non-allergic individuals that is both in the absence and presence of IgE antibodies in the serum and/or on the IgE-receptors of basophils, mast cells and other cell types.

According to this hypothesis summarized in Figure 4, there are several types of interactions between complement activation products and the IgE mediated type 1 hypersensitivity reaction. Allergen-induced complement activation results in generation C5a and C3a that affect sensitization stage of the type 1 hypersensitivity reactions to opposite direction: C3a facilitates while C5a inhibits formation of Th2 type cytokines and IgE antibodies. On the other hand in the effector phase of allergic reaction both C3a and C5a (and maybe other complement activation products such as C5b-9), which are generated on the allergen-exposed mucosa, may affect the basic IgE-mediated processes of the type 1 hypersensitivity reactions. These findings are in accordance with the results of the animal experiments. The very potent inflammatory mediators that are formed from the complement proteins can amplify several processes mostly degranulation triggered by the interaction of allergen with IgE antibodies attached to the IgE receptors of different

cells. In addition, complement activation products were found to exert their
effect in a concerted action with some lymphokines. E.g. presentation of the
human basophilic granulocytes with IL-3 significantly increased the
sensitivity of the cells to C3a (38). Furthermore, TNFα was found to
efficiently prime neutrophils to the response to C5a (39). According to the
studies of Carlson et al. (40) IL-5 selectively primes human eosinophils and
neutrophils for C3b-induced degranulation.

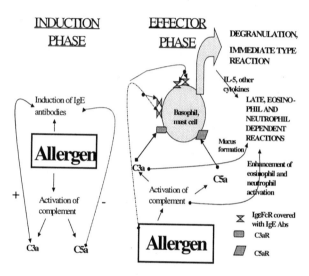

Figure 4. Interactions between the basic IgE-mediated processes and the allergen-induced
complement activation products in the development and effector stage of type 1
hypersensitivity reaction. C5a has a dual effect: inhibits sensitisation and production of IgE
antibodies and binds to IgE-FcR and inhibits in this way allergen-induced degranulation of
the mast cells. C3a has only enhancing effects: facilitates sensitisation and production of IgE
type antibodies, and in the effector phase may bind to C3aR on mast cells and basophil
leukocytes and increases degranulation of these cells.

In persons not allergic to RW, complement activation alone does not
result in inflammatory symptoms. Binding of allergens to IgE fixed to IgE-
Fc receptors of basophils and mast cells and the consequential degranulation
of these cells is an absolute prerequisite of the development of the
symptoms. On pollen-exposed mucosa of the RW-allergic individuals
interactions depicted in Figure 4 occur. According to the findings detailed
above, the severity of the allergic symptoms is related to the extent of
complement activation that is the extent of complement activation acts as a
fine-tuner of IgE-mediated type 1 hypersensitivity reaction. Complement
activation products may enhance the basic, IgE-dependent early and/or late
pathological mechanisms e.g. degranulation of mast cells or the chemotaxis
and activation of eosinophil leukocytes. Therefore in RW-allergic subjects

with a high individual reactivity of complement to RWA the symptoms will be more frequent and/or severe than in the allergic subjects with low complement reactivity. The intensity of this activation, that is the individual reactivity of complement to RWA and possibly to other allergens, is regulated by some yet unidentified factors, with probable involvement of natural antibodies. It would be most important to disclose the factors that are responsible for the low and high complement reactivity of different allergic and non-allergic individuals.

7. CONCLUSIONS

Both animal experiments and observations obtained in patients support the important modulating role of complement activation in the allergy and asthma. Most recently Nakano et al (41) detected elevated C3a in plasma from patients with severe asthma. These findings may have clinical implications and open new avenues for the treatment of allergic patients. According to the very recent results of Taube et al. (42) inhibition of complement activation decreases, indeed, airway inflammation and hyperresponsiveness in mice. Since the development of complement inhibitors is in progress and several of these substances are in phase I or even phase II clinical trials, the first attempts to apply these drugs in the clinical practice may be expected in the near future. Only the results of these experimental trials may decide if the hypothesis on the essential modulating effect of the complement system is correct.

8. REFERENCES

1. Walker, I.C. Complement fixation and precipitin reactions with the serum of broncial asthmatics who are sensitive to the proteins of wheat, horse dandruff, cat hair, and bacteria, using these proteins as antigens, and the cutaneous reaction as an index of sensitization. J Med Res 1917; 36:243-246
2. Albus, G. Beinflussung der Antikörperkonzentration durch spezifische Desensibilierung bei Pollenallergie. Z Ges Exp Med 1935; 95:703-707
3. Cavelti, P.A. Complement fixation studies in allergy. J Allergy 1950; 21:532-544
4. Berrens, L., Van Rijswijk-Verbeek, J., Guikers, C.L.H. Characteristics of complement consumption by atopic allergens. Immunochemistry 1976; 13:367-372
5. Berrens, L., Guikers, C.L.H., van Dijk, A.G. Studies in serum factors mediating complement consumption by house dust allergens Monographs in Allergy. 1979; 14:150-154
6. Nagata, S., Glovsky, M. 1987. Activation of human serum complement with allergens I. Generation of C3a, C4a, and C5a and induction of human neutrophil aggregation. J Allergy Clin Immunol 1987; 80:24-32

7. van der Zee, J.S., van Swieten, P., Aalberse, R.C. Activation of the classical pathway of human complement in vitro by house-dust extracts is caused by IgM antibodies to polysaccharide antigen(s) and is not related to atopy. Mol Immunol 1988; 4:345-354

8. Hidvégi, T., Schmidt, B., Varga, L., Dervaderics, M., Lantos, Á., Gönczi, Zs., Barok, J., Kirschfink, M., Spath, P., Füst, G. In vitro complement activation by ragweed allergen extract in the sera of ragweed allergic and non-allergic persons. Immunol Letts 1995; 48:65-71

9. Varga, L., Szilágyi, K., Lőrincz, Zs., Berrens, L., Thiel, S., Závodszky, P., Daha, M.R., Thielens, N.M., Arlaud, G.J., Nagy, K., Späth, P., Füst, G. Studies on the mechanisms of allergen-induced activation of the classical and lectin pathways of complement. Mol Immunol 2003; 39:839-846.

10. Castro, F.F.M., Schmitz-Schuman, M.,Rother, U., Kirschfink, M. Complement activation by house dust: reduced reactivity of serum complement in patients with bronchila asthma. Int.Arch.Allegy. Appl.Immunol. 1991; 96:305-310

11. Berrens, L. Complement activation by allergeneic house dust fractions is related to IgE binding and is not mediated by IgM antibody. Schweitz med Wschr. Suppl. 1991; 40:II,47-52

12. Berrens, L., de la Cuedra, B. Complement activating agents in allergenic extracts. Inflammation Res 1997; 46:455-460

13. Berrens, L., de la Cuadra, B., Gallego, M.T. Complement inactivation by allergenic plant pollen extracts. Life Sci 1997; 60:1497-1503

14. Karp, C.l., Grupe, A.,Schadt, E., Ewart, S.L., Leena-Moore, M., Cuomo, P.J., Kohl, J., Wahl, L., Kuperman, D., Germer, S. Aud, D., Peltz, G., Wills-Karp, M. Identification of complement factor 5 as a susceptibility locus for experimental allergic asthma. Nat Immunol 2000;1:221-226

15. The Collaborative Study on the Genetics of Asthma (CSGA). A genome-wide search for asthma-susceptibility loci in ethnically diverse populations. Nat genet 1997; 15:389-392

16. Ober, C., Cox, N.J., Abney, M., Di Rienzo A., Lander, E.S., Changyaleket, B., Gidley, H., Kurtz, B., Lee, J., Nance, M., Pettersson, A., Prescott, J., Richardson, A., Schlenker, E., Summerhill, E., Willadsen, S., Parry, R. Genome-wide search for asthma susceptibility loci in a founder population. The Collaborative Study on the Genetics of Asthma. Hum Mol Genet 1998; 7:1393-1398.

17. Wjst, M., Fischer, G., Immervoll, T., Jung, M., Saar, K., Reushendorf, F., Reis, A., Ulbrecht, M, Gomolka, M., Weis, E.H., Jaeger, L., Nickel, R., Richter, K., Kjellman, N.I., Griese, M., von Berg A., Gappa, M., Riedel, F., Boehle, M., van Koningsbruggen, S., Schoberth, P., Szczepanski, R., Dorsch, W., Silbermann, M., Wichmann, H.E. A genome-wide search for linkage to asthma. German Asthma Genetic Group. Genomics 1999; 58:1-8.

18. Drouin, S.M., Corry, D.B., Kildsgaard, J., Wetsel, R.A. Cutting Edge: The absence of C3 demonstrates a role for complement in Th2 effector functions in a murine model of pulmonary allergy. J Immunol 2001; 167:4141-4145

19. Drouin, S.M., Corry, D.B., Hollman, T.J., Kidsgaard, J., Wetsel, R.A. Absence of complement anaplylatoxin C3a receptor suppresses Th2 effector functions in a murine model of pulmonary allergy J Immunol 2002; 169:5926-5933.

20. Marom, Z., Shelhamer, J., Berger, M., Frank, M., Kaliner, M. Anaphylatoxin C3a enhances mucus glycoprotein release from human airways in vitro. J. Exp. Med. 1985; 161:657-668

21. Haeffner-Cavaillon, N., Cavaillon, J.M., Laude, M., Kazatchkine, M.D. C3a(C3adesArg) induces production and release of interleukin 1 by cultured human monocytes J. Immunol. 1987; 139: 794-799.

22. Fraser, D.G., Regal, J.F., Arndt, M.L. Trimellitic anhydride-induced allergic response in the lung: role of the complement system in the cellular changes. J.Pharmacol.Exp.Ther. 1995;273:793-801
23. Gerard, N.P., Gerard, C. Complement in Allergy and asthma. Current Opinion Immunol 2002; 14:705-708
24. Abe, M., Shibata, K., Akatsu, H., Shimuzu, N., Sakata, N., Katsuragi, T., Okada, H. Contribution of anaphylatoxin C5a to late airway responses after repeated exposure of antigen to allergic rats. J Immunol 2001; 167:4651-4660
25. Humbles, A.A., Lu, B., Nilsson, C.A., Lilly, C., Israel, E., Fujiwara, Y., Gerard, N.P., Gerard C. A role for the C3a anaphylatoxin receptor in the effector phase of asthma. Nature 2000; 406:998-1001
26. Bautsch, W., Hoymann, H.G., Zhang, Q., Meier-Wiedenbach, I., Raschke, U., Ames, R.S., Sohns, B., Flemme, N., Meyer, Z.U., Vilsendorf, A. Cutting edge: guinea pigs with a natural C3a-receptor defect exhibit decreased bronchocostriction in allergic airway disease: evidence for an involvment of the C3a anaphylatoxin in the pathogenesis of asthma. J Immunol 2000; 165:5401-5405
27. Varga, L., Dervaderics, M., Zsiray, M., Kárpáthy, J., Füst, G. Granulocyte aggregating activity in sera of workers exposed to textile dust inhalation. Diagn Immunol 1986; 4:140-144
28. Durham, S.R., Lee, T.H., Cromwell, O., Shaw, R.J., Merrett, T.G., Merrett, J., Cooper, P., Kay, A.B. immunological studies in allergen-induced late-phase asthmatic reaction. J Allergy Clin Immunol 1984; 74:49-56
29. Ballow, M., Donshik, P.C., Mendelson, L. Complement proteins and C3 anaphylatoxin in the tears of patients with conjunctivitis. J. Allergy Clin.Immunol. 1985; 76:473-476.
30. Andersson, M., Michel, L., Llull, J.B., Pipkorn, U. Complement activation on the nasal mucosal surface - a feature of the immediate allergic reaction in the nose. Allergy 1994;49: 242-245
31. Mezei, Gy., Varga, L., Veres, A., Füst, G., Cserháti, E. Complement activation in the nasal mucosa following nasal ragweed-allegen challange. Pediatr Allergy Immunol 2001; 12:201-207
32. Teran, L.M., Campos, M.G., Begishvilli, B.T., Schroder, J-M., Djukanovic, R., Schute, J.K., Church, M.K., Hológate, S.T., Davies, D.E. Identification of neutrophil chemotactic factors in brochoalveolar lavage fluid of asthmatic patients. Clin Exp Allergy 1997; 27:396-405
33. Krug, N., Tschernig, T., Erpenbeck, V.J., Hohlfeld, J.M., Köhl, J. Complement factors C3a and C5a are increased in brochoalveolar lavage fluid after segmental allergen provocation in subjects with asthma. Am J Respir Crit Care Med 2001;164:1841-1843
34. Gönczi, Zs., Varga, L., Hidvégi, T., Schmidt, B., Pánya, A., Kókai, M., Füst, G. The severity of clinical symptoms in ragweed-allergic patients is related to the extent of ragweed-induced complement activation in their sera. Allergy 1997; 52: 1110-1114
35. Dervaderics, M., Hidvégi, T., Schmidt, B., Füst, G., Varga, L.: Ragweed allergy: correlation between skin reactivity and in vitro complement activation. Immunol Letts 1998; 64:119-123
36. Hidvégi, T., Berrens, L., Varga, L., Maranon, F., Schmidt, B., Kirschfink, M., Füst G. Comparative study of the complement-activating and specific IgE-binding properties of ragweed pollen allergen. Clin exp Immunol 1997; 108:122-127
37. Berrens, L., Marañón, F. IgE - binding trypsin inhibitors in plant pollen extracts. Experientia 1995; 51: 953-955.
38. Elsner, J., Oppermann, M., Czech, W., Dobos, G., Schöpf, E., Norgauer, J., Kapp, A. C3a activates reactive oxygen radical species production and intracellular calcium transients in human eosinophils. Eur J Immunol. 1994; 24:518-522
39. Crouch, S., Fleischer, J. The priming effect of stimulated mononuclear cells on the response of neutrophils to C5a des arg. Br.J.Hematol. 1991; 74:158-164

40. Carlson, M., Peterson, C., Venge, P. The infuence of IL-3, Il-5 and GM-CSF on normal human eosinophil and neutrophil C3b-induced degranulation. Allergy 1993; 48:437-442.

41. Nakano, Y., Morita, S., Kawamoto, A., Suda, T., Chida, K., Nakamura, H. Elevated complement C3a in plasma from patients with severe acute asthma. J Allergy Clin Immunol 2003; 112:525-530

42. Taube, C., Rha, Y.H., Takeda, K., Park, J.W., Joetham, A., Balhorn, A., Dakhama, A., Giclas, P.C., Holers, V.M., Gelfand, E.W. Inhibition of complement activation decreases airway inflammation and hyperresponsiveness. Am J Respir Crit Care Med 2003;168:1333-1341

Complement Activation-Related Pseudoallergy
Mechanism of Anaphylactoid Reactions to Radiocontrast Media and Drug Carrier Liposomes and Micelles

Janos Szebeni

Department of Membrane Biochemistry, Walter Reed Army Institute of Research, Silver Spring, MD 20910, USA

Abstract: There are numerous drug-induced immediate hypersensitivity reactions (HSRs) that do not fit in Gell and Coombs's Type I category of drug allergies, characterized by a pivotal role of allergen-specific IgE. Such non-IgE-mediated reactions, also referred to as "anaphylactoid, pseudoallergic or idiosyncratic", are caused, among others, by radiocontrast agents, liposomal drugs and micellar solvent systems containing amphiphilic lipids or synthetic block-copolymers. A common feature of the latter agents is that they activate the complement (C) system, and that the reactions they cause can be explained with anaphylatoxin action. This chapter surveys the experimental and clinical evidence for the involvement of C activation in HSRs caused by agents in the above three categories. Further subjects include a proposal to update the classification of Type I allergy to according to the mechanism of mast cell (and basophil) activation, to direct and receptor-mediated reactions, with the latter category divided to IgE-mediated true allergy, C activation-related pseudoallegy (CARPA) and mixed IgE/C-triggered HSRs. The review also surveys the risk factors, laboratory prediction and pharmacological prevention of CARPA.

Key words: allergy, anaphylatoxins, anaphylactoid reaction; micelles, radiocontrast agents, cancer chemotherapy, Taxol, Cremophor EL

1.   INTRODUCTION

It has been estimated that as many as 30% of hospitalized patients may have a drug reaction of some type, with the incidence of severe and fatal reactions being approximately 7% and 0.3 %, respectively (1). These statistics imply roughly 2 million serious reactions per year with ~100,000 fatalities, making adverse drug reactions the fourth to sixth leading cause of death in the USA (1).

Another recent analysis pointed out that about 25% of all adverse drug reactions are of allergic nature (2). These allergic drug reactions were classified by Coombs and Gell in four groups referred to types I to IV (3). Type I reactions were defined as IgE-mediated acute hypersensitivity reactions (HSRs), while the type II-IV categories enclosed those subacute or chronic reactions that are mediated by IgG, immune complexes or lymphocytes, respectively (3). While this categorization certainly accommodated all kinds of HSRs known at the time of its conception, some 60 years ago, recent estimates suggest that the majority of acute HSRs is not IgE mediated, and therefore cannot fit formally in the Type I category. According to Demoly et al. (2) these non-IgE-mediated acute reactions may represent as high as 77% of all immune-mediated immediate HSRs, implying that approximately 20 % of all adverse drug reactions, ~400,000 severe and ~20,000 fatal reactions each year in the USA (1) are excluded from Coombs and Gell's classical scheme. The symptoms of these non-IgE-mediated reactions overlap, but at the same time also differ from those mediated by IgE (Table 1).

Table 1. Symptoms of IgE-mediated type I allergy and pseudoallergy

Ig-E-mediated	Non-IgE-mediated
Common symptoms	
Anaphylactic shock, angioedema, asthma attack, bronchospasm, chest pain, chill, choking, confusion, conjunctivitis, coughing, cyanosis, death, dermatitis, diaphoresis, dispnoea, edema, erythema, feeling of imminent death, fever, flush, headache, hypertension, hypotension, hypoxemia, low back pain,lumbar pain,metabolic acidosis, nausea, pruritus, rash, rhinitis, skin eruptions, sneezing, tachypnea, tingling sensations, urticaria, wheezing	
Unique symptoms	
• Reaction arises after repeated exposure to the allergen • Reaction is stronger upon repeated exposures • Reaction does not ceases without treatment • Reaction rate is low (<2%)	• Reaction arises at first treatment (no prior exposure to allergen) • Reaction is milder or absent upon repeated exposures • Spontaneous resolution High reaction rate (up to 45%), average 7%, severe 2%

At present most immunology and allergy textbooks refer to non-IgE-mediated HSRs as "anaphylactoid, pseudoallergic or idiosyncratic" without defining their pathomechanism. Thus, reactions caused by radiocontrast media (RCM), nonsteroidal anti-inflammatory drugs, analgetics, morphine, insect venoms, liposomal drugs and many other agents are enlisted within this vaguely defined category. Although the exact underlying mechanism probably differs in each of these drug categories, there is overwhelming evidence that the reactions caused by RCM, liposomes and micellar solvents, such as Cremophor EL in Taxol, have a common trigger mechanism: complement (C) activation. Hence, these reactions have been called "C activation-related pseudoallergy (CARPA)". The goal of the present chapter was to review the evidence supporting the CARPA concept, to discuss the mechanism of C activation by pseudoallergic agents and to highlight some diagnostic and therapeutic approaches that might alleviate these reactions.

2.   COMPLEMENT ACTIVATION-RELATED PSEUDOALLERGY CAUSED BY RADIOCONTRAST MEDIA (RCM)

2.1   RCM Reactions: Prevalence and Critical Factors

Radiographic procedures using water-soluble RCM represents routine medical practice today in all developed countries. In the USA, for example, more than 10 million tests are performed yearly with various RCM (4, 5). Nevertheless, intravenous use of RCM still carries a significant risk for HSRs, also referred to as "RCM reactions". The manifestations include those listed in Table 1 under the pseudoallergy category, although true IgE-mediated acute reactions to RCM (6) and non-acute, delayed-type HSRs (7) have also been reported.

RCMs can be classified according to their iodine content, osmolarity (hyper-, low- and iso-osmolar), level of ionization (ionic and non-ionic), and level of polymerization (monomeric and dimeric) (8).   Earlier RMC preparations were mono- or diiodinated compounds (e.g. pyridones), while the structure of current RCMs is based on fully substituted benzoic acid with 3 iodines at positions 2, 4 and 6 on the benzene ring. The ionic monomers are sodium or meglumine salts of the anionic triiodinated benzene ring; these are the high osmolarity RCMs (>1400 mOsm/kg).   Their dimerized derivatives have lower osmolarity (e.g., 600 mOsm/kg), while further derivatization with hydroxyl groups or other hydrophilic conjugates results in non-ionic, lower-osmolarity (500-700 mOsm/kg) or iso-osmotic RCMs (5).

Hypersensitivity reactions have been a concern ever since the first organic, iodinated compound was used for i.v. pyelography in 1928 by Swick, an American urologist (9).   Subsequent development of new-generation RCMs, characterized by a transition from hyperosmolar to isosmolar, ionic to nonionic and monomeric to dimeric preparations, was driven by the need to reduce the reactogenicity while maintaining or improving the opacity of products. Thus, the initial hyperosmolar, ionic, monomeric class of RCM (e.g. diatrizoate, iothathalamate) was outdated in the early 1980s by lower-osmolar, ionic, dimeric RCMs (e.g., ioxaglate). Progress than continued by the introduction of non-ionic, monomeric, lower-osmolar RCM (iopamidol, iohexol, ioversol, iopromide, ioxilan), and finally, in 1996, the US FDA approved iodixanol, the non-ionic, dimeric, iso-osmolar RCM (5).

Table 2 lists the best-known RCMs with specification of their above-discussed physicochemical properties. It should be noted that in addition to categorization according to molecular and physicochemical properties, earlier   classifications   also   considered   the   severity   and   clinical manifestations of HSRs (non-reactogenic, mildly or severely reactogenic RCM, anaphylactoid, vasomotor RCM), the diagnostic procedure for which they were used (i.e., myelography, angiography, arteriography, venography, urography, arthrography, computed tomography, etc) and the pathogenesis of HSRs (C activation, IgE-binding, direct degranulation of mast cells and basophils)

Table 2. Some physicochemical properties of RCM that influence hypersensitivity reactions (8)

Generic name	Osmolarity	Ionization	Polymerization
diatrizoate	Hyper	Ionic	Monomeric
iodixanol	Iso	Non-ionic	dimeric
iohexol	Low	Non-ionic	Monomeric
iopamidol	Low	Non-ionic	Monomeric
iopromide	Low	Non-ionic	Monomeric
iothalamate	Hyper	Ionic	Monomeric
ioversol	Low	Non-ionic	Monomeric
ioxaglate	Low	Ionic	Dimeric
ioxilan	Low	Non-ionic	Monomeric

In addition to the physicochemical properties of RCM, the main factors influencing the rate and extent of RCM reactions include the amount of agent infused, route (site) and speed of administration, premedication status of patients and criteria for positive reaction. With all these variables it is perhaps not surprising that the reported incidence rate of different types of RCM reactions span a range as broad as 0.0004% and 60%. According to comprehensive estimates applied for all kinds of symptoms with all procedures and all types of RCM, the overall incidence rate of RCM reactions is 2.1-12.7% (5). The frequency of severe anaphylactoid reactions is approximately 1-2% (5), while that of non-severe cutaneous, vasomotor, pulmonary, cardiovascular or gastrointestinal symptoms is in the 5-8% range (4). However, to illustrate the critical dependence of these statistics on details, life-threatening RCM reactions during coronary angiography occur only in 0.0004% to 0.002% of patients (4).

As for the relationship between RCM properties and HSRs, it has been proposed in several studies that nonionic, low-osmolality RCM (LO-RCM) are safer than ionic, high-osmolality agents (HO-RCM) (5, 10, 11, 12, 13). Barrett et al. (11), for example, enrolled 1856 patients for comparing the reactogenicity of LO vs. HO RCM used in cardiac angiography. The overall incidence of HSRs requiring treatment was 9% vs. 29% in these groups, respectively, and hemodynamic deterioration and severe or prolonged reactions also occurred more frequently in the HO group (2.9 % vs. 0.8%) (11).

2.2　Pathomechanism of RCM Reactions

The pathogenesis of radiocontrast media-related immediate HSRs cannot be explained by a unique mechanism. As illustrated by the scheme in Fig. 1, major triggering factors implicated are 1) activation of the C system with consequent activation of mast cells and basophils via C5a and C3a receptors; 2) activation of mast cells and basophils via IgE receptors; 3) direct secretory effects on mast cells and basophils due to local changes in osmolality and ion (mainly sodium and calcium) concentrations; and 4) activation of plasma proteolytic systems, in particular the coagulation and kinin-kallikrein systems, entailing additional C activation by various crossover amplifications and depletion of C1INH (8, 14, 15).

As for the effector arm, the best known secondary mediators of anaphylaxis are histamine, tryptase, PAF, LTB_2, LTB_4, LTC_4, LTD_4, LTE_4, TXA_2, PGD_2 and TXD_4 (10, 16, 17) (Fig.1).

The effects of histamine are mediated both by H1 and H2 receptors. Specifically, activation of H1 receptors leads to vasoconstriction and vascular leakage, and is responsible for the cardiovascular and cutaneous symptoms of anaphylaxis. H2 receptors, in turn, increase cellular cAMP levels and cause vasodilation, increased heart rate and pulse pressure (18).

Direct secretory effects on mast cells and basophils involves non-receptor-mediated stimulation of mast cells and basophils for immediate release of preformed allergic mediators, such as PAF, histamine and tryptase, but not those that are de novo synthesized in response to activation of these cells via IgE or C5a receptors (i.e., LTB_1, LTC_4, LTD_4, LTE_4, TXA_2 and PGD_2). The release reaction was shown to be Ca^{++}-dependent and similar to the effects of Ca^{++} ionophores, however RCM (diatrizoate) had a more complex effect on cell function as it rendered basophils refractory to subsequent release reactions (19). Another important detail concerning the secretory response of mast cells and basophils is that these cells display differential response to different RCM or other stimuli. For example, mast cells from the skin may not respond to certain RCM, while pulmonary and cardiac mast cells are triggered for strong release reaction (20). Likewise, mannitol, an osmotic stimulus, may induce the release of histamine from human basophils, but to a lesser extent from mast cells (20).

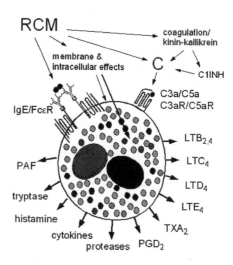

Figure 1. Mechanism of RCM reactions. The scheme illustrates the various triggering mechanisms and secretion products of mast cells and basophils during RCM reactions.

2.3   Complement Activation as Underlying Cause of RCM Reactions

Activation of the C system as the main underlying cause of RCM reactions has been studied since the 1970s with numerous in vitro, in vivo and clinical studies pursuing this concept. Nevertheless, the picture emerged is far from being consistent and the question whether C activation is the major cause of HSRs, or it is a contributing factor, or only an epiphenomenon, is still open. In reviewing the in vitro data it is clear that RCMs have multiple different effects both within the C cascade and in its regulatory system, and that charge, viscosity, iodine number, hydrophilicity and osmotic pressure are all critical variables in these interactions (17, 21). C activation by RCM was demonstrated to proceed both via the classical and the alternative pathways (17, 21), as well as via unusual mechanisms, such as 1) nonspecific, non-sequential cleavage of C proteins (22), 2) suppression of natural inhibitors of C, such as Factor H and I (17) and 3) direct action on the thioester bonds of C4 and C3. Yet a further activation mechanism implicated is an electrolit imbalance in serum (23).

What causes some uncertainty in this field is that some of the in vitro studies contradict to C activation as the underlying cause of HSRs, or at least the authors interpret their data as arguing against the C concept. Vik et al., for example, found no increase in serum SC5b-9 levels following the addition of iodixanol to serum, leading to the conclusion that C activation was unlikely responsible for iodixanol-induced anaphylactoid reactions in man (23). Lieberman et al. suggested that depletion of C proteins in human serum was not due to true C activation in human serum but rather to nonspecific binding of C proteins to RCM, without anaphylatoxin liberation (17). At the extreme, Mikkonen et al. (24) suggested inhibition of C activation by RCM on the basis that iohexol, ioxaglate, iodixanol and meglumin amidotriz solutions effectively blocked inulin-induced generation of C3a-desArg in normal human serum. The authors claimed that these molecules, particularly the ionic ones, inhibited the binding of factor B to surface-associated C3b, interfering with alternative pathway amplification.

Among the animal studies attesting to a causal role of C activation in RCM reactions Lasser et al. reported severe "idiosyncratic" response of a dog to the injection of sodium iothalamate, manifested in vomiting, hypotension, and hyperreflexia. The authors found significant depletion of C during the symptoms, suggesting that C activations was causally involved in the reaction (25). In further dog studies by Lang et al. serial daily injections of RCM (metrizamide, iothalamate, diatrizoate, acetrizoate, iodipamide and iopanoate) caused substantial declines of serum C over several days (26). In rats, Napolovlu et al. proved that various RCM in the 0.5-2.0 g iodine/kg range activated the C system via the alternative pathway, with efficacy in the following order: triombrast > hexabrics > ultravist $\geq$ melitrast = omnipac (21, 27).

Human data on C activation during RCM reactions include case reports, for example on a severe anaphylactoid reaction to a pyelographic RCM, manifested in a precipitous fall in plasma hemolytic C, C3, C4 and C1 esterase inhibitor (C1INH) levels, with a rise of C3 conversion products (28). This patient also developed consumption coagulopathy (28). Vandenplas et al. (29) reported the case of a 29-year-old woman who developed fulminant pulmonary edema following i.v. administration of RMC. The study showed a slight decrease of several C components (C3, C4 and factor B) and a transient consumption coagulopathy. Of particular interest in the latter paper, the authors presented direct hemodynamic and laboratory evidence for pulmonary capillary leakage as the underlying cause of edema, a process known to arise as a consequence of C activation-related sequestration of granulocytes and platelets in the pulmonary microcirculation (30, 31, 32). Yet another case report postulated that C activation was responsible for the death of a patient undergoing i.v. pyelography with diatrizoate (17). Consistent with the key role of anaphylatoxin liberation, the autopsy showed a picture typical of ARDS, including the presence of granulocytic aggregates in the pulmonary microcirculation (17). As is known, C activation plays a key role in the development of ARDS (33, 34, 35, 36, 37, 38).

Among the more extensive clinical studies looking at the role of C activation in RCM reactions, Small et al. (39) analyzed HSRs and C activation in 220 patients undergoing i.v. pyelography. Nineteen % of patients displayed HSRs, while depressed serum CH_{50} levels, indicating C activation, occurred in 49%. The RCM-induced decline of CH_{50}/mL was apparent within 90 sec after starting the infusion and returned to normal after about 30 min. This study highlighted an important fact regarding the relationship between C activation and HSRs, namely, that more people display signs of C activation than HSRs. Hence, C activation may be present in patients without clinically manifest reaction, suggesting that anaphylatoxin liberation does not necessarily cause HSRs. C activation may therefore be a precondition, or contributing factor to HSRs, but it does not solely explain the phenomenon. Other factors or preconditions may also need to be present in people who develop HSR. This point was reinforced in the studies by Westaby et al. (40), who demonstrated significant elevation of the anaphylatoxin C3a in the peripheral blood of 7/11 patients receiving RCM for coronary angiography. In 3/7 patients C3a was increased between four and tenfold, yet only one of these patients developed symptoms, which were mild. It should be noted that C activation has not been a consistent finding in all clinical studies reporting C measurements in patients injected RCM. Kolb et al. (22), for example, found no significant changes in CH_{50} and hemolytic C3 activity in serum samples obtained from 40 patients before and 30 min after undergoing i.v. pyelography with methylglucamine diatrizoate or iothalamate.

3. COMPLEMENT ACTIVATION-RELATED PSEUDOALLERGY CAUSED BY DRUG CARRIER LIPOSOMES AND LIPID COMPLEXES

Phospholipid liposomes and other types of lipid-based molecular assemblies, such as micelles, are increasingly used in medicine for targeted delivery or controlled release of various drugs and diagnostic agents. These vehicles can substantially affect the biodistribution, and, hence, the efficacy and toxicity of associated agents. Table 2 lists the liposome- or lipid-based products that are marketed or in clinical development today. Out of these, Doxil (Caelyx) (41-46), AmBisome (47-51), Abelcet (50), Amphocil (50) and DaunoXome (52-60) have been reported to cause unusual HSRs corresponding to pseudoallergy. Actually, the first report of HSRs to i.v. infusion of liposomes was published as early as 1986 (61), in one of the pioneer studies on the use of liposomes in cancer chemotherapy. The frequency of HSRs to liposomal drugs vary between 3-45% (15, 46, 62).

Table 2. Liposome- or lipid-based products in market or in clinical development

Encapsulated drug	Trade name	Indications	Developer/Producer/ Distributor	Status of development
Doxorubicin (Adriamycin)	Doxil	Ovarian cancer, Kaposi's sarcoma, Metastatic breast cancer	Alza Co./Ortho Biotech, East Bridgewater, NJ	marketed
	Caelyx		Essex Pharma GmBH, Munich, GE	
	Myocet		Elan Corp, Dublin, Ireland	
Daunorubicin	DaunoXome	advanced HIV-associated Kaposi's sarcoma	Gilead Sciences Inc., Foster City, CA	
Amphotericin B	AmBisome	Systemic fungal infections		
	Abelcet		Elan Co/Enzon Inc., Piscataway, New Jersey, USA	
	Amphotec		Intermune Inc., Brisbane, CA	
Verteporfin	Visudyne	subfoveal neovascularization due to macular degeneration, pathologic myopia and ocular histoplasmosis	QLT Inc., Vancouver, BC, CA	
all-*trans*-retinoic acid (ATRA)	ATRA-IV	Non-Hodgkin lymphoma, acute promyelocytic leukaemia, etc.	Antigenics Inc., New York, NY	Phase I-II
Oxeliplatin	Aroplatin	Colorectal and other solid tumors		

Encapsulated drug	Trade name	Indications	Developer/Producer/ Distributor	Status of development
Vincristine	Onco TCS	Lymphoma, acute lymphoblastic leukaemia, Hodgkin's disease lung cancer, pediatric malignancies	Inex Pharm. Co., Burnaby, BC, Canada	Phase III
Topotecan	Topotecan TCS*	Various cancers		Preclinical
Vinorelbine	Vinorelbine TCS*			
Doxorubicin	LED	Advanced cancers, including breast		
Paclitaxel	LEP-ETU**	Advanced cancers, including breast, lung and ovarian		
Mitoxantrone	LEM-ETU**	Advanced cancers, including prostate	NeoPharm Lake Forest, Illinois	Phase I/II
c-raf antisense oligonucleotide	LErafAON	Advanced cancers including pancreatic		
CPT-11 (irinotecan, Camptosar™)	LE-SN38	Advanced cancers including colorectal and lung		

* TCS, Transmembrane Carrier System
** ETU, easy-to-use

3.1 Experimental Evidence for a Role of C activation in Liposome Reactions

3.1.1 In Vitro Studies

In vitro detection of C activation by drugs and biomaterials in human serum has been used as a biocompatibility assay to predict adverse clinical reactions (63-67). The fact that liposomes can activate C has been known since the late sixties (68-71). To date more than 60 publications reported C activation in vitro by various liposomes, highlighting the universality of this phenomenon. Nevertheless, the qualitative and quantitative aspects of liposome-induced C activation greatly vary in different systems and are influenced by a numerous known and unknown factors (15, 62).

Fig. 2A illustrates the basic bilayer structure of liposome membranes, while Fig 2B-E demonstrate the large variety of liposome structures that can lead to C activation. Thus, large multilamellar vesicles in the 5-15 μm size range (B) (81), large unilamellar, hemoglobin-containing liposomes in the 200-400 nm range (75-80) and small, unilamellar, uniformly 90-100-nm doxorubicin-containing liposomes (C) (46, 72, 82) are equally potent activators of C.

Of particular relevance with regard to the role of C activation in liposome-induced HSRs, the author and his collegues reported that incubation of Doxil with 10 different normal human sera led to significant rises in C terminal complex (SC5b-9) levels over PBS control in 7 sera, with rises exceeding 100-200% (relative to PBS control) in 4 subjects (72). While providing evidence for activation of the whole C cascade by Doxil in a majority of humans, these data also highlight the significant individual variation of responses. Further experiments showed that in addition to the quantitative variation in SC5b-9 response, Doxil-induced C activation also varied in different individuals in terms of sensitivity to inhibition by 10 mM EGTA/2.5 mM Mg^{++}, which distinguishes classical vs. alternative pathway activation (72). The minimum effective C-activating concentration of Doxil was 0.05-0.10 mg/mL, and there was near linear dose-effect relationship up to about 0.5 mg/mL. The activation curve reached its plateau at doses ≥ 0.6 mg/mL, suggesting saturation of response (72). Doxil also caused variable liberation of Bb, a specific marker of alternative pathway activation, providing further evidence for a role of alternative pathway activation and/or amplification (72).

These and other studies from our laboratories (73-82) revealed some basic structure-function relationships on liposomal C activation. Most importantly, it appears that positive or negative surface charge, size, and

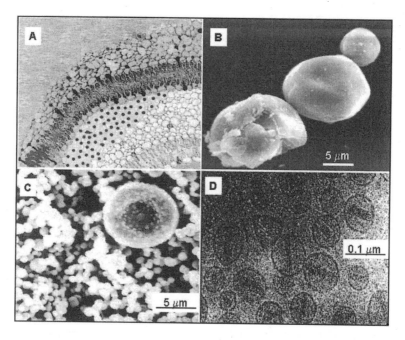

Figure 2. Complement activating liposomes. A) Schematic illustration of liposomes consisting of one or more phospholipid bilayers enclosing an aqueous space with or without water soluble drug therein; B, Scanning electron micrographs of large multilamellar liposomes in the multimicron size range. These are potent C activators regardless of lipid composition. C, Scanning electron micrographs of large unilamellar hemoglobin-containing liposomes (LEH) that were shown to activate C despite their relatively homogeneous size distribution. The picture, courtesy of A.S. Rudolph, shows a red blood cell for size comparison. D) Electron micrograph of Doxil, a potent C activator mall unilamellar liposome preparation. The figure demonstrates the highly homogeneous size distribution of vesicles with doxorubicin gelified within the aqueous space. Courtesy of Y. Barenholz.

polydispersity promote, whereas neutrality and small uniform size reduce the proneness of liposomes for C activation. As for the mechanism of activation, it may involve both the classical and alternative pathways, with the latter acting either as the only activation mechanism, or as a positive feedback mechanism amplifying C activation at the level of C3 convertase. The involvement of immunoglobulins varies from system to system and it does not seem to be a prerequisite for C activation, although the presence of natural anti-liposomal antibodies clearly promote the process. Liposomal C activation, furthermore, sensitively depends on the phospholipid composition and cholesterol content of the vesicles.

3.1.2   In Vivo Evidence

Studies from the author and his colleagues described that minute amounts (5-10 mg) of large multilamellar vesicles (MLV) caused significant hemodynamic changes in pigs, including a massive rise in pulmonary arterial pressure (PAP) with declines of systemic arterial pressure, cardiac output and left ventricular end-diastolic pressure (80, 81). Similar changes were observed with Doxil and the ^{99m}Tc-chelator (HYNIC-PE)-containing pegylated small unilamellar liposomes (82) demonstrating that the phenomenon was not restricted to the use of MLV. In addition to the above hemodynamic changes we also reported massive ECG changes in pigs treated with HYNIC-PEG liposomes and Doxil (82), attesting to severe transient myocardial ischemia with bradyarrhythmia, ventricular fibrillation and other ECG abnormalities.

We suggested that the above MLV-induced hemodynamic and cardiac changes in pigs may represent an amplified model for liposome-induced HSRs in man on the following basis: 1) hypotension is one of the major symptoms of acute HSRs in general and of Doxil reactions, in particular; 2) pulmonary hypertension with consequent decrease of left ventricle filling and coronary perfusion can explain the dyspnea with chest and back pain in man, i.e., typical symptoms of HSRs; 3) the ECG changes observed in the pig exactly correspond to the cardiac electric abnormalities reported in HSRs to liposomes (Ambisome) (83); and 4) the vasoactive dose of Doxil (6-840 µg/kg) corresponds to the dose that triggers HSR in humans (45) suggesting that the pigs' sensitivity to Doxil corresponds to the that of hypersensitive human subjects.

C activation-related pulmonary hypertension in pigs was highly reproducible, quantitative and specific. The high reproducibility of the reaction is illustrated by the remarkably low variation in the rise of PAP in response to a same dose of liposomes (5 mg lipid corresponding to the ED_{50}) in 27 pigs, or within one animal, after 8 consecutive injections (80). The quantitative nature of this "large animal bioassay" (82a) was shown by the linear relationship between liposome dose and submaximal rises of PAP (80), whereas its specificity to C activation became evident from the observations that 1) small unilamellar liposomes, which had negligible C activating effect in vitro, also failed to cause hemodynamic changes in vivo (81) and 2) non-liposomal C activators (zymosan, xenogeneic immunoglobulins) induced pulmonary pressure changes that were indistinguishable from those caused by LMV (80). These data provide validation of the model in terms of quantifying C-mediated cardiopulmonary reactions with high sensitivity and specificity.

3.1.3   Clinical Evidence

In addition to the experimental data delineated above, there is ample clinical support for a causal role of C activation in liposome-induced HSRs. The first indirect evidence appeared as early as in 1983, when Coune et. al (84) reported that that intravenous infusion of liposomes containing NSC 251635, a water-insoluble cytostatic agent, led to increased C3d/C3 ratios in the plasma of cancer patients. This study, however, did not address the presence or absence of HSRs. Another -also still indirect- proof is a paper by Skubitz et al. (85), reporting transient neutropenia with signs of leukocyte activation in patients who displayed HSRs to Doxil. Neutropenia with leukocyte activation are classical hallmarks of anaphylatoxin action (86-88), yet C activation was not considered in the above study. To the authors' knowledge the first direct evidence for the causal relationship between C activation and HSRs to liposomes was provided by Brouwers et al. (89), who reported 16-19% decrease of plasma C3, C4 and factor B in the blood of a patient developing HSR to $^{Tc-99m}$HYNIC-PE-containing pegylated liposomes applied for the scintigraphic detection of infection and inflammation (90). The facts that both C4 and factor B were involved in the consumption of C suggest that C activation proceeded on both the classical and alternative pathways. In a subsequent study by the same group it was reported that 3 out of 9 patients reacted to pegylated HYNIC liposomes (89). Despite clear benefits in imaging inflammatory bowel disease, the presence of HSRs was considered as unacceptable from a diagnostic agent and the Dutch team temporarily abandoned human trials with pegylated HYNIC liposomes.

Activation of C as cause of HSRs to Doxil was the subject of a recent clinical study correlating C activation (formation of C terminal complex, SC5b-9) with the frequency and severity of HSRs in cancer patients infused with Doxil for the first time (46). Forty-five percent (13/29) of patients in the study showed grade 2 or 3 HRS, with reactions occurring in men and women in approximately equal proportions. The reactions were not related to the age of patients. Doxil caused C activation in 21 out of 29 patients (72%) as reflected by significant elevations of plasma SC5b-9 levels following infusion of the drug.

In addition to these surprising statistics on C activation and HSRs caused by Doxil, the study provided several quantitative details regarding these phenomena. One new observation is the time course of SC5b-9 increase in blood following Doxil injection (Fig. 3). The kinetics showed substantial individual variation, including rapid elevations within 10 min with gradual return to near baseline within 2 h (A), rapid elevation without return within 2 h (B), and moderately rapid elevation until about 30 min, followed by partial return to baseline during 2 h (C). The lack of SC5b-9 response is demonstrated in Fig 3D.

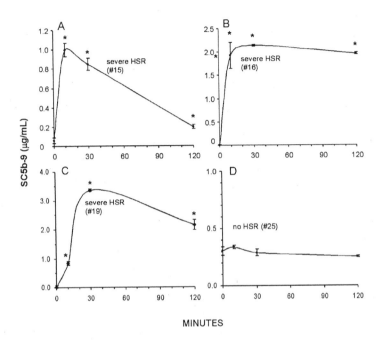

Figure 3. Time course of Doxil induced changes in plasma SC5b-9 in cancer patients and its individual variation. Panels A-D demonstrate data from 4 subjects displaying different patterns of response. Data are mean ± SD for triplicate determinations. *Significantly different from baseline, P<0.05. Reproduced from (46) with permission.

Considering the baseline and 10 minutes post-infusion SC5b-9 values in clinical reactors and non-reactors, the study reported significant increase of SC5b-9 in 9/10 reactor patients in contrast to 9/16 in the non-reactor group (Fig. 4). Thus, 92% of clinical reactors were also laboratory reactors, while only 56% of clinical non-rectors were laboratory reactors. These data led to the conclusion that C activation and HSR show significant (P< 0.05) correlation.

A closer scrutiny of the quantitative relationship between SC5b-9 values at 10 min and severity of HSR also revealed that the SC5b-9 assay is highly sensitive in predicting HSRs (Table 3), although the specificity and positive predictive value of the test was relatively low, particularly in patients in whom the rise of SC5b-9 at 10 minutes remained below 2-times the upper limit of normal SC5b-9 (Table 3, raw 2). However, restricting the criteria for laboratory reactivity to 10-min SC5b-9 values exceeding 2- or 4-fold the upper threshold of normal (Table 3, raw 3), the specificity and positive predictive value of the C assay remarkably increased with relatively less decrease in sensitivity. Thus, the extent of SC5b-9 elevation was proportional with the specificity and positive predictive value of the C assay with regards to HSRs.

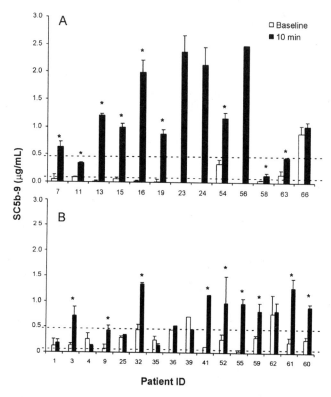

Figure 4. Plasma SC5b-9 levels at baseline and at 10 min post-infusion of Doxil in cancer patients displaying (A) or not displaying (B) HSRs to Doxil. Data are mean ± SD for triplicate or duplicate determinations. The dashed lines indicate the normal range of SC5b-9, i.e., the normal mean ± 2 SD. *, significantly different from baseline ($P<0.05$). The numbers under the bars are the patient ID. Reproduced from (46) with permission.

As for the relationships among Doxil dose rate, C activation and HSRs. Fig. 5 shows the 10-minutes SC5b-9 values of clinical reactors (filled circles) and non-reactors (empty circles) plotted against the initial rate of Doxil administration. Regression analysis revealed significant correlation between dose rate and SC5b-9 ($P<0.01$), indicating that C activation at 10 min was Doxil dose dependent. Consistent with the correlation among Doxil dose, C activation and HSRs, the upper right quadrant of the plot contained readings obtained exclusively from clinical reactors.

Table 3. The SC5b-9 assay as predictor of HSRs to Doxil

10-min SC5b-9 (μg/mL)	Sensitivity tp/(tp+fn)	Specificity tn/(fp+tn)	Positive predictive value tp/(tp+fp)	Negative predictive value tn/(fn+tn)
Significant Increase* (SC5b-9, no limit)	0.92	0.44	0.57	0.88
Significant Increase* SC5b-9 ≤ 0.98	0.83	0.54	0.45	0.88
0.98 ≤ SC5b-9 ≤ 1.96 (≥2X, ≤ 4X normal)	0.80	0.70	0.57	0.88
SC5b-9 ≥ 1.96 (≥ 4X normal)	0.75	1.00	1.00	0.88

Patients were classified into 4 groups according to the concurrent presence (+) or absence (-) of HSR and C reactivity, as follows: true positive (tp: HSR+, C+), false positive (fp: HSR-, C+), true negative (tn: HSR-, C-) and false negative (fn: HSR+, C-). In addition, laboratory reactors were stratified to 3 categories on the basis of 10-min SC5b-9 values, as specified in column 1. The 0.98 and 1.96 μg/mL cut-off values represent 2 and 4-times the upper limit of normal SC5b-9 levels (0.49 μg/mL), respectively, and were chosen arbitrarily. The sensitivity, specificity, and positive and predictive values of the SC5b-9 assay with regard to HSRs were computed as described (46). *Significant increase refers to significant ($P< 0.05$) increase of 10-min SC5b-9 relative to baseline. Reproduced from (46) with permission.

By providing evidence that Doxil caused C activation in a large majority of cancer patients although HSRs was manifested in a smaller portion, the above study confirmed a previous report by Small et al. (39) wherein 19 % of patients infused with a RCM displayed HSR, although C activation was detectable in 49 %.

Taken together, these data strongly suggest that C activation may be an important factor, or precondition in eliciting HSRs, but its presence is not sufficient to actually precipitate the reaction. Thus, C activation may be a triggering, but not rate-limiting factor in the pathogenesis of "pseudoallergy" to RCM, Doxil and other pseudoallergens. A plausible hypothesis explaining this relationship is that reactors differ from nonreactors in at least two conditions: 1) they develop a C reaction to the drug, and 2) their mast cells and basophils have a lower than normal threshold for secretory response to anaphylatoxins. Consistent with this proposal, proneness for HSRs is known to correlate with the presence of other allergies, i.e., with atopic constitution. Also, C5a-induced thromboxane production by leukocytes in vitro was shown to be significantly greater in atopic subjects than in normal controls. In short, CARPA may develop with high probability in those atopic subjects who respond to the drug with C activation and whose mast cells have a low threshold for C5a-induced release reaction.

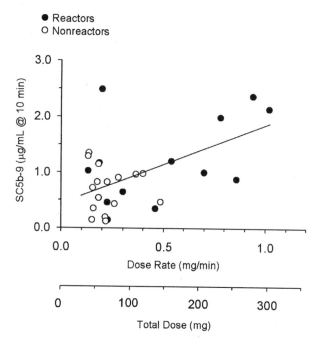

Figure 5. Dependence of C activation and HSRs on Doxil dose rate. The 10-min SC5b-9 levels were plotted against the initial rate of Doxil administration (total dose/60 min x 1/5) in cancer patients displaying (filled circles) or not displaying (empty circles) HSRs. The regression line correlates Doxil dose rate with C activation, R2 = 0.25, n = 29, P<0.01. The probability of developing HSRs at different dose rates were quantified by serial computation of odd's ratios in the 0.2-0.5 mg/min range. Reproduced from (46) with permission.

3.2 Solvent Systems Containing Amphiphilic Emulsifiers

Hypersensitivity reactions represent a longstanding problem with certain water insoluble drugs or other agents (i.e., red cell substitutes) that are delivered in solutions that contain amphiphilic emulsifiers, such as the semisynthetic Cremophor EL (CrEL), emulphor (91-93) or the synthetic block copolymers of the pluronic series.

3.2.1 Semisynthetic Emulsifiers

3.2.1.1 Cremophor EL
Cremophor EL has been used to solubilize many water insoluble drugs, including paclitaxel (Taxol), cyclosporine, the antineoplastic agents

Teniposide, Echinomycin and Didemnin E, the anaesthetic agents propanidid and althesin, steroids and vitamins (A, D, E, K) (94). It is a non-ionic detergent, a complex mixture of unmodified castor (ricinus) oil and a large variety of polyethylene glycols and amphiphilic polyethoxylated glycerols, polyethoxylated fatty acids (mostly ricinoleic acid) and polyethoxylated glycerol esters differing in acyl chain and/or polyethyleneoxide length (95, 96).

While all the abovementioned drugs dissolved in CrEL have been reported to cause HSRs (94, 97) the best known manifestation of hypersensitivity to CrEL is the reactions caused by Taxol, one of the best known anticancer drugs today (98, 99, 100). Reactions to Taxol were reported soon after the beginning of Taxol trials in the early eighties (101) and kept attracting attention ever since, as 2-7% of patients still develop HSRs despite their intense premedication with corticosteroids (mostly dexamethason) and antihistamines (diphenhydramine, cimetidine, ranitidine) (98, 102-117, 119). These reactions are severe, life-threatening in up to 1-3% of patients with occasional deaths mostly due to cardiac arrest (108, 115, 118). Fitting in the CARPA category (Table 1), HSRs to Taxol usually arise within minutes after starting the infusion and include common, as well as unusual allergic symptoms that are explainable with C activation.

In addition to the patients' hardship, the unpredictability and often dramatic picture of Taxol reactions cause substantial anxiety for doctors and caretakers, and they also represent a significant logistic and financial burden on hospitals, the latter estimated to be US$ 2,900-4,900/cycle (119). Most importantly, these reactions exclude some 2% of patients from obtaining a therapy that is considered as state-of-art in extending life in certain cancers.

Attempts to develop Taxol formulations without CrEL (120, 121, 122) have not been successful to date, at least in reaching clinical use. The omission or replacement of CrEL may not be preferential, in any way, in light of its suppressive influence on P-glycoprotein-mediated multidrug resistance (123, 124) that deteriorates the therapeutic efficacy of Taxol. These facts lend substantial importance to understanding the mechanism of HSRs to Taxol.

The concept that C activation could underlie Taxol, i.e., CrEL reactions was proposed by the author and his colleagues on the basis that 1) Taxol and CrEL activate C in vitro, and 2) through release of anaphylatoxins (C3a and C5a), C activation can explain the symptoms of Taxol reactions (30, 95, 125). We presented evidence for significant elevation of SC5b-9 and Bb in the sera of normal as well as cancer patients following incubation with therapeutically relevant concentrations of Taxol or corresponding amount of CrEL/50% ethanol (i.e., the exact composition of Taxol vehicle). We also showed that this C activation could be inhibited by soluble C receptor type 1 (95).

As for the mechanism of C activation by CrEL, we considered that it is a non-ionic emulsifier consisting of a mixture of amphiphilic molecules that form micelles in water (126, 127, 128). Micelles are multimolecular aggregates in the nanometer size range, and those formed from amphiphilic polymers usually apperar as spherical "core-shell" or star-like structures with a dense nucleus surrounded by a less electrodense halo (insert in Fig 6A) (129). Thus, micelles represent a particulate substance satisfying two basic conditions for becoming a C activator; 1) they provide surface for protein deposition and 2) they lack surface-bound C regulatory proteins (e.g., CR1, DAF, MCP) that normally protect self cells from C activation (130). It was, however, unclear whether micelles are present in Taxol solutions under the conditions of infusion therapy, and even if the answer is yes, whether they could cause C activation in vivo?

To address the former question, we utilized various physicochemical and imaging techniques to explore and characterize particles in clinically relevant aqueous solutions of Taxol (96). As shown in Fig 6A and B, cryo-transmission electron microscopy (Cryo-TEM) showed 8-20 nm spherical structures in aqueous solutions of Taxol mimicking the drug infused in patients, typical "star" micelles that are formed from amphiphilic polymers (129). As for the question, whether these micelles can cause C activation, we demonstrated that filtration of aqueous solutions of Taxol or pure CrEL via 30-kDa-cutoff filters eliminated, while the filter retentate restored C activation in human serum (96). Thus, the effect was due to particles with MW > 30 kDa, which is consistent with a causal role of micelles. However, there was still a problem with the implication of micelles in C activation as the surface of even the largest, ~20 nm micelle appears to be too small to allow deposition of C3 convertases, at least as it occurs in the case of C activating cell membranes and other surfaces. Specifically, the molecular dimensions of CrEL micelles are comparable to the classical and/or alternative pathway C3 convertases (for example, C3bBb is about 14 x 8 nm (131). A possible solution to this puzzle was provided by the observation (96) that CrEL micelles underwent massive structural transformation in human plasma, forming microdroplets of varying size up to about 300 nm (Fig 6 C,D).

Although we had no experimental data supporting the claim that these microdroplets were in fact formed from CrEL micelles, a previous study by Kessel et al (124) provided strong indirect support for this proposition. Namely, in studying the effect of Taxol on plasma lipoproteins in cancer patients, these authors noted an increase in size, as well as a decrease in the electrophoretic mobility of HDL and/or LDL relative to pre-treatment values.

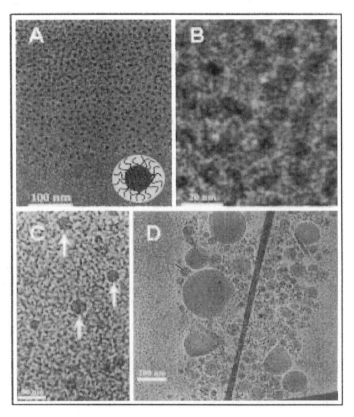

Figure 6. Cryo-TEM images of vitrified specimens of Cremophor EL in saline (PBS) and in human serum. A) Taxol vial-equivalent CrEL/ethanol stock solution was diluted 10-fold in PBS. The dark spots represent "star" micelles, schematically depicted in the insert. B) Larger amplification of CrEL micelles. C) Vitrified specimens of a normal human serum, demonstrating some lipoprotein particles in the chylomicron size range. D) CrEL was incubated with the same serum for 10 min at 37°C, leading to the formation of numerous particles of varying size. Reproduced from (96) with permission.

They also noted that the originally sharp HDL and LDL bands became smeared, and that a new, highly sudanophililic band was formed which slightly migrated towards the cathode (124). Clearly, CrEL and plasma lipoproiteins underwent substantial interaction, which is not surprising in light of the fact that CrEL is a mixture of lipids. In particular, the above data suggest incorporation of CrEL lipids into HDL and LDL, as well as the formation of positively charged particles from apolar molecules in CrEL that does not associate with lipoproteins. Based on these data it seems possible that some of the dense, small structures in our cryo-TEM image of human plasma incubated with Taxol (Fig 6 C,D) are CrEL enriched, enlarged lipoproteins, whereas the large lipid droplets may correspond to the newly formed structures composed of hydrophobic CrEL molecules with some charged amphiphilic components at the water-oil interface.

As for the question, how these newly formed CrEL particles in blood activate C, one possibility is that they bind C3 in a fashion similar to that described for the nonionic block copolymer surfactants, L101 and L121 (95). The latter particles were shown to activate C via the alternative pathway, due to the binding of C3 to their hydrophilic adhesive surface (132-135). In strong support of this proposal, the length of the hydrophilic (polyethoxylated) chains in many amphiphilic molecules in CrEL is remarkably similar to those found in L10 (95). Furthermore, positively charged particles (liposomes) were reported to induce C activation via the alternative pathway (136).

Fig 7 summarizes the above-described complex physicochemical, biochemical and immune processes that may underlie Taxol-induced C activation. Also shown in Fig 7 yet another possible pathway of C activation by Taxol, by crystalline paclitaxel, that forms upon the dilution of Taxol concentrate in water (96). In analyzing Taxol infusion liquids using differential interference contrast (DIC) microscopy we observed needle-like structures extending to the multimicron range (Fig 7, inserts A-D). These were not present in aqueous solutions of CrEL, they were shown by electron diffraction to be crystalline paclitaxel, and they too activated C. However, because the infusion of Taxol is usually carried out via a central line containing a filter, it is not clear to what extent crystalline paclitaxel formed in the infusion liquid can enter the blood. It will be interesting to look for paclitaxel needles in the blood of Taxol-treated patients, as recrystallization of at least a small portion of paclitaxel in blood cannot be *a priori* excluded.

In addition to the above in vitro evidence, some animal and clinical studies provide support for C activation underlying HSRs to CrEL. Among these, Lorenz, Gaudy and others have shown that dogs develop HSR to CrEL, and that that the associated massive histamine release is due to the presence of oxethylated oleic acid in CrEL (137, 138). The studies by Theis, Liau-Chu and others suggest that physical changes, or improper mixing of CrEL-containing infusion liquids, might play a role in the genesis of HSRs to CrEL (139, 140).

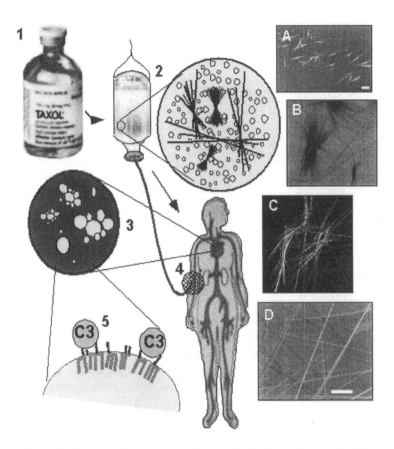

Figure 7. Hypothetical mechanism of C activation by Taxol, illustrating the physical changes of paclitaxel and CrEL during the course of infusion therapy. 1) Taxol injection concentrate containing paclitaxel fully dissolved in CrEL/50% ethanol. 2) Dilution of the concentrate in physiological salt solutions results in the formation of CrEL micelles and paclitaxel crystals. 3) After infusion into the blood CrEL micelles interact with plasma lipoproteins and fuse in large microdroplets. 4) Paclitaxel crystals may be trapped by the inline filter, if used. 5) C3 binds to the hydrophilic adhesive layer on microdroplets formed from amphiphilic components of CrEL. This binding triggers C activation. Insert photos A-D; Light micrographs of paclitaxel needles using differential interference contrast (DIC) optics. One such picture following artistic color enhancement (C). D, Larger amplification showing individual crystal fibers. Bars in A and D correspond to 40 μm.

3.2.1.2 Synthetic amphiphilic polymers

Like the semisynthetic emulsifier molecules discussed above, synthetic amphiphilic polymers have also been used as solvent systems for water insoluble drugs. Some of these polymers have also been used as vaccine adjuvants or as pharmacokinetics-modifier drug conjugates. Examples for synthetic amphiphilic polymers include poloxamers, poloxamines, other copolymers of hydrophilic and hydrophobic blocks, such as polyoxyethylene (PEO) and polyoxypropylene (PPO), and polyethyleneglycols (PEG) attached to phospholipids or to low molecular acyl chains (129). These solvents can also cause HSRs, the best-known example of which is the reaction to poloxamer 188, also known as Pluronic F-68, used as an additive in Fluosol DA, a perfluorocarbon-based blood substitute. Perfluorocarbons have shown promise as clinical blood substitutes. Although early experience in Japan with one such product, Fluosol-DA, has been uncomplicated, serious pulmonary reactions in the US trials led to the abandonment of this perfluorocarbon emulsion as a blood substitute. It was found that the pulmonary complications were due to C activation by Pluronic F-68, the nonionic emulsifier used to maintain the stability of Fluosol-DA (141-144).

In vitro evidence for C activation by block copolymers of the poloxamer and poloxamine series was provided by Norman et al. (145), by SDS-PAGE demonstration of the deposition of C proteins on polystyrene microspheres coated with these polymers. Among the in vivo evidence, Fluosol DA was infused into rabbits, which produced hypoxemia, neutropenia, thrombocytopenia and pulmonary leukostasis, mimicking abnormalities previously demonstrated in rabbits receiving infusions of zymosan-activated plasma (141). These deleterious responses to Fluosol DA were entirely reproduced with pure Pluronic F-68, while they were diminished by premedicating the rabbits with corticosteroids (141). In another in vivo study the cardiorespiratory responses of dogs to 2 ml intravenous doses of different fluorocarbon emulsions, Faithfull and Cain (146) have shown significant decreases in systemic pressure, cardiac output and limb blood flow, as well as a significant elevation of pulmonary artery pressures in 7 of 11 dogs treated with Fluosol-DA and in 24 of 28 dogs treated with Oxypherol (FC-43). Pulmonary and systemic vascular resistances were increased and body and limb muscle oxygen delivery and oxygen consumption were decreased. Also, the reactions were associated with acute myocardial depression. These changes were maximal at 3-4 minutes after fluorocarbon administration, with return to normal values usually by 40-60 minutes. The authors attributed the reactions to C activation and embolisation of the microvasculature (146). It is notable that the above physiological changes are exactly the same as the liposome-induced cardiopulmonary response in pigs (72, 80, 81), as detailed earlier in the section on HSRs to liposomal drugs.

As for the mechanism of poloxamer-induced C activation, Vercellotti et al. found that the Fluosol DA-induced C3 conversion, C consumption and C5a generation in rabbit plasma was prevented by EDTA, but not by EGTA, suggesting alternative pathway C activation (141). The involvement of the alternative pathway in poloxamer 188-induced C activation in human plasma was confirmed in a recent study by Moghimi et al. as well (147). The latter study also provided evidence that poloxamer 188-mediated C activation is an intrinsic property of the polymer, and that it is independent of the degree of sample polydispersity or trace amounts of nonpolymeric contaminants in the preparation, such as organic volatiles (acetaldehyde and propionaldehyde). C activation was triggered at submicellar concentrations of the polymer and was partially due to the presence of double bonds therein. Consistent with the idea that an interaction with plasma lipoproteins plays a key role in polymer-induced C activation, quasi-elastic light scattering established major changes in lipoprotein size following the addition of poloxamer to plasma (147). Interestingly, poloxamer-induced rise in SC5b-9 was significantly suppressed when serum HDL and LDL cholesterol levels were increased above normal levels, suggesting that lipoprotein binding can impact C activation by poloxamer in a complex, dose-related fashion (147).

4.   THEORETICAL IMPLICATIONS OF CARPA

Apart from better understanding the pathomechanism of HSRs, the CARPA concept may represent a step forward in an age-old quandary in theoretical immunology; the classification of HSRs. Gell and Coomb's system of four categories (types I to IV) has serious limitations, including the fact that pseudoallergy cannot be fitted in any of the four types of HSRs. However, no consensus has been reached to date, how to replace this obsolete, yet deeply rooted classification. A recent study by Descotes and Choquet-Kastylevsky (148) proposed to use three major types, namely, immunoglobulin-mediated and cell-mediated HSRs and pseudoallergy. While this scheme is clearly less arbitrary than the old classification, it does not seem to reflect the fact that both pseudoallergy and cell mediated HSRs can be initiated by immunoglobulins. In particular, C activation related reactions, which, by definition, represent a type of pseudoallergy, can be triggered by natural antiphospholipid and anti-cholesterol antibodies (76, 77, 78) which would qualify these reactions in the second group and not in the first. On the other hand, the inflammatory cellular responses to cellular antigens or immune complexes, classified as Types II and III according to Gell and Coombs, or as cell mediated HSRs, according to Descotes and Choquet-Kastylevsky (148) are also antibody triggered. An alternative approach to re-classify HSRs on the basis of dose dependence and predictability was suggested by Rawlins and Thompson (149), while more recently Aronson and Ferner (150) proposed to specify and graphically characterize HSRs according to their time course, susceptibility and dose dependence. However, these classifications appear to be either too narrow or too refined for every-day use. In addition, Aronson and Ferner's system fails to consider the differences in the underlying mechanisms of these reactions.

In an attempt to resolve some of the shortcomings of HSR classifications we proposed in an earlier review (15) a new functional nomenclature that differentiates acute (Type I) HSRs according to the underlying mechanism of mast cell and basophil release reactions. The scheme differentiates 2 major subclasses: 1) direct cell activation and 2) allergomedin receptor-mediated activation, with the latter category encompassing three subcategories: a) IgE-triggered and FCεIII receptor mediated IgE allergy "IGEA", b) anaphylatoxin-triggered and C3a/C5a receptor-mediated "CARPA", and c) mixed type, "DUAL" reactions, triggered by both IgE and anaphylatoxins (Fig. 8).

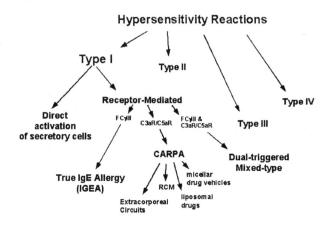

Figure 8. Proposal for a new classifiction of hypersensitivity reactions

The unique advantages of the above classification include the coverage of many previously uncategorized, C-mediated reactions that arise upon the use of extracorporeal circuits, RCM and various liposomal and micellar carriers of intravenous drugs. The practical significance of the CARPA concept lies in the large number of these reactions, as discussed in the introduction, and the conscienciousness of the involvement of C activation in these HSRs, that will hopefully lead to the identification of new preventive and/or therapeutic approaches against these reactions by using C inhibitors.

5. CONCLUDING REMARKS

The causal role of C activation in the HSRs to RCM has been known, or at least suspected since the nineteen thirties, ever since such agents have been used (17, 151). Liposomal activation of the C system was recognized more than 30 years ago (70, 71), and the same applies to the profound hemodynamic actions of anaphylatoxins (30, 125). These facts, taken together with the virtual identity of RCM reactions with those caused by i.v. liposomes and micellar solvent systems raises the intriguing question, why C activation has not been considered and explored for the latter reactions beyond the level described in the studies reviewed here? One factor appears to be, at least with liposomes, the short time (~10 years) since these reactions came to light. Another likely factor is that the C system is perceived as a part of immunology and not of pharmacology, toxicology or allergology, a C mechanism is therefore out of the sight of most current paradigms in the latter disciplines. The role of C in Type I reactions is not unheard of, but is certainly not in the forefront of awareness. Finally, the major applications of liposomal drugs and micellar solvents are in cancer chemotherapy, where risk/benefit considerations mandate the use of these drugs regardless of their short-term side effects. In these applications HSR is not a major issue, nor is its mechanism. Because of the large number of CARPA reactions and the possible benefit of using C inhibitors against them, further studies in this area confirming or refuting the C mechanism seems to be of great medicinal importance.

The opinions contained herein are the private ones of the author and are not to be construed as official policy or reflecting the views of the Department of Defense.

6. REFERENCES

1. Lazarou J., Pomeranz B.H., Corey P.N. Incidence of adverse drug reactions in hospitalized patients. A meta-analysis of prospective studies. JAMA 1998;279:1200-1205
2. Demoly P., Lebel B., Messaad D., Sahla H., Rongier M., Daures J.P., Godard P., Bousquet J. Predictive capacity of histamine release for the diagnosis of drug allergy. Allergy 1999;54:500-506.
3. Coombs R.R.A., Gell P.G.H. (1968). Classification of allergic reactions responsible for drug hypersensitivity reactions. Clinical Aspects of Immunology, 2nd Ed. R. R. A. Coombs and P. G. H. Gell. Philadelphia, PA, Davis: 575-596.
4. Kumar S., Mahalingam R. Anaphylactoid reactions to radiocontrast agents. Pediatrics in review 2001;22:356

5. Hong S.J., Wong J.T., Bloch K.J. Reactions to radiocontrast media. Allergy and Asthma Proc. 2002;23:347-351
6. Laroche D., Aimone-Gastin I., Dubois F., Huet H., G,rard P., Vergnaud M.C., Mouton-Faivre C., Gu,ant J.L., Laxenaire M.C., Bricard H. Mechanisms of severe, immediate reactions to iodinated contrast material. Radiology 1998;209:183-190
7. Courvoisier S., Bircher A.J. Delayed-type hypersensitivity to a nonionic, radiopaque contrast medium. Allergy 1998;53:1221-1224
8. Szebeni J. Hypersensitivity reactions to radiocontrast media: the role of complement activation. Curr Allergy Asthma Rep 2004;4:25-30
9. Grainger R.G. (2001). Intravascular radiologic iodinated contrast media. Diagnostic Radiology: A Textbook of Medical Imaging. R. G. Grainger, Allison, D.J. Oxford, UK, Churchill Livingstone: 27-41.
10. Westhoff-Bleck M., Bleck J.S., Jost S. The adverse effects of angiographic radiocontrast media. J Allergy Clin Immunol. 1990;86:684-686
11. Barrett B.J., Parfrey P.S., Vavasour H.M., O'Dea F., Kent G., Stone E. A comparison of nonionic, low-osmolality radiocontrast agents with ionic, high-osmolality agents during cardiac catheterization. Med J Aust. 1991;154:766-772
12. Katayama H., Spinazzi A., Fouillet X., Kirchin M., Taroni P., Davies A. Iomeprol: current and future profile of a radiocontrast agent. Invest. Radiol. 2001;36:87-96
13. Henry D.A., Evans D.B., Robertson J. The safety and cost-effectiveness of low osmolar contrast media. Can economic analysis determine the real worth of a new technology? Drug Saf. 1991;28-36
14. Fattori R., Piva R., Schicchi F., Pancrazi A., Gabrielli G., Marzocchi A., Piovaccari G., Blandini A., Magnani B. Iomeprol and iopamidol in cardiac angiography: a randomised, double-blind parallel-group comparison. N Engl J Med 1992;326:431-436
15. Szebeni J. Complement activation-related pseudoallergy caused by liposomes, micellar carriers of intravenous drugs and radiocontrast agents. Crit. Rev. Ther. Drug Carr. Syst. 2001;18:567-606
16. Greenberger P.A. Contrast media reactions. J Allergy. Clin. Immunol. 1984;74:600-605
17. Lieberman P. Anaphylactoid reactions to radiocontrast materia. Clin. Rev. Allergy 1991;9:319-338
18. Lieberman P. The use of antihistamines in the prevention and treatment of anaphylaxis and anaphylactoid reactions. Singapore Med J. 1989;30:290-293
19. Younger R.E., Herrod H.G., Lieberman P.L., Trouy R., Crawford L.V. Characteristics of diatrizoate-induced basophil histamine release. 1986;
20. Genovese A., Stellato C., Patella V., Lamparter-Schummert B., de Crescenzo G., Adt M., Marone G. Contrast media are incomplete secretagogues acting on human basophils and mast cells isolated from heart and lung, but not skin tissue. Eur J Radiol. 1994;18, Suppl 1:S61-66
21. Napolovlu K., Bolotova E.N., Shimanovskii N.L. The complement-activating action of modern x-ray contrast agents. J. Eksp. Klin. Farmakol. 1998;61:60-64
22. Kolb W.P., Lang J.H., Lasser E.C. Nonimmunologic complement activation in normal human serum induced by radiographic contrast media. J. Immunol. 1978;1232-1238
23. Vik H., Froysa A., Sonstevold A., Toft K., Stov P.S., Ege T. Complement activation and histamine release following administration of roentgen contrast media. Acta Radiol. Suppl. 1995;399:83-89
24. Mikkonen R., Lehto T., Koistinen V., Aronen H.J., Kivisaari L., Meri S. Suppression of alternative complement pathway activity by radiographic contrast media. Scand. J. Immunol. 1997;45:371-377

25. Lasser E.C., Sovak M., Lang J.H. Development of contrast media idiosyncrasy in the dog. J. Radiology 1976; 119: 91-95

26. Lang J.H., Lasser E.C., Kolb W.P. Activation of serum complement by contrast media. Invest. Radiol. 1976;303-308

27. Napolovlu K. The effect of epsilon-aminocaproic acid and prednisolone on the activation of the complement system due to x-ray contrast agents in rats in vitro. Eksp. Klin. Farmakol. 1997;62-64

28. Lasser E.C., Lang J.H., A Lyon S.G., Hamblin A.E. Changes in complement and coagulation factors in a patient suffering a severe anaphylactoid reaction to injected contrast material: some considerations of pathogenesis. Invest. Radiol. 1980;15:S6-12

29. Vandenplas O., Hantson P., Dive A., Mahieu P. Fulminant pulmonary edema following intravenous administration of radiocontrast media. Acta Clin. Belg. 1990;45:334-339

30. Marceau F., Lundberg C., Hugli T.E. Effects of anaphylatoxins on circulation. Immunopharmacol 1987;14:67-84

31. Schmid E., Piccolo M.T., Friedl H.P., Warner R.L., Mulligan M.S., Hugli T.E., Till G.O., Ward P.A. Requirement for C5a in lung vascular injury following thermal trauma to rat skin. *Shock* 1997;8:119-124

32. Heideman M., Hugli T.E. Anaphylatoxin generation in multisystem organ failure. J Trauma 1984;24:1038-1043

33. Hammerschmidt D.E., Hudson L.D., Weaver L.J., Craddock P.R., Jacob H.S. Association of complement activation and elevated plasma-C5a with adult respiratory distress syndrome. Lancet 1980;May 3,:947-949

34. Hohn D.C., Meyers A.J., Gherini S.T., Beckmann A., Markison R.E., Churg A.M. Production of acute pulmonary injury by leukocytes and activated complement. Surgery 1980;88:48-58

35. Fein A., Wiener-Kronish J.P., Niederman M., Matthay M.A. Pathophysiology of the adult respiratory distress syndrome. What have we learned from human studies? Crit Care Clin 1986;2:429-453

36. Zimmermann T., Laszik Z., Nagy S., Kaszaki J., Joo F. The role of the complement system in the pathogenesis of multiple organ failure in shock. Prog Clin Biol Res 1989;308:291-297

37. Bengtsson A. Cascade system activation in shock. Acta Anaesthesiol Scand Suppl 1993;98:7-10

38. Kearney M.L. Adult respiratory distress syndrome following thoracic trauma. Crit Care Nurs Clin North Am 1993;5:723-734

39. Small P., Satin R., Palayew M.J., Hyams B. Prophylactic antihistamines in the management of radiographic contrast reactions. Clin. Allergy 1982;12:289-294

40. Westaby S., Dawson P., Turner M.W., Pridie R.B. Angiography and complement activation. Evidence for generation of C3a anaphylatoxin by intravascular contrast agents. Cardiovasc. Res. 1985;19:85-88

41. Uziely B., Jeffers S., Isacson R., Kutsch K., Wei-Tsao D., Yehoshua Z., Libson E., Muggia F.M., Gabizon A. Liposomal doxorubicin: antitumor activity and unique toxicities during two complementary phase I studies. J Clin Oncol 1995;13:1777-1785

42. Alberts D.S., Garcia D.J. Safety aspects of pegylated liposomal doxorubicin in patients with cancer. Drugs 1997;54, Suppl. 4:30-45

43. Dezube B.J. (1996). Safety assessment: DoxilR (Doxorubicin HCl liposome injection) in refractory AIDS-related Kaposi's sarcoma. Doxil Clinical Series. Califon, NJ, Gardiner-Caldwell SynerMed. 1: 1-8.

44. Gabizon A., Martin F. Polyethylene glycol-coated (pegylated) liposomal doxorubicin. Rationale for use in solid tumours. Drugs 1997;54:15-21

45. Gabizon A.A., Muggia F.M. (1998). Initial clinical evaluation of pegylated liposomal doxorubicin in solid tumors. Long-Circulating Liposomes: Old Drugs, New Therapeutics. M. C. Woodle and S. G. Austin, TX, Landes Bioscience: 155-174.

46. Chanan-Khan A., Szebeni J., Savay S., Liebes L., Rafique N.M., Alving C.R., Muggia F.M. Complement activation following first exposure to pegylated liposomal doxorubicin (Doxil): possible role in hypersensitivity reactions. Ann Oncol 2003;14:1430-1437

47. Levine S.J., Walsh T.J., Martinez A., Eichacker P.Q., Lopez-Berstein G., Natanson C. Cardiopulmonary toxicity after liposomal amphotericin B infusion. Annals Int Med 1991;114:664-666

48. Laing R.B.S., Milne L.J.R., Leen C.L.S., Malcolm G.P., Steers A.J.W. Anaphylactic reactions to liposomal amphotericin. Lancet 1994;344:682

49. Ringdén O., Andström E., Remberger M., Svahn B.M., Tollemar J. Allergic reactions and other rare side effects of liposomal amphotericin. Lancet 1994;344:1156-1157

50. de Marie S. Liposomal and lipid-based formulations of amphotericin B. Leukemia 1996;10, Suppl. 2.:S93-S96

51. Schneider P., Klein R.M., Dietze L., Sohngen D., Leschke M., Heyll A. Anaphylactic reaction to liposomal amphotericin (AmBisome). Br. J. Haematol. 1998;102:1108

52. Cabriales S., Bresnahan J., Testa D., Espina B.M., Scadden D.T., Ross M., Gill P.S. Extravasation of liposomal daunorubicin in patients with AIDS-associated Kaposi's sarcoma: a report of four cases [see comments]. Oncol Nurs Forum 1998;25:67-70

53. Eckardt J.R., Campbell E., Burris H.A., Weiss G.R., Rodriguez G.I., Fields S.M., Thurman A.M., Peacock N.W., Cobb P:, Rothenberg M.L., al e. A phase II trial of DaunoXome, liposome-encapsulated daunorubicin, in patients with metastatic adenocarcinoma of the colon. Am J Clin Oncol 1994;17:498-501

54. Fossa S.D., Aass N., Paro G. A phase II study of DaunoXome in advanced urothelial transitional cell carcinoma. Eur J Cancer 1998;34:1131-1132

55. Gill P.S., Espina B.M., Muggia F., Cabriales S., Tulpule A., Esplin J.A., Liebman H.A., Forssen E., Ross M.E., Levine A.M. Phase I/II clinical and pharmacokinetic evaluation of liposomal daunorubicin. J Clin Oncol 1995;13:996-1003

56. Gill P.S., Wernz J., Scadden D.T., Cohen P., Mukwaya G.M., von Roenn J.H., Jacobs M., Kempin S., Silverberg I., Gonzales G., Rarick M.U., Myers A.M., Shepherd F., Sawka C., Pike M.C., Ross M.E. Randomized phase III trial of liposomal daunorubicin versus doxorubicin, bleomycin, and vincristine in AIDS-related Kaposi's sarcoma. J Clin Oncol 1996;14:2353-2364

57. Girard P.M., Bouchaud O., Goetschel A., Mukwaya G., Eestermans G., Ross M., Rozenbaum W., Saimot A.G. Phase II study of liposomal encapsulated daunorubicin in the treatment of AIDS-associated mucocutaneous Kaposi's sarcoma. AIDS 1996;10:753-757

58. Guaglianone P., Chan K., DelaFlor-Weiss E., Hanisch R., Jeffers S., Sharma D., Muggia F. Phase I and pharmacologic study of liposomal daunorubicin (DaunoXome). Invest New Drugs 1994;12:103-110

59. Money-Kyrle J.F., Bates F., Ready J., Gazzard B.G., Phillips R.H., Boag F.C. Liposomal daunorubicin in advanced Kaposi's sarcoma: a phase II study. Clin Oncol (R Coll Radiol) 1993;5:367-371

60. Richardson D.S., Kelsey S.M., Johnson S.A., Tighe M., Cavenagh J.D., Newland A.C. Early evaluation of liposomal daunorubicin (DaunoXome, Nexstar) in the treatment of relapsed and refractory lymphoma. Invest New Drugs 1997;15:247-253

61. Sculier J.P., Coune A., Brassinne C., Laduron C., Atassi G., Ruysschaert J.M., Fruhling J. Intravenous infusion of high doses of liposomes containing NSC 251635, a water-

insoluble cytostatic agent. A pilot study with pharmacokinetic data. J. Clin. Oncol. 1986;4:789-797

62. Szebeni J. The interaction of liposomes with the complement system. Crit Rev Ther Drug Carrier Syst 1998;15:57-88

63. Hugli T.E., Chenoweth D.E. (1980). Biologically active peptides of complement. Techniques and significance of C3a and C5a measurements. Laboratory and Research Methods in Biology and Medicine. R. M. Nakamura, W. R. Dito and E. S. Tucher. New York, Alan R. Liss: 443.

64. Labarre D., Montdargent B., Carreno M.-P., Maillet F. Strategy for in vitro evaluation of the interactions between biomaterials and complement system. J Appl Biomat 1993;4:231-240

65. Brett T. The laboratory assessment of biocompatibility: the role of complement activation testing. Medical Device Technol. 1992;(March):26-30

66. Chang T.M.S., Lister C.W. Use of finger-prick human blood samples as a more convenient way for in-vitro screening of modified hemoglobin blood substitutes for complement activation: a preliminary report. Biomat. Art. cells & Immob. Biotech. 1993;21:685-690

67. Janatova J. Activation and control of complement, inflammation, and infection associated with the use of biomedical polymers. ASAIO J 2000;46:S53-62.

68. Haxby J.A., Kinsky C.B., Kinsky S.C. Immune response of a liposomal model membrane. *Proc. Natl. Acad. Sci. US.* 1968;61:300-307

69. Haxby J.A., Gotze O., Muller-Eberhard H.J., Kinsky S.C. Release of trapped marker from liposomes by the action of purified complement components. *Proc. Natl. Acad. Sci. USA* 1969;64:290-295

70. Kinsky S.C., Haxby J.A., Zopf D.A., Alving C.R., Kinsky C.B. Complement-dependent damage to liposomes prepared from pure lipids and Forssman hapten. Biochemistry 1969;8:4149-4158

71. Alving C.R., Kinsky S.C., Haxby J.A., Kinsky C.B. Antibody binding and complement fixation by a liposomal model membrane. *Biochemistry* 1969;8:1582-1587

72. Szebeni J., Baranyi B., Savay S., Lutz L.U., Jelezarova E., Bunger R., Alving C.R. The role of complement activation in hypersensitivity to pegylated liposomal doxorubicin (Doxil®). J. Liposome Res. 2000;10:347-361

73. Szebeni J., DiIorio E.E., Hauser H., Winterhalter H.K. Encapsulation of hemoglobin in phospholipid liposomes: characterization and stability. Biochemistry 1985;24:2827-2832

74. Szebeni J., Hauser H., Eskelson C.D., Watson R.R., Winterhalter H.K. Interaction of hemoglobin derivatives with liposomes. Membrane cholesterol protects against the changes of hemoglobin. Biochemistry 1988;27:6425-6434

75. Szebeni J., Wassef N.M., Spielberg H., Rudolph A.S., Alving C.R. Complement activation in rats by liposomes and liposome-encapsulated hemoglobin: evidence for anti-lipid antibodies and alternative pathway activation. Biochem Biophys Res Comm 1994;205:255-263

76. Szebeni J., Wassef N.M., Rudolph A.S., Alving C.R. Complement activation in human serum by liposome-encapsulated hemoglobin: the role of natural anti-phospholipid antibodies. Biochim Biophys Acta 1996;1285:127-130

77. Szebeni J., Wassef N.M., Hartman K.R., Rudolph A.S., Alving C.R. Complement activation in vitro by the red blood cell substitute, liposome-encapsulated hemoglobin: Mechanism of activation and inhibition by soluble complement receptor type 1. Transfusion 1997;37:150-159

78.   Szebeni J., Spielberg H., Cliff R.O., Wassef N.M., Rudolph A.S., Alving C.R. Complement activation and thromboxane A2 secretion in rats following administration of liposome-encapsulated hemoglobin: Inhibition by soluble complement receptor type 1. Art Cells Blood Subs and Immob Biotechnol 1997;25:379-392

79.   Szebeni J., Alving C.R. Complement-mediated acute effects of liposome-encapsulated hemoglobin. Artif Cells Blood Substit Immobil Biotechnol 1999;27:23-41

80.   Szebeni J., Fontana J.L., Wassef N.M., Mongan P.D., Morse D.S., Dobbins D.E., Stahl G.L., Bünger R., Alving C.R. Hemodynamic changes induced by liposomes and liposome-encapsulated hemoglobin in pigs: a model for pseudo-allergic cardiopulmonary reactions to liposomes. Role of complement and inhibition by soluble CR1 and anti-C5a antibody. Circulation 1999;99:2302-2309

81.   Szebeni J., Baranyi B., Savay S., Bodo M., Morse D.S., Basta M., Stahl G.L., Bunger R., Alving C.R. Liposome-induced pulmonary hypertension: Properties and mechanism of a complement-mediated pseudoallergic reaction. Am. J. Physiol. 2000;279:H1319-H1328

82.   Szebeni J., Baranyi L., Savay S., Milosevits J., Bunger R., Laverman P., Metselaar J.M., Storm G., Chanan-Khan A., Liebes L., Muggia F.M., Cohen R., Barenholz Y., Alving C.R. Role of complement activation in hypersensitivity reactions to Doxil and HYNIC-PEG liposomes: experimental and clinical studies. J. Liposome Res. 2002; 12:165-172

82a. Szebeni J, Baranyi L, Savay S, Milosevits J, Bodo M, Bunger R, Alving CR. The interaction of liposomes with the complement system: in vitro and in vivo assays. Methods Enzymol. 2003;373:136-154

83.   Aguado J.M., Hidalgo M., Moya I., Alcazar J.M., Jimenez M.J., Noriega A.R. Ventricular arrhythmias with conventional and liposomal amphotericin. Lancet 1993;342 (8881):1239

84.   Coune A., Sculier J.P., Frühling J., Stryckmans P., Brassine C., Ghanem G., Laduron C., Atassi G., Ruysschaert J.M., Hildebrand J. Iv administration of a water-insoluble antimitotic compound entrapped in liposomes. Preliminary report on infusion of large volumes of liposomes to man. Cancer Treat. Rep. 1983;67:1031-1033

85.   Skubitz K.M., Skubitz A.P. Mechanism of transient dyspnea induced by pegylated-liposomal doxorubicin (Doxil). Anticancer Drugs 1998;9:45-50

86.   Cheung A.K., Parker C.J., Hohnholt M. Soluble complement receptor type 1 inhibits complement activation induced by hemodialysis membranes in vitro. Kidney Int 1994;46:1680-1687

87.   Skroeder N.R., Jacobson S.H., Lins L.E., Kjellstrand C.M. Acute symptoms during and between hemodialysis: the relative role of speed, duration, and biocompatibility of dialysis. Artif Organs 1994;18:880-887

88.   Skroeder N.R., Kjellstrand P., Holmquist B., Kjellstrand C.M., Jacobson S.H. Individual differences in biocompatibility responses to hemodialysis. Int J Artif Organs 1994;17:521-530

89.   Brouwers A.H., De Jong D.J., Dams E.T., Oyen W.J., Boerman O.C., Laverman P., Naber T.H., Storm G., Corstens F.H. Tc-99m-PEG-Liposomes for the evaluation of colitis in Crohn's disease. *J Drug Target* 2000;8:225-233

90.   Dams E.T., Oyen W.J., Boerman O.C., Storm G., Laverman P., Kok P.J., Buijs W.C., Bakker H., van der Meer J.W., Corstens F.H. 99mTc-PEG liposomes for the scintigraphic detection of infection and inflammation: clinical evaluation. J. Nucl. Med. 2000;41:622

91. Blum R.H., Garnick M.B., Israel M., Canellos G.P., Henderson I.C., Frei III E. Initial clinical evaluation of N-trifluoroacetyladriamycin-14-valerate (AD-32), an adriamycin analog. Cancer Treat Rep 1979;63:919-928

92. O'Dwyer P.J., Weiss R. Hypersensitivity reactions induced by etoposide. Cancer Treat Rep 1984;68:959-961

93. Athanassiou A.E., Bafaloukos D., Pectasidis D., al. e. Acute vasomotor response- a reaction to etoposide. J Clin Oncol 1988;6:1204-1205

94. Lassus M., Scott D., Leyland-Jones B. Allergic reactions associated with cremophor-containing antineoplastics (abstract). Proc Annu Meet Am Soc Clin Oncol 1985;4:268

95. Szebeni J., Muggia F.M., Alving C.R. Complement activation by Cremophor EL as a possible contributor to hypersensitivity to paclitaxel: an in vitro study. J Natl Cancer Inst 1998;90:300-306

96. Szebeni J., Alving C.R., Savay S., Barenholz Y., Priev A., Danino D., Talmon Y. Formation of complement-activating particles in aqueous solutions of Taxol: Possible role in hypersensitivity reactions. Intern. Immunopharm. 2001;1:721-735

97. Nolte H., Carstensen H., Hertz H. VM-26 (teniposide)-induced hypersensitivity and degranulation of basophils in children. Am J Ped Hematol-Oncol 1988;10:308-312

98. Rowinsky E.K., Onetto N., Canetta R.M., Eisenhauer E.A., Arbuck S.G. Taxol: the first of the taxanes, an important new class of antitumor agents. Semin Oncol 1992;19:646-662

99. Rowinsky E.K., Donehower R.C. Paclitaxel (Taxol). New Engl J Med 1995;332:1004-1014

100. Rowinsky E.K. The development and utility of the taxane class of antimicrotubule chemotherapy agents. Ann. Rev. Med. 1997;48:353-374

101. Kris M.G., O'Connell J.P., Gralla R.J. A phase I trial of Taxol given as 3-hour infusions every 21 days. Cancer Treat Rep 1986;70:605-607

102. Weiss R.B., Donehower R.C., Wiernik P.H., Ohnuma T., Gralla R.J., Trump D.L., Baker J.R., VanEcho D.A., VonHoff D.D., Leyland-Jones B. Hypersensitivity reactions from Taxol. J Clin Oncol 1990;8:1263-1268

103. Guchelaar H.J., ten Napel C.H., de Vries E.G., Mulder N.H. Clinical, toxicological and pharmaceutical aspects of the antineoplastic drug taxol: a review. Clin Oncol 1994;6:40-48

104. Tsavaris N.B., Kosmas C. Risk of severe acute hypersensitivity reactions after rapid paclitaxel infusion of less than 1-h duration. Cancer Chemother Pharmacol 1998;42:509-511

105. Del Priore G., Smith P., Warshal D., Dubeshter B., Angel C. Paclitaxel-associated hypersensitivity reaction despite high-dose steroids and prolonged infusions. Gynecol Oncol 1995;56:316-318

106. Bookman M.A., Kloth D.D., Kover P.E., Smolinski S., Ozols R.F. Intravenous prophylaxis for paclitaxel-related hypersensitivity reactions. Semin Oncol 1997;24, Suppl 19:S19-13-S19-15

107. Bookman M.A., Kloth D.D., Kover P., Smolinski S., Ozols R.F. Short-course intravenous prophylaxis for paclitaxel-related hypersensitivity reactions. Ann Oncol 1997;8:611-614

108. Rowinsky E.K., McGuire W.P., Guarnieri T. Cardiac disturbances during the administration of Taxol. J Clin Oncol 1991;9:1704-1712

109. Rowinsky E.K. Clinical pharmacology of Taxol. Monogr Natl Cancer Inst 1993;15:25-37

110. Rowinsky E.K., Eisenhauer E.A., Chaudhry V., Arbuck S.G., Donehower R.C. Clinical toxicities encountered with paclitaxel (Taxol). Semin Oncol 1993;20:1-15

111. Rowinsky E.K., Donehower R.C. The clinical pharmacology of paclitaxel (Taxol). Semin Oncol 1993;20:16-25

112. Rowinsky E.K., Wright M., Monsarrat B., Donehower R.C. Clinical pharmacology and metabolism of Taxol (paclitaxel): update 1993. Ann Oncol 1994;5:S7-16

113. Ramanathan R.K., Reddy V.V., Holbert J.M., Belani C.P. Pulmonary infiltrates following administration of paclitaxel. Chest 1996;110:289-292

114. Essayan D.M., Kagey-Sobotka A., Colarusso P.J., Lichtenstein L.M., Ozols R.F., King E.D. Successful parenteral desensitization to paclitaxel. J Allerg Clin Immunol 1996;97:42-46

115. Laher S., Karp S.J. Acute myocardial infarction following paclitaxel administration for ovarian carcinoma. Clin Oncol 1997;9:124-126

116. Nannan Panday V.R., Huizing M.T., Ten Bokkel Huinink W.W., Vermorken J.B., Beijnen J.H. Hypersensitvity reactions to the taxanes paclitaxel and docetaxel. Clin Drug Invest 1997;14:418-427

117. Ciesielski-Carlucci C., Leong P., Jacobs C. Case report of anaphylaxis from cisplatin/paclitaxel and a review of their hypersensitivity reaction profiles. Am J Clin Oncol 1997;20:373-375

118. Markman M., Kennedy A., Webster K., Kulp B., Peterson G., Belinson J. Paclitaxel administration to gynecologic cancer patients with major cardiac risk factors. J Clin Oncol 1998;16:3483-3485

119. Grosen E., Siitari E., Larrison E., C. T., Roecker E. Paclitaxel hypersensitivity reactions related to bee sting allergy. Lancet 1999;354:288-289

120. Terwogt J.M., Nuijen B., Huinink W.W., Beijnen J.H. Alternative formulations of paclitaxel. Cancer Treat Rev 1997;23:87-95

121. Lundberg B.B. A submicron lipid emulsion coated with amphipathic polyethylene glycol for parenteral administration of paclitaxel (Taxol). J Pharm Pharmacol 1997;49:16-21

122. Paradis R., Page M. New active paclitaxel amino acids derivatives with improved water solubility. Anticancer Res 1998;18:2711-2716

123. Webster L., Linsenmeyer M., Millward M., Morton C., Bishop J., Woodcock D. Measurement of cremophor EL following taxol: plasma levels sufficient to reverse drug exclusion mediated by the multidrug-resistant phenotype. J Natl Cancer Inst 1993;85:1685-1690

124. Kessel D., Woodburn K., Kecker D., Sykes E. Fractionation of Cremophor EL delineates components responsible for plasma lipoprotein alterations and multidrug resistance reversal. Oncol Res 1995;7:207-212

125. Hugli T.E. Structure and function of anaphylatoxins. Spring Semin Immunopathol 1984;7:193-219

126. Kessel D. Properties of cremophor EL micelles probed by fluorescence. Photochem Photobiol 1992;56:447-451

127. Nerurkar M.M., Ho N.F.H., Burton P.S., Vidmar T.J., Borchardt R.T. Mechanistic roles of neutral surfactants on concurrent polarized and passive membrane transport of a model peptide in Caco-2 cells. J. Pharm. Sci. 1997;86:813-821

128. Trissel L.A. Pharmaceutical properties of paclitaxel and their effects on preparation and administration. Pharmacotherapy 1997;17:133S-139S

129. Kwon G.S. Polymeric micelles for delivery of poorly water-soluble compounds. Crit Rev Ther Drug Carrier Syst. 2003;20:357-403

130. Liszewski K., Atkinson J.P. (1993). The complement system. Fundamental Immunology, Third Edition. W. E. Paul. New York, Raven Press, Ltd.: 917-939.

131. Smith C.A., Vogel C.V., Muller-Eberhard H.J. Ultrastructure of cobra venom factor-dependent C3/C5 convertase and its zymogen, factor B of human complement. J. Biol. Chem. 1982;257:9879-9882
132. Hunter R.L., Bennett B. The adjuvant activity of nonionic block polymer surfactants. II. Antibody formation and inflammation related to the structure of triblock and octablock copolymers. J Immunol 1984;133:3167-3175
133. Hunter R.L., Bennett B. Modulation of antigen presentation and host mediators by block copolymer adjuvants. Prog Leuk Biol 1987;6:181-190
134. Hunter R.L. (1990). Nonionic block polymers: new preparations and review of the mechanism of action. New Generation Vaccines. G. C. Woodrow and M. M. Levine. New York, Marcel Decker.
135. Hunter R.L., McNicholl J., Lal A.A. Mechanisms of action of nonionic block copolymer adjuvants. AIDS Res Hum Retroviruses 1994;10 Suppl 2:S95-S98
136. Chonn A., Cullis P.R., Devine D.V. The role of surface charge in the activation of the classical and alternative pathways of complement by liposomes. J Immunol 1991;146:4234-4241
137. Lorenz W., Riemann H.J., Schmal A. Histamine release in dogs by Cremophor EL and its derivatives: oxyethylated oleic acid is the most effective constituent. Agents Actions 1977;7:63-67
138. Gaudy J.H., Sicard J.F., Lhoste F., Boitier J.F. The effects of cremophor EL in the anaesthetized dog. Can J Anaesth 1987;34:122-129
139. Theis J.G., Liau-Chu M., Chan H.S., Doyle J., Greenberg M.L., Koren G. Anaphylactoid reactions in children receiving high-dose intravenous cyclosporine for reversal of tumor resistance: the causative role of improper dissolution of Cremophor EL. J Clin Oncol 1995;13:2508-2516
140. Liau-Chu M., Theis J.G., Koren G. Mechanism of anaphylactoid reactions: improper preparation of high-dose intravenous cyclosporine leads to bolus infusion of Cremophor EL and cyclosporine. Ann Pharmacother 1997;31:1287-1291
141. Vercellotti G.M., Hammerschmidt D.E., Craddock P.R., Jacob H.S. Activation of plasma complement by perfluorocarbon artificial blood: probable mechanism of adverse pulmonary reactions in treated patients and rationale for corticosteroids prophylaxis. Blood 1982; 59:1299-1304
142. Fukushima K., Nakamura M., Hinuma K. Influence of Fluosol-DA infusion on the complement activation and on the blood level of histamine in man. J. Prog. Clin. Biol. Res. 1983;122:291-298
143. Tremper K.K., Vercellotti G.M., Hammerschmidt D.E. Hemodynamic profile of adverse clinical reactions to Fluosol-DA 20%. Crit. Care Med. 1984;12:428-431
144. Vercellotti G.M., Hammerschmidt D.E. Immunological biocompatibility in blood substitutes. Int. Anesthesiol. Clin. 1985;23:47-62
145. Norman M.E., Williams P., Illum L. Influence of block copolymers on the adsorption of plasma proteins to microspheres. *Biomaterials* 1993;14(3)::193-202
146. Faithfull N.S., Cain S.M. Cardiorespiratory consequences of fluorocarbon reactions in dogs. Biomater. Artif. Cells Artif. Organs 1988;16:463-472
147. Moghimi M.S., Hunter C., Dadswell C.M., Savay S., Alving C., Szebeni J. Causative factors behind poloxamer 188 (Pluronic F68, Flocor™)-induced complement activation in human sera. A protective role against poloxamer-mediated complement activation by elevated serum lipoprotein levels. Biochim. Biophys Acta 2004;In press:
148. Descotes J., Choquet-Kastylevsky G. Gell and Coombs's classification: is it still valid? *Toxicology* 2001;158:43-49

Complement in Health and Disease

149. Rawlins M.D. Clinical pharmacology: adverse reactions to drugs. Br. Med. J. 1981;282:974-976
150. Aronson J.K., Ferner R.E. Joining the DoTS: new approach to classifying adverse drug reactions. British Med J 2003;327:1222-1225
151. Lieberman P., Siegle R.L., Treadwell G. Radiocontrast reactions. Clin. Rev. Allergy 1986;4:229-245

18

The Role of Complement in Transplantation

Michael Kirschfink[1] and Tom Eirik Mollnes[2]

[1]Institute of Immunology, University of Heidelberg, Germany and [2]Institute of Immunology, Rikshospitalet University Hospital, Oslo, Norway

Abstract: Organ transplantation is an established therapy for patients with end-stage organ disease. In the past years, a growing understanding of physiology and pathophysiology, refinement of tissue typing, better surgical techniques and more effective immunosuppressive strategies has progressively favoured prolonged graft survival. However, still a significant proportion of grafts fail within the first months and years after transplantation because of a progressive and irreversible immune response of the recipient. The pathogenesis of graft rejection comprises complex immunological and non-immunological mechanisms. Humoral as well as cell-mediated immune reactions have been implicated in graft rejection. Although primarily driven by T-cell response the role of complement activation in acute graft rejection has become evident in recent years. Here, modern complement analysis as an integral part of posttransplantation monitoring may contribute to early recognition of impeding graft rejection. Hyperacute graft rejection is a rare occurrence in the clinic. It may occur immediately after allotransplantation due to preexisting blood group directed or anti-HLA antibodies. In xentransplantation, hyperacute rejection is a major barrier to organ survival. The binding of pre-existing, so-called natural antibodies, mostly of the IgM class, to donor cells leads to fulminant activation of the complement and clotting systems with rapid loss of graft function. Therapeutic substitution of appropriate complement regulators appears to be a reasonable approach to reduce undesirable complement-mediated inflammatory reactions in the grafted organ.

Key words: Complement, transplantation, ischemia-reperfusion, organ preservation, rejection, allotransplantation, xenotransplantation, therapy

1.   INTRODUCTION

Transplantation is defined as replacement of cells, tissue or whole organs and is divided into four categories dependent on the donor to recipient relationship. *Autotransplantation* is when the graft originates from the same individual, such as bone marrow stem cells, skin or bone. *Isotransplantation* occurs between genetically identical animals or identical twins.

Allotransplantation refers to individuals of the same species and in *Xenotransplantation* the organ is transplanted into a different species. In the first two cases there are no antibody- or cell-mediated immunological response to be expected, whereas upon allotransplantation and xenotransplantation rejection may vary from mild, which can be controlled by immunosuppression, to vigorous when preformed antibodies are present.

Activation of complement in transplantation is based on two different mechanisms: 1) a direct and immediate activation occurs if components of the initial pathways are exposed to foreign surfaces and/or damaged endothelium, and 2) antibody-mediated classical pathway activation is initiated by preformed or elicited antibodies to the graft. Thus, complement is of potential importance in all four types of transplantation described above, particularly of vascularized grafts. The ischemia-reperfusion injury is considered a key event in whole organ transplantation independent of the source of the organ. The role of complement in xenotransplantation is undisputed, and naturally occurring antibodies and complement are accepted as the major triggers of the hyperacute rejection. In allotransplantation, the role of complement has been more controversial, but increasing evidence points to complement as an important factor for long-time allograft survival. Thus, specific inhibition of complement has been put on the agenda for future therapy to increase transplant survival.

2.   TRANSPLANTATION OF NON-VASCULAR GRAFTS

Complement activation is usually not a problem in transplantation of autologous cells and tissues, like bone marrow cells, skin and bone. Allo- and xenotransplantation of skin and bone is usually intended for transient treatment, until the recipient's own tissue is regenerated. Strategies to avoid complement activation in these situations may not be crucial. Xeno-tissue used as bioscaffolds for remodelling seems to be relatively protected from rejection in contrast to whole organs (1). Cell allotransplants, like insulin-producing pancreatic islet cells, are principally subjected to rejection, but since these are non-vascularized grafts the typical rejection phases as described for whole organs do not occur. Allotransplantation of pancreatic islet cells has already reached clinical trials. Here, a major challenge seems to be the prevention of tissue factor induced hemostasis (2). The main problem arises from primary loss of function of the engrafted cells, which is even greater in transplantation of xenogeneic cells. Activation of complement by such cells appears not to be induced by anti-Gal antibodies (3). Probably more important is a direct activation of complement by the cell surface in the absence of antibodies (4-6). Expression of human complement regulatory proteins on porcine islet cells confers protection against human complement-mediated lysis (7).

Various encapsulation strategies are under development to protect the cells from the recipient's immune response (8). A main challenge is to prepare membranes that allow selective diffusion of essential substances, such as insulin, but exclude access of complement proteins. Microencapsulation of porcine islet cells has been shown to protect against human antibody-induced and complement-mediated destruction (9). A second challenge is to make the material used for encapsulation biocompatible and inert with respect to complement activation. Alginate, which is a frequently used substance for this purpose, has been shown to activate complement (10) and to induce an antibody-mediated immune reaction (11).

Techniques for the transplantation of stem cells intended for differentiation into organ-specific cells are rapidly approaching the clinic. If autologous, such cells should not activate complement, unless undesired modifications occur during culture. Stem cells obtained by cloning techniques should also be well tolerated, although it should be noted that mitochondrial DNA from the enucleated ovum still persists in the cloned cell.

Transplantation of embryonic tissue in the form of immature organs is an alternative to stem cell transplantation. Experimental data from transplantation of metanephroi, the embryonic kidney precursor, are encouraging (12). These structures are invaded by the recipients' endothelial cells forming autologous vessels and the metanephroi differentiate into functional kidneys with glomerular and excretory function. Since the vessels are originating from the recipient, there will be no complement-dependent endothelial cell activation, although a possible reaction against the foreign cells may be suspected. Thus, in case of xenotransplantation of such tissue it has been suggested that animals transgenic for human complement membrane regulators would be most suitable.

Bioartificial organs are technical devices containing human or animal cells intended for extracorporeal treatment of end stage organ failure. Bioartificial livers have been developed and even come to preclinical use. The interphase between the patient's blood and the cells of the device is a semipermeable membrane which partly protects the cells from immunologic attack, but some form of rejection reactions may still occur, in which complement may be of importance (13-15).

Transplantation of vascular organs differs principally from that of cells and of non-vascular tissue in two ways. First, reperfusion of the organ after a certain time of ischemia induces an inflammatory reaction which may develop to ischemia-reperfusion injury (IRI), independent of the source of the organ. Second, the fate of the transplant will depend on the type and strength of the subsequent immunologic reaction. The complement system is critically involved in both these processes, as outlined in the following part of this chapter.

3.   THE ISCHEMIA-REPERFUSION INJURY

Occlusion of arteries leading to distal impairment of blood supply causes ischemia with subsequent tissue damage and infarction. If reperfusion occurs, either spontaneously or therapeutically, the infarction area may be reduced, but a paradoxically and partially oxygen-mediated injury may occur. Preventing ischemia-reperfusion injury will certainly further improve tissue survival. Complement is known to play a key role in IRI, e.g. in myocardial-, renal-, intestinal- and skeletal muscle infarction (16-18). Here, a characteristic property of complement becomes evident, namely to discriminate not only between self and non-self (19), but also between normal self and altered self, e.g. in disrupted homeostasis of the endothelium which normally protects tissue against homologous complement attack (20).

Several mechanisms of complement activation have been proposed for the IRI, including activation through any of the three initial pathways. There are two lines of evidence for the role of classical pathway activation in ischemia-reperfusion injury: the presence of naturally occurring complement-fixing antibodies binding to damaged endothelium (21, 22), and the beneficial effect on tissue damage by specifically blocking the classical pathway (23). The alternative pathway may be activated directly or as an amplification of classical or lectin pathway activation. In early studies performed before the lectin pathway was discovered, its activation may have been misinterpreted as alternative pathway activation. The efficacy of the lectin pathway is also likely to depend on the amplification by the alternative pathway (24). In fact, recent studies have highlighted the role of the lectin pathway in ischemia-reperfusion injury. Hypoxia and reoxygenation of human endothelial cells induced MBL-dependent complement activation (25) and inhibition of MBL markedly reduced rat myocardial ischemia-reperfusion injury (26).

Transplantation-related IRI differs from endogenous IRI in several aspects. First, the condition is artificial and performed under controlled conditions, enabling precautions in order to reduce the injury. Second, reperfusion of the donor organ with recipient blood will potentially activate complement by somehow other means than during autologous reperfusion. It should be emphasized that the initial and crucial event in IRI is endothelial cell activation (27). It has become gradually clear that this initial endothelial cell activation is important not only for immediate graft function, but also for long-time survival (28). Furthermore, it has been shown experimentally by comparing iso- and allografts that the renal IRI is independent on the immunological background (29). Notably, complement activation contributes to graft dysfunction after lung isotransplantation (30) and autotransplantation (31), further supporting a role for complement in transplantation-associated IRI, independent on the source of the graft. Thus, strategies are needed to minimize IRI, including the optimization of organ harvesting and preservation.

Preservation solutions used for immediate perfusion and subsequent storage of the donor organ are composed for optimal maintenance of tissue and cell homeostasis aiming at to reduce ischemia-related damage (32). Particular attention has been paid to preserve endothelial cell function (33). Routinely, organs are stored cold and attempts are made to reduce the time between harvesting and transplantation, since the ischemia time influences the outcome (34). Although time and temperature are critical factors for complement activation in general, the possible impact of complement inhibition during organ preservation is largely unknown. Recent data, however, have demonstrated a beneficial effect of adding C1-inhibitor to the preservation solution in experimental *ex vivo* liver perfusion both with respect to complement activation and inflammatory reaction in the liver (35). *In vitro*, C1-inhibitor was found to bind to endothelial cells under cold storage conditions maintaining its regulatory function (36).

4.   ALLOGRAFT REJECTION

Recent data are shedding new light on the role of the innate immune system in general (37), and of complement in particular (38), in the complex processes of allograft rejection. Rejection of allografts is traditionally considered either as humoral or cellular. Hitherto unknown interactions between complement and adaptive immunity have become evident over the last decade, which also seem to take place in experimental renal allograft rejection (39-41). A prolonged survival of renal allografts was observed in C3-deficient animals where failure of local C3 synthesis was obviously associated with an impaired T-cell response (42).

Hyperacute rejection may occur immediately after allotransplantation due to anti-A or -B blood group antibodies or if a presensitized recipient presents high titers of anti-HLA antibodies at the time of transplantation. This reaction is largely complement-dependent and usually leads to rapid loss of graft function. Due to consequent pretansplantation serology testing including "cross-match", this clinically severe condition fortunately became rare. Precautions like plasmapheresis and immunosuppression are taken when ABO incompatible organs are transplanted.

Acute vascular rejection is still a major clinical problem in allotransplantation. The role of complement activation in this condition has become evident in recent years, both from a diagnostic and prognostic point of view (43). Peritubular capillary deposition of C4d, a marker of classical and lectin pathway activation, has emerged as a useful marker of acute vascular or antibody-mediated rejection of kidneys (44, 45) (Fig. 1).

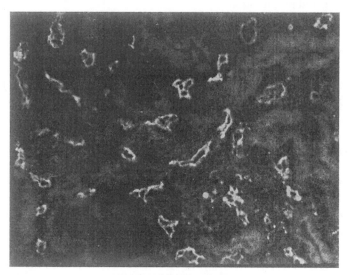

Figure 1. Activation of complement in acute vascular renal graft rejection is reflected by positive C4d staining in peritubular capillaries (kindly provided by Prof. Dr. Rüdiger Waldher, Heidelberg).

It was shown to correlate with future graft dysfunction (46-56), and may be an independent long-term prognostic factor (57, 58). C4d deposition closely correlates with the presence of anti-donor antibodies (47, 59), supporting a humoral mechanism of this rejection (60, 61). On the other hand, several studies could not confirm a regular capillary presence of immunoglobulin (62-65) or C1q (62, 65) in acute humoral rejection. The reason for this is unclear, but may be explained by the fact that C4d, in contrast to antibodies and C1q, is covalently bound to the cell surface during complement activation, thereby enabling longer detection. Furthermore, although not yet investigated in detail, in the absence of antibody and C1q C4d deposition may be derived from lectin pathway activation. In fact, in a recent case of acute vascular rejection glomerular deposition of MASP-1, a component of the lectin pathway, was found together with C4d and C3, in the absence of C1q (66). This study, performed on protocol biopsies one week after transplantation, also indicated a higher risk of graft loss when C4d was co-deposited with C3.

In plasma, high levels of C1rs-C1-inhibitor appear to be of prognostic value as an early indicator of impeding renal graft failure (67). In other studies, the urinary levels of C5a (68) and C4d (69) were favoured to better reflect renal allograft rejection, in comparison to levels of complement activation markers in plasma. Urinary measurement of complement activation has, however, not yet reached clinical utility in diagnosis of renal rejection, in contrast to immunohistochemical evaluation of kidney biopsies.

Although much less investigated than in kidneys, deposition of C4d in heart capillaries also appears to predict organ dysfunction after human allotransplantation (70, 71). Animal models of heart allotransplantation point to the pathogenetic importance of the terminal pathway with formation of the C5b-9 complex for allograft rejection (72-74) as well as for the development of chronic graft sclerosis (75). In further support of complement as a mediator of heart graft dysfunction, intra-coronary application of C1-inhibitor led to improved ventricular function in a pig allotransplantation model (76).

Lung allotransplantation is the only condition where complement inhibition has come to clinical application. A multicenter trial using soluble complement receptor 1 (sCR1, TP-10) demonstrated improved postoperative pulmonary function (77). In a case report, two transplanted patients suffering from severe pulmonary graft failure recovered upon systemic C1-inhibitor treatment (78). Another patient with pulmonary graft failure due to ABO incompatibility recovered after receiving sCR1 (TP10) as adjuvant therapy (79). Several animal studies using either complement deficient strains or specific complement inhibitors underline the important role of complement in the rejection of pulmonary allografts (80-84).

Upon liver transplantation the recipient complement protein phenotypes disappear and, with variations in kinetics, are replaced by the respective donor phenotypes (85, 86). A combined kidney and liver transplantation in a child with haemolytic uremic syndrome (HUS) associated with factor H mutation restored the defective complement regulator with hitherto no recurrence of the disease (87). Activation of complement during orthotopic liver transplantation (OLT) has been assessed in various studies, either reflected by increased plasma levels of complement activation products, such as C3a, C3d, C5a and/or SC5b-9 (88, 89) or by demonstration of C5b-9 precipitation in liver biopsies (90, 91). From a longitudinal study in liver transplant patients Pfeifer et al (88) concluded that even subclinical rejection episodes may be detected by inclusion of complement activation products in posttransplantation immune monitoring. Heparinization of veno-venous bypass circuits (92) or high dose aprotinin treatment (93) appears to have no impact on complement activation.

Serial posttransplantation measurements revealed that also decreased plasma levels of sCR1 (not produced by hepatocytes) correlated with liver dysfunction (94). It has also been suggested that reduced expression of CD59 in liver tissue (91) or a general defective expression of membrane regulators CD55 and CD59 (95) may favour MAC deposition and subsequent liver damage. However, in contrast to those observations by Scoazec et al (95) we were able to clearly identify the presence of all mCRP on primary liver hepatocytes (Halme and Kirschfink (personal communication). Based on studies in a rat model, Chiang et al. (96) suggested that the complement regulator clusterin may play a role in liver allograft tolerance. Therapeutic complement inhibition by recombinant soluble CR1 (TP10) (97) or C1-inhibitor (98) significantly improved liver microcirculation in a rat model of liver transplantation. Treatment with C1-inhibitor was successful in a patient suffering from septic shock after liver transplantation (99).

5.   XENOGRAFT REJECTION

Transplantation of vascular xenografts faces a number of challenges different from those known from allografts, including anatomical and physiological differences, functional molecular incompatibilities, potential risk of xenoses, as well as accompanying legal and ethical aspects (100-108). On the other hand, if successful, xenotransplantation could solve the problem of organ deficit and transplantation could be planned logistically with a minimum of ischemic time. The organ size could be adapted to the recipient even for newborns. Currently, the pig is regarded to be the candidate of choice for xenotransplantation (109); breading is easy and economically favourable, anatomy and physiology are similar to that in humans, species distance reduces the risk of pathogen transmission, and ethical aspects are generally regarded less problematic than with higher primates.

In principal, the same immunological hurdles exist for xenotransplantation as for allotransplantation (110), but in case of discordant transplants, as pig-to-human, a massive hyperacute rejection (111, 112) regularly occurs within minutes due to preformed 'naturally occurring' antibodies directed to the carbohydrate antigen Galα(1-3)Gal (113, 114). The Gal antigen, originating from the galactosyl transferase gene, is present in all animals except Old World monkeys, apes and humans. The antigen resembles the H structure of the ABO blood group system, which is coded by the analogous fucosyl transferase gene. Gal is present on a number of glycoproteins including adhesion molecules and more than 80% of the complement-fixing xeno-reactive antibodies in human serum recognize the Gal epitope (115). Anti-Gal antibodies are potent complement activators and complement is a prerequisite for the induction of hyperacute rejection. Thus, prevention of hyperacute rejection relies on strategies to neutralize the effect of either anti-Gal antibodies or complement.

Anti-Gal antibodies can be neutralized by injection of Gal antigen (116), by plasmapheresis (117), or by immunoadsoption (118) of immunoglobulins or more specifically of anti-porcine (119) or anti-Gal antibodies (120). The effect is, however, transient, since antibodies are continuously produced. Efforts have therefore been made to reduce or remove the Gal antigen, like enzymatic treatment displacing the Gal moiety from the surface (121), by neutralizing intracellular galactosyl transferase by antibodies (122, 123), by genetic modifications of the donor or by making the recipient tolerant. Genetic modifications have been achieved in principally two different ways, either transgenic by introducing the human fucosyl transferase gene into the pig genome, or by knocking out the glucosyl transferase gene followed by cloning. The first approach led to suppression of the Gal antigen in favour of the human H antigen (124-127). Although attenuating experimental HAR, its suppression was not complete. Gal knock-out pigs have recently been cloned and are considered to be promising as future xenotransplant candidates (128, 129). Small amounts of Gal are, however, still present in these animals (130). Furthermore, concerns have been risen with respect to deleting the Gal antigen since it may be of importance in protection against certain viruses (131). Finally, the approach of tolerizing the recipient against Gal has attracted attention. Attempts have been made by destruction of anti-Gal producing B-cells (132) and recently tolerance was obtained in Gal knock-out mice by injecting syngeneic peripheral mononuclear cells containing Gal (133). The latter observations are of potential importance since tolerance was obtained without using bone marrow cells and without any immunosuppressive regimen.

The second way of preventing hyperacute rejection is to neutralize complement. The role of complement in hyperacute rejection is undisputed, which is reflected by more than one thousand references published over the last decades. Intervention strategies have been focused on inhibition of complement activation either by supply of soluble inhibitors or by generating transgenic animals expressing human complement regulatory molecules in their tissues. Both approaches have definitely documented the pivotal role of complement in hyperacute rejection (134).

Inhibition of complement in the fluid phase has clearly verified not only that complement is crucial for hyperacute rejection, but also that the antibody-mediated classical pathway activation is the critical mode of activation (135). However, the pathogenic role of complement seems to depend on the terminal pathway since blocking C5 activation or a deficiency in terminal components seem to equally well protect against hyperacute rejection as blocking complement at an earlier stage (136, 137). Only occasionally, a terminal pathway independent hyperacute rejection has been described (138).

Complement is controlled by a number of membrane regulatory molecules, of which several show homologous restriction, indicating a species specificity of this regulation (139-141). A number of successful attempts have been made to produce pigs transgenic for human complement regulatory proteins, including decay accelerating factor (DAF, CD55) (142), membrane cofactor protein (MCP, CD46) (143), protectin (CD59) (144, 145), or combinations thereof (146). Organs from such animals do not undergo hyperacute rejection when transplanted to primates, even in the presence of anti-Gal antibodies, underscoring the potency of complement in accomplishing the hyperacute rejection. Notably, data indicate that increased expression of pig CD59, which is normally modestly expressed, on donor endothelial cells protect the cells equally well as human CD59 (147), indicating that homologous restriction may not be critical, but rather the amount of regulator expressed. The fact that organs from pigs transgenic for human complement regulatory proteins are protected against hyperacute rejection does not imply that vascular endothelial cells of the graft are not activated, a process that may have consequences for the fate of the organ. Such activation may take place due to an insufficient density or clustering of regulator proteins on the surface. Thus, the application of soluble complement inhibitors may be beneficial as adjuvant therapy even if the transplanted organ is transgenic for complement regulators.

Although the problem of hyperacute rejection is principally solved by interventions as described above, an acute vascular rejection (148), alternatively called delayed xenograft rejection (149), occurs after hours to a few days. The molecular mechanisms of acute vascular xenograft rejection (AVR) are only partly understood, but the impact of antibodies, naturally occurring and elicited, is well documented (150, 151). Furthermore, cumulative data support a role for macrophages and natural killer cells in this process (152-154). Until recently, it has been questioned if complement is of any importance in acute vascular rejection. This view is currently being revisited by several recent studies. In a porcine-to-primate transplantation experiment using human DAF transgenic kidneys, acute vascular rejection was associated with binding of elicited antibodies and a substantial classical pathway activation (155). In a similar model acute vascular rejection was reversed by treating the recipient with C1-inhibitor (156). Inhibition of complement by soluble complement receptor type 1 (sCR1) combined with immunosuppression delayed the occurrence of AVR of porcine hearts transplanted to cynomolgus monkeys (157). Furthermore, hDAF-transgenic porcine kidneys transplanted to cynomolgus monkeys were to some extent protected against AVR (158). In contrast to hyperacute rejection, acute vascular rejection is characterized by type II endothelial cell activation with induction of E-selectin expression and release of various chemo- and cytokines. Terminal complement pathway activation induces such changes in porcine endothelial cells exposed to human serum (159, 160). This endothelial cell activation was found to be efficiently inhibited using various specific complement inhibitors (161). In a recent review, Dorling summarized the pathogenesis of acute vascular rejection as follows: antibodies are always involved and antibody-mediated rejection may be either complement-dependent or complement-independent. In contrast, the role for antibody- and complement-independent cellular reactions are still uncertain since the observations are derived from experiments with small animal models (162).

Cellular and chronic graft rejections are well known from allotransplantation, the former usually being restrained by immunosuppressive regimens, whereas the latter is related to an intractable and slowly progressing vasculopathy. Analogous rejections are likely to occur in xenotransplantation, but for obvious reasons limited amounts of data are available. Classical immunosuppressive regimens have resulted in experimental long-time organ survival in pig-to-primate models, but are still limited to a few months observation period (163). The future ultimate goal for success in xenotransplantation, as in allotransplantation, will be the achievement of specific tolerance of the recipient to the donor tissue. This will prevent elicited immunological reactions leading to acute and chronic rejection. However, the hyperacute antibody- and complement-mediated xenograft rejection mediated by naturally occurring antibodies cannot be prevented by tolerization and needs to be dealt with by other regimens, as discussed above.

Accommodation is a peculiar phenomenon, first realised after ABO-incompatible allotransplantation, where the graft was accepted despite the reoccurrence of antibodies and a functional complement system. Accommodation is different from immunological tolerance, although the net effect is similar. Achievement of accommodation has been a goal for xenotransplantation research to enable long-time survival (164). The endothelial cell is crucial in the achievement of accommodation and different underlying mechanisms have been postulated (165). Whether accommodation will be an alternative or a supplement to tolerance to achieve successful xenotransplatation remains to be clarified.

6.   CONCLUDING REMARKS

There is compelling evidence that complement, although to different degrees, contributes to post-transplantation graft rejection. However, despite convincing studies on the value of complement diagnosis in early recognition of rejection episodes, complement analysis still lacks acceptance to be generally included in post-transplantation immune monitoring, except for renal C4d deposition. Numerous animal models and first clinical trials demonstrate the potential value of therapeutic complement inhibition in the management of rejection episodes. Although our knowledge on the role of complement in xenograft rejection has substantially increased, leading to powerful intervention strategies, e.g. by generation of animals transgenic for human mCRP, risk of infection, lack of anatomical and metabolic compatibilities and ethical issues have raised concerns which need to be carefully addressed before realizing xenotransplantation.

7.   REFERENCES

1. Raeder RH, Badylak SF, Sheehan C, Kallakury B, Metzger DW. Natural anti-galactose alpha 1,3 galactose antibodies delay, but do not prevent the acceptance of extracellular matrix xenografts. Transpl Immunol 2002;10:15-24.
2. Moberg L, Johansson H, Lukinius A, Berne C, Foss A, Kallen R, Ostraat O, Salmela K, Tibell A, Tufveson G, Elgue G, Ekdahl KN, Korsgren O, Nilsson B. Production of tissue factor by pancreatic islet cells as a trigger of detrimental thrombotic reactions in clinical islet transplantation. Lancet 2002;360:2039-45.
3. Mckenzie IFC, Koulmanda M, Mandel TE, Sandrin MS. Pig islet xenografts are susceptible to "anti-pig" but not Gal alpha(1,3)Gal antibody plus complement in gal o/o mice. J Immunol 1998;161:5116-9.
4. Schaapherder AFM, Wolvekamp MCJ, Tebulte MTJW, Bouwman E, Gooszen HG, Daha MR. Porcine islet cells of Langerhans are destroyed by human complement and not by antibody-dependent cell-mediated mechanisms. Transplantation 1996;62:29-33.
5. Mirenda V, Lemauff B, Cassard A, Huvelin JM, Boeffard F, Faivre A, Soulillou JP, Anegon I. Intact pig pancreatic islet function in the presence of human xenoreactive natural antibody binding and complement activation. Transplantation 1997;63:1452-62.
6. Bennet W, Sundberg B, Lundgren T, Tibell A, Groth CG, Richards A, White DJ, Elgue G, Larsson R, Nilsson B, Korsgren O. Damage to porcine islets of Langerhans after exposure to human blood in vitro, or after intraportal transplantation to cynomologus monkeys - Protective effects of sCR1 and heparin. Transplantation 2000;69:711-9.
7. Schmidt P, Goto M, Lemauff B, Anegon I, Korsgren O. Adenovirus-mediated expression of human CD55 or CD59 protects adult porcine islets from complement-mediated, cell lysis by human serum. Transplantation 2003;75:697-702.
8. deVos P, Hamel AF, Tatarkiewicz K. Considerations for successful transplantation of encapsulated pancreatic islets. Diabetologia 2002;45:159-73.

9. Rayat GR, Rajotte RV, Ao ZL, Korbutt GS. Microencapsulation of neonatal porcine islets: Protection from human antibody/complement-mediated cytolysis in vitro and long-term reversal of diabetes in nude mice. Transplantation 2000;69:1084-90.

10. Darquy S, Pueyo ME, Capron F, Reach G. Complement activation by alginate-polylysine microcapsules used for islet transplantation. Artif Organs 1994;18:898-903.

11. Kulseng B, SkjakBraek G, Ryan L, Andersson A, King A, Faxvaag A, Espevik T. Transplantation of alginate microcapsules - Generation of antibodies against alginates and encapsulated porcine islet-like cell clusters. Transplantation 1999;67:978-84.

12. Hammerman MR. Transplantation of embryonic kidneys. Clin Sci 2002;103:599-612.

13. Hughes RD, Nicolaou N, Langley PG, Ellis AJ, Wendon JA, Williams R. Plasma cytokine levels and coagulation and complement activation during use of the extracorporeal liver assist device in acute liver failure. Artif Organs 1998;22:854-8.

14. Esch JSA, Hamann D, Soltau M, Zante B, Jungbluth M, Sputek A, Nierhaus A, Hillert C, Broering DC, Rogiers X. Human antibody deposition, complement activation, and DNA fragmentation are observed for porcine hepatocytes in a clinically applied bioartificial liver assist system. Transplant Proc 2002;34:2321

15. Nyberg SL, Yagi T, Matsushita T, Hardin J, Grande JP, Gibson LE, Platt JL. Membrane barrier of a porcine hepatocyte bioartificial liver. Liver Transpl 2003;9:298-305.

16. Lucchesi BR, Kilgore KS. Complement inhibitors in myocardial ischemia/reperfusion injury. Immunopharmacology 1997;38:27-42.

17. Dong J, Pratt JR, Smith RAG, Dodd I, Sacks SH. Strategies for targeting complement inhibitors in ischaemia/reperfusion injury. Mol Immunol 1999;36:957-63.

18. Monsinjon T, Richard V, Fontaine M. Complement and its implications in cardiac ischemia/reperfusion: strategies to inhibit complement. Fundam Clin Pharmacol 2001;15:293-306.

19. Atkinson JP, Farries T. Separation of self from non-self in the complement system. Immunol Today 1987;8:212-5.

20. Matsuo S, Ichida S, Takizawa H, Okada N, Baranyi L, Iguchi A, Morgan BP, Okada H. In vivo effects of monoclonal antibodies that functionally inhibit complement regulatory proteins in rats. J Exp Med 1994;180:1619-27.

21. Weiser MR, Williams JP, Moore FD, Kobzik L, Ma MH, Hechtman HB, Carroll MC. Reperfusion injury of ischemic skeletal muscle is mediated by natural antibody and complement. J Exp Med 1996;183:2343-8.

22. Williams JP, Pechet TTV, Weiser MR, Reid R, Kobzik L, Moore FD, Carroll MC, Hechtman HB. Intestinal reperfusion injury is mediated by IgM and complement. J Appl Physiol 1999;86:938-42.

23. Buerke M, Murohara T, Lefer AM. Cardioprotective effects of a C1 esterase inhibitor in myocardial ischemia and reperfusion. Circulation 1995;91:393-402.

24. Zhang Y, Suankratay C, Zhang XH, Lint TF, Gewurz H. Lysis via the lectin pathway of complement activation: minireview and lectin pathway enhancement of endotoxin-initiated hemolysis. Immunopharmacology 1999;42:81-90.

25. Collard CD, Vakeva A, Morrissey MA, Agah A, Rollins SA, Reenstra WR, Buras JA, Meri S, Stahl GL. Complement activation after oxidative stress - Role of the lectin complement pathway. Am J Pathol 2000;156:1549-56.

26. Jordan JE, Montalto MC, Stahl GL. Inhibition of mannose-binding lectin reduces postischemic myocardial reperfusion injury. Circulation 2001;104:1413-8.

27. Boyle EM, Pohlman TH, Cornejo CJ, Verrier ED. Ischemia-reperfusion injury. Ann Thorac Surg 1997;64:S24-S30

28. Nagano H, Tilney NL. Chronic allograft failure: the clinical problem. Am J Med Sci 1997;313:305-9.

29. Dragun D, Hoff U, Park JK, Qun Y, Schneider W, Luft FC, Haller H. Ischemia-reperfusion injury in renal transplantation is independent of the immunologic background. Kidney Int 2000;58:2166-77.

30. Naka Y, Marsh HC, Scesney SM, Oz MC, Pinsky DJ. Complement activation as a cause for primary graft failure in an isogeneic rat model of hypothermic lung preservation and transplantation. Transplantation 1997;64:1248-55.

31. Scherer M, Demertzis S, Langer F, Moritz A, Schafers HJ. C1-esterase inhibitor reduces reperfusion injury after lung transplantation. Ann Thorac Surg 2002;73:233-8.

32. Nydegger UE, Carrel T, Laumonier T, Mohacsi P. New concepts in organ preservation. Transpl Immunol 2002;9:215-25.

33. Parolari A, Rubini P, Cannata A, Bonati L, Alamanni F, Tremoli E, Biglioli P. Endothelial damage during myocardial preservation and storage. Ann Thorac Surg 2002;73:682-90.

34. Roodnat JI, Mulder PGH, vanRiemsdijk IC, Izermans JNM, vanGelder T, Weimar W. Ischemia times and donor serum creatinine in relation to renal graft failure. Transplantation 2003;75:799-804.

35. Bergamaschini L, Gobbo G, Gatti S, Caccamo L, Prato P, Maggioni M, Braidotti P, Di Stefano R, Fassati LR. Endothelial targeting with C1-inhibitor reduces complement activation in vitro and during ex vivo reperfusion of pig liver. Clin Exp Immunol 2001;126:412-20.

36. Bergamaschini L, Gatti S, Caccamo L, Prato P, Latham L, Trezza P, Maggioni M, Gobbo G, Fassati LR. C1 inhibitor potentiates the protective effect of organ preservation solution on endothelial cells during cold storage. Transplant Proc 2001;33:939-41.

37. Baldwin WM, Larsen CP, Fairchild RL. Innate immune responses to transplants: A significant variable with cadaver donors. Immunity 2001;14:369-76.

38. Baldwin WM, III, Qian Z, Ota H, Samaniego M, Wasowska B, Sanfilippo F, Hruban RH. Complement as a mediator of vascular inflammation and activation in allografts. J Heart Lung Transplant 2000;19:723-30.

39. Pratt JR, Harmer AW, Levin J, Sacks SH. Influence of complement on the allospecific antibody response to a primary vascularized organ graft. Eur J Immunol 1997;27:2848-53.

40. Pratt JR, Abe K, Miyazaki M, Zhou W, Sacks SH. In situ localization of C3 synthesis in experimental acute renal allograft rejection. Amer J Pathol 2000;157:825-31.

41. Marsh JE, Farmer CKT, Jurcevic S, Wang Y, Carroll MC, Sacks SH. The allogeneic T and B cell response is strongly dependent on complement components C3 and C4. Transplantation 2001;72:1310-8.

42. Pratt JR, Basheer SA, Sacks SH. Local synthesis of complement component C3 regulates acute renal transplant rejection. Nature Med 2002;8:582-7.

43. Regele H, Bohmig GA. Tissue injury and repair in allografts: novel perspectives. Curr Opin Nephrol Hypertens 2003;12:259-66.

44. Kato M, Morozumi K, Takeuchi O, Oikawa T, Koyama K, Usami T, Shimano Y, Ito A, Horike K, Otsuka Y, Toda S, Takeda A, Uchida K, Haba T, Kimura G. Complement fragment C4d deposition in peritubular capillaries in acute humoral rejection after ABO blood group-incompatible human kidney transplantation. Transplantation 2003;75:663-5.

45. Feucht HE. Complement C4d in graft capillaries -- the missing link in the recognition of humoral alloreactivity. Am J Transplant 2003;3:646-52.

46. Feucht HE, Schneeberger H, Hillebrand G, Burkhardt K, Weiss M, Riethmuller G, Land W, Albert E. Capillary deposition of C4d complement fragment and early renal graft loss. Kidney Int 1993;43:1333-8.

47. Crespo M, Pascual M, TolkoffRubin N, Mauiyyedi S, Collins AB, Fitzpatrick D, Farrell ML, Williams WW, Delmonico FL, Cosimi AB, Colvin RB, Saidman SL. Acute humoral rejection in renal allograft recipients: I. Incidence, serology and clinical characteristics. Transplantation 2001;71:652-8.

48. Mauiyyedi S, Crespo M, Collins AB, Schneeberger EE, Pascual MA, Saidman SL, Tolkoff-Rubin NE, Williams WW, Delmonico FL, Cosimi AB, Colvin RB. Acute humoral rejection in kidney transplantation: II. Morphology, immunopathology, and pathologic classification. J Am Soc Nephrol 2002;13:779-87.

49. Magil AB, Tinckam K. Monocytes and peritubular capillary C4d deposition in acute renal allograft rejection. Kidney Int 2003;63:1888-93.

50. Haas M, Ratner LE, Montgomery RA. C4D staining of perioperative renal transplant biopsies. Transplantation 2002;74:711-7.

51. Regele H, Bohmig GA, Habicht A, Gollowitzer D, Schillinger M, Rockenschaub S, Watschinger B, Kerjaschki D, Exner M. Capillary deposition of complement split product C4d in renal allografts is associated with basement membrane injury in peritubular and glomerular capillaries: A contribution of humoral immunity to chronic allograft rejection. J Amer Soc Nephrol 2002;13:2371-80.

52. Platt JL. C4d and the fate of organ allografts. J Amer Soc Nephrol 2002;13:2417-9.

53. Watschinger B, Pascual M. Capillary C4d deposition as a marker of humoral immunity in renal allograft rejection. J Amer Soc Nephrol 2002;13:2420-3.

54. Nickeleit V, Zeiler M, Gudat F, Thiel G, Mihatsch MJ. Detection of the complement degradation product C4d in renal allografts: Diagnostic and therapeutic implications. J Amer Soc Nephrol 2002;13:242-51.

55. Lederer SR, Kluth-Pepper B, Schneeberger H, Albert E, Land W, Feucht HE. Impact of humoral alloreactivity early after transplantation on the long-term survival of renal allografts. Kidney Int 2001;59:334-41.

56. Bohmig GA, Exner M, Watschinger B, Regele H. Acute humoral renal allograft rejection. Curr Opin Urol 2002;12:95-9.

57. Herzenberg AM, Gill JS, Djurdjev O, Magil AB. C4d deposition in acute rejection: An independent long- term prognostic factor. J Amer Soc Nephrol 2002;13:234-41.

58. Bohmig GA, Exner M, Habicht A, Schillinger M, Lang U, Kletzmayr J, Saemann MD, Horl WH, Watschinger B, Regele H. Capillary C4d deposition in kidney allografts: a specific marker of alloantibody-dependent graft injury. J Am Soc Nephrol 2002;13:1091-9.

59. Mauiyyedi S, Colvin RB. Humoral rejection in kidney transplantation: new concepts in diagnosis and treatment. Curr Opin Nephrol Hypertens 2002;11:609-18.

60. Halloran PF, Schlaut J, Solez K, Srinivasa NS. The significance of the anti-class I response. II. Clinical and pathologic features of renal transplants with anti-class I-like antibody. Transplantation 1992;53:550-5.

61. Trpkov K, Campbell P, Pazderka F, Cockfield S, Solez K, Halloran PF. Pathologic features of acute renal allograft rejection associated with donor-specific antibody. Analysis using the Banff grading schema. Transplantation 1996;61:1586-92.

62. Feucht HE, Felber E, Gokel MJ, Hillebrand G, Nattermann U, Brockmeyer C, Held E, Riethmuller G, Land W, Albert E. Vascular deposition of complement-split products in kidney allografts with cell-mediated rejection. Clin Exp Immunol 1991;86:464-70.

63. Collins AB, Schneeberger EE, Pascual MA, Saidman SL, Williams WW, Tolkoff-Rubin N, Cosimi AB, Colvin RB. Complement activation in acute humoral renal

allograft rejection: Diagnostic significance of C4d deposits in peritubular capillaries. J Amer Soc Nephrol 1999;10:2208-14.

64. Svalander C, Hedman L, Nyberg G, Eggertsen G, Nilsson B, Nilsson U. Local C3 activation and macrophage accumulation in renal allografts with early vascular rejection. Transplant Proc 1992;24:305-6.

65. Eggertsen G, Nyberg G, Nilsson B, Nilsson U, Svalander CT. Complement deposition in renal allografts with early malfunction. APMIS 2001;109:825-34.

66. Sund S, Hovig T, Reisæter AV, Scott H, Bentdal Ø, Mollnes TE. Complement activation in early protocol kidney graft biopsies after living-donor transplantation. Transplantation 2003;75:1204-13.

67. Kirschfink M, Wienert T, Rother K, Pomer S. Complement Activation in Renal Allograft Recipients. Transplant Proc 1992;24:2556-7.

68. Muller TF, Kraus M, Neumann C, Lange H. Detection of renal allograft rejection by complement components C5A and TCC in plasma and urine. J Lab Clin Med 1997;129:62-71.

69. Bechtel U, Scheuer R, Landgraf R, Konig A, Feucht HE. Assessment of soluble adhesion molecules (sICAM-1, sVCAM-1, sELAM-1) and complement cleavage products (sC4d, sC5b-9) in urine - Clinical monitoring of renal allograft recipients. Transplantation 1994;58:905-11.

70. Behr TM, Feucht HE, Richter K, Reiter C, Spes CH, Pongratz D, Uberfuhr P, Meiser B, Theisen K, Angermann CE. Detection of humoral rejection in human cardiac allografts by assessing the capillary deposition of complement fragment C4d in endomyocardial biopsies. J Heart Lung Transplant 1999;18:904-12.

71. Baldwin WM, Samaniego-Picota M, Kasper EK, Clark AM, Czader M, Rohde C, Zachary AA, Sanfilippo F, Hruban RH. Complement deposition in early cardiac transplant biopsies is associated with ischemic injury and subsequent rejection episodes. Transplantation 1999;68:894-900.

72. Brauer RB, Baldwin WM, Ibrahim S, Sanfilippo F. The contribution of terminal complement components to acute and hyperacute allograft rejection in the rat. Transplantation 1995;59:288-93.

73. Qian ZP, Wasowska BA, Behrens E, Cangello DL, Brody JR, Kadkol SS, Horwitz L, Liu JH, Lowenstein C, Hess AD, Sanfilippo F, Baldwin WM. C6 produced by macrophages contributes to cardiac allograft rejection. Amer J Pathol 1999;155:1293-302.

74. Qian Z, Jakobs FM, Pfaff-Amesse T, Sanfilippo F, Baldwin WM3. Complement contributes to the rejection of complete and class I major histocompatibility complex--incompatible cardiac allografts. J Heart Lung Transplant 1998;17:470-8.

75. Qian ZP, Hu WM, Liu JH, Sanfilippo F, Hruban RH, Baldwin WM. Accelerated graft arteriosclerosis in cardiac transplants - Complement activation promotes progression of lesions from medium to large arteries. Transplantation 2001;72:900-6.

76. Klima U, Kutschka I, Warnecke G, Kim P, Struber M, Kirschfink M, Haverich A. Improved right ventricular function after intracoronary administration of a C1 esterase inhibitor in a right heart transplantation model. Eur J Cardiothorac Surg 2000;18:321-7.

77. Zamora MR, Davis RD, Keshavjee SH, Schulman L, Levin J, Ryan U, Patterson GA. Complement inhibition attenuates human lung transplant reperfusion injury - A multicenter trial. Chest 1999;116:46S

78. Struber M, Hagl C, Hirt SW, Cremer J, Harringer W, Haverich A. C1-esterase inhibitor in graft failure after lung transplantation. Intensive Care Med 1999;25:1315-8.

79. Pierson RN, Loyd JE, Goodwin A, Majors D, Dummer JS, Mohacsi P, Wheeler A, Bovin N, Miller GG, Olson S, Johnson J, Rieben R, Azimzadeh A. Successful management of an ABO-mismatched lung allograft using antigen-specific immunoadsorption, complement inhibition, and immunomodulatory therapy. Transplantation 2002;74:79-84.

80. Magro CM, Deng A, PopeHarman A, Waldman WJ, Collins AB, Adams PW, Kelsey M, Ross P. Humorally mediated posttransplantation septal capillary injury syndrome as a common form of pulmonary allograft rejection: A hypothesis. Transplantation 2002;74:1273-80.

81. Nakashima S, Qian ZP, Rahimi S, Wasowska BA, Baldwin WM. Membrane attack complex contributes to destruction of vascular integrity in acute lung allograft rejection. J Immunol 2002;169:4620-7.

82. Stammberger U, Hamacher J, Hillinger S, Schmid RA. sCR1sLe(X) ameliorates ischemia/reperfusion injury in experimental lung transplantation. J Thorac Cardiovasc Surg 2000;120:1078-84.

83. Salvatierra A, Velasco F, Rodriguez M, Alvarez A, Lopez-Pedrera R, Ramirez R, Carracedo J, Lopez-Rubio F, Lopez-Pujol A, Guerrero R. C1-esterase inhibitor prevents early pulmonary dysfunction after lung transplantation in the dog. Am J Respir Crit Care Med 1997;155:1147-54.

84. Kallio EA, Lemstrom KB, Hayry PJ, Ryan US, Koskinen PK. Blockade of complement inhibits obliterative bronchiolitis in rat tracheal allografts. Amer J Respir Crit Care Med 2000;161:1332-9.

85. Wolpl A, Robin-Winn M, Pichlmayr R, Goldmann SF. Fourth component of complement (C4) polymorphism in human orthotopic liver transplantation. Transplantation 1985;40:154-7.

86. Koskimies S, Lokki ML, Hockerstedt K. Changes in plasma complement C4 and factor B allotypes after liver transplantation. Complement Inflamm 1991;8:257-60.

87. Remuzzi G, Ruggenenti P, Codazzi D, Noris M, Caprioli J, Locatelli G, Gridelli B. Combined kidney and liver transplantation for familial haemolytic uraemic syndrome. Lancet 2002;359:1671-2.

88. Pfeifer PH, Brems JJ, Brunson M, Hugli TE. Plasma C3a and C4a levels in liver transplant recipients: a longitudinal study. Immunopharmacology 2000;46:163-74.

89. Ronholm E, Tomasdottir H, Runeborg J, Bengtsson A, Bengtson JP, Stenqvist O, Friman S. Complement system activation during orthotopic liver transplantation in man - Indications of peroperative complement system activation in the gut. Transplantation 1994;57:1594-7.

90. Scoazec JY, BorghiScoazec G, Durand F, Bernuau J, Pham BN, Belghiti J, Feldmann G, Degott C. Complement activation after ischemia-reperfusion in human liver allografts: Incidence and pathophysiological relevance. Gastroenterology 1997;112:908-18.

91. Lautenschlager I, Hockerstedt K, Meri S. Complement membrane attack complex and protectin (CD59) in liver allografts during acute rejection. J Hepatol 1999;31:537-41.

92. Scholz T, Solberg R, Okkenhaug C, Videm V, Gallimore MJ, Mathisen O, Mollnes TE, Bergan A, Soreide O, Klintmalm GB, Aasen AO. The significance of heparin-coated veno-venous bypass circuits in liver transplantation. Perfusion 2002;17:45-50.

93. Segal H, Sheikh S, Kallis P, Cottam S, Beard C, Potter D, Townsend E, Bidstrup BP, Yacoub M, Hunt BJ. Complement activation during major surgery: the effect of extracorporeal circuits and high-dose aprotinin. J Cardiothorac Vasc Anesth 1998;12:542-7.

94. Sadallah S, Giostra E, Mentha G, Schifferli JA. Increased levels of soluble complement receptor 1 in serum of patients with liver diseases. Hepatology 1996;24:118-22.
95. Scoazec JY, Delautier D, Moreau A, Durand F, Degott C, Benhamou JP, Belghiti J, Feldmann G. Expression of complement-regulatory proteins in normal and UW-preserved human liver. Gastroenterology 1994;107:505-16.
96. Chiang KC, Goto S, Chen CL, Lin CL, Lin YC, Pan TL, Lord R, Lai CY, Tseng HP, Hsu LW, Lee TH, Yokoyama H, Kunimatsu M, Chiang YC, Hashimoto T. Clusterin may be involved in rat liver allograft tolerance. Transpl Immunol 2000;8:95-9.
97. Lehmann TG, Koeppel TA, Kirschfink M, Gebhard MM, Herfarth C, Otto G, Post S. Complement inhibition by soluble complement receptor type 1 improves microcirculation after rat liver transplantation. Transplantation 1998;66:717-22.
98. Lehmann TG, Heger M, Munch S, Kirschfink M, Klar E. In vivo microscopy reveals that complement inhibition by C1-esterase inhibitor reduces ischemia/reperfusion injury in the liver. Transpl Int 2000;13 Suppl 1:S547-S550
99. Marx G, Nashan B, Cobas MM, Vangerow B, Schlitt HJ, Ziesing S, Leuwer M, Piepenbrock S, Rueckoldt H. Septic shock after liver transplantation for Caroli's disease: clinical improvement after treatment with C1-esterase inhibitor. Intensive Care Med 1999;25:1017-20.
100. Sachs DH, Sykes M, Robson SC, Cooper DKC. Xenotransplantation. Advances in Immunology, 2001;79:129-223.
101. Hammer C, Thein E. Physiological aspects of xenotransplantation, 2001. Xenotransplantation 2002;9:303-5.
102. Samstein B, Platt JL. Physiologic and immunologic hurdles to xenotransplantation. J Amer Soc Nephrol 2001;12:182-93.
103. Platt JL. Xenotransplantation - New risks, new gains. Nature 2000;407:27-30.
104. Hammer C, Linke R, Wagner F, Diefenbeck M. Organs from animals for man. Int Arch Allergy Immunol 1998;116:5-21.
105. Bach FH. Xenotransplantation: Problems and prospects. Annu Rev Med 1998;49:301-10.
106. Auchincloss H, Sachs DH. Xenogeneic transplantation. Annu Rev Immunol 1998;16:433-70.
107. Lawson JH, Platt JL. Molecular barriers to xenotransplantation. Transplantation 1996;62:303-10.
108. Dorling A, Riesbeck K, Warrens A, Lechler R. Clinical xenotransplantation of solid organs. Lancet 1997;349:867-71.
109. Cooper DKC, Gollackner B, Sachs DH. Will the pig solve the transplantation backlog? Annu Rev Med 2002;53:133-47.
110. Dorling A. Strategies for preventing porcine xenograft rejection: recent progress and future developments. Expert Opin Ther Patents 1997;7:1307-19.
111. Daniels LJ, Platt JL. Hyperacute xenograft rejection as an immunologic barrier to xenotransplantation. Kidney Int 1997;58:S28-S35
112. Malassagne B, Calmus Y, Houssin D, Weill B. Xenotransplantation: pathophysiology of hyperacute rejection and therapeutic perspectives. Pathol Biol 2000;48:377-82.
113. Galili U. Evolution and pathophysiology of the human natural anti-alpha- galactosyl IgG (anti-Gal) antibody. Springer Semin Immunopathol 1993;15:155-71.
114. Galili U. The alpha-gal epitope (Gal alpha 1-3Gal beta 1-4GlcNAc-R) in xenotransplantation. Biochimie 2001;83:557-63.
115. Parker W, Bruno D, Holzknecht ZE, Platt JL. Characterization and affinity isolation of xenoreactive human natural antibodies. J Immunol 1994;153:3791-803.

116. Byrne GW, Schwarz A, Fesi JR, Birch P, Nepomich A, Bakaj I, Velardo MA, Jiang C, Manzi A, Dintzis H, Diamond LE, Logan JS. Evaluation of different alpha-galactosyl glycoconjugates for use in xenotransplantation. Bioconjugate Chemistry 2002;13:571-81.

117. Kobayashi T, Yokoyama I, Morozumi K, Nagasaka T, Hayashi S, Uchida K, Takagi H, Nakao A. Comparative study of the efficacy of removal of anti-ABO and anti-gal antibodies by double filtration plasmapheresis. Xenotransplantation 2000;7:101-8.

118. Brenner P, Reichenspurner H, Schmoeckel M, Wimmer C, Rucker A, Eder V, Meiser B, Hinz M, Felbinger T, Hammer C, Reichart B. Prevention of hyperacute xenograft rejection in orthotopic xenotransplantation of pig hearts into baboons using immunoadsorption of antibodies and complement factors. Transpl Int 2000;13 Suppl 1:S508-S517

119. Lucchiari N, Azimzadeh A, Wolf P, Regnault V, Cinqualbre J. In vivo and in vitro optimization of depletion of IgM and IgG xenoantibodies by immunoadsorption using cell membrane proteins. Artif Organs 1997;21:278-86.

120. Xu Y, Lorf T, Sablinski T, Gianello P, Bailin M, Monroy R, Kozlowski T, Awwad M, Cooper DKC, Sachs DH. Removal of anti-porcine natural antibodies from human and nonhuman primate plasma in vitro and in vivo by a Gal alpha 1- 3Gal beta 1-4 beta Glc-X immunoaffinity column. Transplantation 1998;65:172-9.

121. Ogawa H, Kobayashi T, Yokoyama I, Nagatani N, Mizuno M, Yoshida J, Kadomatsu K, Muramatsu H, Nakao A, Muramatsu T. Reduction of alpha-galactosyl xenoantigen by expression of endo-beta-galactosidase C in pig endothelial cells. Xenotransplantation 2002;9:290-6.

122. Vanhove B, Charreau B, Cassard A, Pourcel C, Soulillou JP. Intracellular expression in pig cells of anti-alpha 1,3galactosyltransferase single-chain Fv antibodies reduces Gal alpha 1,3Gal expression and inhibits cytotoxicity mediated by anti-Gal xenoantibodies. Transplantation 1998;66:1477-85.

123. Sepp A, Farrar CA, Dorling T, Cairns T, George AJT, Lechler RI. Inhibition of expression of the Gal alpha 1-3Gal epitope on porcine cells using an intracellular single-chain antibody directed against alpha 1,3Galactosyltransferase. J Immunol Method 1999;231:191-205.

124. Chen CG, Fisicaro N, Shinkel TA, Aitken V, Katerelos M, vanDenderen BJW, Tange MJ, Crawford RJ, Robins AJ, Pearse MJ, Dapice AJF. Reduction in Gal-alpha 1,3-Gal epitope expression in transgenic mice expressing human H-transferase. Xenotransplantation 1996;3:69-75.

125. Sharma A, Okabe J, Birch P, McClellan SB, Martin MJ, Platt JL, Logan JS. Reduction in the level of Gal(alpha 1,3)Gal in transgenic mice and pigs by the expression of an alpha(1,2)fucosyltransferase. Proc Natl Acad Sci USA 1996;93:7190-5.

126. Osman N, Mckenzie IFC, Ostenried K, Ioannou YA, Desnick RJ, Sandrin MS. Combined transgenic expression of alpha-galactosidase and alpha 1,2-fucosyltransferase leads to optimal reduction in the major xenoepitope Gal alpha(1,3)Gal. Proc Natl Acad Sci USA 1997;94:14677-82.

127. Costa C, Zhao L, Burton WV, Rosas C, Bondioli KR, Williams BL, Hoagland TA, Dalmasso AP, Fodor WL. Transgenic pigs designed to express human CD59 and H-transferase to avoid humoral xenograft rejection. Xenotransplantation 2002;9:45-57.

128. Lai LX, KolberSimonds D, Park KW, Cheong HT, Greenstein JL, Im GS, Samuel M, Bonk A, Rieke A, Day BN, Murphy CN, Carter DB, Hawley RJ, Prather RS. Production of alpha-1,3-galactosyltransferase knockout pigs by nuclear transfer cloning. Science 2002;295:1089-92.

128. Lai LX, KolberSimonds D, Park KW, Cheong HT, Greenstein JL, Im GS, Samuel M, Bonk A, Rieke A, Day BN, Murphy CN, Carter DB, Hawley RJ, Prather RS. Production of alpha-1,3-galactosyltransferase knockout pigs by nuclear transfer cloning. Science 2002;295:1089-92.
129. Phelps CJ, Koike C, Vaught TD, Boone J, Wells KD, Chen SH, Ball S, Specht SM, Polejaeva IA, Monahan JA, Jobst PM, Sharma SB, Lamborn AE, Garst AS, Moore M, Demetris AJ, Rudert WA, Bottino R, Bertera S, Trucco M, Starzl TE, Dai YF, Ayares DL. Production of alpha 1,3-galactosyltransferase-deficient pigs. Science 2003;299:411-4.
130. Sharma A, Naziruddin B, Cui C, Martin MJ, Xu H, Wan H, Lei Y, Harrison C, Yin J, Okabe J, Mathews C, Stark A, Adams CS, Houtz J, Wiseman BS, Byrne GW, Logan JS. Pig cells that lack the gene for alpha 1-3 galactosyltransferase express low levels of the gal antigen. Transplantation 2003;75:430-6.
131. Welsh RM, ODonnell CL, Reed DJ, Rother RP. Evaluation of the Gal alpha 1-3Gal epitope as a host modification factor eliciting natural humoral immunity to enveloped viruses. J Virol 1998;72:4650-6.
132. Tanemura M, Ogawa H, Yin DP, Chen ZC, DiSesa VJ, Galili U. Elimination of anti-Gal B cells by alpha-Gal ricin. Transplantation 2002;73:1859-68.
133. Ogawa H, Yin DP, Shen JK, Galili U. Tolerance induction to a mammalian blood group-like carbohydrate antigen by syngeneic lymphocytes expressing the antigen. Blood 2003;101:2318-20.
134. Dorling A. Graft specific inhibition of complement activation after xenotransplantation; genetically modified pig organs versus systemic anticomplement strategies. Transplantation 2000;69:1033-4.
135. Roos A, Daha MR. Antibody-mediated activation of the classical complement pathway in xenograft rejection. Transpl Immunol 2002;9:257-70.
136. Wang H, Rollins SA, Gao ZH, Garcia B, Zhang Z, Xing JJ, Li L, Kellersmann R, Matis LA, Zhong R. Complement inhibition with an anti-C5 monoclonal antibody prevents hyperacute rejection in a xenograft heart transplantation model. Transplantation 1999;68:1643-51.
137. Brauer RB, Baldwin WM, Daha MR, Pruitt SK, Sanfilippo F. Use of C6-deficient rats to evaluate the mechanism of hyperacute rejection of discordant cardiac xenografts. J Immunol 1993;151:7240-8.
138. Alwayn IPJ, vanBockel HJ, Daha MR, Scheringa M. Hyperacute rejection in the guinea pig-to-rat model without formation of the membrane attack complex. Transpl Immunol 1999;7:177-82.
139. Kinoshita T. Protection of host from its own complement by membrane- bound complement inhibitors: C3 convertase inhibitors vs membrane attack complex inhibitors. Res Immunol 1996;147:100-3.
140. Liszewski MK, Farries TC, Lublin DM, Rooney IA, Atkinson JP. Control of the complement system. Adv Immunol 1996;61:201-83.
141. Asghar SS. Biology of disease - Membrane regulators of complement activation and their aberrant expression in disease. Lab Invest 1995;72:254-71.
142. Cozzi E, White DJG. The generation of transgenic pigs as potential organ donors for humans. Nature Med 1995;1:964-6.
143. Adams DH, Kadner A, Chen RH, Farivar RS. Human membrane cofactor protein (MCP, CD 46) protects transgenic pig hearts from hyperacute rejection in primates. Xenotransplantation 2001;8:36-40.
144. Fodor WL, Williams BL, Matis LA, Madri JA, Rollins SA, Knight JW, Velander W, Squinto SP. Expression of a functional human complement inhibitor in a transgenic pig

as a model for the prevention of xenogeneic hyperacute organ rejection. Proc Natl Acad Sci USA 1994;91:11153-7.

145. Diamond LE, Mccurry KR, Martin MJ, McClellan SB, Oldham ER, Platt JL, Logan JS. Characterization of transgenic pigs expressing functionally active human CD59 on cardiac endothelium. Transplantation 1996;61:1241-9.

146. Byrne G, Mccurry KR, Martin M, Platt J, Logan J. Development and analysis of transgenic pigs expressing the human complement regulatory proteins CD59 and DAF. Transplant Proc 1996;28:759

147. Maher SE, Pflugh DL, Larsen NJ, Rothschild MF, Bothwell ALM. Structure/function characterization of porcine CD59 - Expression, chromosomal mapping, complement-inhibition, and costimulatory activity. Transplantation 1998;66:1094-100.

148. Platt JL, Lin SS, McGregor CGA. Acute vascular rejection. Xenotransplantation 1998;5:169-75.

149. Bach FH, Winkler H, Ferran C, Hancock WW, Robson SC. Delayed xenograft rejection. Immunol Today 1996;17:379-84.

150. Lin SS, Weidner BC, Byrne GW, Diamond LE, Lawson JH, Hoopes CW, Daniels LJ, Daggett CW, Parker W, Harland RC, Davis RD, Bollinger RR, Logan JS, Platt JL. The role of antibodies in acute vascular rejection of pig- to- baboon cardiac transplants. J Clin Invest 1998;101:1745-56.

151. Sato K, Takigami K, Miyatake T, Czismadia E, Latinne D, Bazin H, Bach FH, Soares MP. Suppression of delayed xenograft rejection by specific depletion of elicited antibodies of the IgM isotype. Transplantation 1999;68:844-54.

152. Candinas D, Belliveau S, Koyamada N, Miyatake T, Hechenleitner P, Mark W, Bach FH, Hancock WW. T cell independence of macrophage and natural killer cell infiltration, cytokine production, and endothelial activation during delayed xenograft rejection. Transplantation 1996;62:1920-7.

153. Fryer JP, Chen S, Johnson E, Simone P, Sun LH, Goswitz JJ, Matas AJ. The role of monocytes and macrophages in delayed xenograft rejection. Xenotransplantation 1997;4:40-8.

154. Wu GS, Korsgren O, Vanrooijen N, Wennberg L, Tibell A. The effect of macrophage depletion on delayed xenograft rejection: studies in the guinea pig-to-C6-deficient rat heart transplantation model. Xenotransplantation 1999;6:262-70.

155. Loss M, Vangerow B, Schmidtko J, Kunz R, Jalali A, Arends H, Przemeck M, Ruckholt H, Leuwer M, Kaup FJ, Rensing S, Cozzi E, White DJ, Klempnauer J, Winkler M. Acute vascular rejection is associated with systemic complement activation in a pig-to-primate kidney xenograft model. Xenotransplantation 2000;7:186-96.

156. Vangerow B, Hecker JM, Lorenz R, Loss M, Przemeck M, Appiah R, Schmidtko J, Jalali A, Rueckoldt H, Winkler M. C1-inhibitor for treatment of acute vascular xenograft rejection in cynomolgus recipients of h-DAF transgenic porcine kidneys. Xenotransplantation 2001;8:266-72.

157. Davis EA, Pruitt SK, Greene PS, Ibrahim S, Lam TT, Levin JL, Baldwin WM, Sanfilippo F. Inhibition of complement, evoked antibody, and cellular response prevents rejection of pig-to-primate cardiac xenografts. Transplantation 1996;62:1018-23.

158. Zaidi A, Schmoeckel M, Bhatti F, Waterworth P, Tolan M, Cozzi E, Chavez G, Langford G, Thiru S, Wallwork J, White DJG, Friend P. Life-supporting pig-to-primate renal xenotransplantation using genetically modified donors. Transplantation 1998;65:1584-90.

159. Selvan RS, Kapadia HB, Platt JL. Complement-induced expression of chemokine genes in endothelium: Regulation by IL-1-dependent and -independent mechanisms. J Immunol 1998;161:4388-95.

160. Saadi S, Holzknecht RA, Patte CP, Platt JL. Endothelial cell activation by pore-forming structures - Pivotal role for interleukin-1 alpha. Circulation 2000;101:1867-73.

161. Sølvik UO, Haraldsen G, Fiane AE, Boretti E, Lambris JD, Fung M, Thorsby E, Mollnes TE. Human serum-induced expression of E-selectin on porcine aortic endothelial cells in vitro is totally complement mediated. Transplantation 2001;72:1967-73.

162. Dorling A. Are anti-endothelial cell antibodies a pre-requisite for the acute vascular rejection of xenografts? Xenotransplantation 2003;10:16-23.

163. Cozzi E, Bhatti F, Schmoeckel M, Chavez G, Smith KGC, Zaidi A, Bradley JR, Thiru S, Goddard M, Vial C, Ostlie D, Wallwork J, White DJG, Friend PJ. Long-term survival of nonhuman primates receiving life-supporting transgenic porcine kidney xenografts. Transplantation 2000;70:15-21.

164. Winkler H, Ferran C, Bach FH. Accomodation of xenografts: a concept revisited. Xenotransplantation 1995;2:53-6.

165. Platt JL. Recent Advances in Xenotransplantation. Presse Med 1992;21:1932-8.

PART 6

ROLE OF COMPLEMENT IN ACUTE CATASTROPHIC ILLNESSES

19

Role of Complement in Myocardial Ischemia and Infarction

Mary C. Walsh*, Melanie L. Hart*, Todd Bourcier, Deepak Bhole, Minoru Takahashi and Gregory L. Stahl
Center for Experimental Therapeutics and Reperfusion Injury,Department of Anesthesiology, Perioperative & Pain Medicine, Brigham and Women's Hospital, Boston, MA 02115

* co-authorship

Abstract: The complement system is involved in several aspects of the pathophysiology of myocardial ischemia and infarction. Initially a role for complement in ischemic heart disease was inferred from the deposition of complement components within the myocardium of experimental models of myocardial infarction. Further animal models demonstrated that depletion or inhibition of complement prior to myocardial ischemia/reperfusion (MI/R) can reduce complement-mediated tissue injury. Recently, in vivo examination of naturally occurring complement inhibitors and monoclonal antibodies directed at specific complement components has confirmed complement dependent injury following MI/R. Current research provides intriguing evidence on the initiating pathways and the possible methods of complement regulation in the management of MI/R injury. This chapter focuses on many of the studies demonstrating complement activation and deposition in MI/R, the functional consequences of complement activation following MI/R, the initial and recent anti-complement therapies used in vivo and the current insight of the mechanisms of complement activation following MI/R.

Key words: myocardial ischemia and reperfusion injury, complement, infarction, cardiovascular function

1. INTRODUCTION

Ischemic heart disease (IHD), including myocardial infarction and angina pectoris, account for 20% of all cardiovascular diseases (CVD), but disproportionately account for 54% of deaths from CVD. Despite a 25% decline in patient mortality over the past decade, IHD remains the number one cause of death in America (1). The evolution of reperfusion therapies has had a substantial impact on the effective treatment of IHD (2,3). The interventional tools of thrombolytics, bypass grafting and angioplasty efficiently reestablish coronary blood flow and alleviate ischemia, thus salvaging at-risk myocardium. The earlier coronary flow is reestablished, the greater the benefit in terms of limiting myocardial damage and infarct size. The clinical utility of reperfusion therapies has been tempered, however, by a host of events referred to as myocardial reperfusion injury (MI/R). Clinical manifestations of MI/R include the 'no-reflow' phenomena, myocardial stunning, and the onset of ventricular arrhythmias (4). There is evidence of 'lethal' MI/R, or reperfusion-induced death of cardiomyocytes that were initially viable at the time of reperfusion (5-7). MI/R also elicits a robust inflammatory response that may further expand tissue injury and adversely affect recovery of left ventricular (LV) function (8). Thus targeting the mechanisms of MI/R holds the promise of reducing ischemic myocardial injury, enhancing the efficacy of reperfusion therapy and improving post-ischemic myocardial function.

Considerable evidence supports the hypothesis that complement contributes to several aspects of the pathophysiology of MI/R (reviewed (9,10)). The complement system is a network of proteases, conserved through evolution, that execute innate immune responses and also participates in non-immune inflammatory processes (reviewed (11)). Several studies have shown complement deposition on damaged tissue in myocardial infarctions (12-15). Complement components induce proinflammatory genes, promote leukotaxis and transmigration, regulate apoptotic processes and cause direct cellular injury, all events associated with MI/R. However, the relative contribution of the classical, lectin, and alternative pathways of complement activation to MI/R, and the factors that trigger complement activation in MI/R, are still not completely understood. Nevertheless, results from experimental models of MI/R predict clinical benefits of inhibiting complement in the setting of interventional reperfusion. Results from ongoing clinical trials of cardiac surgery patients indeed validate complement as a viable target in the treatment of MI/R injury.

2. COMPLEMENT ACTIVATION AND DEPOSITION IN MI/R

The first studies to link the complement system in MI/R were performed by Hill and Ward who demonstrated in a rat model of permanent coronary artery occlusion that the ischemic heart produced a protease that cleaved C3 and stimulated leukocyte activation and chemotaxis (12,16). A subsequent study demonstrated that human serum levels of complement components C1, C2, C4 and C3 were significantly reduced within 24 to 48 hours after myocardial infarction (17). This reduction was likely due to the consumption of complement components following myocardial injury, since in vitro studies showed that complement was activated by heart subcellular membranes, especially mitochondrial membranes (18,19). Many investigators have since shown in both human and animal experimental models of myocardial ischemia that MBL, C1q, C3, C4, C5 and C5b-9 deposit within the myocardium (12,13,20-28). Time course analysis of deposition of the C1, C3, C8 and C9 components in post-ischemic myocardium indicated that complement components could be detected by immunofluorescence as early as 2-4 hours after ischemia (29). Deposition of the membrane attack complex (MAC), or C5b-9, has also been demonstrated in areas of cardiac damage in autopsy material derived from patients with myocardial infarctions (13). Furthermore, this finding was supported by a study which showed that CD59, an inhibitor of the MAC, was lost from the infarcted areas of the myocardium (24). Depletion or inhibition of complement has also been shown to attenuate MI/R injury (14,15,30). Complement activation in myocardial infarction is thus not a passive event, but indeed may be a critical mediator of inflammation and injury resulting from reperfusion of ischemic myocardium. Additionally, in human hearts, upregulation of both mRNAs and proteins for C1q, C1r, C1s, C2, C3, C4, C5, C6, C7, C8 and C9 were demonstrated in areas of both recent and old myocardial infarctions (31). Thus, local myocardial production of complement components may also contribute to MI/R.

3. FUNCTIONAL CONSEQUENCES OF COMPLEMENT ACTIVATION FOLLOWING MI/R

Complement-mediated injury in MI/R is predominately mediated by the direct and indirect activities of the anaphylatoxins C3a and C5a and by cytolytic C5b-9 (MAC) (32,33). Cleavage of C3 and C5 by convertases, results in the formation of local (34) and systemic (22,35) release of C3a and C5a. These anaphylatoxins increase smooth muscle tone and induce the release of mediators such as histamine and platelet-activating factor, thereby causing an increase in vascular permeability with subsequent cellular edema (36-39). Furthermore, elevated C3a and C5a following MI/R promote neutrophil activation and aggregation, whereas only C5a mediates neutrophil chemotaxis, release of reactive oxygen species, arachidonic acid metabolites and proteases (32,34,36,40-44). In addition to stimulating PMNs and chemotaxis, C5a may further amplify the inflammatory response by inducing production of macrophage inflammatory protein (MIP)-2, MIP-1α, MIP-1β, monocyte chemoattractant protein (MCP)-1, tumor necrosis factor-α (TNF-α), interleukin (IL)-1 and IL-6 (45-49).

Additionally, several lines of evidence suggest that the terminal complement complex, also known as MAC or C5b-9, plays an important role in myocardial ischemia. First, direct injury may be induced via assembly and deposition of the MAC on cell membranes in the ischemic myocardium after reperfusion (50). Other studies provide evidence that the MAC is a predominant factor causing myocardial injury via direct cell lysis by forming a pore in cellular membranes (51), and by eliciting a sudden influx of Ca^{2+} (52-54). An increase in intracellular Ca^{2+} during MI/R may be harmful to cardiomyocytes due to increased ATPase activity and uncoupling of oxidative phosphorylation in mitochondria (55,56). This rapid increase of calcium ions in the cytoplasm may also lead to cell signaling by the activation of calcium-dependent phospholipases and protein kinase C (57).

Second, the MAC promotes PMN activation and chemotaxis by inducing secretion of proinflammatory cytokines, IL-1α, IL-8 and MCP-1 (58). The MAC also initiates nuclear translocation of nuclear factor-κB (NF-κB) to stimulate the production of these proinflammatory cytokines as well as expression of adhesion molecules like ICAM-I (59,60). ICAM-1 expression in ischemic myocardium is upregulated during reperfusion and may promote the adherence and cytotoxic activity of PMNs (61-63). The MAC has also been shown to induce NF-κB activation on cardiac myocytes in vitro as well as transcription, translation and secretion of TNF-α (64). Elevated serum levels of circulating TNF-α have been demonstrated in patients with congestive heart failure and TNF-α is reported to exert negative inotropic effects on the myocardium (65,66). Moreover, TNF-α triggers apoptosis in cardiomyocytes (67-69) and terminal complement components are reported to mediate myocardial apoptosis following ischemia-reperfusion (26).

Third, C5b-9 may alter vascular tone by inhibiting endothelium-dependent relaxation of smooth muscle (70,71) and by decreasing endothelial cyclic guanosine monophosphate (72), thereby potentially further compromising blood flow to an already ischemic myocardium (9). Thus, complement activation may alter vascular homeostasis and blood flow by inhibiting endothelium-dependent relaxation in addition to promoting PMN activation and adhesion.

4. ANTI-COMPLEMENT THERAPY IN MI/R

Many early in vivo studies of MI/R used cobra venom factor (CVF) to deplete complement as a therapeutic approach to reducing inflammation and injury. CVF acts as a constitutive C3 convertase, leading to continual consumption of C3 in animals (73). Depletion of C3 by administration of CVF reduces infiltration of neutrophils after MI/R in rats (12). Depleting complement with CVF also significantly reduces myocardial necrosis in dogs, rats and baboons (14,20,74).

Other inhibitors of the complement cascade are based on the powerful complement regulatory proteins (CRPs) naturally present in vivo. CRPs act to control excessive amplification of the complement cascade, thus preventing the unwarranted destruction of healthy tissue during inflammatory responses. The soluble form of complement receptor type one (sCR1-TP10) is an example of a potential therapeutic based on a naturally occurring CRP. The membrane bound form of CR1 is found on many phagocytic cells where it controls the complement cascade at the level of the C3 and C5 convertases (15). Blocking these convertases prevents the production of inflammatory anaphylatoxins and prevents the formation of the MAC. Soluble CR1, a truncated form of the membrane bound CR1, retains the ability to inhibit these events in vivo. Distinct regions of sCR1 bind C4b or C3b components of the C3 and C5 convertases and displace these subunits from their respective catalytic complexes (15). In addition, sCR1 assists in the factor I mediated cleavage of both C4b and C3b. sCR1 administered prior to ischemia in rats undergoing MI/R demonstrated attenuated myocardial infarction associated with decreased deposition of C5b-9 complexes along the endothelium and decreased leukocyte infiltration after 24 hours of reperfusion (15). In a similar study, administration of sCR1 prior to MI/R decreased infarct size and the infiltration of PMNs into the area at risk (AAR) (75). Interestingly, the study by Smith et. al. also demonstrated significant attenuation of myocardial infarction when sCR1 was administered immediately before reperfusion of the ischemic myocardium (75). In a rat MI/R model examining an alternatively glycosylated form of sCR1 (TP20), which possesses the sialyl Lewis x ligand for P-, E- and L-selectin adhesion molecules (76,77), there was no significant difference in the cardioprotection mediated by sCR1sLe^x in comparison to sCR1, as measured by infarct size and production of cardiac troponin T (cTnT marker for cardiac damage) (78). However, there was significant attenuation of PMN infiltration into the infarct zone in the sCR1sLe^x treatment group in comparison to rats treated with sCR1(79), suggesting that the cardioprotection afforded during MI/R in this sCR1/ sCR1sLe^x model may be independent of PMN blockade. Recently, a re-analysis of data from Phase II clinical trials using sCR1 (TP10) male patients from a high risk population undergoing open-heart procedures demonstrated decreased mortality and a reduction in the size of infarctions, although this significant decrease in both endpoints was not seen in female subjects (80).

Thus, the potential benefits of sCR1 as a treatment for IHD must await the results from additional clinical trials.

Another naturally occurring moiety, which controls excessive complement activation in vivo, is the C1 esterase inhibitor (C1-INH). This plasma-derived protein has also been adapted for the therapeutic inhibition of complement during MI/R. C1-INH covalently binds the serine proteases C1s and C1r of the classical complement pathway and the MASP-1 and MASP-2 proteases of the lectin pathway (81,82). In a feline model of MI/R, administration of C1-INH (15 mg/kg) prior to reperfusion attenuated infarction, decreased neutrophil infiltration, increased recovery of myocardial contractility and preserved endothelial function (30). In a rat model of MI/R, Buerke et al. demonstrated decreased myocardial injury and adhesion molecule expression associated with attenuated neutrophil accumulation in ischemic myocardium following administration of C1-INH (10-100 U/kg) prior to reperfusion (83). Similar cardioprotection was evident in a pig model of MI/R following application of 20 IU/kg of C1-INH five minutes prior to reperfusion (84).

Human clinical trials have substantiated the cardioprotective effects of C1-INH administration during cardiopulmonary bypass (CPB) or myocardial infarction accompanied with thrombolytic therapy (85-87). It has since been demonstrated, however, that the protective effects of C1-INH during MI/R are dose dependent and excess administration of C1-INH may have severe consequences during a cardiac event. In an attempt to prevent capillary leakage, administration of C1-INH (500 IU/kg) during CPB in a group of thirteen newborn babies caused great vein thrombosis in all patients and resulted in nine deaths (88,89). Another study analyzing the dose response of C1-INH administered intravenously 5 to 10 minutes before coronary reperfusion at a dose of 40, 100, and 200 IU/kg body weight, demonstrated that when C1-INH was applied at the correct dose, it significantly protected ischemic tissue from reperfusion damage (90). However, high doses (>/=100 IU/kg) of C1-INH provoked detrimental side effects (91). Therefore, C1-INH is a promising candidate for protection against MI/R injury, however continued dose-response analysis profiles are required to demonstrate appropriate safety and continued efficacy in the clinical setting.

Finally, other members belonging to the group of naturally derived inhibitors include sCR1[des-LHR-A] (92), C1s-INH-248 (93) and CGS 32359 (94). sCR1[des-LHR-A] is an alternative form of sCR1, which lacks the C4b binding domain, and is thus specific for the alternative pathway. Both forms of soluble CR1 demonstrated equal capabilities to abrogate cardiac damage and decrease PMN infiltration into the AAR during MI/R (95). The small molecule inhibitor C1s-INH-248 binds the serine protease C1s of the classical complement pathways with high specificity. The extent of C1s-INH-248 interaction with the early components of the lectin pathway remains unclear. Administration of C1s-INH-248 prior to reperfusion caused a significant reduction in infarct size-associated cardiac damage as measured by cardiac creatine kinase (CK) activity and a reduction in neutrophil infiltration into the infarct zone (96). CGS 32359, a C5a receptor antagonist, is a recombinant form of C5a which binds to the C5 receptor without activating subsequent inflammatory functions of neutrophils(97). In a porcine model of MI/R, animals treated prior to reperfusion with CGS 32359 demonstrated a significant reduction in infarct size and PMN infiltration (98). To date, there are no clinical data available on the efficacy or safety of CGS 32359 or the other complement inhibitors addressed in this paragraph.

In addition to applications of naturally occurring complement inhibitors during MI/R, there has also been success with monoclonal antibodies (mAb) directed at specific complement components as a therapy to prevent MI/R injury. In a porcine model of MI/R, our lab demonstrated that animals treated with mAb to the anaphylatoxin C5a prior to reperfusion showed attenuated infarction, although this protection was not accompanied by a decrease in PMN infiltration (99). However, rats treated with C5 mAb (which blocks both C5a and C5b-9) prior to MI/R demonstrated attenuated infarct size, neutrophil infiltration and apoptosis in the myocardium (26). Importantly, administration of a humanized anti-C5 scFv (pexelizumab) to patients requiring concomitant coronary artery bypass grafting (CABG) plus CPB significantly reduces myocardial injury and accompanying disorders during a phase IIa clinical trial (9,100) and decreased overall patient mortality associated with acute myocardial infarction during a phase IIb clinical trial (101). Thus, anti-C5 mAb is a promising candidate for MI/R therapy and is currently in phase III clinical trials (PRIMO-CABG).

5. THE MECHANISMS OF COMPLEMENT ACTIVATION FOLLOWING MI/R

Substantial information supports a role for complement in exacerbation of myocardial injury during ischemia and reperfusion. However, there is still one unanswered question: which pathway is responsible for complement initiation in this particular injury? Current complement inhibitors outlined in this chapter generally do not fully discriminate between the classical, lectin, and alternative pathways of complement activation, and therefore cannot directly address the issue of mechanism. However, recent studies using specific inhibitors of the lectin pathway have shed new light on our understanding of the mechanisms of complement activation during myocardial reperfusion injury. One early study suggests that subcellular fractions of cardiomyocyte mitochondria activates the classic and alternative pathways in vitro (102). Further studies in a canine model of MI/R demonstrated that ischemic tissues release mitochondrial membranes and cardiolipin, which can bind to C1q and activate the classical complement pathway (22). Similar findings were observed in humans, whereby sera from a large percentage of patients with documented myocardial infarction contained abnormally large quantities of molecules that formed complexes with C1q (103). However, none of these studies could exclude the potential involvement of the lectin pathway of complement activation.

Anoxic human endothelial cells were recently shown to activate complement in the absence of immunoglobulin binding, suggesting antibody-independent complement activation (26). Depleting or inhibiting mannose-binding lectin (MBL) decreased complement activation following oxidative stress (104-107) and our lab has shown that MBL and C3 co-localize in an in vivo rat model of MI/R (108). Moreover, specifically blocking the lectin complement pathway with anti-MBL inhibitory mAbs protects rat hearts from ischemia-reperfusion injury, reduces neutrophil infiltration and attenuates proinflammatory gene expression (109).

Based on this evidence, we propose that the lectin pathway initiates complement activation in MI/R, and is thus the key pathway leading to myocardial damage and inflammation associated with MI/R. The proposal that C1q initiates complement activation in MI/R is not sufficient to explain robust C3 deposition and infarction in C1q knockout animals (devoid of the classical pathway) subjected to experimental MI/R (unpublished data). Additionally, analysis of infarct size following MI/R in wild type and C1q knockout mice shows no protection from injury in the absence of C1q (Figure 1A and B) unless C1q$^{-/-}$ mice are treated with anti-C5 prior to the ischemic event (Figure 1C).

Thus, the classical pathway may not initiate complement activation nor mediate acute myocardial injury, but rather serve an as-yet unidentified role in the myocardial response to ischemia/reperfusion. Further studies are needed to fully dissect the relative roles of the three complement pathways in MI/R. Moreover, it will indeed be interesting to see how genetically altered animals supplement our understanding of MI/R injury. Ultimately, these studies will lead to the development of more specific inhibitors of complement activation that may prove to be beneficial in the treatment of IHD.

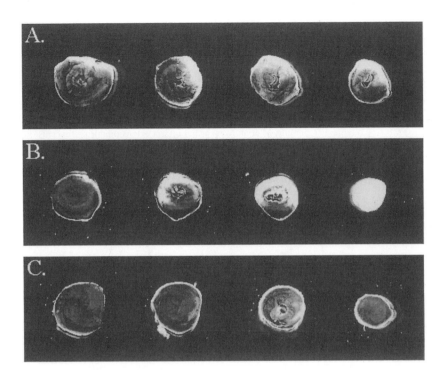

Figure 1. Infarct size using Evans blue/TTC staining of wild type (WT) or C1q-/- hearts following myocardial ischemia and reperfusion. The LAD of WT mice (A), C1q-/- mice (B), or C1q-/- mice plus anti-C5 (C; BB5.1) was occluded for 30 minutes followed by 3 hours of reperfusion. Following reperfusion, the LAD was occluded again, the aorta cannulated with PE-10 tubing, and hearts perfused with Evans blue dye. Hearts were then removed, sectioned and stained with TTC. Areas stained blue with Evans blue represent healthy non-ischemic tissue, and the remaining area represents the area that was at risk for ischemia. The red area represents TTC positive staining or non-infarcted tissue. White tissue represents infarction. Notice that compared to WT hearts, C1q -/- mice display as much, if not more, infarcted area; suggesting that C1q is not involved in ischemia/reperfusion injury and tissue infarction. On the other hand, inhibition of mouse C5 in C1q -/- mice with BB5.1 mAb clearly demonstrates that following myocardial ischemia/reperfusion 1) complement is activated in the C1q -/- mouse, 2) inhibition of C5 protects the C1q -/- heart from infarction, and 3) the classical pathway (i.e., C1q) is not involved in tissue injury.

6.   REFERENCES

1.   American Heart Association. Heart Disease and Stroke Statistics - 2003 Update. American Heart Association . 2002.

2. Ribichini F, Wijns W. Acute myocardial infarction: reperfusion treatment. *Heart.* 2002;88:298-305.
3. Braunwald E, Zipes DP, Libby P. Heart Disease. 6th. 2001.
4. Kloner RA. Does reperfusion injury exist in humans? *J Am Coll Cardiol.* 1993;21:537-545.
5. Ganz W. Direct Demonstration in Dogs of the Absence of Lethal Reperfusion Injury. *J Thromb Thrombolysis.* 1997;4:105-107.
6. Farb A, Kolodgie FD, Jenkins M et al. Myocardial infarct extension during reperfusion after coronary artery occlusion: pathologic evidence. *J Am Coll Cardiol.* 1993;21:1245-1253.
7. Matsumura K, Jeremy RW, Schaper J et al. Progression of myocardial necrosis during reperfusion of ischemic myocardium. *Circulation.* 1998;97:795-804.
8. Frangogiannis NG, Smith CW, Entman ML. The inflammatory response in myocardial infarction. *Cardiovasc Res.* 2002;53:31-47.
9. Shernan SK, Collard CD. Role of the complement system in ischaemic heart disease: potential for pharmacological intervention. *BioDrugs.* 2001;15:595-607.
10. Riedemann NC, Ward PA. Complement in ischemia reperfusion injury. *Am J Pathol.* 2003;162:363-367.
11. Walport MJ. Complement. First of two parts. *N Engl J Med.* 2001;344:1058-1066.
12. Hill JH, Ward PA. The phlogistic role of C3 leukotactic fragments in myocardial infarcts in rats. *J Exp Med.* 1971;133:885-900.
13. Schafer H, Mathey D, Hugo F et al. Deposition of the terminal C5b-9 complement complex in infarcted areas of human myocardium. *J Immunol.* 1986;137:1945-1949.
14. Maroko PR, Carpenter CB, Chariello M. Reduction by cobra venom factor of myocardial necrosis after coronary artery occlusion. *J Clin Invest.* 1978;61:661-670.
15. Weisman HF, Bartow T, Leppo MK et al. Soluble human complement receptor type 1: in vivo inhibitor of complement suppressing post-ischemic myocardial inflammation and necrosis. *Science.* 1990;249:146-151.
16. Hill JH, Ward PA. C3 leukotactic factors produced by a tissue protease. *J Exp Med.* 1969;130:505-518.
17. Pinckard RN, Olson MS, Giclas PC et al. Consumption of classical complement components by heart subcellular membranes in vitro and in patients after acute myocardial infarction. *J Clin Invest.* 1975;56:740-750.
18. Pinckard RN, Olson MS, Giclas PC et al. Consumption of classical complement components by heart subcellular membranes in vitro and in patients after acute myocardial infarction. *J Clin Invest.* 1975;56:740-750.
19. Giclas PC, Pinckard RN, Olson MS. In vitro activation of complement by isolated human heart subcellular membranes. *J Immunol.* 1979;122:146-151.
20. Pinckard RN, O'Roarke RA, Crawford MH. Complement localization and mediation of ischemic injury in baboon myocardium. *J Clin Invest.* 1980;66:1050-1056.
21. McManus LM, Kolb WP, Crawford MH et al. Complement localization in ischemic baboon myocardium. *Lab Invest.* 1983;48:436-447.
22. Rossen RD, Swain JL, Michael LH. Selective accumulation of the first component of complement and leukocytes in ischemic canine heart muscle. A possible initiator of an extra myocardial mechanism of ischemic injury. *Circ Res.* 1985;57:119-130.
23. Crawford MH, Grover FL, Kolb WP et al. Complement and neutrophil activation in the pathogenesis of ischemic myocardial injury. *Circ Res.* 1988;78:1449-1458.
24. Vakeva A, Laurila P, Meri S. Loss of expression of protectin (CD59) is associated with complement membrane attack complex deposition in myocardial infarction. *Lab Invest.* 1992;67:608-616.

25. Väkevä A, Laurila P, Meri S. Co-deposition of clusterin with the complement membrane attack complex in myocardial infarction. *Immunology*. 1993;80:177-182.

26. Vakeva A, Agah A, Rollins SA et al. Myocardial infarction and apoptosis after myocardial ischemia and reperfusion. Role of the terminal complement components and inhibition by anti-C5 therapy. *Circulation*. 1998;97:2259-2267.

27. Buerke M, Prüfer D, Dahm M et al. Blocking of classical complement pathway inhibits endothelial adhesion molecule expression and preserves ischemic myocardium from reperfusion injury. *Journal of Pharmacology and Experimental Therapeutics*. 1998;286:429-438.

28. Collard CD, Vakeva A, Morrissey MA et al. Complement activation after oxidative stress: role of the lectin complement pathway. *Am J Pathol*. 2000;156:1549-1556.

29. Väkevä A, Morgan BP, Tikkanen I et al. Time course of complement activation and inhibitor expression after ischemic injury of rat myocardium. *Am J Pathol*. 1994;144:1357-1368.

30. Buerke M, Murohara T, Lefer AM. Cardioprotective effects of a C1 esterase inhibitor in myocardial ischemia and reperfusion. *Circulation*. 1995;91:393-402.

31. Yasojima K, Schwab C, McGeer EG et al. Human heart generates complement proteins that are upregulated and activated after myocardial infarction. *Circ Res*. 1998;83:860-869.

32. Kilgore KS, Friedrichs GS, Homeister JW et al. The complement system in myocardial ischaemia/reperfusion injury. *Cardiovasc Res*. 1994;28:437-444.

33. Gardinali M, Conciato L, Cafaro C et al. Complement system in coronary heart disease: A review. *Immunopharmacology*. 1995;30:105-117.

34. Dreyer WJ, Michael LH, Nguyen T et al. Kinetics of C5a release in cardiac lymph of dogs experiencing coronary artery ischemia-reperfusion injury. *Circ Res*. 1992;71:1518-1524.

35. McManus LM, Kolb WP, Crawford MH et al. Complement localization in ischemic baboon myocardium. *Lab Invest*. 1983;48:436-447.

36. Chenoweth DE. The properties of human C5a anaphylatoxin. The significance of C5a formation during hemodialysis. *Contr Nephrol*. 1987;59:51-71.

37. Daffern PJ, Pfeifer PH, Ember JA et al. C3a is a chemotaxin for human eosinophils but not for neutrophils. I. C3a stimulation of neutrophils is secondary to eosinophil activation. *J Exp Med*. 1995;181:2119-2127.

38. Takafuji S, Tadokoro K, Ito K et al. Degranulation from human eosinophils stimulated with C3a and C5a. *Int Arch Allergy Immunol*. 1994;104 Suppl 1:27-29.

39. Chakraborti T, Mandal A, Mandal M et al. Complement activation in heart diseases: Role of oxidants. *Cell Signal*. 2000;12:607-617.

40. Ito BR, Roth DM, Engler RL. Thromboxane A_2 and peptidoleukotrienes contribute to the myocardial ischemia and contractile dysfunction in response to intracoronary infusion of complement C5a in pigs. *Circ Res*. 1990;66:596-607.

41. Stahl GL, Amsterdam EA, Symons JD et al. Role of thromboxane A_2 in the cardiovascular response to intracoronary C5a. *Circ Res*. 1990;66:1103-1111.

42. Entman ML, Michael L, Rossen RD et al. Inflammation in the course of early myocardial ischemia. *FASEB J*. 1991;5:2529-2537.

43. Dreyer WJ, Smith CW, Entman ML. Invited letter concerning: neutrophil activation during cardiopulmonary bypass. *J Thorac Cardiovasc Surg*. 1991;102:318-320.

44. Sacks T, Moldow CF, Craddock PR et al. Endothelial damage provoked by toxic oxygen radicals released from complement-triggered granulocytes. *Prog Clin Biol Res*. 1978;21:719-26.:719-726.

45. Schindler R, Gelfand JA, Dinarello CA. Recombinant C5a stimulates transcription rather than translation of interleukin-1 (IL-1) and tumor necrosis factor: Translational signal provided by lipopolysaccharide or IL-1 itself. *Blood*. 1990;76:1631-1638.
46. Scholz W, McClurg MR, Cardenas GJ et al. C5a-mediated release of interleukin 6 by human monocytes. *Clin Immunol Immunopathol*. 1990;57:297-307.
47. Cavaillon JM, Fitting C, Haeffner-Cavaillon N. Recombinant C5a enhances interleukin 1 and tumor necrosis factor release by lipopolysaccharide-stimulated monocytes and macrophages. *Eur J Immunol*. 1990;20:253-257.
48. Moon R, Parikh AA, Szabo C et al. Complement C3 production in human intestinal epithelial cells is regulated by interleukin 1beta and tumor necrosis factor alpha. *Arch Surg*. 1997;132:1289-1293.
49. Buerke M, Prüfer D, Dahm M et al. Blocking of classical complement pathway inhibits endothelial adhesion molecule expression and preserves ischemic myocardium from reperfusion injury. *Journal of Pharmacology and Experimental Therapeutics*. 1998;286:429-438.
50. Mathey D, Schofer J, Schafer H et al. Early accumulation of the terminal complement-complex in the ischemic myocardium after reperfusion. *Eur Heart J*. 1994;15:418-423.
51. Homeister JW, Satoh P, Lucchesi BR. Effects of complement activation in the isolated heart. Role of the terminal complement components. *Circ Res*. 1992;71:303-319.
52. Kim SH, Carney DF, Hammer CH et al. Nucleated cell killing by complement: effects of C5b-9 channel size and extracellular Ca2+ on the lytic process. *J Immunol*. 1987;138:1530-1536.
53. Nicholson-Weller A, Halperin JA. Membrane signaling by complement C5b-9, the membrane attack complex. *Immunol Res*. 1993;12:244-257.
54. Berger H-J, Taratuska A, Smith TW et al. Activated complement directly modifies the performance of isolated heart muscle cells from guinea pig and rat. *Am J Physiol Heart Circ Physiol*. 1993;265:H267-H272.
55. Becker LC, Ambrosio G. Myocardial consequences of reperfusion. *Prog Cardiovasc Dis*. 1987;30:23-44.
56. Hoerter JA, Miceli MV, Renlund DG et al. A phosphorus-31 nuclear magnetic resonance study of the metabolic, contractile, and ionic consequences of induced calcium alterations in the isovolumic rat heart. *Circ Res*. 1986;58:539-551.
57. Wiedmer T, Ando B, Sims PJ. Complement C5b-9-stimulated platelet secretion is associated with a Ca2+-initiated activation of cellular protein kinases. *J Biol Chem*. 1987;262:13674-13681.
58. Saadi S, Holzknecht RA, Patte CP et al. Endothelial cell activation by pore-forming structures: pivotal role for interleukin-1alpha. *Circulation*. 2000;101:1867-1873.
59. Collard CD, Agah A, Reenstra W et al. Endothelial nuclear factor-kappaB translocation and vascular cell adhesion molecule-1 induction by complement: inhibition with anti-human C5 therapy or cGMP analogues. *Arterioscler Thromb Vasc Biol*. 1999;19:2623-2629.
60. Kilgore KS, Schmid E, Shanley TP et al. Sublytic concentrations of the membrane attack complex of complement induce endothelial interleukin-8 and monocyte chemoattractant protein-1 through nuclear factor-kappaB activation. *Am J Pathol*. 1997;150:2019-2031.
61. Entman ML, Youker K, Shoji T et al. Neutrophil induced oxidative injury of cardiac myocytes. A compartmented system requiring CD11b/CD18-ICAM-1 adherence. *J Clin Invest*. 1992;90:1335-1345.
62. Kukielka GL, Hawkins HK, Michael L et al. Regulation of intercellular adhesion molecule-1 (ICAM-1) in ischemic and reperfused canine myocardium. *J Clin Invest*. 1993;92:1504-1516.

63. Youker K, Smith CW, Anderson DC et al. Neutrophil adherence to isolated adult cardiac myocytes. Induction by cardiac lymph collected during ischemia and reperfusion. *J Clin Invest.* 1992;89:602-609.

64. Zwaka TP, Manolov D, Ozdemir C et al. Complement and dilated cardiomyopathy: a role of sublytic terminal complement complex-induced tumor necrosis factor-alpha synthesis in cardiac myocytes. *Am J Pathol.* 2002;161:449-457.

65. Meldrum DR, Dinarello CA, Shames BD et al. Ischemic preconditioning decreases postischemic myocardial tumor necrosis factor-alpha production. Potential ultimate effector mechanism of preconditioning. *Circulation.* 1998;98:II214-II218.

66. Meldrum DR. Tumor necrosis factor in the heart. *Am J Physiol.* 1998;274:R577-R595.

67. Ceconi C, Cargnoni A, Curello S et al. Recognized molecular mechanisms of heart failure: approaches to treatment. *Rev Port Cardiol.* 1998;17 Suppl 2:II79-II91.

68. Meldrum DR, Dinarello CA, Shames BD et al. Ischemic preconditioning decreases postischemic myocardial tumor necrosis factor-alpha production. Potential ultimate effector mechanism of preconditioning. *Circulation.* 1998;98:II214-II218.

69. Doyama K, Fujiwara H, Fukumoto M et al. Tumour necrosis factor is expressed in cardiac tissues of patients with heart failure. *Int J Cardiol.* 1996;54:217-225.

70. Stahl GL, Reenstra WR, Frendl G. Complement mediated loss of endothelium-dependent relaxation of porcine coronary arteries. Role of the terminal membrane attack complex. *Circ Res.* 1995;76:575-583.

71. Lennon PF, Collard CD, Morrissey MA et al. Complement-induced endothelial dysfunction in rabbits: mechanisms, recovery, and gender differences. *Am J Physiol Heart Circ Physiol.* 1996;270:H1924-H1932.

72. Collard CD, Agah A, Reenstra W et al. Endothelial nuclear factor-kappaB translocation and vascular cell adhesion molecule-1 induction by complement: inhibition with anti-human C5 therapy or cGMP analogues. *Arterioscler Thromb Vasc Biol.* 1999;19:2623-2629.

73. Lucchesi BR, Kilgore KS. Complement inhibitors in myocardial ischemia/reperfusion injury. *Immunopharmacology.* 1997;38:27-42.

74. MacLean D, Fishbein MC, Braunwald E et al. Long-term preservation of ischemic myocardium after experimental coronary artery occlusion. *J Clin Invest.* 1978;61:541-551.

75. Smith EF, III, Griswold DE, Egan JW et al. Reduction of myocardial reperfusion injury with human soluble complement receptor type 1 (BRL 55730). *Eur J Pharmacol.* 1993;236:477-481.

76. Zacharowski K, Otto M, Hafner G et al. Reduction of myocardial infarct size with sCR1sLe(x), an alternatively glycosylated form of human soluble complement receptor type 1 (sCR1), possessing sialyl Lewis x. *Br J Pharmacol.* 1999;128:945-952.

77. Foxall C, Watson SR, Dowbenko D et al. The three members of the selectin receptor family recognize a common carbohydrate epitope, the sialyl Lewis(x) oligosaccharide. *J Cell Biol.* 1992;117:895-902.

78. Zacharowski K, Otto M, Hafner G et al. Reduction of myocardial infarct size with sCR1sLe(x), an alternatively glycosylated form of human soluble complement receptor type 1 (sCR1), possessing sialyl Lewis x. *Br J Pharmacol.* 1999;128:945-952.

79. Zacharowski K, Otto M, Hafner G et al. Reduction of myocardial infarct size with sCR1sLe(x), an alternatively glycosylated form of human soluble complement receptor type 1 (sCR1), possessing sialyl Lewis x. *Br J Pharmacol.* 1999;128:945-952.

80. AVANT Pharmaceuticals. AVANT TP-10 clinical trial press release. 4-29-2003.

81. Sahul A, Lambris JD. Complement inhibitors: a resurgent concept in anti-inflammatory therapeutics. *Immunopharmacology.* 2000;49:133-148.

82. Matsushita M, Thiel S, Jensenius JC et al. Proteolytic activities of two types of mannose-binding lectin- associated serine protease. *J Immunol*. 2000;165:2637-2642.
83. Buerke M, Prüfer D, Dahm M et al. Blocking of classical complement pathway inhibits endothelial adhesion molecule expression and preserves ischemic myocardium from reperfusion injury. *Journal of Pharmacology and Experimental Therapeutics*. 1998;286:429-438.
84. Horstick G, Heimann A, Gotze O et al. Intracoronary application of C1 esterase inhibitor improves cardiac function and reduces myocardial necrosis in an experimental model of ischemia and reperfusion. *Circulation*. 1997;95:701-708.
85. Horstick G, Berg O, Heimann A et al. Application of C1-esterase inhibitor during reperfusion of ischemic myocardium: dose-related beneficial versus detrimental effects. *Circulation*. 2001;104:3125-3131.
86. Horstick G. C1-esterase inhibitor in ischemia and reperfusion. *Immunobiology*. 2002;205:552-562.
87. de Zwaan C, Kleine AH, Diris JH et al. Continuous 48-h C1-inhibitor treatment, following reperfusion therapy, in patients with acute myocardial infarction. *Eur Heart J*. 2002;23:1670-1677.
88. Horstick G, Berg O, Heimann A et al. Application of C1-esterase inhibitor during reperfusion of ischemic myocardium: dose-related beneficial versus detrimental effects. *Circulation*. 2001;104:3125-3131.
89. Shwerwiegende Thrombenbildung nach Berinert HS. Arzneimittelkommission der Deutschen Aerzteschaft. Dtsch Aerztebl. 97, B-684. 2002.
90. Horstick G, Berg O, Heimann A et al. Application of C1-esterase inhibitor during reperfusion of ischemic myocardium: dose-related beneficial versus detrimental effects. *Circulation*. 2001;104:3125-3131.
91. Horstick G, Berg O, Heimann A et al. Application of C1-esterase inhibitor during reperfusion of ischemic myocardium: dose-related beneficial versus detrimental effects. *Circulation*. 2001;104:3125-3131.
92. Scesney SM, Makrides SC, Gosselin ML et al. A soluble deletion mutant of the human complement receptor type 1, which lacks the C4b binding site, is a selective inhibitor of the alternative complement pathway. *Eur J Immunol*. 1996;26:1729-1735.
93. Buerke M, Schwertz H, Seitz W et al. Novel small molecule inhibitor of C1s exerts cardioprotective effects in ischemia-reperfusion injury in rabbits. *J Immunol*. 2001;167:5375-5380.
94. Pellas TC, Boyar W, Van Oostrum J et al. Novel C5a receptor antagonists regulate neutrophil functions in vitro and in vivo. *J Immunol*. 1998;160:5616-5621.
95. Murohara T, Guo JP, Delyani JA et al. Cardioprotective effects of selective inhibition of the two complement activation pathways in myocardial ischemia and reperfusion injury. *Meth and Find Exptl Clin Pharmacol*. 1995;17:499-507.
96. Buerke M, Schwertz H, Seitz W et al. Novel small molecule inhibitor of C1s exerts cardioprotective effects in ischemia-reperfusion injury in rabbits. *J Immunol*. 2001;167:5375-5380.
97. Pellas TC, Boyar W, Van Oostrum J et al. Novel C5a receptor antagonists regulate neutrophil functions in vitro and in vivo. *J Immunol*. 1998;160:5616-5621.
98. Riley RD, Sato H, Zhao ZQ et al. Recombinant human complement C5a receptor antagonist reduces infarct size after surgical revascularization. *J Thorac Cardiovasc Surg*. 2000;120:350-358.
99. Amsterdam EA, Stahl GL, Pan H-L et al. Limitation of reperfusion injury by a monoclonal antibody to C5a during myocardial infarction in pigs. *Am J Physiol Heart Circ Physiol*. 1995;268:H448-H457.

100. Fitch JCK, Rollins SA, Matis LA et al. Pharmacology and biological efficacy of a recombinant, humanized, single chain antibody, C5 complement inhibitor in patients undergoing coronary artery bypass graft surgery utilizing cardiopulmonary bypass. *Circulation*. 1999;100:2499-2509.
101. American Heart Association. AHA Scientific Sessions 2002 - COMMA and COMPLY. American Heart Association . 2002.
102. Giclas PC, Pinckard RN, Olson MS. In vitro activation of complement by isolated human heart subcellular membranes. *J Immunol*. 1979;122:146-151.
103. Rossen RD, Michael LH, Kagiyama A et al. Mechanism of complement activation after coronary artery occlusion: Evidence that myocardial ischemia in dogs causes release of constituents of myocardial subcellular origin that complex with human C1q in vivo. *Circ Res*. 1988;62:572-584.
104. Collard CD, Vakeva A, Morrissey MA et al. Complement activation after oxidative stress: role of the lectin complement pathway. *Am J Pathol*. 2000;156:1549-1556.
105. Collard CD, Montalto MC, Reenstra WR et al. Endothelial oxidative stress activates the lectin complement pathway: role of cytokeratin 1. *Am J Pathol*. 2001;159:1045-1054.
106. Montalto MC, Collard CD, Buras JA et al. A keratin peptide inhibits mannose-binding lectin. *J Immunol*. 2001;166:4148-4153.
107. Lekowski R, Collard CD, Reenstra WR et al. Ulex europaeus agglutinin II (UEA-II) is a novel, potent inhibitor of complement activation. *Protein Sci*. 2001;10:277-284.
108. Collard CD, Vakeva A, Morrissey MA et al. Complement activation after oxidative stress: role of the lectin complement pathway. *Am J Pathol*. 2000;156:1549-1556.
109. Jordan JE, Montalto MC, Stahl GL. Inhibition of mannose-binding lectin reduces postischemic myocardial reperfusion injury. *Circulation*. 2001;104:1413-1418.

20

Role of Complement in Intestinal Ischemia/Reperfusion Induced Injury

Sherry D. Fleming and George C. Tsokos
Walter Reed Army Institute of Research, Silver Spring, MD 20910 and Department of Medicine, Uniformed Services University of the Health Sciences, Bethesda, MD 20814

Abstract: Complement activation occurs during tissue injury and inappropriate or excessive activation contributes to the expression of pathology becoming a double-edged sword. Understanding the role of complement and its natural regulatory molecules will enable the development of therapeutic interventions to prevent excessive damage during mesenteric ischemia/reperfusion (IR). In this chapter, we briefly review the mechanism of complement activation during intestinal IR and discuss the results and significance of mesenteric IR injury in animal models with altered complement activation. Finally we focus on the use of complement inhibitors in IR injury.

Key words: mesenteric, intestine, ischemia, complement, reperfusion, therapeutics

1. ISCHEMIA/REPERFUSION INTESTINAL DAMAGE

The splanchnic circulation is a large vascular bed that receives as much as 25-30% of the total blood flow bringing oxygen and nutrients to the intestine. As blood flow to the intestine decreases, the flow to the various circuits is not decreased equally resulting in more blood shunted to the mucosa than to other networks. The rapid turnover of the mucosa makes it extremely sensitive to hypoxia. Therefore, loss of blood flow to this tissue for a limited amount of time, as little as 20 min, results in damage to the mucosal surfaces with villi disruption. However, reperfusion induces pathological changes to the tissue that are greatly enhanced compared to that of ischemia alone. These alterations of reperfusion injury following mesenteric ischemia cause additional local inflammation characterized by complement activation and deposition, neutrophil infiltration and eicosanoid generation that coincides with mucosal injury (1-3). The role of complement in mediating this injury and the possibilities of inhibiting complement activation are the focus of current research.

2.   COMPLEMENT ACTIVATION IN INTESTINAL DAMAGE

Complement is a complex cascade of over 30 proteins that are activated in an orderly manner. The cascade has 3 initiating arms, including the classical, lectin and alternative pathways that each produce enzymatic complexes, C3 and C5 convertases (Fig.1).

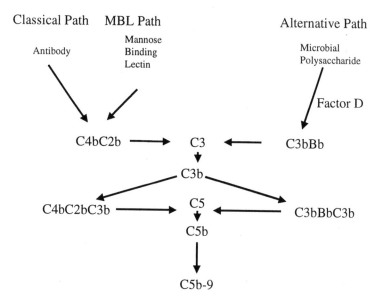

Figure 1. Simplified complement activation cascade

The cascade continues with the cleavage of C3 and C5 and all 3 pathways culminate in a common terminal pathway. The terminating complex, the membrane attack complex, is a lytic complex that inserts into the membrane forming a pore in the cell. Since the complement pathway is capable of extreme cell and tissue damage, complement regulatory molecules that control the rate of its activation are essential and occur naturally at multiple points within the cascade. However, in many clinical conditions, unregulated complement activation results in additional tissue injury. Inappropriate complement activation and subsequent tissue damage occurs during intestinal ischemia, blunt trauma and hemorrhagic shock.

Many of the clinical conditions associated with inappropriate complement activation also reduce blood volume and lead to subsequent mesenteric vasoconstriction resulting in functional intestinal ischemia (4). When organs such as the intestine are subjected to severe vascular ischemia followed by reperfusion of blood into the site, local as well as remote tissue inflammation and injury ensues. Intestinal damage as a result of ischemia and subsequent reperfusion varies by the region of the intestine. However, the extremes of the IR-induced injury apply to the entire intestine. In other words, the intestine can tolerate short periods of ischemia without severe injury but long periods of mesenteric ischemia followed by reperfusion results in death. Mesenteric ischemia triggers an inflammatory reaction, characterized by neutrophil infiltration, activation and local mucosal injury, in which complement activation plays a pivotal role. Reperfusion of the ischemic gut is believed to lead to another surge of complement activation and further mucosal injury (5).

Using rodent models, the mechanism of IR-induced intestinal damage has been shown to involve complement activation. The exact mechanism of complement activation during intestinal IR remains unclear as there is evidence that more than one complement pathway (classical, alternative or lectin) may be activated and enhance tissue injury (6-8). Further evidence that complement activation is directly involved in the effector phases of intestinal IR injury has been provided by studies showing that inhibition of the complement pathway at the point of C3 or C5 activation can either prevent or substantially attenuate intestinal injury (1, 2, 8-11). In addition, inflammatory mediators generated during complement pathway activation, such as the anaphylatoxin C5a and the membrane attack complex (MAC), are known to be able to directly cause cellular activation and injury as well (11-13). The specifics of each complement initiating pathway, the terminal complex and the anaphylatoxins will be discussed below.

3. INDICATIONS OF COMPLEMENT INVOLVMENT

The essential role of complement in mesenteric ischemia/reperfusion induced tissue injury has been shown in numerous animal models. We have established the mesenteric IR model in mice and confirmed the role of complement in intestinal IR using cobra venom factor (CVF) to deplete C3. The intestinal mucosa of the sham-operated animals remained normal as indicated by an injury score of 0.68 (Fig. 2).

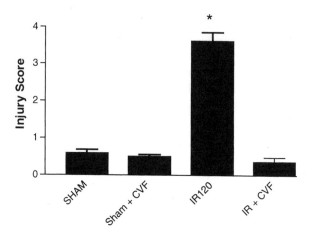

Figure 2. Complement depletion inhibits IR-induced intestinal injury. Balb/c mice were treated with CVF for 24 hr prior to subjecting the animals to either sham treatment or IR. After 2 hr reperfusion, intestinal sections were collected and immediately formalin fixed. Gimsa stained intestinal sections from each treatment groups were scored for mucosal injury (0-6). Each bar is the average ± SEM from 6-8 animals/group. * indicates significant difference from sham group, p<0.05.Using ANOVA with Neuman Keuls post-hoc test,

Mice subjected to IR had significant intestinal injury as indicated macroscopically by swollen and edematous with areas of red streaks. Microscopically, the injury ranged from shortened and vacuolated villi to complete destruction of normal mucosal architecture with frank hemorrhage. In contrast, mice subjected to sham procedure or IR after treatment with CVF had no significant intestinal mucosal injury (Fig. 1). Thus, similar to the rat model, complement has a role in the local injury induced by IR in mice.

Activation of complement 5 (C5) leads to the production of a potent anaphylotoxin, C5a, along with C5b, the initiator of the membrane attack complex. The use of C5 deficient mice showed that either the membrane attack complex, the anaphylatoxin, C5a or a combination of both could prevent or substantially attenuate intestinal injury (9, 14). In additional studies, anti-C5 monclonal antibodies have been administered to mice to prevent C5 activation and subsequent local and remote tissue damage (11, 14, 15). Inhibition of C5 activation by an anti-C5 antibody administered to wild type mice subjected to mesenteric IR, prevents C5a generation, PMN infiltration and deposition of the terminal complement complex on the damaged issues in a manner similar to that observed in C5 deficient mice (14, 16-20). These studies however, do not distinguish between the actions of C5a and C5b-9 terminal complex or address the initiating pathways.

4.   EVIDENCE FOR THE INITIATING PATHWAY

It is known that complement is activated immediately after injury and the severity of the trauma is directly proportional to the level of complement activation (21). The complement cascade can be activated by contact with microbes but, during short periods of intestinal IR, the alternative and classical pathways are both over-activated in the absence of microbial infection. It is well known that the clotting cascade activates complement. Some possible alternative complement activators include: reactive oxygen or nitrogen metabolites, exposed collagen, mitochondrial membranes and extracellular ATP (22-24). In addition, in vitro data shows that damage to the endothelium activates the alternative pathway and recent data show that the absence of Factors D or B protects mice from IR-induced damage (7, 25). It is possible that multiple pathways are involved in the complex mechanisms of mesenteric ischemia reperfusion induced damage. Although the exact method of complement activation may differ with the nature of the traumatic insult, the down-stream events of excessive complement activation results in an inflammatory reaction.

The ability to design logical therapeutics to prevent complement action depends on our understanding of the complement pathways that are involved and the initiating factors for the specific pathway(s). The availability of a mouse model and mice engineered to be genetically deficient in a specific complement factor has aided our understanding of the role of complement components in mesenteric injury. These studies are summarized in Fig. 3 and detailed below.

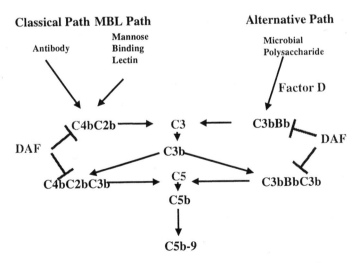

Figure 3. Mesenteric IR studies using complement deficient mice

4.1   Role of Classical Complement Pathway

Three observations have strongly implicated the classical pathway in the IR-induced injury process. The first is that intestinal IR injury is significantly decreased in *RAG-1-/-* mice, and reconstitution of these Ig deficient mice with normal levels of purified IgM natural antibody (8) restores IR-induced injury. The second is that mice that have normal levels of natural antibody, but which also have the gene encoding complement C4 inactivated (*C4-/-*), are protected from injury (8). The importance of natural IgM antibody and the classical complement pathway in mediating IR injury of skeletal muscle has also been shown using a similar experimental strategy with C3, C4 and Ig deficient mice (26). From these and other findings, it has been proposed that natural antibodies bind to antigen(s) revealed on the surface membrane of cells subjected to ischemia and subsequently activate complement by recruiting C1 and then cleaving C4 (8). This is followed by the generation of complement C3 and C5 activation fragments with ensuing increases in adhesion molecule expression and release of a cascade of inflammatory mediators, including leukotriene B4 and others (1, 2, 6). Finally, mice deficient in complement receptors 1 and 2 (CR2-/-) are also resistant to local IR induced damage (6, 27). Injection of IgM and IgG from wildtype mice restored all measured parameters of IR-induced injury, indicating that antibody and the classical complement pathway are important in initiating complement activation in these mice as well.

4.2   Role of Lectin Pathway

The studies discussed above using C3 and C4 deficient mice, suggest that either the classical or the lectin pathways have a role in local IR-induced injury. There is a lack of intestinal ischemia studies using lectin pathway deficient mice or lectin specific inhibitors. However, Stahl's group has shown deposition of MBL on hypoxic endothelial cells in vitro (28). In additional studies, anti-mannose binding lectin antibodies were used to determine the role of MBL in myocardial IR-induced injury (29). These studies indicate that the lectin pathway is activated during the oxidative stress associated with ischemia. Further studies will be needed to show the pathway's role in intestinal IR-induced injury.

4.3   Role of Alternative Pathway

There is recent data indicating that the alternative complement pathway is also involved in intestinal IR injury. Factor D, of the alternative pathway, forms the alternative pathway C3 convertase by cleaving Factor B. Factor D deficient mice, lacking the alternative C3 convertase, are resistant to IR-induced intestinal and pulmonary damage. Mesenteric IR-induced complement deposition is prevented in both the intestine and the lungs. Additionally, administration of Factor D restored the IR-induced decrease in intestinal lactate dehydrogenase. This restoration was prevented by treatment with anti-Factor D antibodies. Thus, it appears that the alternative complement pathway is actively involved in the complex mechanism of mesenteric IR injury.

5. ROLE OF THE LYTIC COMPLEX OR ANAPHYLATOXINS

C5a, a small, glycosylated peptide, is a potent chemoattractant for PMN, monocytes and T cells (reviewed in (13, 30)). In vitro studies have shown that C5a induces degranulation and respiratory burst, increases adhesion molecule expression and delays apoptosis in PMN (31-33). In addition, *in vivo* studies using anti-C5a antibodies have indicated that C5a alters vascular permeability and neutrophil activation during cardiopulmonary bypass (34), hind limb IR (35), sepsis (36-39) and inflammatory lung injury (40). C5a receptors (C5aR) are expressed on the surface of intestinal cells under inflammatory conditions, as well as on bronchial epithelial cells (41). Blockade of these receptors using C5aR antagonists (C5aRa) indicates a role for C5a in systemic activation of neutrophils in multiple animal models (42-45). To distinguish the role of C5a from that of C5b-9 on local and remote tissue injury, we inhibited the actions of C5a during mesenteric IR by treating wildtype mice with a cyclic hexapeptide C5a receptor antagonist (C5aRa) and we administered C5a to C5 deficient ($C5^{-/-}$) mice subjected to mesenteric IR. These experiments showed that during IR, C5a is sufficient to induce limited local damage and eicosanoid production but not systemic PMN activation (15). In addition, systemic C5a administered during IR can induce VCAM-1 expression on remote organs such as the lung without inducing increased vascular permeability (11).

This inflammation involves anaphylatoxin recruitment and subsequent activation of granulocytes as well as upregulation of endothelial adhesion molecules, the local release of other inflammatory mediators and cytokines. Together these potent mediators may result in local damage or may activate the inflammatory response (and complement) systemically. Extensive systemic complement activation can lead to a whole body inflammatory reaction such as adult respiratory distress syndrome, systemic inflammatory response syndrome, and multiple organ failure.

6.   EFFECTS OF COMPLEMENT INHIBITORS

Because this cascade of proteins results in cell lysis and tissue destruction, the complement system includes multiple regulatory proteins that prevent non-specific complement activation. Some of these regulatory proteins are cellular receptors for the breakdown products of the components of the system. The understanding of natural regulatory proteins and receptors and their involvement in protection of mesenteric damage has allowed the design and development of therapeutic interventions that inhibit complement activation and prevent inflammatory tissue damage. Complement inhibitors are currently being studied to determine their ability to inhibit tissue damage as a result of mesenteric IR (summarized in Fig.4).

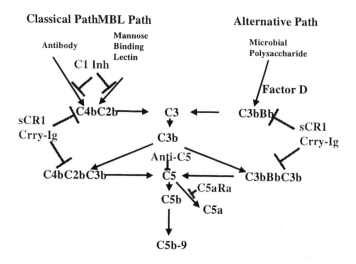

Figure 4. Mesenteric IR studies using complement inhibitors

Using a rat model of intestinal IR, several groups showed that administration of sCR1, a regulator of both classical and alternative pathways, significantly reduced rat local and systemic injury, PMN infiltration, and leukotriene B_4 (LTB_4) production (2, 10).

In mice, complement receptor 1-related gene/protein y (Crry) is a membrane regulatory protein altering the activity of both the classical and alternative complement pathways. Using a recombinant soluble form of Crry fused to the hinge, CH2, and CH3 domains of mouse IgG_1 (Crry-Ig), mice were pretreated either 5 min prior to, or 30 min after, the initiation of the reperfusion phase of mesenteric IR (1). IR-induced injury was reduced after Crry-Ig was administered. Pre-treatment with Crry-Ig reduced the local intestinal mucosal injury and decreased generation of LTB$_4$. When given 30 min after the beginning of the reperfusion phase, Crry-Ig resulted in a decrease in IR-induced intestinal mucosal injury comparable to when it was given 5 min prior to initiation of the reperfusion phase. Despite the presence of substantial number of neutrophils, Crry-Ig administered 30 min after the initiation of the reperfusion prevented the IR-induced tissue injury damage. This indicates that although neutrophils may have a role in the damage, complement inhibition is beneficial.

C1 inhibitor (C1 Inh) inhibits the earliest steps of the classical and the mannose binding lectin pathways. When C1 Inh was administered to mice prior to mesenteric IR, mucosal injury and was effectively inhibited in a dose dependent manner (51). These findings emphasize the importance of complement activation in ischemia/reperfusion and highlight the potential therapeutic use of C1 Inh in limiting and/or preventing damage.

Because the local damage itself is not believed to be life threatening, other groups have focused on C5a as a cause of the excessive systemic inflammatory response. Using a small peptide C5a receptor antagonist that binds the human C5a receptor, it has been shown that serum markers of systemic inflammation, neutrophil activation and remote organ injury can be prevented even when the peptide is given during the ischemic period, prior to beginning reperfusion (11, 15, 45).

Recently, IVIg (high-doses of immunoglobulins modified for intravenous use (46)) have successfully blocked complement mediated tissue injury in a rat model of mesenteric ischemia/reperfusion (47-49). Therefore, although the exact mechanism of complement activation has not been elucidated, it is apparent that complement plays a substantial role in both local and systemic tissue injury during ischemia of multiple organs.

7.   DEVELOPMENT OF THERAPEUTICS TO PREVENT COMPLEMENT MEDIATED INTESTINAL INJURY

As indicated above, complement activation is part of the pathogenic process in mesenteric IR. The complement activation process appears to involve each of the three initiation channels as well as the common terminal pathway and anaphylatoxin in the damage process. As discussed above, animal models of mesenteric IR have clearly shown that inhibition of complement activation can prevent, improve or reverse the disease pathology. Naturally occurring inhibitors control the amount of injury induced by the cascade of complement activation and may become useful therapeutics. However prior to the therapeutic use of these inhibitors, a number of important questions must be answered. First, is complement central in pathology of mesenteric IR? Second, which pathway is the primary initiator of the activation? Third, is general complement inhibition associated with side effects such as suppression of the innate immunity and the appearance of overwhelming infections?

Complement inhibitors for therapeutic use in mesenteric IR are being designed in a logical fashion. First, using molecular engineering, monoclonal antibodies that block activation of central complement factors can be humanized and used in the treatment of disease. An anti-C5 antibody is in human trials for use in other diseases. Second, the half-life of natural complement activation inhibitors such as DAF, CD59, CR1 can be extended by genetically fusing with the Fc portion of IgG. Third, fusing of multiple complement inhibitors that act at different stages of the activation cascade may act at different phases resulting in more effective complement inhibition. Fourth, recently, peptide inhibitors blocking the action of convertases have emerged as a new promising approach. Compstatin represents such an example as it inhibits complement activation by blocking C3 convertase-mediated cleavage of C3 (50). Fifth, and lastly, in response to the consideration that the use of complement inhibitors may cause systematic inhibition and unwanted side effects, from the complete lack of complement, such as overwhelming infection, investigators have considered the fusion of complement inhibitors to molecules that will direct it to the site of inflammation. For example, complement inhibitors can be conjugated to selectin ligands that will direct them to sites of increased selectin expression, i.e., inflammation or delivered via targeted liposomes to a specific location where the inhibitor is released in a concentrated region.

The opinions contained herein are the private ones of the authors and are not to be construed as official policy or reflecting the views of the Department of Defense.

8.   REFERENCES

1. Rehrig, S., S. D. Fleming, J. Anderson, J. M. Gutheridge, J. Rakstang, C. McQueen, V. M. Holers, G. C. Tsokos, and T. Shea-Donohue. 2001. Complement inhibitor, Crry-Ig attenuates intestinal damage after the onset of mesenteric ischemia/reperfusion injury in mice. *J. Immunol. 167:5921-5927.*

2. Eror, A. T., A. Stojadinovic, B. W. Starnes, S. C. Makrides, G. C. Tsokos, and T. Shea-Donohue. 1999. Anti-inflammatory effects of soluble complement receptor type 1 promote rapid recovery of ischemia/reperfusion injury in rat small intestine. *Clin. Immunol. 90:266-275.*

3. Conner, W. C., C. M. Gallagher, T. J. Miner, H. Tavaf-Motamen, K. M. Wolcott, and T. Shea-Donohue. 1999. Neutrophil priming state predicts capillary leak after gut ischemia in rats. *J. Surg. Res. 84:24-30.*

4. Kilgore, K. S., R. F. Todd, and B. R. Lucchesi. 1999. Reperfusion injury. In *Inflammation:basic principles and clinical correlates.* J. I. Gallin, and R. Snyderman, eds. Lippincott Williams and Wilkins, Philadelphia, p. 1047-1060.

5. D'Ambrosio, A. L., D. J. Pinsky, and E. S. Connolly. 2001. The role of the complement cascade in ischemia/reperfusion injury: implications for neuroprotection. *Mol. Med. 7:367-382.*

6. Fleming, S. D., S. T. Rehrig, J. M. Guthridge, T. Shea-Donohue, G. C. Tsokos, and V. M. Holers. 2000. Role of CR2- and CD19-regulated natural antibodies in intestinal ischemia reperfusion-induced injury. *Immunopharmacol. 49:22.*

7. Stahl, G. L., Y. Xu, L. Hao, M. Miller, J. A. Buras, M. Fung, and H. Zhao. 2003. Role for the alternate complement pathway in ischemia/reperfusion injury. *Am. J. Pathol. 162:449-455.*

8. Williams, J. P., T. T. V. Pechet, M. R. Weiser, R. Reid, L. Kobzik, F. D. Moore, M. C. Carroll, and H. B. Hechtman. 1999. Intestinal reperfusion injury is mediated by IgM and complement. *Journal of Applied Physiology 86:938-942.*

9. Austen, W. G., C. Kyriakides, J. Favuzza, Y. Wang, L. Kobzik, F. D. Moore, and H. B. Hechtman. 1999. Intestinal ischemia-reperfusion injury is mediated by the membrane attack complex. *Surgery 126:343-348.*

10. Hill, J., T. F. Lindsay, F. Ortiz, C. G. Yeh, H. B. Hechtman, and F. D. Moore. 1992. Soluble complement receptor type 1 ameliorates the local and remote organ injury after intestinal ischemia-reperfusion in the rat. *J. Immunol. 149:1723-1728.*

11. Fleming, S. D., J. Anderson, F. Wilson, T. Shea-Donohue, and G. C. Tsokos. 2003. C5 is required for CD49d expression on neutrophils and VCAM expression on vascular endothelial cells following mesenteric ischemia/reperfusion. *Clin. Immunol. 105:55-64.*

12. Ward, D. T., S. A. Lawson, C. M. Gallagher, W. C. Conner, and T. Shea-Donohue. 2000. Sustained nitric oxide production via L-Arginine administration ameliorates effects of intestinal ischemia-reperfusion. *J. Surg. Res. 89:13-19.*

13. Kohl, J. 2001. Anaphylatoxins and infections and non-infectious inflammatory diseases. *Mol. Immunol. 38:175-187.*

14. Wada, K., M. C. Montalto, and G. L. Stahl. 2001. Inhibition of complement C5 reduces local and remote organ injury after intestinal ishcmenia/reperfusion in the rat. *Gastroent. 120:126-133.*

15. Fleming, S. D., D. Mastellos, G. Karpel-Massler, T. Shea-Donohue, J. D. Lambris, and G. C. Tsokos. 2003. C5a-mediated mesenteric ischemia/reperfusion injury is independent of polymorphonuclear neutrophils. *Clin. Immunol 108:263-273.*

16. Wang, Y., S. A. Rollins, J. A. Madri, and L. A. Matis. 1995. Anti-C5 monoclonal antibody therapy prevents collagen-induced arthritis and ameliorates established disease. *Proceeding of the National Academy of Sciences USA 92:8955-8959.*

17. Vakeva, A. P., A. Agah, S. A. Rollins, L. A. Matis, L. Li, and G. L. Stahl. 1998. Myocardial infarction and apoptosis after myocardial ischemia and reperfusion: role of the terminal complement components and inhibition by anti-C5 therapy. *Circulation 97:2259-2267.*

18. Vakeva, A., and S. Meri. 1998. Complement activation and regulator expression after anoxic injury of human endothelial cells. *APMIS 106:1149-1156.*

19. Rinder, C. S., H. M. Rinder, B. R. Smith, J. C. K. Fitch, M. J. Smith, J. B. Tracey, L. A. Matis, S. P. Squinto, and S. A. Rollins. 1995. Blockade of C5a and C5b-9 generation

inhibits leukocyte and platelet activation duringextracorporeal circulation. *J. Clin. Invest.* *96:1564-1572.*

20. Fleming, S. D., T. Shea-Donohue, J. M. Guthridge, L. Kulik, T. J. Waldschmidt, M. G. Gipson, G. C. Tsokos, and V. M. Holers. 2002. Mice deficient in complement receptors 1 and 2 lack a tissue injury-inducing subset of the natural antibody repertoire. *J. Immunol. 169:2126-2133.*

21. Fosse, E., J. Pillgram-Larsen, J. Svennevig, C. Nordby, A. Skulberg, T. E. Mollnes, and M. Abdelnoor. 1998. Complement activation in injured patients occurs immediately and is dependent on the severity of the trauma. *Injury 29:509-514.*

22. Goris, R. J. A. 2000. Pathophysiology of shock in trauma. *Eur. J. Surg. 166:100-111.*

23. Gallinaro, R., W. G. Cheadle, K. Applegate, and H. C. Polk. 1992. The role of the complement system in trauma and infection. *Surgery 174:435-440.*

24. Mollnes, T. E., H.-J. Haga, J. G. Brun, E. W. Nielsen, A. Sjoholm, G. Sturfeldt, U. Martensson, K. Bergh, and O. P. Rekvig. 1999. Complement activation in patients with sytemic lupus erythematosus without nephritis. *Rheumatology 38:933-940.*

25. Fruchterman, T. M., D. A. Spain, M. A. Wilson, P. D. Harris, and R. N. Garrison. 1998. Complement inhbition prevents gut ischemia and endothelial cell dysfunction after hemorrhage/resuscitation. *Surgery 124:782-792.*

26. Weiser, M. R., T. T. Pehet, J. P. Williams, M. Ma, P. S. Frenette, F. D. Moore, L. Kobzik, R. O. Hines, D. D. Wagner, M. C. Carroll, and H. B. Hechtman. 1997. Experimental murine acid aspiration injury is mediated by neutrophils and the alternative complement pathway. *Journal of Applied Physiology 83:1090-1095.*

27. Zhou, W., C. A. Farrar, K. Abe, J. R. Pratt, J. E. Marsh, Y. Wang, G. L. Stahl, and S. H. Sacks. 2000. Predominant role of C5b-9 in renal ischemia/reperfusion injury. *J. Clin. Invest. 105:1363-1371.*

28. Collard, C. D., R. Lekowski, J. E. Jordan, A. Agah, and G. L. Stahl. 1999. Complement activation following oxidative stress. *Mol. Immunol. 36:941-948.*

29. Jordan, J. E., M. C. Montalto, and G. L. Stahl. 2001. Inhibition of mannose-binding lectin reduces postischemic myocardial reperfusion injury. *Circulation 104:1413-1418.*

30. Wetsel, R. A., J. Kildsgaard, and D. L. Haviland. 2000. Complement anaphylatoxins (C3a, C4a, C5a) and their receptors (C3aR, C5aR/CD88) as therapeutic targets in inflammation. In *Therapeutic interventions in the complement system.* J. D. Lambris, and V. M. Holers, eds. Humana Press, Totowa, NJ, p. 113-153.

31. Perianayagam, M. C., V. S. Balakrishnan, A. J. King, B. J. G. Pereira, and B. L. Jaber. 2002. C5a delays apoptosis of human neutrophils by a phosphatidylinositol 3-kinase-signaling pathway. *Kidney International 61:456-463.*

32. Tyagi, S., L. B. Klickstein, and A. Nicholson-Weller. 2000. C5a-stimulated human neutrophils use a subset of $\beta 2$ integrins to support the adhesion-dependent phase of superoxide production. *Journal of Leukocyte Biology 68:679-686.*

33. Binder, R., A. Kress, G. Kan, K. Hermann, and M. Kirschfink. 1999. Neurtophil priming by cytokines and vitamin D binding protein (Gc-globulin): impact on C5a-mediated chemotaxis, degranulation and respiratory burst. *Mol. Immunol. 36:885-892.*

34. Tofukuji, M., G. L. Stahl, C. Metais, M. Tomita, A. Agah, c. Bianchi, M. P. Fink, and F. W. Sellke. 2000. Mesenteric dysfunction after cardiopulmonary bypass: role of complement C5a. *Ann Thorac. Surg. 69:799-807.*

35. Bless, N. M., R. L. Warner, V. A. Padgaonkar, A. B. Lentsch, B. J. Czermak, H. Schmal, H. P. Friedl, and P. A. Ward. 1999. Roles for C-X-C chemokines and C5a in lung injury after hindlimb ischemia-reperfusion. *Am. J. Physiol. 276:L57-L63.*

36. Huber-Lang, M. S., J. V. Sarma, S. R. McGuire, K. T. Lu, R. F. Guo, V. A. Padgaonkar, E. M. Younkin, I. J. Laudes, N. C. Riedemann, J. G. Younger, and P. A. Ward. 2001.

Protective effects of anti-C5a peptide antibodies in experimental sepsis. *FASEB Journal 15:568-570.*

37. Huber-Lang, M., J. V. Sarma, K. T. Lu, S. R. McGuire, V. A. Padgaonkar, R. F. Guo, E. M. Younkin, R. G. Kunkel, J. Ding, R. Erickson, J. T. Curnutte, and P. A. Ward. 2001. Role of C5a in multiorgan failure during sepsis. *J. Immunol. 166:1193-1199.*

38. Riedemann, N. C., and P. A. Ward. 2003. Complement in ischemia reperfusion injury. *Am. J. Pathol. 162:363-367.*

39. Riedemann, N. C., R. F. Guo, T. A. Neff, I. J. Laudes, K. A. Keller, J. V. Sarma, M. M. Markiewski, D. Mastellos, C. W. Strey, C. L. Pierson, J. D. Lambris, F. S. Zetoune, and P. A. Ward. 2002. Increased C5a receptor expression in sepsis. *J. Clin. Invest. 110:101-108.*

40. Mulligan, M. S., E. Schmid, B. Beck-Schimmer, G. O. Till, H. P. Friedl, R. Brauer, T. E. Hugli, M. Miyasaka, R. L. Warner, K. J. Johnson, and P. A. Ward. 1996. Requirement and role of C5a in acute lung inflammatory injury in rats. *J. Clin. Invest. 98:503-512.*

41. Rothermel, E., O. Gotze, S. Zahn, and G. Schlaf. 2000. Analysis of the tissue distribution of the rat C5a receptor and inhibition of C5a-mediated effects through the use of two MoAbs. *Scand. J. Immunol. 52:401-410.*

42. Pellas, T. C., W. Boyar, J. V. Oostrum, J. Wasvary, L. R. Fryer, G. Pastor, M. Sills, A. Braunwalder, D. R. Yarwood, R. Kramer, E. Kimble, J. Hadala, W. Haston, R. Moreira-Ludewig, S. Uziel-Fusi, P. Peters, K. Bill, and L. Wennogle. 1998. Novel C5a receptor antagonists regulate neutrophil functions in vitro and in vivo. *Journal of Immunologyl 160:5616-5621.*

43. Heller, T., M. Hennecke, U. Baumann, J. E. Gessner, A. Meyer zu Vilsendorf, M. Baensch, F. Boulay, A. Kola, A. Klos, W. Bautsch, and J. Kohl. 1999. Selection of a C5a receptor antagonist from phage libraries attenuating the inflammatory response in immune complex disease and ischemia/reperfusion injury. *J. Immunol. 163:985-994.*

44. Haynes, D. R., D. G. Harkin, L. P. Bignold, M. J. Hutchens, S. M. Taylor, and D. P. Fairlie. 2000. Inhibition of C5a-induced neutrophil chemotaxis and macrophage cytokine production in vitro by a new C5a receptor antagonist. *Biochemical Pharmacology 60:729-733.*

45. Arumugam, T. V., I. A. Shiels, T. M. Woodruff, R. C. Reid, D. P. Fairlie, and S. M. Taylor. 2002. Protective effect of a new C5a receptor antagonist against ischemia-reperfusion injury in the rat small intestine. *J. Surg. Res. 103:260-267.*

46. Basta, M. 1996. Modulation of complement-mediated immune damage by intravenous immune globulin. *Clin. Exp. Immunol. 104 Suppl.1:21-25.*

47. Anderson, J., S. Fleming, M. Basta, G. Tsokos, and T. Shea-Donohue. 2001. Intravenous immunoglobulin (IVIG) attenuates mesenteric ischemia/reperfusion injury in rats. *Gastroenterology 120:A195.*

48. Anderson, J., S. Fleming, G. Tsokos, C. Swiecki, and T. Shea-Donohue. 2002. Intravenous immunoglobulin (IVIG) protects against the development of systemic injury following mesenteric ischemia/reperfusion. *Gastroent. (in press).*

49. Anderson., J., S. Rehrig, S. Fleming, M. Basta, G. Tsokos, and T. Shea-Donohue. 2001. Intravenous immunoglobulin attenuates mesenteric ischemia-reperfusioninjury. *Clin. Immunol. 99:170.*

50. Sahu, A., D. Morikis, and J. D. Lambris. 2003. Compstatin, a peptide inhibitor of complement, exhibits species specific binding to complement component C3. *Mol. Immunol. 39:557-566.*

51. Karpel-Massler, G., S.D. Fleming, M. Kirschfink, and G.C. Tsokos, 2003. Human C1 esterase inhibitor attenuates murine mesenteric ischemia/reperfusion induced local organ injury. *J. Surg. Res. 115:247-256.*

21

Role of C5a and C5a Receptor in Sepsis

F.S. Zetoune[*], P.A. Ward[*], M. S. Huber-Lang[#]
Department of Pathology, University of Michigan Medical School, Ann Arbor, MI. 48109
#Department of Trauma, Hand and Reconstructive Surgery, University of Ulm, Ulm, Germany

Abstract: In experimental sepsis (after cecal ligation and puncture, CLP) there is convincing evidence of complement activation, as there is in human sepsis. In addition, in sepsis involving rodents and humans, blood neutrophils have lost innate immune functions (chemotaxis, phagocytosis, the ability to produce H_2O_2). In CLP, and in neutrophils exposed to the complement anaphylatoxin, C5a, there is defective activation of MAPK (mitogen activated protein kinase), phosphorylation of p47, and inability to assemble NADPH oxidase. In experimental sepsis, the consumptive coagulopathy can be prevented by anti-C5a. Sepsis is also associated with loss of C5a receptor (C5aR) on neutrophils. In sepsis, thymocytes undergo apoptosis that is C5a mediated. All of these abnormalities occurring in experimental sepsis can be reversed by treatment with anti-C5a, with C5aR antagonist, with anti-C5aR, or with anti-IL-6, which causes upregulation of C5aR. These data suggest that generation of C5a during sepsis is harmful and that its interception or blockade of C5aR is beneficial.

Key words: TNFα, C3a, C4a, C5a, C5b, C5aR, PMN, CARS

1.   INTRODUCTION

Sepsis in humans is a daunting clinical problem that has, in general, defied effective therapy. At present, therapy is largely supportive, although recent clinical trials with moderate steroid dosage (1) or with activated protein C (2) have provided some evidence for encouragement. Over the past decade, clinical trials with a variety of anti-inflammatory interventions (e.g. antibodies to LPS or TNFα, use of interleukin-1 receptor antagonist, anti-thrombin interventions, kinin antagonists, etc.) have been therapeutically unsuccessful (reviewed, 3). Such interventions have been based on an assumption that the sepsis syndrome represents an uncontrolled systemic inflammatory response (4). These failed clinical trials suggest that we are still some distance from an accurate understanding of the nature of the sepsis syndrome. In as much as in the U.S. there are approximately 750,000 cases of sepsis per year with a mortality rate higher than 25% (5), there is an urgent need to secure a better understanding of the pathophysiology of sepsis.

2.   EXPERIMENTAL MODELS OF SEPSIS

The appropriate use of animal models of sepsis is key to developing more effective therapeutic interventions for the treatment of sepsis in humans. Up to the present, rodent models have been frequently employed as surrogates for human sepsis. The intravenous infusion of LPS into mice results in an early peak in plasma levels of TNFα, as well as IL-1β and IL-6 (reviewed, 6). Pretreatment of mice with antibodies to TNFα effectively protects these animals from lethality (7). This became the basis for the design of human clinical trials in sepsis (8). Other models of sepsis in rodents and subhuman primates have included the intravenous infusion of live bacteria (*E. coli* or *Pseudomonas aeruginosa*), which eventually results in cardio-vascular collapse and death (9-11). However, these models have been criticized as not being representative of human sepsis in as much as massive infusions of live bacteria were employed, which does not reflect the pathophysiological changes seen in human sepsis. Such approaches have been described as models of "intoxication" (12).

The cecal ligation/puncture (CLP) model has been widely used in rodents and has many features of sepsis in humans (Table 1).

Table 1. Cecal ligation/puncture (CLP) as a model of sepsis

- Used in rodents (rats, mice).
- Simulates the clinical course of human sepsis (a hyperdynamic followed by a hypodynamic phase).
- Simulates the pattern of pro- and anti-inflammatory mediators in human sepsis (cytokine/chemokine network).
- Lethality can be calibrated by needle size and number of cecal punctures.
- Extensive literature describing the CLP model.
- Knockout" mice can be used to define mediator pathways

This model can be calibrated to produce lower or higher rates of lethality based on the size of the ligated cecum, the number of needle-induced punctures, and the needle size (reviewed, 13). CLP animals develop an early hyperdynamic phase characterized by increased cardiac output and tachycardia, fever, leukocytosis and hypercapnia. As sepsis progresses over the next 12-24 hr, these features evolve into bradycardia, falling cardiac output, hypothermia, and an overt shock-like syndrome, along with the development multi-organ failure (liver, heart, kidneys, lungs) (14). As such, these features closely mimic the clinical progression of sepsis observed in humans, with the exception that the events in septic rodents appear to be occurring within a compressed frame of time as compared to the usual 4-5 day time frame in humans treated in intensive care units. The CLP model in rats and mice currently is probably the most widely used and accepted model of experimental sepsis.

3. EVIDENCE FOR COMPLEMENT ACTIVATION IN SEPSIS

There is compelling evidence that in sepsis (both in animals and in humans), complement activation and consumption have occurred (Table 2).

Table 2. Evidence for complement activation in sepsis

- Falling serum CH50/mL values
- Presence in plasma of C3a, C4a, C5a and C5b-9
- Reduced levels of C5aR on blood PMN
- Correlation of plasma C3a, C4a and C5a with clinical outcome

Falling levels of complement hemolytic activity (CH50) have been observed frequently in experimental sepsis and in humans with sepsis (15,16). In the CLP model, rat CH50 levels fall by about 50% during the first 24 hr of sepsis and then gradually return towards normal levels in survivors (15). The complement activation products, including the anaphylatoxins (C3a, C4a, C5a) and the membrane attack complex (C5b-9) have been detected in the plasma of subhuman primates and humans with sepsis (11,17). The ability to detect the anaphylatoxins, especially C5a, is technically difficult because of the presence of high affinity C5a receptors (C5aR) on circulating neutrophils (PMN). These receptors, which number approximately 50,000/PMN, will absorb C5a, which can only be detected in serum after C5aR saturation on leukocytes has occurred. While it might be argued that C5a detection on blood PMN could be an effective alternative to measuring plasma C5a, it is known that once C5a is bound to C5aR, the receptor-ligand is rapidly internalized, with subsequent C5aR recycling via the Golgi apparatus, with return of C5aR to the cell surface. Accordingly, measurement of leukocyte-bound C5a is technically not a reliable strategy for estimates of C5a generation *in vivo*.

There are data that indirectly suggest C5a generation in humans with sepsis. While more extensive accumulation of data in humans is required, the information to date indicates an early reduction in C5aR content on surfaces of blood PMN in the first 24-36 hr of sepsis, with a gradual restoration during subsequent days (18). As described below, in rats with CLP there are substantial reductions in C5aR content in blood PMN in the first 36 hr, in a manner that is predictive of survival or lethality. C5aR internalization in CLP rodents is also associated with the loss of innate immune functions (chemotaxis, phagocytosis, H_2O_2 production) (19, see below for details).

4.   SEPSIS AND LOSS OF REGULATION OF THE INFLAMMATORY RESPONSE

It is well established that sepsis is associated with the systemic inflammatory response syndrome (SIRS), defined by the main presence of pro-inflammatory mediators in the plasma (e.g. TNFα, IL-1, IL-6, IL-8, etc.).   The phenomenon could be due to excessive local generation of mediators or loss of control in the generation of inflammatory mediators. In fact, both appear to be responsible for SIRS.   The compensatory anti-inflammatory response syndrome (CARS) features increased levels of anti-inflammatory interleukins (IL-4, IL-10, IL-13, etc.), which can function to inhibit the inflammatory response during sepsis (4,20) (Fig. 1).

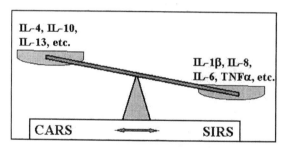

Figure 1. Perturbed inflammatory response during sepsis

In CLP-induced sepsis, generation of inflammatory proteins is indicated by the presence of inflammatory mediators in the peritoneal cavity (21,22), presumably caused by local activation of macrophages.   In addition, organ and plasma levels of the anti-inflammatory interleukins, IL-4, IL-10 and IL-13, are altered, for reasons unknown (23,24). IL-4 and IL-10 are potent anti-inflammatory mediators that suppress generation of pro-inflammatory mediators by blocking activation of NFκB or by modulating both the transcription and stability of specific mRNAs (25). The disturbance of these anti-inflammatory interleukins implies that gene activation leading to production of pro-inflammatory mediators is relatively uncontrolled, resulting in unregulated expression of these powerful mediators. It has been suggested that the sepsis syndrome is in part due to the lack of CARS, i.e., generation of regulatory interleukins with anti-inflammatory potency (20). There is no doubt that the "unhindered" presence in plasma of potent pro-inflammatory mediators such as TNFα and IL-1 during sepsis is an indication that control of the inflammatory response has been lost, resulting in a serious compromise of homeostasis (Figure 1).

4.1 COMPLEMENT-DEPENDENT LOSS OF INNATE IMMUNE FUNCTIONS

Recent studies suggest that CLP-induced sepsis in rats leads to loss of innate immune functions (15,19). Innate immunity is defined as protective shield against invading micro-organisms or pathogens, with protective cell functions that do not require induction of an immune response, a "primed" cellular defense or a secondarily enhanced humoral immune response. It is well established during sepsis that leukocyte function is perturbed (reviewed, 3). Our own studies indicate that, in CLP rats, blood PMN is functionally defective (Table 3).

Table 3. Loss of innate immune functions in PMN during sepsis

- Defective binding of C5a
- Defective chemotactic responses
- Defective phagocytosis
- Defective H_2O_2 production

PMN lose their ability to phagocytize IgG opsonized zymosan particles (19), which implies that phagocytic functions of leukocytes (including PMN) are impaired. This would suggest that the ability of PMN to phagocytize and kill bacteria is also lost, which would represent a fundamental loss of innate host defense function. In addition, blood PMN obtained from CLP rats demonstrate a striking loss (nearly 90%) in C5a binding. This defect appears to be rather specific since binding of the bacterial chemotactic peptide, formyl-Met-Leu-Phe (fMLP) via their specific receptors (C5aR or fMLP-R, respectively) is not affected (14).

Nevertheless, chemotactic responses of blood PMN from CLP rats are greatly depressed to both C5a and fMLP, implying the development of a defect in a common signaling pathway that is engaged after receptor interaction with either C5a or fMLP. This C5a-related defect in chemotactic responsiveness of blood PMN is correlated with several abnormalities in the common signaling pathways of PMN in response to agonists such as C5a, fMLP or PMA, loss in the ability to phosphorylate p42 of MAPK and loss of phosphorylation of the protein, p47^{phox}, which is key subunit in the cytosol required for assembly of NADPH oxidase on the surface of PMN (Table 4). (Please check sentence, too complex)

Table 4. Signaling defects in PMN exposed to C5a
- Defective MAPK activation (reduced phosphorylation of p42 (ERK ½)
- Defective phosphorylation of p47^{phox}
- Defective translocation of p47^{phox} to cell membrane

The inability to phosphorylate cytoplasmic p47^{phox} causes defective translocation of p47^{phox} from the cytosol to the cell membrane. Under these conditions, assembly of NADPH oxidase is blocked, and the ability of blood PMN stimulated with PMA to generate H_2O_2 is greatly impaired. The inability of PMN to generate H_2O_2 results in a loss of their intrinsic capacity to kill ingested bacteria in an oxygen-dependent manner. These defects appear to explain why during CLP phagocytic cells lose innate immune functions that are necessary for bacterial clearance.

The above mentioned studies indicate that loss of innate immune function (chemotaxis, phagocytosis and H_2O_2 production) in phagocytic cells is related to excessive systemic production of C5a. Treatment of CLP rats with antibodies to C5a greatly improves survival and preserves innate immune functions that are described above (15,19,26). *In vitro* studies confirm that exposure of PMN to C5a impairs the ability of PMN to respond to PMA with generation of H_2O_2. This process is time-dependent and related to the concentration of C5a used for PMN exposure (19). The concentrations of C5a (10-100 nM) that will induce these defects are those that have been found in the sera of human patients with sepsis (16,27,28).

5.   EVIDENCE FOR C5A-DEPENDENT CHANGES IN SEPSIS

As indicated above, reduction of CH50/mL in sera/plasma obtained from animals with sepsis has been described, as has the enhanced presence in serum of C5a. Our own experiments have indicated the loss of C5aR on blood PMN during CLP-induced sepsis. As demonstrated by flow cytometry, blood PMN lost nearly 90% of C5aR protein during the first 36 hr of CLP-induced sepsis in rats (29). This closely correlates with a companion loss in binding of ^{125}I-C5a to blood PMN under the same conditions (19). Loss of C5aR on blood PMN is probably due to internalization of C5a-C5aR complexes on the surfaces of PMNs during sepsis-induced generation of C5a. There appears to be a close correlation between C5aR loss, loss of innate immune functions and lethal outcomes of sepsis (19,29).

While CLP-induced sepsis is associated with loss of C5aR on PMN and loss of innate immune functions of these cells (see above), there is an interesting inverse finding with changes in C5aR content in organs (liver, lung, kidneys, heart) during sepsis. In this case, C5aR content, as defined by mRNA and protein for C5aR (detected by binding of ^{125}I-anti-C5aR), is considerably increased 6 hr after CLP (29,30). This increase is associated, as would be expected, with increased binding of ^{125}I-C5a to these organs. The increase in CLP-induced C5aR expression appears to be dependent on the appearance of IL-6 during CLP (30). IL-6 is an acute phase protein, which peaks early (within 6 hr) after CLP-induced sepsis. IL-6 has been described to be able to induce C5aR on rat hepatocytes (31). Our own studies indicate that *in vitro* exposure of microvascular endothelial or alveolar epithelia cells to IL-6, LPS or IFN-γ induces increased binding of C5a (32). As well, increased C5aR expression (both RNA and protein) during CLP is suppressed by infusion of anti-IL-6. This intervention also provides considerably enhanced protection of mice after CLP, supporting the linkage between increased expression of C5aR in various organs during sepsis and susceptibility to organ injury and lethality (30). However, direct evidence that exposure of organs to C5a during sepsis leads to organ dysfunction has yet to be demonstrated.

6. C5A-SENSITIVE CHANGES IN COAGULATION/FIBRINOLYSIS DURING SEPSIS

In CLP rats treated with control (pre-immune) rabbit IgG, there was, as expected, increased evidence of procoagulant activity (prolongation of the activated partial thromboplastin time and prothrombin time, reduced platelet counts, and increased plasma levels of fibrinogen (33), (reviewed, Table 5). Evidence indicating thrombin formation was shown by early consumption of factor VII:C, consumption of factors IX:C, and IX:C and anti-thrombin. In addition, the plasma showed elevated levels of thrombin-anti-thrombin complexes and D-dimer. These plasma samples also showed evidence for fibrinolysis as indicated by increased plasma levels of plasminogen activator together with reduced levels of plasminogen. Collectively, these data suggest that, during CLP-induced sepsis, activation of both the clotting and fibrinolytic cascades occurs, as shown by appearance of activated factors, consumptive depletion of others, and presence of protein complexes indicative of these changes. Almost without exception, all of the perturbations in the clotting and fibrinolytic systems were reversed in CLP rats that had been infused with rabbit IgG targeting C5a (anti-C5a) at the beginning of CLP. In addition, treatment of CLP rats with anti-C5a (using the same animals as those used for the blood parameters described in Table 5) showed an improvement in survival (see below). The precise mechanisms for the protective effects of anti-C5a are not known. They could be due to the attenuated bacteremia occurring in CLP rats treated with anti-C5a in as much as this treatment preserves innate immune function of PMN (see above). Alternatively, improved outcome might be due to the fact that C5a has a variety of stimulatory effects on endothelial cells, including induction and release of von Willebrand factor (vWF) and tissue factor (TF) (34), both of which could lead to activation of the coagulation system and expression of endothelial P-selectin, which would cause adherence of PMN (35).

Table 5. C5a-dependent changes in clotting and fibrinolytic cascades during experimental sepsis

- Increased procoagulant activity.
- Prolonged activated partial thromboplastin time.
- Prolonged activated prothrombin time.
- Reduced platelet counts in blood.
- Increased plasma fibrinogen.
- Thrombin activation.
- Early consumption of factor VII: C.
- Consumption of factors XI:C, IX:C.
- Consumption of anti-thrombin.
- Presence of thrombin-anti-thrombin complexes and D-dimer.
- Activation of fibrinolysis.
- Reduced plasminogen.
- Increased tissue plasminogen activator and plasminogen activator inhibitor.

Whatever the mechanisms may be, treatment of CLP with control IgG was associated with survival at 12, 24 and 36 hr of 87%, 40% and 31%, respectively, while at the same intervals of time mortality rates in anti-C5a treated CLP rats were 92%, 72% and 63%, respectively. These data confirm our earlier reports describing the protective effects of anti-C5a in CLP rats.

7.   APOPTOSIS DURING SEPSIS

It has been suggested that sepsis causes apoptosis, which may result in organ dysfunction. Apoptosis in CLP mice has been reported to occur in lymphoid organs (36), resulting in acute immunodeficiency, which is linked to lethality (37,38). Mice which transgenically express the apoptosis inhibitor, Bcl2 are protected from the lethal effects of CLP-induced sepsis (39) as are CLP mice treated with caspase inhibitors (caspase 3-inhibitor or polycaspase inhibitor) (40). As expected, during experimental sepsis, CLP rats show a nearly 66% loss of thymic mass within the first 24 hr of CLP (41) (Table 6).

Table 6. Apoptosis during experimental sepsis

- Reduced lymphoid mass (spleen, lymph nodes, Peyers patches, thymus).
- Increased expression of mRNA and protein for C5aR on thymocytes.
- Increased binding of C5a to thymocytes.
- Activation of caspases 3,6,8, leading to apoptosis.

This is associated with activation of caspases 3, 6, and 9. Such findings are consistent with the caspase pathway of activation involving mitochondrial release of cytochrome C, its interaction with Apaf-1, and subsequent caspase activation, which leads to breakdown of nuclear DNA. In rats, CLP causes increased expression of mRNA for C5aR in thymocytes, increased binding of C5a, and C5a-dependent induction of apoptosis, as quantitated by increased binding of annexin-V (41,42). Treatment of CLP rats with anti-C5a protects against the loss of thymic mass and greatly reduces apoptosis of thymocytes (41). Whether enhanced expression of C5aR in lungs, liver, kidneys and heart is also associated with C5a dependent apoptosis during CLP-induced sepsis is not presently known. Those findings indicate that CLP-induced sepsis in rats leads to C5a-dependent loss of innate immune function of phagocytic cells and also results in apoptosis of thymocytes, both of which would appear to be inimical to survival of these animals.

8. PROTECTIVE INTERVENTIONS IN EXPERIMENTAL SEPSIS

As reviewed in Table 7 and described above, interventions that directly block C5a or C5aR are highly protective in rodents undergoing CLP. In a dose-dependent manner, polyclonal rabbit IgG to rat C5a greatly attenuates the lethal outcomes of sepsis (14,26,43). These protective effects are dependent on the dose of anti-C5a as well as the time of administration of anti-C5a. Administration of anti-C5a simultaneously with induction of CLP is highly protective, whereas delayed infusion of the antibody (6 and 12 hr after CLP) has progressively diminished protective effects (26). The specificity of the anti-C5a preparation in relation to the resulting *in vivo* effect (such as cellular, organ- and immune functions or survival of animals with sepsis) is also important. Antibody directed against the N-terminal region (residues 1-16) of C5a is poorly protective whereas antibodies directed against the middle (residues 17-36) and C-terminal (residues 58-77) regions of rat C5a are highly protective (26).

Antibody to C5aR has been shown to be a particularly protective intervention in CLP mice (29). The antibody is a polyclonal rabbit IgG directed towards the N-terminal extracellular peptide region of C5aR. When infused at time 0 of CLP, mice were significantly protected (survival at 5 days improving from 0% to 70%). Although the mechanism of these protective effects is not known, it is presumed that infusion of the antibody prevents interaction of C5a with C5aR, protecting innate immune functions of phagocytic cells that otherwise would deteriorate during sepsis (as described above). Another protective intervention aimed at blocking interactions of C5a with C5aR is treatment of CLP mice with the recently developed C5aR antagonist (C5aRa), F[OPdChaWR] (44). This cyclic peptide is resistant to hydrolysis and prevents binding of C5a to C5aR. When infused into CLP mice, the survival rate at 7 days is also greatly improved, from 0% to 60% (45).

Finally, as indicated above, during CLP IL-6 appears to cause upregulation of C5aR in a variety of organs (lung, liver, heart, kidney). Infusion of antibody against IL-6 (anti-IL-6) at the time of induction of CLP improved the survival rate at day 7 from 0% to 60% (30). It was demonstrated that this treatment prevented or delayed expression of mRNA for C5aR in lungs, liver, kidneys and heart and reduced C5aR protein expression in organs back to control levels. In accord with the effect of anti-C5a and anti-C5aR, anti-IL-6 was protective because of its ability to suppress upregulation of C5aR during sepsis.

Table 7. Protective interventions in sepsis

1) Blockade of C5a by antibodies
   a. antibodies against the whole C5a molecule
   b. antibodies against specific (synthetic) peptide regions of C5a (representing the amino- or middle- or carboxy-terminal region of the C5a molecule)
2) Blockade of C5aR by:
   a. antibodies,
   b. C5aR antagonist (C5aRa),
   c. blockade of IL-6.

9.   CONCLUSIONS

Based upon the use of the CLP model of sepsis in rodents, there appears to be strong evidence that activation of complement in the course of the development of sepsis is harmful, probably because excessive C5a has been generated.   This leads to direct harmful impacts especially on blood neutrophils which under such conditions lose their innate immune functions (chemotaxis, phagocytosis, H_2O_2 production).   Concomitantly, the systemic inflammatory response syndrome (SIRS) develops, associated with the presence of cytokines and chemokines in the circulation, suggesting that there has been loss of control and containment of the inflammatory response. These changes result in a greatly diminished ability of the phagocytic cell system to clear and destroy bacteria.   Excessive production of C5a during sepsis also appears to be associated with extensive consumption of coagulation and fibrinolytic pathways, resulting in consumptive depletion of these factors and loss of homeostatic control of the coagulation system. All of these adverse consequences can be largely attenuated and survival can be greatly improved if C5a is blocked, if C5aR is blocked or if IL-6 is blocked; the last appears to be an important inducer of C5aR.   Collectively, these studies suggest that excessive activation of the complement system during sepsis goes beyond the protective functions of complement and, with excess of C5a generation greatly compromises host defenses.   The studies in rodents suggest the possibility that similar mechanisms may pertain to humans with sepsis.

10.   REFERENCES

1.   Annane, D., Sebille, V., Charpentier, C., Bollaert, P.E., Francois, B., Korach, J.M., Capellier, G., Cohen, Y., Azoulay, E., Troche, G., Chaumet-Riffaut, P., Bellisant, E. Effects of treatment with low doses of hydrocortisone and fludrocortisone on mortality in patients with septic shock. JAMA 2002; 288:862-871.
2.   Bernard, G.R. Vincent, J.L., Laterre, P.F., LaRosa, S.P., Dhainaut, J.F., Lopez-Rodriguez, A., Steingrub, J.S., Garber, G.E., Helterbrand, J.D., Ely, E.W., Fisher, C.J. Jr. Efficacy and safety of recombinant human activated protein C for severe sepsis. N Engl J Med 2001; 344:366-709.
3.   Hotchkiss, R.S., Karl, I.E. The pathophysiology and treatment of sepsis. N Engl J Med 2003; 348:138-150.
4.   American College of Chest Physicians/Society of Critical Care Medicine Consensus Conference. Definitions for sepsis and organ failure and guidelines for the use of innovative therapies in sepsis. Crit Care Med 1992; 20:864-874.
5.   Angus, D.C., Linde-Zwirble, W.T., Lidicker, J., Clermont, G., Carcillo, J., Pinsky, M.R. Epidemiology of sever sepsis in the United States: analysis of incidence, outcome, and associated cost of care. Crit Care Med 2001; 29:1303-1310.

6.   Ertel, W., Morrison, M.H., Wang, P., Ba, Z.F., Ayala, A., Chaudry, I.H. The complex pattern of cytokines in sepsis. Ann Surg 1991; 214:141-148.
7.   Beutler, G., Milsark, I.W., Cerami, A. Passive immunization against cachectin/tumor necrosis factor protects mice from lethal effects of endotoxin. Science 1985; 229:869-871.
8.   Abraham, E., Wunderink, R., Silverman, H., Perl, T.M., Nasraway, S., Levy, H., Bone, R., Wenzel, R.P., Balk, R., Allred, R., et al. Efficacy and safety of monoclonal antibody to human tumor necrosis factor alpha in patients with sepsis syndrome: a randomized, controlled, double-blind, multicenter clinical trial. JAMA 1995; 273:934-41.
9.   Mohr, M., Hopken, U., Oppermann, M., Mathes, C., Goldmann, K., Siever, S., Gotze, O., Burchardi, H. Effects of anti-C5a monoclonal antibodies on oxygen use in a porcine model of severe sepsis. Eur J Clin Invest 1998; 28(3):227-234.
10. Stevens, J.H., O'Hanley, P., Shapiro, J.M., Mihm, F.G., Satoh, P.S., Collins, J.A., Raffin, T.A. Effects of anti-C5a antibodies on the adult respiratory distress syndrome in septic primates. J Clin Invest 1986; 6:1812-1816.
11. Hangen, D.H., Stevens, J.H., Satoh, P.S., Hall, E.W., O'Hanley, P.T., Raffin, T.A. Complement levels in septic primates treated with anti-C5a antibodies. J Surg Res 1989; 46(3):195-199.
12. Deitch, E.A. Animal models of sepsis and shock: a review and lessons learned. Shock 1997; 9:1-11.
13. Wichterman, K.A., Baue, A.E., Chaudry, I.H. Sepsis and septic shock – a review of laboratory models and a proposal. J Surg Res 1980; 29:189-201.
14. Huber-Lang, M., Sarma, V.J., Lu, K.T., McGuire, S.R., Padgaonkar, V.A., Guo, R.F., Younkin, E.M., Kunkel, R.G., Ding, J., Erickson, R., Curnutte, J.T., Ward, P.A. Role of C5a in multiorgan failure during sepsis. J Immunol 2001; 166:1193-1199.
15. Czermak, B.J., Breckwoldt, M., Ravage, Z.B., Huber-Lang, M., Schmal, H., Bless, N.M., Friedl, H.P., Ward, P.A. Mechanism of enhanced lung injury during sepsis. Am J Pathol 1999; 154:1057-1065.
16. Nakae, H., Endo, S., Inada, K., Yoshida, M. Chronological changes in the complement system in sepsis. Surg Today 1996; 26:225-229.
17. Bengtson, A., Heideman, M. Anaphylatoxin formation of sepsis. Arch Surg 1988; 123(5):645-649.
18. Furebring, M., Hakansson, L.D., Venge, P., Nilsson, B., Sjolin, J. Expression of the C5a receptor (CD88) on granulocytes and monocytes in patients with severe sepsis. Crit Care 2002; 6:363-370.
19. Huber-Lang, M., Younkin, E.M., Sarma, V.J., McGuire, S.R., Lu, K.T., Guo, R.F., Padgaonkar, V.A., Curnutte, J.T., Erickson, R., Ward, P.A. Complement-induced impairment of innate immunity during sepsis. J Immunol 2002; 169:3223-3231.
20. Bone, R.C., Grodzin, C.J., Balk, R.A. Sepsis: a new hypothesis for pathogenesis of the disease process. Chest 1997; 112:235-243.
21. Matsukawa, A., Hogaboam, C.M., Lukacs, N.W., Lincoln, P.M., Strieter, R.M., Kunkel, S.L. Endogenous monocyte chemoattractant protein-1 (MCP-1) protects mice in a model of acute septic peritonitis: cross-talk between MCP-1 and leukotriene B4. J Immunol 1999; 163:6148-6154.
22. Qiu, G., Wang, C., Smith, R., Harrison, K., Yin, K. Role of IFN-gamma in bacterial containment in a model of intra-abdominal sepsis. Shock 2001; 16:425-429.
23. Matsukawa, A., Hogaboam, C.M., Lukacs, N.W., Lincoln, P.M., Evanoff, H.L., Strieter, R.M., Kunkel, S.L. Expression and contribution of endogenous IL-13 in an experimental model of sepsis. J Immunol 2000; 164:2738-2744.

24. Ayala, A., Deol, Z.K., Lehman, D.L., Herdon, C.D., Chaudry, I.H. Polymicrobial sepsis but not low-dose endotoxin infusion causes decreased splenocyte IL-2/IFN-gamma release while increasing IL-4/IL-10 production. J Surg Res 1994; 56:579-585.

25. Hamilton, T.A., Ohmori, Y., Tebo, J. Regulation of chemokine expression by antiinflammatory cytokines.Immunol Res 2002; 25:229-245.

26. Huber-Lang, M., Sarma, V.J., McGuire, S.R., Lu, K.T., Guo, R.F., Padgaonkar, V.A., Younkin, E.M., Laudes, I.J., Riedemann, N.C., Younger, J.G., Ward, P.A. Protective effects of anti-C5a peptide antibodies in experimental sepsis. FASEB J 2001; 15:568-570.

27. McCabe, W.R. Serum complement levels in bacteremia due to gram negative organisms. N Engl J Med 1973; 288:21-23.

28. Hecke, F., Schmidt, U., Kola, A., Bautsch, W., Klos, A., Kohl, J. Circulating complement proteins in multiple trauma patients--correlation with injury severity, development of sepsis, and outcome. Crit Care Med 1997; 12:2015-2024.

29. Riedemann, N.C., Guo, R.F., Neff, T.A., Laudes, I.J., Keller, K.A., Sarma, V.J., Markiewski, M.M., Mastellos, D., Strey, C.W., Pierson, C.L., Lambris, J.D., Zetoune, F.S., Ward, P.A. Increased C5a receptor expression in sepsis. J Clin Invest 2002; 110:101-108.

30. Riedemann, N.C., Neff, T.A., Guo, R.F., Bernacki, K.D., Laudes, I.J., Sarma, J.V., Lambris, J.D., Ward, P.A. Protective effects of IL-6 blockade in sepsis are linked to reduced c5a receptor expression. J Immunol 2003; 170:503-507.

31. Schieferdecker, H.L., Schlaf, G., Koleva, M., Gotze, O., Jungermann, K. Induction of functional anaphylatoxin C5a receptors on hepatocytes by in vivo treatment of rats with IL-6. J Immunol 2000; 164:5453-5458.

32. Laudes, I.J., Chu, J.C., Huber-Lang, M., Gou, R.F., Riedemann, N.C., Sarma, J.V., Mahdi, F., Murphy, H.S., Speyer, C., Lu, K.T., Lambris, J.D., Zetoune, F.S., Ward, P.A. Expression and function of C5a receptor in mouse microvascular endothelial cells. J Immunol, 2002; 169:5962-5970.

33. Laudes, I.J., Chur, J.C., Sikranth, S., Huber-Lang, M., Guo, R.F., Riedemann, N., Sarma, J.V., Schmair, A.H., Ward, P.A. Anti-C5a ameliorates coagulation/fibrinolytic protein changes in a rat model of sepsis. Am J Pathol 2002; 160:1867-1875.

34. Ikeda, K., Nagasawa, K., Horiuchi, T., Nishizaka, H., Niho, Y. C5a induces tissue factor activity on endothelial cells. Thromb Haemost 1997; 77:394-398.

35. Foreman, K.E., Vaporciyan, A.A., Bonish, B.K., Jones, M.L., Johnson, K.J., Glovsky, M.M., Eddy, S.M., Ward, P.A. C5a-induced expression of P-selectin in endothelial cells. J Clin Invest 1994; 94:1147-1155.

36. Hiramatsu, M., Hotchkiss, R.S., Karl, I.E., Buchman, T.G. Cecal ligation and puncture (CLP) induces apoptosis in thymus, spleen, lung, and gut by an endotoxin and TNF-independent pathway. Shock 1997; 7:247-253.

37. Ayala, A., Herdon, C.D., Lehman, D.L., Ayala, C.A., Chaudry, I.H. Differential induction of apoptosis in lymphoid tissues during sepsis: variation in onset, frequency, and the nature of the mediators. Blood 1996; 87:4261-4275.

38. Hotchkiss, R.S., Swanson, P.E., Cobb, J.P., Jacobson, A., Buchman, T.G., Karl, I.E. Apoptosis in lymphoid and parenchymal cells during sepsis: findings in normal and T- and B-cell-deficient mice. Crit Care Med 1997; 25:1298-1307.

39. Coopersmith, C.M., Chang, K.C., Swanson, P.E., Tinsley, K.W., Stromberg, P.E., Buchman, T.G., Karl, I.E., Hotchkiss, R.S. Overexpression of Bcl-2 in the intestinal epithelium improves survival in septic mice. Crit Care Med 2002; 30:195-201.

40. Hotchkiss, R.S., Chang, K.C., Swanson, P.E., Tinsley, K.W., Hui, J.J., Klender, P., Xanthoudakis, S., Roy, S., Black, C., Grimm, E., Aspiotis, R., Han, Y., Nicholson,

D.W., Karl, I.E. Caspase inhibitors improve survival in sepsis: a critical role of the lymphocyte. Nat Immunol 2000; 1(6):496-501.

41. Guo, R.F., Huber-Lang, M., Wang, X., Sarma, V., Padgaonkar, V.A., Craig, R.A., Riedemann, N.C., McClintock, S.D., Hlaing, T., Shi, M.M., Ward, P.A. Protective effects of anti-C5a in sepsis-induced thymocyte apoptosis. J Clin Invest 2000; 106:1271-1280.

42. Riedemann, N.C., Guo, R.F., Laudes, I.J., Keller, K., Sarma, V.J., Padgaonkar, V., Zetoune, F.S., Ward, P.A. C5a receptor and thymocyte apoptosis in sepsis. FASEB J 2002; 16:887-888.

43. Czermak, B.J., Sarma, V., Pierson, C.L., Warner, R.L., Huber-Lang, M., Bless, N.M., Schmal, H., Friedl, H.P., Ward, P.A. Protective effects of C5a blockade in sepsis. Nature Med 1999; 5:788-792.

44. Strachan, A.J., Woodruff, T.M., Haaima, G., Fairlie, D.P., Taylor, S.M. A new small molecule C5a receptor antagonist inhibits the reverse-passive Arthus reaction and endotoxic shock in rats. J Immunol 2000; 164:6560-6565.

45. Huber-Lang, M., Riedemann, N.C., Sarma, V.J., Younkin, E.M., McGuire, S.R., Laudes, I.J., Lu, K.T., Guo, R.F., Neff, T.A., Padgaonkar, V.A., Lambris, J., Spruce, L., Mastellos, D., Zetoune, F.S., Ward, P.A. Protection of innate immunity by C5aR antagonist in septic mice. FASEB J 2002; 16:1567-1574.

22

Role of Complement in Multi-Organ Dysfunction Syndrome

Markus S. Huber-Lang[*,1], J. Vidya Sarma[*], Firas S. Zetoune[*], Peter A. Ward[*]

[*]Department of Pathology, University of Michigan Medical School, Ann Arbor, Michigan, 48109, [1]Department of Trauma, Hand and Reconstructive Surgery, University of Ulm, Ulm, Germany

Abstract: In critically ill humans with manifestation of a systemic inflammatory response syndrome (SIRS), the onset of multi-organ dysfunction syndrome (MODS) is a well known complication that is associated with a high mortality rate. Clinical and experimental evidence increasingly suggests, a disturbance of innate immunity, linked to the uncontrolled activation of the complement system, which results in excessive generation of anaphylatoxins (C3a, C4a, C5a) and impairment of the cellular defense system (especially neutrophil-dysfunction). Such changes may play a central role in the development of MODS. In experimentally-induced MODS, complement depletion, absence of C5 (C5-/- mice), specific blockade of the complement system by C1-inhibitor (C1-INH), soluble complement receptor-1 (sCR-1), blockade of C5a or its C5a receptor (C5aR), all appear to prevent the development of MODS and improve survival. Therefore, irrespective of the initial insult, early inhibition of excessive complement activation during SIRS might be a promising approach for preventing development of the deathly spiral of MODS

Key words: Complement, C3a, C4a, C5a, MAC, SIRS, MODS, MOF

1. INTRODUCTION

For more than a decade, it has been known that various severe insults or diseases can lead to a process of progressive dysfunction and failure of several interdependent organ systems. This so-called "multi-organ dysfunction syndrome" (MODS) (1) can be initiated either directly by tissue-damaging forces or indirectly as a consequence of a generalized inflammatory host response. Despite a concerted scientific and clinical effort to understand and interrupt the deathly spiral of the cell- and organ derangement, MODS is still poorly understood and worldwide is one of the major causes for a fatal outcome in patients during intensive care treatment (2,3). The development of MODS in both humans and animals appears to emerge as a consequence of progressive tissue hypoxia, complement activation and an unregulated release into the blood of a variety of pro-inflammatory mediators (interleukins, cytokines, chemokines) (3,4,5). In humans with systemic inflammatory response and MODS, there is well-established evidence for the appearance in plasma of complement activation products, especially the anaphylatoxins C3a, C4a, and C5a and the complement membrane attack complex (C5b-9) (6,7,8). In the tissue of lungs, liver, small intestine and kidneys of patients with developing MODS, deposition of C3a and C3b has been described (9). Furthermore, C5b-9 was found in capillary walls during MODS (10). Persistent elevation of C3a, C4a and C5a in plasma appears to be strongly correlated with development of MODS and is inversely correlated with survival (7,11,12). In children undergoing cardiopulmonary bypass surgery, increased C3 conversion (activation) with an increased ratio of C3d/C3 has been detected in patients who developed multi-organ failure (MOF) after surgery (13), suggesting increased generation of complement activation products during development of MODS.

Although MODS has long been looked upon as a sequel of sepsis, it is now evident that MODS can be considered as a separate entity, can develop in the absence of any invasive bacteria (14), and can occur exclusively as a consequence of excessive activation of the innate immune system (15) (eg. after ischemia, severe trauma, haemorrhage, acute pancreatitis, etc.). Once initiated, the apocalyptic path of progressive cellular- and organ dysfunction follows almost the same pathophysiologic and clinic patterns, irrespective of the nature of the initial insult. There is increasing evidence that the long missing link between the various initial triggers and the ultimate clinical appearance of MODS may be related to unregulated activation of the complement system.

2.   PATHOPHYSIOLOGY OF MODS

In critically ill patients (especially in patients with multiple-injury or after major surgery) there is a complex immune-modulation, usually with coexistence of pro-inflammatory events for host defenses and anti-inflammatory events in order to contain harmful effects of these inflammatory responses. It is now commonly understood that the development of MODS occurs mainly based on the following pathophysiologic sequel (1,15) (Figure 1).

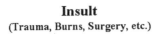

Insult

(Trauma, Burns, Surgery, etc.)

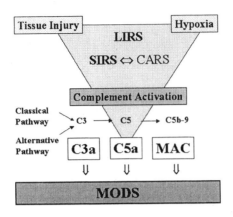

Figure 1. Pathophysiology of multi-organ dysfunction syndrome (MODS).
(LIRS, local inflammatory response; SIRS, systemic inflammatory response syndrome;
CARS, compensatory anti-inflammatory response syndrome; MAC, membrane attack
complex, C5b-9)

After the initial insult (induced by physical, biological or chemical injury) there is a local inflammatory response at the site of injury or infection. If the injured and/or hypoxic "microenvironment" cannot control the initial insult, there is an accentuated inflammatory response. If the impact of the injury is too extensive (e.g. during polytrauma, after major surgery, etc.) or if the host's immune system is weakened (e.g. advanced age, drug induced immunosuppression, etc.), there may occur a systemic inflammatory response (SIRS) resulting in excessive activation of the complement and cellular defense systems. Furthermore, there may also follow a dysregulation of the coagulation cascade and profound dysfunction of the endothelium with persistent vasodilatation. At this stage, clinical signs of MODS appear, as reflected by lung dysfunction (impairment of arterial oxygenation), renal dysfunction (azotemia, oliguria), liver dysfunction (increasing transaminases with hyperbilirubinemia), cardiac dysfunction (altered cardiac output), hypercoagulation (thrombocytopenia), to name just a few aspects of physiological dysfunction. If the compensatory anti-inflammatory response (CARS) is too dominant or if the immune system is impaired because of lymphocyte apoptosis, an "immune paralysis" with suppressed humoral- and cellular responses will appear (15-17). Clinically, this may be reflected by vulnerability to bacteria that are usually easily contained. The final stage of MODS has been called "immunological dissonance" (15), indicating an imbalance of the immune system, all of which is clinically manifest as progressive MODS.

During such events, there is evidence for excessive activation of the complement system which may be the "first trumpet of apocalyptic events" leading to MODS, organ failure and death (17-20).

3.   ROLE OF COMPLEMENT IN EXPERIMENTALLY-INDUCED MODS

To study the role of complement in MODS, different animal models have been established, all of which finally lead to a failing innate immune system with organ dysfunction or complete failure (Figure 2).

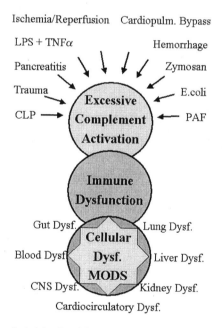

Figure 2. Various animal models of multi-organ dysfunction (MODS) lead via complement activation to immunological dysfunction and consequently to cellular and organ dysfunction. (dysf., dysfunction; LPS, lipopolysaccharides; TNFα, tumor necrosis factor alpha; CLP, cecal ligation and puncture; PAF, platelet activating factor.)

Since MODS is usually triggered by bacteria or bacterial products, it is not surprising that intravenous injection of bacterial wall products such as lipopolysaccharides (LPS) into mice induces some signs found in MODS (21,22), (e.g. activation of complement, accumulation of platelets in the lungs, intravascular fibrin deposition and cardio-respiratory changes). When C1-esterase inhibitor in combination with antithrombin III was administered to rabbits following LPS-induced lung and liver dysfunction, there was a significant decrease in intravascular clot formation in lungs and liver and improved cardiovascular function (22). In dogs, infusion of LPS induced endotoxic shock and resulted in MODS. However, dogs with genetically based C3 deficiency had decreased clearance of LPS and intensified organ damage when compared to complement-sufficient littermates, suggesting that C3 plays a beneficial role in the development of MODS (23).

Another important trigger for MODS is hypoxia occurring during ischemia (I). Occlusion of the superior mesenteric artery (SMA) for 1 hr has been shown subsequently to induce reperfusion (R) injury, bacterial translocation and finally, MODS (24). Increased plasma levels of C5a and thromboxane B2 were detected after the beginning of the reperfusion phase. The authors concluded that the anaphylatoxin, C5a, may be a potential factor in the development of gut barrier failure and MODS (24). Lower torso ischemia (2h) in mice also led during reperfusion (3h) to multi-organ injury. The remote organ injury was linked to increased lung vascular permeability and elevated transaminase levels (reflecting hepatocellular dysfunction) and increased neutrophil sequestration in various organs. Complement inhibition with soluble complement receptor type 1 (sCR1) demonstrated decreased lung and liver injury after I/R. Furthermore, mice deficient in C5 (C5$^{-/-}$ mice) exhibited nearly normal functional parameters during I/R, whereas lung and liver injury developed in C5$^{-/-}$ mice reconstituted with wild-type serum (from C5$^{+/+}$ mice), indicating that remote organ injury is complement C5-dependent (25).

Another experimental model in rats is massive blood loss which triggers MODS. In this hemorrhagic model, the presence of C1-inhibitor (C1-INH) abrogated enhanced leukocyte adhesion and rolling in the mesenteric microcirculation, which represents pathophysiologically an important mechanism related to induction of gut barrier failure during MODS (26). If in addition to hemorrhage, animals are also subjected to a simultaneous application of endotoxin (at a low dose), enormous intravascular activation of complement including C5a formation occurs and deposition of C3a and C3b in various tissues was observed (9). The severity of organ dysfunction in this "double hit" model is closely correlated with the extent of complement deposition. Microvascular lesions and infiltration of neutrophils into tissues were intense in lungs and liver, and to a lesser degree in the kidneys and gut. This is similar to clinical observations in which lungs and liver are usually the organs to fail (9).

If complement-intact mice were primed intravenously by tumor necrosis factor alpha (TNFα), followed 30 min later by infusion of LPS, all animals developed severe tissue injury (eg. bowel injury) and shock symptoms and ultimately died, whereas C5-deficient mice were protected against these fatal consequences (27) suggesting that TNFα and LPS act synergistically to activate the complement system in ways that are harmful. The same group showed in follow-up experiments that application of an antagonist to platelet-activating factor (PAF) prevented the TNFα/LPS-induced MODS. The injection of PAF alone (3 μg/kg body weight) was able to induce substantial signs of MODS. $C5^{-/-}$ mice were protected from these fatal effects, indicating that PAF leads via complement activation to shock and tissue injury (28).

The zymosan-induced mouse model of MODS (29) (induced by intraperitoneal injection of zymosan particles), which is a very effective and highly reproducible model, histologically exhibited an early neutrophil infiltration into lungs and spleen and an increasing number of blood neutrophils, the latter being decreased in $C5^{-/-}$ mice. Furthermore, the lack of C5 lead to a fourfold decrease in mortality in comparison to the complement-intact littermates (30).

Development of MODS can also be induced in association with severe acute pancreatitis (31), which is associated with increased plasma levels of C3a and C5a. Both C3a and C5a plasma levels correlated with severity of the MODS. The highest and most persistent anaphylatoxin levels were found in the MODS group, suggesting once again an important role of complement during MODS development.

In previous studies using the cecal ligation/puncture (CLP) model of sepsis in rats, which simulates human sepsis very closely, MODS occurred during the first 48 hr as reflected by a development of pulmonary, liver and renal dysfunction (see above). In this model an early respiratory alkalosis developed, followed by a metabolic acidosis with increased levels of blood lactate. If CLP-animals were treated with antibodies to rat C5a, the indicators of MODS and lactate acidosis were greatly attenuated (19).

As indicated above, various animal models may mimic development of MODS. Early activation of the complement system (especially involving C3 and C5) may be a common event leading to development of MODS.

4.   ROLE OF COMPLEMENT IN CELLULAR DYSFUNCTION

The development of MODS usually is the clinical mirror of "multi-cellular dysfunction" with perturbed intracellular and intercellular communication. With increasing hypoxemia there is overt or occult reduction in systemic oxygen supply, leading to cell dysfunction, associated with ATP depletion, failure of membrane ion pumps, calcium influx activating multiple enzymes, and sodium influx causing cell swelling, all of which results in cellular failure and in cell death. Common to hypoxic effects is the activation of the immuno-inflammatory cascade. Responses of cells which form the "first line of defense" of innate immunity no longer seem to be regulated (32). Neutrophil recruitment via endothelial activation seems to be essential to this process. Cytokines, chemokines and activated complement products (especially C5a) activate neutrophils and promote their adhesion and migration through the vascular endothelium. C5a is known to upregulate adhesion molecules on the endothelium via P-selectin, ICAM-1 and counter-receptors (such as β2 integrins) on the inflammatory cells (33). After recruitment, neutrophils do not appear to re-enter the circulation and apparently remain trapped in the tissue, putting the tissue at further risk of injury. Release from neutrophils of proteases and toxic oxygen species as well as enhanced adhesion of neutrophils to endothelial cells is thought to be associated with local or remote tissue injury that occurs in SIRS and MODS (16). There is now evidence that, during MODS development in sepsis, defective functions of neutrophils occurs. Neutrophils from patients with sepsis-induced multi-organ failure exhibited a loss of *in vitro* chemotactic responsiveness to C5a (16,17), this functional deficit being correlated with a loss of the ability of neutrophils to bind C5a (17). Our recent studies of CLP-induced MODS in rats have demonstrated an "immune paralysis" of neutrophils during developing sepsis, as evident by: substantial inhibition of blood neutrophils to migrate in vitro to chemotactic attractants, impaired phagocytotic activity, and significant reduction of the oxidative burst response (18,19). The cellular mechanisms are described in this volume by F.S. Zetoune, et. al. (Chapter 21). Thus, activated complement may be central for development of cellular dysfunction and, ultimately, organ failure.

5. ROLE OF COMPLEMENT IN ORGAN DYSFUNCTION

Based on these findings at the cellular level, excessive activation of the complement system occurs, followed by dysfunction of cellular defense involving the innate immune system. This constellation of events seems to be ultimately linked to initiation and progression of organ injury.

5.1   Immune Failure

As a "first line of defense", recruited neutrophils with their antimicrobial arsenal of proteases and reactive oxygen species, may contain invading bacteria but may also harm host tissues (34). Neutrophils also participate independently of remote organ injury by "transferring" the initial localized inflammatory response to other organs. It is well known, especially in the early stage of the systemic inflammatory response, that excessively generated complement factors, C3a and C5a, can "prime" and stimulate neutrophils and the monocyte/macrophage system to cause enhanced release of proteases, oxygen radicals and pro-inflammatory chemokines.   The terminal complement complex, C5b-9, is also deposited on invading bacteria.   When assembled, on mammalian cells, C5b-9 might also contribute to the cell and organ damage (10). In concert with hypoxia, complement has been shown to play an important role in ARDS (35). After hyperactivation of the immuno-inflammatory cascades, substantial immuno-suppression may follow (15).   Again, the complement system seems to be crucially involved in this development. Uncontrolled generation of C3a is known to be associated with an immuno-suppressive outcome affecting B-cell function, leading to diminished production of antibodies (36). Not only the humoral branch of the immune system but also the cellular branch appears to be altered by complement. For example, excessive production of C5a leads to: neutrophil dysfunction with loss of bacterial killing (18), platelet activation (37), and direct or indirect microvascular damage (38). Disturbances of the complement system seem to be closely related to the late "immunologic dissonance" (15) or "immune failure", resulting in the loss of ability to contain bacteria in tissues, putting all organs at risk of increased vulnerability, dysfunction and failure.

5.2   Lung Failure

MODS in humans is usually coincident with development of the "adult respiratory distress syndrome" (ARDS), which frequently represents a fatal complication of the systemic inflammatory response (39).   Several factors have been implicated in the pathogenesis of ARDS, including neutrophils, chemokines, cytokines and activation products of complement. In humans, an increased C3a/C3 ratio has been described to be a predictor of ARDS (40).   There is also a strong association between elevated plasma C5a and the onset of ARDS, with elevated plasma levels of C5a being observed 8-72 hr before the clinical recognition of ARDS (41). In the early stages of ARDS, development of a mild respiratory alkalosis is caused by hyperventilation, at which time normal oxygenation is occurring.   In contrast, in the later stages there is a fall in oxygenation (decreased pO_2/F_iO_2) followed by the onset of metabolic acidosis (lactate acidosis, Figure 3D) (42) often in combination with respiratory acidosis caused by hypoventilation. In the CLP-model of MODS, these time-dependent patterns of lung failure occur with a relatively late onset of hypoxemia (60 hr after CLP), but not in those animals with antibody-induced blockade of C5a (19) (Figure 3A). In early sepsis (4-6 hr), pigs or monkeys challenged with very high doses of live *E. coli* and treated with an antibody to porcine or human C5a showed partial improvement in some functional parameters, such as oxygenation, lung edema, oxygen uptake and an improvement in the oxygen extraction ratio, accompanied by an attenuated increase in lactate levels (43-45), suggesting that C5a may be involved in the development of lung failure during *E. coli* bacteremia.

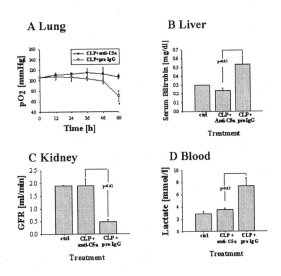

Figure 3. Blockade of complement activation product C5a exhibits protective effects on various organ functions during experimentally induced MODS. (A) Respiratory dysfunction; (B) Hepatic dysfunction; (C) Renal dysfunction; (D) Blood dysfunction. (CLP, cecal ligation and puncture; anti-C5a, antibodies to C5a; pre-IgG, preimmune immunoglobulin G; GFR, glomerular filtration rate.)

5.3   Liver Failure

For multi-organ dysfunction scores in humans, hepatic failure (HF) is defined by elevated levels of serum bilirubin and transaminases (46). This pattern has been clearly seen in rats with CLP-induced MODS. Other studies using the CLP model have revealed an early onset of a neutrophil-dependent hepatocellular dysfunction (47) and late onset of liver endothelial cell dysfunction, associated with elevated serum levels of LDH (48). In the CLP-induced MODS in rats, the biochemical changes defining hepatic failure were greatly attenuated by anti-C5a treatment of CLP rats (19), suggesting a link between C5a and depressed liver function (Figure 3B). In perfused rat livers, C3a and C5a have been shown to stimulate hepatic stellatae cells and Kupffer cells via the presence of the C3a receptor (C3aR) and C5a receptor (C5aR), resulting in prostaglandin release, increased hepatic glucose output and reduced blood flow through the liver (49). Thus, complement activation products may be linked to development of hepatic failure during systemic inflammation.

5.4   Kidney Failure

Acute renal failure (ARF) as complication of the systemic inflammatory response is a clinical entity characterized by an abrupt decline in the glomerular filtration rate (GFR), resulting in oliguria and azotemia, all of which have been detected in the CLP-induced MODS rats, but not in those with blockade of C5a (19) (Figure 3C). Though the presence of C5aR has been described on human glomerular mesangial cells and more recently on renal tubular cells, the linkage between C5a and development of ARF during MODS is obscure. There are suggestions that infusion of C5a leads to a significant fall in renal blood flow by increasing the vascular resistance in the afferent and efferent arterioles (50). Proteinuria was observed in CLP-induced MODS, reflective of the presence in urine of proteins larger than the glomerular filtration barrier of 60 kDa. In CLP rats there were morphological changes in podocytes, including fusion of their foot processes and flattening of their cell surfaces, and necrosis of proximal convoluted tubular cells (19). In an ARF model in dogs induced by norepinephrine infusion into the renal artery, similar morphological changes of podocytes were found together with development of tubular necrosis, mainly involving the proximal convoluted tubules (51). The morphological changes in kidneys of CLP-induced MODS rats were absent in rats treated with anti-C5a antibody (19). In a model of immunological glomerulonephritis in mice, a genetic deficiency of C5 was associated with reduced glomerular injury when compared to C5-intact mice (52), suggesting that activated complement products may be linked to development of glomerular injury.

5.5   Hemodynamic Failure

Excessive generation of complement activation products may be involved directly or indirectly in progressive organ failure or by induction of apoptotic events (53). Excessive generation of both C3a and C5a can lead to massive release from phagocytic cells or mast cells of mediators such as histamine, the result of which could be a compromise of the cardiovascular and hemodynamic function. During cardiopulmonary bypass surgery, it has been shown that anti-C5a reduces ischemic injury of the porcine myocardium (54), suggesting that during cardiopulmonary bypass C5a can be detrimental to tissues. When C5a was injected into dogs there was an immediate decrease of the venous return, cardiac output and arterial pressure, all of which indicate failing hemodynamic performance (55). When purified human C3a was administered into coronary arteries in isolated guinea pig hearts, C3a caused in a dose-dependent manner tachycardia, impairment of arterioventricular conduction, left ventricular contractile failure and coronary vasoconstriction, all of which resulted in manifestation of cardiac dysfunction (56). The data suggest possible hemodynamic interferences in the course of MODS by excessively produced complement activation products, C3a and C5a.

6.   NOVEL IMMUNO-MODULATORY APPROACHES

Once cellular and organ damage has occurred, the pathophysiological events become increasingly complex and, sometimes self-sustaining. Therefore, prevention of MODS remains its best treatment. Classical therapy with rapid volume resuscitation, adequate nutrition, appropriate antibiotic usage, and aggressive pulmonary management are exceedingly important for preventing the downward pathophysiological spiral that leads to MODS and death. Once MODS is clinically manifest, it is not clear if there is any treatment which will move back the situation from the "point of no return". However, during the early stages of the systemic inflammatory response often leading to MODS, there are hints for some interesting and novel therapeutic approaches. Recently, several clinical trials have demonstrated a modest reduction in mortality during the systemic inflammatory response by intensified tissue oxygenation, aggressive insulin therapy to keep blood glucose within strict limits, treatment with the antiinflammatory and anticoagulatory protein (activated protein C, APC) (57), and by application of low dose corticosteroids (eg. hydrocortisone 50 mg intravenous bolus four times/24 hr and fludrocortisone 50 ug/24 hr) which may attenuate an exaggerated inflammatory response (for review see 58).

Promising attempts to attenuate or inhibit MODS development by specific complement inhibitors have included the application of endogenous soluble complement inhibitors (C1-inhibitor, recombinant soluble complement receptor 1- sCR1) (22,26,59-61) and the administration of antibodies, either blocking C5a or C5aR (5,18-20,43-45). Another approach to block the harmful effects of excessive amounts of C5a is the application of the recently developed antagonists to C5aR (C5aRa) (62). In experimental sepsis, the progressive onset of MODS and the multifunctional disturbances of neutrophils have recently been documented (18, 19, 63). Furthermore, the ability of anti-C5a (or C5aRa) to preserve chemotactic, phagocytotic and oxidative burst responsiveness of neutrophils, all of which are associated with greatly reduced development of MODS has been demonstrated (19,62,63).

Antibodies interfering with complement receptor 3 (CR3, CD11b/18)-mediated adhesion of inflammatory cells to the vascular endothelium also inhibited development of the inflammatory response. In addition, transfection experiments that incorporated membrane-bound complement regulators (DAF-CD55, MCP [CD64], CD59) showed beneficial alteration of the systemic inflammatory response (64,65). The latter studies still have to prove efficacy under the more complex clinical conditions of SIRS and MODS.

Collectively, these studies suggest that excessive and uncontrolled activation of the complement system during the systemic inflammatory response play a central role in development of immune dysfunction and cellular dysfunction, and is closely associated with the onset and progression of multi-organ dysfunction.

7.   REFERENCES

1. American College of Chest Physicians/Society of Critical Care Medicine Consensus Conference. 1992. Definitions for sepsis and organ failure and guidelines for the use of innovative therapies in sepsis. Crit Care Med 20:864-874.
2. Deitch, E.A. Multiple organ failure. Pathophysiology and potential future therapy. Ann Surg 1992; 216:117-134.
3. Angus, D.C., Linde-Zwirble, W.T., Lidicker, J., Clermont, G., Carcillo, J., Pinsky, M.R. Epidemiology of severe sepsis in the United States: analysis of incidence, outcome, and associated cost of care. Crit Care Med 2001; 29:1303-1310.
4. Faist, E., Wichmann, M.W. Immunology in the severely injured. Chirurg 1997; 68(11):1066-1070.

5. Hopken, U., Mohr, M., Struber, A., Montz, H., Buchardi, H., Gotze, O., Oppermann, M. Inhibition of interleukin-6 synthesis in an animal model of septic shock by anti-C5a monoclonal antibodies. Eur J Immunol 1996; 26(5):1103.

6. Bengtson, A., Heideman, M. Anaphylatoxin formation of sepsis. Arch Surg 1988; 123(5):645-649.

7. Nakae, H., Endo, S., Inada, K., Yoshida, M. Chronological changes in the complement system in sepsis. Surg Today 1996; 26:225-229.

8. Roumen, R.M., Redl, H., Schlag, G., Zilow, G., Sandtner, W., Koller, W., Hendriks, T., Goris, R.J. Inflammatory mediators in relation to the development of multiple organ failure in patients after severe blunt trauma. Crit Care Med 1995; 23:474-480.

9. Zimmermann, T., Laszik, Z., Nagy, S., Kaszaki, J., Joo, F. The role of complement system in the pathogenesis of multiple organ failure in shock. Prog Clin Biol Res 1989; 308:291-297.

10. Helliwell, T.R., Wilkinson, A., Griffiths, R.D., Palmer, T.E., McClelland, P., Bone, J.M. Microvascular endothelial activation in the skeletal muscles of patients with multiple organ failure. J Neuro Sci 1998; 154:26-34.

11. Bengtson, A., Heideman, M. Altered anaphylatoxin activity during induced hypoperfusion in acute and elective abdominal surgery. J Trauma 1986; 26(7):631-637.

12. Heideman, M., Hugli, T.E. Anaphylatoxin generation in multisystem organ failure. J Trauma 1984; 24:1038-1043.

13. Seghaye, M.C., Duchateau, J., Grabitz, R.G., Faymonville, M.L., Messmer, B.J., Buro-Rathsmann, K., von Bernuth, G. Complement activation during cardiopulmonary bypass in infants and children. Relation to postoperative multiple system organ failure. J Thorac Cardiovasc Surg 1993; 106:978-987.

14. Goris, R.J., te Boeckhorst, T.P.A., Nuytinck, J.K., Gimbrere, J.S. Multiple-organ failure: generalized autodestructive inflammation? Arch Surg 1985; 120:1109-1115.

15. Bone, R.C., Grodzin, C.J., Balk, R.A. Sepsis: a new hypothesis for pathogenesis of the disease process. Chest 1997; 112:235-243.

16. Goya, T., Morisaki, T., Torisu, M. Immunologic assessment of host defense impairment in patients with septic multiple organ failure: Relationship between complement activation and changes in neutrophil function. Surgery 1994; 115(2):145-155.

17. Solomkin, J.S., Jenkins, M.K., Nelson, R.D., Chenoweth, D., Simmons, R.L. Neutrophil dysfunction in sepsis. II. Evidence for the role of complement activation products in cellular deactivation. Surgery 1981; 90(2):319-327.

18. Czermak, B.J., Sarma, V., Pierson, C.L., Warner, R.L., Huber-Lang, M., Bless, N.M., Schmal, H., Friedl, H.P., Ward, P.A. Protective effects of C5a blockade in sepsis. Nat Med 1999; 5 (7):788-792.

19. Huber-Lang, M., Sarma, V.J., Lu, K.T., McGuire, S.R., Padgaonkar, V.A., Guo, R.F., Younkin, E.M., Kunkel, R.G., Ding, J., Erickson, R., Curnutte, J.T., Ward, P.A. Role of C5a in multiorgan failure during sepsis. J Immunol 2001; 166:1193-9.

20. Gerard, C. Complement C5a in the sepsis syndrome - too much of a good thing? N Engl J Med 2003; 348:167-169.

21. Zhao, L., Ohtaki, Y., Yamaguchi, K., Matsushita, M., Fujita, T., Yokoc, T., Takada, H., Endo, Y. LPS-induced platelet response and rapid shock in mice: contribution of O-antigen region of LPS and involvement of lectin pathway o the complement system. Blood 2002; 100:3233-3239.

22. Giebler, R., Schmidt, U., Koch, S., Peters, J., Scherer, R. Combined antithrombin III and C1-esterase inhibitor treatment decreases intravascular fibrin deposition and attenuates cardiorespiratory impairment in rabbits exposed to Escherichia coli endotoxin. Crit Care Med 1999; 27:597-604.

23. Quezado, Z.M., Hoffman, W.D., Winkelstein, J.A., Yatsiv, I., Koev, C.A., Cork, L.C., Elin, R.J., Eichacker, P.Q., Natanson, C. The third component of complement protects against Escherichia coli endotoxin-induced shock and multiple organ failure. J Exp Med 1994; 179:569-578.

24. Zhi-Yong, S., Dong, Y.L., Wang, X.H. Bacterial translocation and multiple system organ failure in bowel ischemia and reperfusion. J Trauma 1992; 32:148-153.

25. Kyriakides, C., Austen, W.G., Wang, Y., Favuzza, J., Moore, F.D., Hechtmann, H.B. Neutrophil mediated remote organ injury after lower torso ischemia and reperfusion is selectin and complement dependent. J Trauma 2000; 48:32-38.

26. Horstick, G., Kempf, T., Lauterbach, M., Bhakdi, S., Kopacz, L., Heimann, A., Malzahn, M., Horstick, M., Meyer, J., Kempski, O. C1-esterase inhibitor treatment at early reperfusion of hemorrhagic shock reduces mesentry leukocyte adhesion and rolling. Microcirculation 2001; 8:427-433.

27. Hsueh, W., Sun, X., Rioja, L.N., Gonzalez-Crussi, F. The role of the complement in shock and tissue injury induced by tumor necrosis factor and endotoxin. Immunology 1990; 70:309-314.

28. Sun, X., Hsueh, W. Platelet-activating factor produces shock, in vivo complement activation, and tissue injury in mice. J Immunol 1991; 147:509-514.

29. Goris, R.J., Boekholtz, W.K., van Bebber, I.P., Nuytinck, J.K., Schillings, P.H. Multiple-organ failure and sepsis without bacteria. An experimental model. Arch Surg 1986; 121:897-901.

30. Mahesh, J., Daly, J., Cheadle, W.G., Kotwal, G.J. Elucidation of the early events contributing to zymosan-induced multiple organ dysfunction syndrome using MIP-1alpha, C3 knockout, and C5-deficient mice. Shock 1999; 12:340-349.

31. Roxvall, L., Bengston, A., Heideman, M. Anaphylatoxin generation in acute pancreatitis. J Surg Res 1989; 47:138-143.

32. Hotchkiss, R.S., Karl, I.E. The pathophysiology and treatment of sepsis. N Engl J Med 2003; 348:138-150.

33. Foreman, K.E., Vaporciyan, A.A., Bonish, B.K., Jones, M.L., Johnson, K.J., Glovsky, M.M., Eddy, S.M., Ward, P.A. C5a-induced expression of P-selectin in endothelial cells. J Clin Invest 1994; 94:1147-1155.

34. Elsbach, P., Weiss, J. Oxygen-dependent and oxygen independent mechanisms of microbiological activity of neutrophils. Immunol Lett 1985; 11:159-163.

35. Nuytinck, J.K., Goris, R.J., Weerts, J.G., Schillings, P.H., Stekhoven, J.H. Acute generalized microvascular injury by activated complement and hypoxia: the basis of the adult respiratory distress syndrome and multiple organ failure? Br J Pathol 1986; 67:537-548.

36. Morgan, E.L., Weigle, W.O., Hugli, T.E. Anaphylatoxin-mediated regulation of the immune responses. J Exp Med 1982; 255:1412-1426.

37. Grossklaus, C., Damerau, B., Lemgo, E., Vogt, W. Induction of platelet aggregation by the complement-derived peptides C3a and C5a. Naunyn Schmiedebergs Arch Pharmacol 1976; 12;295(1):71-76.

38. Björk, J., Hugli, T.E., Smedegard, G. Microvascular effects of anaphylatoxins C3a and C5a. J Immunol 1985; 134:1115-1119.

39. Schlag, G., Redl, H. Lung in shock – posttraumatic failure (organ failure) –MOFS. Prog Clin Biol Res. 1989; 308:3-16

40. Zilow, G., Sturm, J.A., Rother, U., Kirschfink, M. Complement activation and the prognostic value of C3a in patients at risk of adult respiratory distress syndrome. Clin Exp Immunol 1990; 79:151-157.

41. Hammerschmidt, D.E., Weaver, L.J., Hudson, L.D., Craddock, P.R., Jacob, H.S. Association of complement activation and elevated plasma-C5a with adult respiratory distress syndrome. Lancet 1980; (8175):947-949.
42. Oda, S., Hirasawa, H., Sugai, T., Shiga, H., Matsuda, K., Ueno, H. Cellular injury score for multiple organ failure severity scoring system. J Trauma 1998; 45(2):304-310.
43. Mohr, M., Hopken, U., Oppermann, M., Mathes, C., Goldmann, K., Siever, S., Gotze, O., Burchardi, H. Effects of anti-C5a monoclonal antibodies on oxygen use in a porcine model of severe sepsis. Eur J Clin Invest 1998; 28(3):227-234.
44. Stevens, J.H., O'Hanley, P., Shapiro, J.M., Mihm, F.G., Satoh, P.S., Collins, J.A., Raffin, T.A. Effects of anti-C5a antibodies on the adult respiratory distress syndrome in septic primates. J Clin Invest 1986; 6:1812-1816.
45. Hangen, D.H., Stevens, J.H., Satoh, P.S., Hall, E.W., O'Hanley, P.T., Raffin, T.A. Complement levels in septic primates treated with anti-C5a antibodies. J Surg Res 1989; 46(3):195-199.
46. Marshall, J.C., Cook, D.J., Christou, N.V., Bernard, G.R., Sprung, C.L., Sibbald, W.J. Multiple organ dysfunction score: a reliable descriptor of a complex clinical outcome. Crit Care Med 1995; 23(10):1638-1652.
47. Molnar, R.G., Wang, P., Ayala, A., Ganey, P.E., Roth, R.A., Chaudry, I.H. The role of neutrophils in producing hepatocellular dysfunction during the hyperdynamic stage of sepsis in rats. J Surg Res 1997; 73:117-122.
48. Wang, P., Ba, Z.F., Chaudry, I.H. Liver endothelial cell function is depressed only during hypodynamic sepsis. J Surg Res 1997; 68:38-43.
49. Schieferdecker, H.L., Pestel, S., Puschel, A., Gotze, O., Jungermann, K. Increase by anaphylatoxin C5a of glucose output in perfused rat liver via prostanoid derived from nonparenchymal cells: direct action of prostaglandins and indirect action of thromboxane A(2) on hepatocytes. Hepatology 1999; 30:454-461.
50. Sekse, I., Iversen, B.M., Daha, M.R., Ofstad, J. Acute effect of passive Heymann nephritis on renal blood flow and glomerular filtration rate in the rat: role of the anaphylatoxin C5a and the alpha-adrenergic nervous system. Nephron 1992; 60:453-459.
51. Cox, J.W., Baehler, R.W., Sharma, H., O'Dorisio, T., Osgood, R.W., Stein, J.H., Ferris, T.F. Studies of the mechanism of oliguria in a model of unilateral acute renal failure. J Clin Invest 1974; 53(6):1546-1558.
52. Falk, R.J., Jennette, J.C. Immune complex induced glomerular lesions in C5 sufficient and deficient mice. Kidney Int 1986; 30:678-686.
53. Guo, R.F., Huber-Lang, M., Wang, X., Sarma, V., Padgaonkar, V.A., Craig, R.A., Riedemann, N.C., McClintock, S.D., Hlaing, T., Shi, M.M., Ward, P.A. Protective effects of anti-C5a in sepsis-induced thymocyte apoptosis. J Clin Invest 2000; 106:1271-1280.
54. Amsterdam, E.A., Stahl, G.L., Pan, H.L., Rendig, S.V., Fletcher, M..P, Longhur, J.C. Limitation of reperfusion injury by a monoclonal antibody to C5a during myocardial infarction in pigs. Am J Physiol 1995; 268:H448-457.
55. Pavek, K., Piper, P.J., Smedegard, G. Anaphylatoxin-induced shock and two patterns of anaphylactic shock: hemodynamics and mediators. Acta Physiol Scand 1978; 105:393-403.
56. Hachfeld del Balzo, U., Levi, R., Polley, M.J. Cardiac dysfunction caused by purified human C3a anaphylatoxin. Proc Natl Acad Sci 1985; 82:886-890.
57. Bernard, G.R., Vincent, J.L., Laterre, P.F., LaRosa, S.P., Dhainaut, J.F., Lopez-Rodriguez, A., Steingrub, J.S., Garber, G.E., Helterbrand, J.D., Ely, E.W., Fisher, C.J. Jr. Efficacy and safety of recombinant human activated protein C for severe sepsis. N Engl J Med 2001; 344:366-709.

58. Cohen, J. The immunpathogenesis of sepsis. Nature 2002; 420:885-891.
59. Caliezi, C., Zeerleder, S., Redondo, M., Regli, B., Rothen, H.U., Zurcher-Zenklusen, R., Rieben, R., Devay, J., Hack, C.E., Lammle, B., Wuillemin, W.A. C1-inhibitor in patients with severe sepsis and septic shock: beneficial effect on renal dysfunction. Crit Care Med 2002; 30:1722-1728.
60. Kirschfink, M., Mollnes, T.E. C1-inhibitor: an anti-inflammatory reagent with therapeutic potential. Expert Opin Pharmacother 2001; 2:1073-1083.
61. Fischer, M.B., Prodeus, A.P., Nicholson-Weller, A., Ma, M., Murrow, J., Reid, R.R., Warren, H.B., Lage, A.L., Moore Jr, F.D., Rosen, F.S., Carroll, M.C. Increased susceptibility to endotoxin shock in complement C3- and C4-deficient mice is corrected by C1 inhibitor replacement. J Immunol 1997; 159(2):976.
62. Huber-Lang, M., Riedemann, N.C., Sarma, V.J., Younkin, E.M., McGuire, S.R., Laudes, I.J., Lu, K.T., Guo, R.F., Neff, T.A., Padgaonkar, V.A., Lambris, J., Spruce, L., Mastellos, D., Zetoune, F.S., Ward, P.A. Protection of innate immunity by C5aR antagonist in septic mice. FASEB J, 2002; 16:1567-1574.
63. Huber-Lang, M.S., Younkin, E.M., Sarma, J.V., McGuire, S.R., Lu, K.T., Guo, R.F., Padgaonkar, V.A., Curnutte, J.T., Erickson, R., Ward, P.A. Complement-induced impairment of innate immunity during sepsis. J Immunol 2002; 169:3223-3231.
64. Kirschfink, M. Controlling the complement system in inflammation. Immunopharmacology 1997; 38:51-62.
65. Kirschfink, M. Targeting complement in therapy. Immunol Rev 2001; 180:177-89.

PART 7

THE COMPLEMENT SYSTEM
AS THERAPEUTICAL
TARGET

23

Therapeutic Manipulation of the Complement System

Tom Eirik Mollnes

Institute of Immunology, Rikshospitalet University Hospital, Oslo, Norway

Abstract: The complement system is essential for host defence and tissue homeostasis. It acts largely by inflammatory reactions mediated directly by activated components and indirectly by other inflammatory systems triggered by complement. A consequence of this inflammation is destruction of micro-organisms, but frequently also damage to host tissues. Thus, complement is a double-edged sward; if activated improperly or excessively, it may cause considerable organ damage. A number of inflammatory diseases are associated with enhanced complement activation and recent data obtained from animal studies indicate that complement is in fact an important mediator in the pathogenesis of many of these conditions. An attractive approach has therefore been to develop complement inhibitors for possible therapeutic use. Such inhibitors include small molecules, naturally occurring and recombinant regulatory proteins, and monoclonal antibodies. The actual component(s) to be inhibited and the mode of application depend on the pathogenesis of the disease. Pro-drugs and targeted inhibition are to be considered for optimal benefit and minimal side effects. Despite the large body of evidence obtained from animal studies showing that complement inhibition markedly improves mortality and morbidity in a number of inflammatory conditions, it remains to be shown whether complement inhibition will be applicable in clinical medicine.

Key words: Complement inhibitors, therapy, sCR1, DAF, C1-INH, antibodies

1.   INTRODUCTION

The complement system is a double-edged sword. An intact complement cascade is required for protection against infection and for maintaining the inflammatory homeostasis in the body, whereas improper, excessive or uncontrolled complement activation is disadvantageous to the host. Thus, there are two main aspects of complement pathophysiology where manipulation of the system is justified. First, genetic complement deficiencies, although rare, are frequently associated with serious diseases and substitution therapy to restore the defect function may be desired. Second, uncontrolled complement activation contributes to tissue damage in a number of disease conditions and its inhibition could be a therapeutic approach for these diseases.

Substitution therapy with purified C1 inhibitor or plasma to treat patients with hereditary angioedema has been used for decades. Double-blind placebo-controlled studies have clearly demonstrated its clinical efficacy both in acute treatment and prevention (1). Other complement deficiencies have occasionally been treated with plasma since purified components for therapeutic use are not available. Factor H deficiency associated with haemolytic uremic syndrome (2) and C2 deficiency with systemic lupus erythemaytosus (3) have been successfully treated with plasma. Recently, a patient with factor H deficiency and hemolytic uremic syndrome with renal failure was treated by combined liver and kidney transplantation, where the defect factor H was restored by a normal protein synthesized by the liver (4). In one case of factor I deficiency, complement function was restored by administration of purified factor I (5). However, except for C1 inhibitor treatment of patients with hereditary angioedema, there are no current established regimens for substitution therapy to patients with other complement deficiencies.

Inhibition of excessive or improper complement activation has appeared to be an attractive approach to treat a number of diseases, which in animal models have been demonstrated to be totally or partly mediated by complement activation. The list of such conditions is growing and the question "In which conditions does complement activation contribute to the pathophysiology?" may be changed to "In which conditions are complement not involved?" Currently, complement activation is implicated in numerous disease conditions, e.g. ischemia-reperfusion (I/R) injury locally manifested as infarctions or systemically as a post-ischemic inflammatory syndrome, systemic inflammatory response syndrome (SIRS) and acute respiratory distress syndrome (ARDS), septic shock, trauma, burns, acid aspiration to the lungs, immune complex diseases like rheumatoid arthritis and systemic lupus erythematosus, various renal diseases, a number of inflammatory diseases in the nervous system, arteriosclerosis and transplant rejection. In principle, when inflammation is involved in the pathogenesis, complement should be considered as a possible mediator in the disease process.

This chapter is focused on therapeutic complement inhibition, with emphasis on different approaches for development of inhibitors, site of action in the cascade, possible disease conditions for complement inhibition based on experimental animal data, and finally the potential side effects of such treatment. Due to the vast amount of data already available in the literature, only parts of it can be included here. For further reading, see (6) and some selected reviews from the last 5 years on this topic (7-34).

2.   GENERAL ASPECTS OF COMPLEMENT INHIBITION THERAPHY

2.1   Complement Inhibition in Human Disease

A general principle for any patient treatment is "primum non nocere" – first of all do not harm. Thus, targeting complement as a therapeutic goal requires detailed knowledge about the activation mechanisms and mediators responsible for the inflammation, enabling optimal inhibitory treatment for the actual condition. Many mechanisms have been experimentally elucidated, particularly in I/R injury, but the field is still in its infancy. Due to species differences, results from animal studies are not necessarily applicable to humans. Results from knock-out mice studies have been very useful in elucidating the pathogenic role of complement in various diseases. Successful treatment with a specific complement inhibitor is the ultimate proof that complement plays an essential role in the actual disease. The design of clinical trials has to rely on the data from the animal disease models. At the end, application of complement inhibitors to patients will reveal to what extent the various diseases will benefit from the treatment. In fact, the latter will be the ultimate concept validation for the role of complement in the pathogenesis of human diseases.

Activation of complement, as detected by increased levels of complement activation products in plasma samples, is known to occur in a number of disease conditions. However, increased complement activation does not necessarily imply that complement is of importance in the pathogenesis. On the other hand, normal systemic levels of activation products is seen in many conditions where local complement activation is likely to play a role in local tissue damage. In such conditions complement activation can be detected in tissue biopsies or body fluids. In general, an ongoing systemic activation is required for increased activation products to be detected in a plasma sample. Whether the complement activation is local or systemic will determine the inhibitor to be used and its route of application.

2.2   Complement and the Inflammatory Network

The pathophysiology of inflammation is complex and diverse, depending on the triggering factors. The role of complement in the inflammatory network may also vary with the different conditions, from being crucial to just epiphenomenonal. Inflammatory mediators mutually interact. The most important issue is whether complement activation, by activation of leucocytes, endothelial cells and platelets, induces secondary inflammatory mediators which may contribute to the tissue damage, like cyto- and chemokines, reactive oxygen species, arachidonic acid metabolites and expression of adhesion molecules. On the other hand, some of these mediators may be primarily induced and activate complement as a secondary mechanism of inflammation. The question frequently raised is what comes first, the chicken or the egg. This has significant implication to the rationale and design of anti-inflammatory therapy in general and for complement inhibition in particular. In principle, it would be most effective to block upstream of the inflammation cascade, e.g. the primary inducer(s). The matter is, however, rather complex since some of the inflammatory mediators may have mainly adverse effects on tissue homeostasis whether others are beneficial. Thus, a major task is to identify and inhibit those mediators contributing to the tissue damage and to spare those which are beneficial. This is vital to designing a clinically optimal therapeutic regimen based on the manipulation of complement activity.

2.3   The Complement Cascade and Sites of its Therapeutic Inhibition

Fig. 1 presents a scheme of the complement cascade with an updated map of sites of inhibition (35). In brief, the complement system comprises more than 30 proteins acting together in a specific manner to protect the host against invading organisms. The *classical pathway* (upper left in Fig. 1) is activated when natural or elicited antibodies bind to antigen. C1q triggers the serine proteases C1r and C1s, the latter cleaving C4 to C4b, which exposes a specific binding site for C2. C1s then cleaves C2 and the resulting C3 convertase C4b2a cleaves C3 to C3b to form the C5 convertase C4b2a3b. Splitting of C5 to the highly potent anaphylatoxin C5a and the C6-binding fragment C5b is the last enzymatic step in the cascade.

Activation of the *lectin pathway* (Fig. 1, upper middle) is initiated by mannose binding lectin (MBL) recognising mannose on bacteria. In addition, this pathway can be activated by IgA and probably by structures exposed by damaged endothelium. MBL is homologous to C1q and triggers the MBL associated serine proteases (MASPs), of which three forms (MASP1, MASP2 and MASP3) have been described. Further lectin pathway activation is virtually identical to classical pathway activation forming the same C3 and C5 convertases. In addition there is some evidence that MASPs under some conditions may activate C3 directly.

The *alternative pathway* (Fig. 1, upper right) activation mechanisms differ from the classical and lectin pathway. Under normal physiological conditions the C3 molecule undergoes a low-grade spontaneous hydrolysis of the internal thiol-ester and thereby binds factor B, which is cleaved by factor D and a C3 convertase is formed containing the whole C3 molecule (C3(H2O)Bb). This complex then cleaves C3 to C3a and C3b. The latter binds factor B, which is cleaved by factor D and the second alternative pathway C3 convertase C3bBb is formed. Properdin (P), the only regulator of complement which amplifies activation, binds to C3bBb and stabilises this complex, which then cleaves C3, binds C3b and the C5 convertase C3b3bBbP is formed and cleaves C5 in the same manner as the classical/lectin pathway C5 convertase.

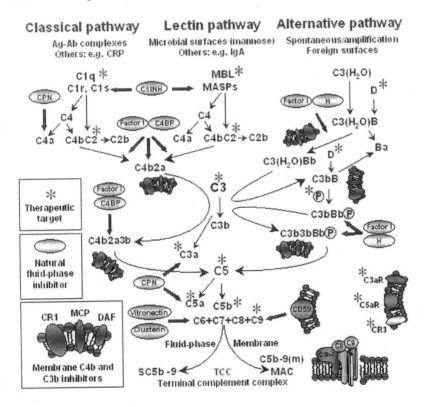

Figure 1. The complement cascade and sites of its therapeutic inhibition. Reprinted from Trends In Immunol., Vol. 23, Mollnes, T.E., Song, W-Ch., and Lambris, J.D., Complement in Inflammatory Tissue damage and Disease, pp. 61-64, Copyright (2002), with permission from Elsevier.

The *terminal pathway* (lower middle) proceeds in the same way irrespective of the initial pathway activation by assembly of C7 to C5b6, forming an amphiphilic complex able to insert into a lipid membrane. One C5b-7 moiety binds one C8 and one or more C9 molecules, creating a physical pore penetrating the membrane (C5b-9(m) or membrane attack complex (MAC)), leading to transmembrane leakage and subsequent cell activation, or more infrequently to lysis (lower right). If the activation occurs in the fluid-phase and there is no membrane present, the C5b-7 complex binds to vitronectin and clusterin (fluid-phase regulators of the terminal pathway) and thus retains hydrophilic properties. Final assembly of a soluble C5b-9 (SC5b-9), the second form of the terminal complement complex (TCC), occurs by binding of C8 and C9.

Complement activation is strictly regulated by inhibitory proteins. In the fluid-phase C1-inhibitor (C1INH) controls C1r, C1s and MASPs whereas carboxypeptidase N (CPN) inactivates the anaphylatoxins C5a, C3a and C4a by splitting off the terminal arginine. Factor I cleaves and inactivates C4b and C3b and uses C4b-binding protein (C4BP) as co-factor in the classical/lectin pathway and factor H in the alternative pathway. The membrane regulators complement receptor 1 (CR1; CD35), membrane co-factor protein (MCP; CD46) and decay accelerating factor (DAF; CD55) regulate complement activation by either acting as co-factors for factor I mediated cleavage of C4b and C3b (CR1 and MCP), or accelerating the decay of the bimolecular C3 and C5 convertases (CR1 and DAF). CD59, also a membrane regulator, prevents the binding of C9 to the C5b-8 complex in the terminal pathway. CR1 and MCP are transmembrane proteins whereas DAF and CD59 attach to the cell membrane via a glycosylphosphatidylinositol anchor. Many of the biological effects induced by complement activation are mediated by membrane receptors such as receptors for C3a (C3aR), C5a (C5aR) and iC3b (CR3; CD11b/CD18). Activated complement is a double-edged sword with undesired effects in many conditions. Thus, various reagents with potential therapeutic applications have been developed to target complement activation and function (indicated by red asterisks in Fig. 1).

The traditional discussion of complement inhibition has focused on two alternatives: blocking at the level of C3 implying a general and broad inhibition of the system, or selective blocking of C5 activation and subsequent inhibition of C5a and C5b-9 (TCC) formation. The main argument for the first approach is that if complement activation is detrimental, it is logical to completely inhibit complement activation. The opposite view is that blocking of the terminal pathway would reduce the adverse effects whereas keeping the C3 activation open would preserve important defense mechanisms against foreign pathogens. This discussion has its background in arguing for either of the two main products developed for clinical use, namely sCR1 and anti-C5. In fact, both arguments oversimplify the situation and have limited clinical validation. The mechanisms of complement activation and the contribution of this activation in the pathophysiology of different clinical conditions are so diverse that a differential approximation to this issue is required and several strategies must be considered.

One such strategy will be to target the initial event in the activation. This will require detailed knowledge on the activation mechanism. Each of the three initial activation pathways can be blocked separately. In the classical pathway (CP) mediated activation inhibition of C1 blocks the very first activation step and prevents the formation of C4 and C2. Similarly, blocking of mannan binding lectin (MBL) will inhibit lectin pathway (LP) activation at the step before C4 activation. A possible role of other proteins like ficolins in activation of the MBL-associated serine proteases (MASPs) must, however, be considered. Inhibition of MASP 2 would probably inhibit any LP-mediated activation. Targeting C2 will block both CP and LP, but will not prevent C4 cleavage. It has been suggested that MASP 1 may activate C3 directly, in which case blocking of C2 would not influence activation via the LP. It is, however, not likely that such a mechanism is operative *in vivo*. Inhibition of factor D, the rate-limiting component in the alternative pathway (AP) is an attractive approach in inhibiting AP activation. It should be noted that AP activation may either be primary or induced by CP or LP activation for amplification. Although inhibition of AP could block the amplification of complement activation, certain CP and LP activity important for normal functions should still be intact. In certain conditions of systemic complement activation the AP amplification loop may be responsible for an uncontrolled and detrimental activation, irrespective of the initial pathway activation mechanism. Inhibition of factor B and properdin are alternative approaches for blocking the alternative pathway. The former will require higher amount of inhibitor and the latter may not be complete, since properdin stabilizes but is not absolutely required for AP convertase activity.

A second strategy will be to inhibit the common components C3 or C5. C3 can be inhibited either by blocking activation of C3 or by inhibiting the C3 convertases. This will give a potent and broad inhibition of the whole cascade irrespective of the initial pathway. Although both C3 and C5 activation are prevented, C1/MBL, C4 and C2 will be activated. The immunomodulatory effects of C3 as well as C3 opsonization will be impaired, but may not be a concern during short-term therapy. Inhibition of C5 activation will leave the C3 functions open but block the formation of C5a and TCC. This may be beneficial in conditions where both of these terminal pathway products are involved in the pathogenesis.

A third strategy will be to target specific activation products or their respective receptors, particularly the anaphylatoxins C3a or C5a. In the case of airway hyper-responsiveness there may be an indication for selective blocking of C3a function, which can be achieved by anti-C3a antibodies or C3aR antagonists, leaving the rest of the C3 functions open. Similarly, if C5a is the main contributor to the pathophysiology of systemic complement activation, C5a function could be blocked, leaving the C5b-9 pathway open for killing of bacteria such as Neisseria.

The main challenge for developing effective and safe anti-complement therapeutics is to balance the beneficial effects obtained by the inhibition with the preservation of sufficient functional activity for microbial protection and for tissue homeostasis.

2.4   Possible Adverse Effects

The adverse effects of inhibition of complement may be directly related to the function of complement, i.e. increased susceptibility to infection and autoimmune- and immune complex diseases, due to impaired opsonisation, antigenic responses, tolerance and handling of immune complexes. To date, such complications have not been observed in animal models. This could be attributed to incomplete inhibition and short duration of the studies. In fact, 60% inhibition of complement activity was sufficient for treatment of collagen-induced arthritis (36). This is most important when considering long-term treatment in chronic diseases. A certain degree of inhibition may be sufficient to reduce detrimental effects of complement activation, though defence mechanisms may still be preserved. The risk of infectious complications is suggested to be highest when blocking C3. The redundancy of the three initial activation pathways would reduce the risk of infection if one pathway is selectively blocked. Furthermore, blocking of C5b-9 formation could lead to increased susceptibility to Neisserial strains. Paradoxically, septic shock is one of the conditions that may benefit from complement inhibition. In these cases the patient would be appropriately treated with antibiotics and thus short-term inhibition of complement may be acceptable.

The inhibitors could be immunogenic, leading to an immune response and loss of function. The risk of antigen response is lowered by use of recombinant human proteins, small molecular inhibitors and humanized antibodies, as discussed below. Recently, a novel role for complement in tissue regeneration has been demonstrated (37). It is unknown whether impairment of this function will be a consequence of long-term complement inhibition.

2.5   Costs

Production of recombinant proteins and antibodies in eukaryotic cells is costly, whereas bacteria-produced products can be produced in large-scale at potentially lower costs. Production of small molecule inhibitors is in general economical. Costs should be considered in the context of the severity of the disease and the duration of treatment. Thus, high-cost short-time intensive treatment to save lives may be acceptable, whereas life-long treatment for chronic diseases will require low-cost regimens.

3.   THERAPEUTIC STRATEGIES

Complement therapy is not only a question of which drug to be given, and at which step it interferes, but also in which form the drug is produced and administered.

3.1   Mode of Administration

The administration route is critical for chronic diseases requiring long-time therapy. Oral, nasal or rectal application is definitely superior to intravenous injection in these cases, whereas acute, severe illness is preferentially treated through the intravenous route. Furthermore, although systemic diseases like sepsis and SIRS may require systemic administration, diseases with organ specific damage, like glomerulonephrtis, central nervous system diseases and rheumatoid arthritis may benefit from local application.

3.2   Clearance and Long-Term Treatment

Recombinant proteins and small molecular inhibitors, in contrast to antibodies, generally have a short half-life and are best suited for treatment of acute conditions. Modifications to increase half-life of recombinant proteins have however been made with considerable success. Thus, conjugating the proteins to human immunoglobulin Fc fragments could increase the half-life considerably (38). This has immediate consequences for the application of the drug in long-term treatment, although the ultimate goal in these cases will be oral administration.

3.3   Targeted Application

The intention of targeted application is to deliver the drug to a specific cite for limiting the potential systemic side effects. This approach is indicated if no systemic fluid phase activation is going on. If activation occurs systemically, inhibition should not be targeted but achieved by an agent kept soluble intravascularly.

Targeting may be nonspecific, directed to any membrane, or specific, directed to certain cells or organs. One approach for nonspecific targeting is the membrane "tagging", obtained by coupling the inhibitor to a lipid tail. This tail will bind to membranes undergoing internal-external changes, as illustrated by the myristoyl-electrostatic switch paradigm where a truncated form of sCR1 (APT070) was used (28, 39). This agent was 100-fold more potent than the parent molecule and has been used for treatment of experimental rheumatoid arthritis (40). Based on the promising experimental results, the agent has been tested in volunteers. Clinical studies in patients with rheumatoid arthritis are underway. sCD59 has also been "tagged" in a similar manner, being 100-fold more potent than sCD59 (39). The rodent complement C3 inhibitor Crry (complement receptor 1 related gene/protein) has been "tagged" using the same approach in experimental animal studies (41).

Another approach for targeted application is antigen-specific direction using antibody-conjugates. DAF was successfully targeted to the surface of Chinese hamster ovary cells by a conjugate of DAF and IgG anti-danasyl antibody (42). A similar antigen-targeted form of sCD59 has been produced (43). Recently conjugates were made between a CR2 fragment, which will recognize sites of C3 activation, and DAF and CD59 (44). These conjugates bound to C3 opsonized cells and were more than 20-fold more efficient than the untargeted molecules in inhibiting complement activation. In a mouse model of lupus nephritis CR2-DAF but not soluble DAF targeted the kidney.

A third approach for targeted inhibition is conjugating the complement inhibitor to another inflammation-modulating molecule, exemplified by the sCR1-sLe(x) (TP20) molecule (45). sLe(x) is a ligand for E- and P-selectin and thus TP20 combines inhibition of complement and leukocyte adhesion (46). TP20 was found to be superior to unconjugated sCR1 (TP10) in reducing the tissue damage in an experimental model of cerebral stroke (47), in immune-complex mediated lung injury (48), and in I/R injury in experimental allogeneic lung transplantation (49). Furthermore, TP20 reduced myocardial (50) and skeletal muscle I/R injury (51) and moderated the acid aspiration injury in mice (52).

3.4   Prodrugs

A prodrug is inactive or has low activity until it reaches a site where it is activated. Fusion of DAF or CD59 with human immunoglobulin Fc domains markedly extend the half-life (38, 53, 54). However it was found that the biological activity was reduced. This principle was utilized to develop a novel fusion protein with virtually no biologic activity. The protein contains a site which is sensitive for enzymatic cleavage by a metalloproteinase. After enzymatic cleavage, restricted to sites of inflammation, the biologic activity of the inhibitor is restored (29, 55).

3.5 Gene Therapy

A transgene strategy for delivery of rat complement regulators using adenovirus vectors has been developed (56). Local production of the complement inhibitor Crry by astrocytes was found to attenuate experimental allergic encephaloymyelitis (57). sCR1 was delivered by retrovirally transfected cells or by naked DNA directly to the joint and prevented progression of collagen-induced arthritis (58). A similar approach was described by Quigg et al., with delivery of the inhibitor systemically (59).

Hyperacute xenotransplant rejection is caused by binding of naturally occurring antibodies and subsequent complement activation. In order to overcome this complement-mediated rejection various transgenic animals expressing human membrane complement regulators have been developed for use in xenotransplantation (see chapter 18 in this book).

4. INHIBITORS

The complement system is normally kept under strict control by fluid-phase and membrane-bound regulatory proteins (figure 1). The need for keeping this system under control is illustrated by the fact that there are as many regulators as there are ordinary components, and that deficiency of a regulatory protein is associated with substantially disturbed homeostasis. All the regulators are inhibitors of activation, except for properdin, which stabilizes the alternative C3 convertase (C3bBbP) and thus enhance activation.

4.1 C1-Inhibitor

C1-inhibitor is a naturally occurring serine protease inhibitor and the only known inhibitor of C1r and C1s. In addition to controlling the classical pathway, C1-inhibitor is also a regulator of MASP-1 and MASP-2 of the lectin pathway (60). Recently a novel inhibitory function on the AP was documented (61). Thus, an effect of C1-inhibitor may principally be mediated through either of the initial pathways. Furthermore, C1-inhibitor is not complement specific but has a broad spectrum of targets including factor XIIa, kallikrein and factor XIa.

C1-inhibitor is available for clinical use as substitution therapy in hereditary angioedema (HAE). Notably, the pathophysiology of HAE is closely related to the release of bradykinin and the main effect of C1-inhibitor is to reduce bradykinin formation through inhibition of the kallikrein/kinin system. From this point of view, HAE is not a complement-mediated disease, and it should be emphasized that the effect of C1-inhibitor, when used for treatment of other diseases than HAE, is not necessarily complement-dependent, but may well be explained by inhibition of other proteins.

C1-inhibitor has been widely used in a number of clinical conditions. The principle of supra-physiological doses to obtain more efficient regulation has been applied, although in some cases the treatment may be regarded as substitution for acquired low concentrations. The conditions treated with C1-inhibitor include sepsis, burns, capillary leak syndrome associated with bone marrow transplantation and IL-2 therapy, myocardial infarction, trauma and transplantation. Recently it was shown in an open-labeled clinical study that C1-inhibitor given 6 hours after thrombolytic therapy markedly reduced the size of infarction compared to matched controls (62). C1-inhibitor will not be discussed further in the present chapter, but it is referred to recent reviews on the application of C1-inhibitor in clinical medicine (63-65).

4.2   Recombinant Proteins

The family of regulators of complement activation (RCA) comprises CR1 (CD35), CR2 (CD21), MCP (CD46), DAF (CD55), factor H and C4BP. They are all powerful inhibitors of C3 and C5 convertases, except for CR2, which may play a minor role in regulation of complement. If an extensive inhibition of complement is required, the RCA proteins are candidates since they all interfere with activity of the C3 and C5 convertases.

4.2.1   C4BP and Factor H

C4b-binding protein (C4BP) and factor H are soluble regulators of the classical and alternative C3/C5 convertases, respectively. Recombinant factor H has been produced (66). Using a glycosyl-phosphatidyl inositol (GPI) anchor, a membrane form of C4BP was constructed which protected porcine endothelial cells against attack by human complement (67). A similar approach was used to bind factors H and I to a xenosurface (68), and binding of factor H to an artificial surface abrogated the surface-induced complement activation and thereby improved biocompatibility (69). C4BP and factor H have not been used clinically. A more likely indication for recombinant factor H would be substitution therapy in factor H deficiency rather than treating enhanced complement activation. Soluble CR1 is much more potent as fluid-phase inhibitor of C3 activation than C4BP and factor H.

4.2.2 Soluble CR1

CR1 is the only member of the RCA family having cofactor activity and decay accelerating activity both in the CP and AP (C4b and C3b). A soluble form of CR1 (sCR1) was constructed by deleting the transmembrane part of the molecule (70). sCR1 inhibited both CP and AP activation in concentrations equivalent to 1% of physiological C4BP and factor H concentration. The protein was first demonstrated to reduce experimental myocardial I/R injury by approximately 50%. The cardioprotective effects have later been confirmed in several studies (71-74).

The half-life of the original sCR1 was only a few hours. A slightly extended half-life was obtained by fusing sCR1 with an albumin-binding receptor (75). An sCR1-F(ab')2 chimeric protein extended the half-life and the technique made targeting possible (76). Improving the culture condition further extended the half-life to approximately 30 hours. Parenteral administration is required.

A variant of sCR1 which specifically inhibits the alternative pathway has been constructed by deleting the C4b binding domain, sCR(desLHR-A) (77). This protein attenuated tissue damage in experimental myocardial infarction (78, 79) and reduced the endothelium-dependent relaxation in rabbit tissue, shown to be mediated by C5b-9 (80).

Human sCR1 is immunogenic in rodents, limiting its application in animal studies. Therefore, the rodent C3 convertase inhibitor Crry, which has both decay accelerating and cofactor activity and therefore resembles CR1, has been used in two different strategies in mouse models. First, a soluble Crry was constructed and coupled to an immunoglobulin tail for injection (Crry-Ig) (53). Second, Crry was over-expressed as a soluble protein in the animal under the control of a widely expressed transgene (59). Both approaches protected mice against experimentally induced acute glomerulonephritis and the Crry protein was not immunogenic. Furthermore, transgenic expression of Crry in mice developing SLE (MRL/lpr mice) prolonged survival and attenuated the renal damage (81), later confirmed by treatment with the soluble Crry-Ig protein (82). Soluble Crry was also shown to inhibit intestinal I/R injury in mice even when administered 30 minutes after start of reperfusion (54). Recently it has become evident that control of complement activation is of crucial importance for the placenta barrier homeostasis and that complement activation may induce fetal loss (see chapter 9 in this volume). Thus, in a mouse model of anti-phospholipid antibody-induced fetal loss, soluble Crry was protective (83).

sCR1 has been used in a number of animal disease models with convincing protective effects against tissue damage. In addition to the beneficial effect on myocardial I/R injury described above, the following I/R injuries have been attenuated by sCR1: local and remote injury in rat intestine (84, 85), gut ischemia and endothelial cell function after hemorrhage and resuscitation in rats (86), liver injury (87), and local and remote (lung) injury in skeletal muscle (88, 89).

The beneficial effect of sCR1 in autoimmune diseases has been demonstrated in the passive reverse Arthus reaction, which is a dermal vascular immune-complex condition (90), in experimental arthritis in rats (91, 92), in immune-complex and complement-mediated lung injuries and thermal trauma in rats (93). Furthermore, allergic reactions (94) and pseudoallergic reaction to infusion of liposomes (95) were attenuated by sCR1. Improvement was obtained in an experimental rodent model of ARDS (96) as well as in a guinea-pig model of asthma (97). The inflammatory reaction induced by acid aspiration to the lungs in a murine model was markedly improved by sCR1 (98).

sCR1 has proved to be efficient in treatment of experimental conditions in kidneys, including glomerulonephritis (99) and in the nervous system, like myasthenia gravis (100), experimental allergic encephalomyelitis (a model for multiple sclerosis) (101), autoimmune neuritis in rats (102) and traumatic brain injury (103).

The role of complement in xenotransplantation has been indisputable and therefore the effects of sCR1 in reducing hyperacute rejection was not surprising (73, 104-106). Coupling a mini-CR1 to a GPI anchor and incorporating it into porcine cells was protective against human complement (107). The role of complement in allotransplant rejection has been less clear, but the beneficial results obtained using sCR1 in various allotransplant models has highlighted complement as an important mechanism in allotransplant rejection as well (108-111).

Extracorporeal circulation, like haemodialysis and cardiopulmonary bypass (CPB), is associated with a complement-dependent systemic inflammatory response. sCR1 reduced lung injury and pulmonary hypertension in pigs undergoing CPB (112) and inhibited complement- and leukocyte activation in a simulated extracorporeal circulation setup (113).

sCR1 (TP-10; Avant Immunotherapeutics Inc, Needham, MA) has been awarded Orphan Drug status by the FDA and has reached clinical studies. It has been tested in patients with ARDS, acute myocardial infarction, lung transplantation and post-cardiopulmonary bypass syndrome (114). Most of the data have been published in abstract form only, but the results of the ARDS study have been published (115). Although sCR1 inhibited complement activation, there was no significant difference between the clinical outcome in the groups and the programme is discontinued.

4.2.3 Soluble DAF and MCP

A recombinant soluble form of DAF (sDAF) was constructed and found to inhibit complement both *in vitro* and *in vivo*. It attenuated the reverse passive Arthus reaction (116), but the lack of factor I cofactor activity may limit its potential for clinical application. Similarly, a recombinant soluble form of MCP (sMCP) has been made (117). sMCP attenuated the reverse passive Arthus reaction (118) and prolonged hyperacute xenograft rejection (117). A fusion protein of sMCP and a soluble form of the low affinity human IgG receptor Fc gamma RII (CD32) was more effective in protection against xenotransplant rejection than the sMCP alone (119). Comparison between sDAF, sMCP and sCR1 showed that sCR1 was more effective than each of the other two in the classical pathway. In the alternative pathway sCR1 and sMCP had almost the same effect (118). Combination of sDAF and sMCP was more effective than each protein alone. A fusion protein of sDAF and sMCP was constructed (CAB-2) which retained both decay acceleration (DAF) and co-factor activity (MCP). CAB-2 was protective in the passive reverse Arthus reaction and in Forssman shock (120), and prolonged pig-to-primate heart xenotransplant survival (121) as well as *ex vivo* porcine-to-human heart transplant graft survival (122).

4.2.4 Soluble CD59

A recombinant soluble form of CD59, sCD59, has been constructed, but is rather inefficient in the fluid phase (123). A fusion protein of sCD59 and sDAF has been constructed (124), with the aim of combining a C3/C5 convertase inhibitor activity with a C5b-9 inhibitor. It remains to be shown whether this molecule has any clinical application. A soluble form of CD59 has been fused with a soluble form of the rodent C3 convertase inhibitor, Crry, enabling inhibition of rodent complement activation both at the C3 and C9 level (125). A selective inhibition of C5b-9 may have limited indications in clinical medicine, but certain forms of glomerulonephritis, arthritis and encephalomyelitis may depend mainly on C5b-9 formation.

4.2.5 Microbial Proteins

Microbes frequently make proteins with high homology to human complement regulatory proteins and thus protect themselves against complement attack. One such protein, vaccinia virus complement control protein, has CR1-like activity and has been studied in detail (126). It has been postulated as a candidate for complement therapy. In addition to the complement-inhibitory function this protein has a binding site for heparin and direct interferes with binding of xenoantibodies to their targets.

4.3   Antibodies

Monoclonal antibodies have the advantage of high specificity, relatively long half-life and amenability for largescale production. A main limitation is the need for parenteral administration and the risk of immunization. The latter can be reduced by humanizing the antibody, or by producing human monoclonal antibodies, as recently described for an anti-C5 antibody isolated from a human phage display library (127).

4.3.1   Anti-MBL, -Factor D and -Properdin

Several recent data indicate that the lectin pathway is of importance in the pathogenesis of I/R injury (128, 129) and in experimental septicaemia where MBL-A deficiency improved survival (130). Anti-MBL antibodies blocking the lectin pathway have been developed (131, 132). A plant lectin, Ulex europaeus agglutinin II (UEA-II), has been identified as a potent inhibitor of MBL binding and thus of lectin pathway activation (133).

Factor D is the rate-limiting component in the alternative pathway and of pivotal importance for the I/R injury in mice (134), either by direct activation or through the amplification loop. An anti-human factor D monoclonal antibody (mAb) (166-32) has been characterized (135, 136) and found to inhibit complement and leukocyte activation in baboons undergoing CPB (137). An alternative approach for inhibition of the AP is blocking of properdin, although this will not lead to complete inhibition. Anti-properdin antibodies have been used *in vitro* and the data underscored the importance of AP as amplification from CP activation (138).

4.3.2 Anti-C5

Since there are no natural inhibitors acting directly on C5, there is a particular need to develop specific C5 inhibitors. Furthermore, it has been shown *in vitro* that C5 can be activated directly by leukocyte enzymes independent of C3 activation (139), but it is unclear whether this can occur *in vivo*. Monoclonal antibodies to mouse C5, like the mAb BB5.1 (140) were important tools to demonstrate the role of the terminal complement pathway in experimental diseases like collagen-induced arthritis (36) and lupus-like nephritis (141). Notably, such treatment of collagen-induced arthritis with anti-C5 antibody not only prevented disease onset, but also ameliorated established disease. An anti-rat C5 mAb was found to be protective in experimental myocardial infarction (142). The human anti-C5 antibody N19/8 described by Würzner et al. (143) was a breakthrough in this field. It was used to demonstrate inhibition of terminal pathway activation in an artificial cardiopulmonary bypass model where leukocyte and platelet activation was also attenuated (144) and it prevented hyperacute graft rejection in a model of porcine-to-human heart transplantation (145). Later several anti-C5 antibodies have been generated. One of these, the scFv fragment h5G1.1-scFv (146) has reached clinical trials as pexelizumab (Alexion Pharmaceuticals, Cheshire, CT). In a study of patients undergoing CPB complement inhibition was obtained with subsequent reduced leukocyte activation and postoperative complications, including cognitive defects, myocardial damage and blood loss (147). Studies in rheumatoid arthritis, idiopathic membranous nephropathy, lupus nephritis and myocardial infraction are underway, but until to date the results have been described only in abstract form.

4.3.3   Anti-C5a

C5a is the biologically most potent fragment formed during complement activation and is therefore regarded as an important target for inhibition (148, 149). In animal studies anti-C5a antibodies reduced myocardial I/R injury (150), reduced neutrophil-mediated impairment of endothelium-dependent relaxation after CPB (151), reduced local and remote injury in intestinal I/R injury (152), improved survival (153, 154) and reduced IL-6 production (155) and oxygen demand (156) in sepsis, inhibited sepsis-related thymic cell apoptosis (157, 158), alleviated symptoms of ARDS in septic primates (159) and reduced lung vascular injury following thermal trauma (160). Recently anti-C5a antibodies were shown to have direct effects on the coagulation and fibrinolytic systems in a rat model of sepsis, emphasizing a possible role of C5a in activation of other plasma cascade systems (161). Anti-guinea pig C5 and anti-C5a mAbs have also been generated for examination of the terminal pathway in experimental xenotransplantation (162).

A novel approach for C5a inhibition was recently demonstrated using a mAb reacting with the C5a moiety of the C5 molecule without inhibiting C5 cleavage (163). Thus, C5a is "pre-neutralized" before it is formed and thereby increases efficacy of C5a neutralization. This antibody has been investigated in a human blood model of Neisseria, with virtually complete inhibition of the inflammatory reaction while bacterial killing was not affected (164).

4.3.4 Anti-C5-9

Anti-C8, which blocks C5b-9 (TCC) formation without interfering with C5 cleavage, was found to reduce tissue damage in rat hearts perfused with human serum (165). Furthermore, anti-C8 inhibited platelet activation during simulated CPB (166).

4.4   Small Molecule Inhibitors

4.4.1   C1 Binding Peptides

Peptides interacting with the function of C1q has been produced form phage display libraries (167, 168). Synthetic peptides interacting with IgG binding to C1 prolonged xenograft survival (169). It should be noted that C1q is not only activated by antibodies, but by several other substances which may be of pathogenic importance in human diseases, like beta-amyloid in Alzheimers disease, and C-reactive protein with possible implications for the pathogenesis of atherosclerosis. Inhibition of C1q has recently been extensively reviewed (26). A novel highly selective small molecule C1s inhibitor (C1s-INH-248, Knoll) was found to protect against experimental myocardial I/R injury (170).

4.4.2   BCX-1470

BCX-1470 is a serine protease inhibitor which was made on the basis of the 3D crystal structure of factor D. It was found to attenuate the reverse-passive Arthus reaction (171). It was found to be safe in animal toxicity studies and was tested in healthy volunteers. BCX-1470 inhibits factor D, but also C1s and several other serine proteases, which is in contrast to the specificity of the anti-factor D mAb described above. In general, serine protease inhibitors which inhibit factor D, also inhibit other serine proteases.

4.4.3   Compstatin

A 13-residue cyclic peptide was isolated using combinatorial peptide libraries to identify C3 binding peptides (172), later characterized in detail and named compstatin (173). This peptide blocks cleavage of C3 and is highly specific for binding to C3. No interaction with other cascade proteins has been demonstrated. It was found to reduce complement and granulocyte activation in an *in vitro* model of extracorporeal circulation (174) and to protect against hyperacute xenograft rejection *ex vivo* (175). Compstatin works only in primates and therefore animal studies are limited. One study showed inhibition of heparin-protamine induced complement activation in a primate *in vivo* model (176).

4.4.4   C3aR Antagonists

A nonpeptide C3aR antagonist (SB 290157) blocking human C3aR also antagonizes rodent C3aR and was found to reduce neutrophil recruitment in LPS-induced airway neutrophilia (177). The C3a/C3aR interaction may be a candidate for therapy in asthma (178, 179). Antibodies neutralizing C3a has also been shown to abolish C3aR mediated function (180). Disrupting the C3aR showed protective anti-inflammatory effects in endotoxic shock (181).

4.4.5   C5aR Antagonists

The first peptide antagonist was the linear *N* MeFKPdCHaWdR (182). Later a cyclic peptide was made, AcF[OPdChaWR] (183), which has been extensively studied in various animal models. It reacts both with primates and rodents. Beneficial effects of this antagonist have been observed in I/R injury in small intestine (184) and in kidneys (185). It attenuated chemotaxis and cytokine production (186), endotoxin-induced neutropenia (187) and the reverse passive Arthus reaction (188). It was effective when given orally to animals with immune-complex mediated dermal inflammation (189) and experimental arthritis (190).

C5aR antagonists were also developed by screening of phage-display libraries and by site directed mutagenesis of C5a, both shown to be effective in reducing complement-mediated inflammation *in vivo* (191, 192). The dimeric recombinant human C5a antagonist, CGS 32359 (191), attenuated neutrophil activation and reduced myocardial infarction size in a porcine model of surgical revascularization (193). Another C5aR antagonist significantly reduced murine renal I/R injury (194). The tertiary structure of a unique C5a receptor antagonist was determined by two-dimensional NMR spectroscopy (195) and an antisense homology box approach was used to design C5a antagonist peptides (196). Recently, a non-peptide C5aR antagonist active in cynomolgus monkeys and gerbils, was shown to inhibit C5a mediated neutropenia after oral administration (197).

4.4.6   RNA Aptamers

Screening of an RNA pool obtained by the SELEX combinatorial chemistry technique revealed several clones binding to and inhibiting activation of human and rat C5 (198). It remains to be shown whether these molecules are possible complement inhibitors *in vivo*.

4.5   Other Inhibitors

Numerous natural and synthetic substances have been documented to inhibit complement, but these are in general not complement specific. Only a few are mentioned here.

Nafamostat mesilate (FUTHAN; FUT-175) and gabexate mesylate (FOY) are synthetic serine potease inhibitors with a broad spectrum of targets. Nafamostate is effective in several animal disease models of I/R injury, pancreatitis, xenotransplantation and cerebral infarction, but is not complement specific. Aprotinin, a complex polypeptide with effects on coagulation and inflammation, reduces postoperative bleedings, has been regarded as a candidate for general cascade inhibition. K-76 monocarboxylic acid (MX-1) is a fungal product found to inhibit several complement components, but in particular C5 (199). Although initially regarded as a promising complement inhibitor (200-202) later studies on xenotransplantation did not show efficient effect on graft survival neither by K-76 nor by FUT-175 (203, 204).

Heparin has a number of effects on complement and coagulation. Modifications to obtain complement-inhibitory heparin without effect on coagulation have been made (205). Dextran potentiates the effects of several complement inhibitory proteins including C1-inhibitor and was found to delay *ex vivo* hyperacute xenograft rejection (206). Coating of artificial devises with heparin improves biocompatibility by reducing complement activation and subsequent inflammatory reaction (207).

High-dose intravenous immunoglobulins (IVIG) are currently used to treat various inflammatory diseases. The list of biological effects of IVIG is long, including several complement modulating activities (see chapter 24 in this volume) In fact, the effect of IVIG on complement is not directly inhibitory. IVIG act as scavenger for C1q, C4b and C3b binding, thus diverting the activation products from the target to the immunoglobulin molecules. Thus, IVIG should not be used as a primary complement inhibitor, but its effect on complement could be an additional benefit to certain inflammatory diseases.

Cobra venom factor (CVF) is frequently on the list of complement inhibitors. It should be noted, however, that CVF is not a complement inhibitor, but a potent complement activator, which depletes C3 from plasma by activating the alternative pathway amplification loop. The activation per se may influence the results obtained, therefore specific complement inhibitors developed to date should replace CVF in animal studies.

5. CONCLUDING REMARKS

Three decades ago the role of complement in human disease was largely unknown. Two decades ago it became evident that complement activation was associated with a number of pathophysiologic conditions, although the role of this activation in the pathogenesis of the diseases was largely unknown. During the last decade studies using specific complement inhibitors or complement knock-out animals have revealed that complement plays a crucial role in the pathogenesis of tissue inflammation in a number of animal disease models. These include local and remote damage after ischemia and reperfusion, immune-complex and autoimmune diseases in general and joint, kidney and central nervous system diseases in particular, ARDS and systemic inflammatory response due to sepsis or extracorporeal circulation, antibody-mediated fetal loss, and allo- and xenotransplantat graft rejections. Based on these encouraging data a great enthusiasm evolved for treatment of human diseases using complement inhibitors. Unfortunately the progress in clinical application has been relatively slow. This may be attributed to several reasons: Human diseases may have a more complex pathophysiology than the animal models. Experimental conditions differ significantly from the clinical with respect to time for and mode of application. The number of drugs for clinical use has been markedly limited compared to those used in animal models. Targeted inhibition has hardly reached clinical application. Finally, the selection of patients and size of test groups may have been inadequate for demonstrating clinical benefit. The approach of complement inhibition for treatment of human diseases is still in its infancy, in fact it has hardly reached delivery. There is a need for more experimental studies, which should focus on the mechanisms of complement-mediated damage. This will provide a rational approach to design and optimize the treatment, i.e. identifying the component(s) needed to be inhibited in the actual condition and targeting the inhibition to the actual site of inflammation. With the advent of numerous novel complement inhibitors, it is hopeful that the potential benefits of complement inhibition in human inflammatory diseases could be validated and realized.

6. REFERENCES

1. Waytes AT, Rosen FS, Frank MM. Treatment of hereditary angioedema with a vapor-heated C1 inhibitor concentrate. N Engl J Med 1996;334:1630-4.
2. Nathanson S, Fremeaux-Bacchi V, Deschenes G. Successful plasma therapy in hemolytic uremic syndrome with factor H deficiency. Pediatr Nephrol 2001;16:554-6.
3. Steinsson K, Erlendsson K, Valdimarsson H. Successful plasma infusion treatment of a patient with C2 deficiency and systemic lupus erythematosus: clinical experience over forty-five months. Arthritis Rheum 1989;32:906-13.
4. Remuzzi G, Ruggenenti P, Codazzi D, Noris M, Caprioli J, Locatelli G, Gridelli B. Combined kidney and liver transplantation for familial haemolytic uraemic syndrome. Lancet 2002;359:1671-2.
5. Ziegler JB, Alper CA, Rosen RS, Lachmann PJ, SheringtonL. Restoration by purified C3b inactivator of complement-mediated function in vivo in a patient with C3b inactivator deficiency. J Clin Invest 1975;55:668-72.
6. Lambris JD and Holers VM, editors. Therapeutic intervention in the complement system. Totowa, NJ. Humana Press; 2000.
7. Makrides SC. Therapeutic inhibition of the complement system. Pharmacol Rev 1998;50:59-87.
8. McGeer EG, McGeer PL. The future use of complement inhibitors for the treatment of neurological diseases. Drugs 1998;55:739-46.
9. Morgan BP, Rushmere NK, Harris CL. Therapeutic uses of recombinant complement receptors. Biochem Soc Trans 1998;26:49-54.
10. Nangaku M. Complement regulatory proteins in glomerular diseases. Kidney Int 1998;54:1419-28.
11. Mathieson PW. Is complement a target for therapy in renal disease? Kidney Int 1998;54:1429-36.
12. Morgan BP. Regulation of the complement membrane attack pathway. Crit Rev Immun 1999;19:173-98.
13. Barnum SR. Inhibition of complement as a therapeutic approach in inflammatory central nervous system (CNS) disease. Mol Med 1999;5:569-82.
14. Marsh JE, Pratt JR, Sacks SH. Targeting the complement system. Curr Opin Nephrol Hypertens 1999;8:557-62.
15. Pellas TC, Wennogle LP. C5a receptor antagonists. Curr Pharm Des 1999;5:737-55.
16. Dong J, Pratt JR, Smith RAG, Dodd I, Sacks SH. Strategies for targeting complement inhibitors in ischaemia/reperfusion injury. Mol Immunol 1999;36:957-63.
17. Linton SM, Morgan BP. Complement activation and inhibition in experimental models of arthritis. Mol Immunol 1999;36:905-14.
18. Sahu A, Lambris JD. Complement inhibitors: a resurgent concept in anti- inflammatory therapeutics. Immunopharmacology 2000;49:133-48.
19. Asghar SS, Pasch MC. Therapeutic inhibition of the complement system. Y2K update. Front Biosci 2000;5:E63-E82
20. Lucchesi BR, Tanhehco EJ. Therapeutic potential of complement inhibitors in myocardial ischaemia. Expert Opin Investig Drugs 2000;9:975-91.

21. Kawano M. Complement regulatory proteins and autoimmunity. Arch Immunol Ther Exp (Warsz) 2000;48:367-72.
22. Kirschfink M. Targeting complement in therapy. Immunol Rev 2001;180:177-89.
23. D'Ambrosio AL, Pinsky DJ, Connolly ES. The role of the complement cascade in ischemia/reperfusion injury: Implications for neuroprotection. Mol Med 2001;7:367-82.
24. Shernan SK, Collard CD. Role of the complement system in ischaemic heart disease: potential for pharmacological intervention. BioDrugs 2001;15:595-607.
25. Monsinjon T, Richard V, Fontaine M. Complement and its implications in cardiac ischemia/reperfusion: strategies to inhibit complement. Fundam Clin Pharmacol 2001;15:293-306.
26. Roos A, Ramwadhdoebe TH, Nauta AJ, Hack CE, Daha MR. Therapeutic inhibition of the early phase of complement activation. Immunobiology 2002;205:595-609.
27. Quigg RJ. Use of complement inhibitors in tissue injury. Trends Mol Med 2002;8:430-6.
28. Smith RAG. Targeting anticomplement agents. Biochem Soc Trans 2002;30:1037-41.
29. Harris CL, Fraser DA, Morgan BP. Tailoring anti-complement therapeutics. Biochem Soc Trans 2002;30:1019-26.
30. Morikis D, Lambris JD. Structural aspects and design of low-molecular-mass complement inhibitors. Biochem Soc Trans 2002;30:1026-36.
31. Gerard NP, Gerard C. Complement in allergy and asthma. Curr Opin Immunol 2002;14:705-8.
32. Bhole D, Stahl GL. Therapeutic potential of targeting the complement cascade in critical care medicine. Crit Care Med 2003;31:S97-104.
33. Pugsley MK, Abramova M, Cole T, Yang X, Ammons WS. Inhibitors of the complement system currently in development for cardiovascular disease. Cardiovasc Toxicol 2003;3:43-70.
34. Hsu SI, Couser WG. Chronic progression of tubulointerstitial damage in proteinuric renal disease is mediated by complement activation: a therapeutic role for complement inhibitors? J Am Soc Nephrol 2003;14 Suppl 2:S186-S191.
35. Mollnes TE, Song WC, Lambris JD. Complement in inflammatory tissue damage and disease. Trends Immunol 2002;23:61-4.
36. Wang Y, Rollins SA, Madri JA, Matis LA. Anti-C5 monoclonal antibody therapy prevents collagen- induced arthritis and ameliorates established disease. Proc Natl Acad Sci USA 1995;92:8955-9.
37. Mastellos D, Lambris JD. Complement: more than a 'guard' against invading pathogens? Trends Immunol 2002;23:485-91.
38. Harris CL, Williams AS, Linton SM, Morgan BP. Coupling complement regulators to immunoglobulin domains generates effective anti-complement reagents with extended half-life in vivo. Clin Exp Immunol 2002;129:198-207.
39. Smith GP, Smith RAG. Membrane-targeted complement inhibitors. Mol Immunol 2001;38:249-55.
40. Linton SM, Williams AS, Dodd I, Smith R, Williams BD, Morgan BP. Therapeutic efficacy of a novel membrane-targeted complement regulator in antigen-induced arthritis in the rat. Arthritis Rheum 2000;43:2590-7.
41. Fraser DA, Harris CL, Smith RAG, Morgan BP. Bacterial expression and membrane targeting of the rat complement regulator Crry: A new model anticomplement therapeutic. Protein Sci 2002;11:2512-21.
42. Zhang HF, Lu SL, Morrison SL, Tomlinson S. Targeting the functional antibody-decay-accelerating factor fusion proteins to a cell surface. J Biol Chem 2001;276:27290-5.

43. Zhang HF, Yu JH, Bajwa E, Morrison SL, Tomlinson S. Targeting of functional antibody-CD59 fusion proteins to a cell surface. J Clin Invest 1999;103:55-61.
44. Song H, He C, Knaak C, Guthridge JM, Holers VM, Tomlinson S. Complement receptor 2-mediated targeting of complement inhibitors to sites of complement activation. J Clin Invest 2003;111:1875-85.
45. Picard MD, Pettey CL, Marsh HC, Thomas LJ. Characterization of N-linked oligosaccharides bearing sialyl Lewis x moieties on an alternatively glycosylated form of soluble complement receptor type I (SCRI). Biotechnol Appl Biochem 2000;31:5-13:5-13.
46. Rittershaus CW, Thomas LJ, Miller DP, Picard MD, GeogheganBarek KM, Scesney SM, Henry LD, Sen AC, Bertino AM, Hannig G, Adari H, Mealey RA, Gosselin ML, Couto M, Hayman EG, Levin JL, Reinhold VN, Marsh HC. Recombinant glycoproteins that inhibit complement activation and also bind the selectin adhesion molecules. J Biol Chem 1999;274:11237-44.
47. Huang J, Kim LJ, Mealey R, Marsh HC, Zhang Y, Tenner AJ, Connolly ES, Pinsky DJ. Neuronal protection in stroke by an sLe(X)-glycosylated complement inhibitory protein. Science 1999;285:595-9.
48. Mulligan MS, Warner RL, Rittershaus CW, Thomas LJ, Ryan US, Foreman KE, Crouch LD, Till GO, Ward PA. Endothelial targeting and enhanced antiinflammatory effects of complement inhibitors possessing sialyl Lewis(X) moieties. J Immunol 1999;162:4952-9.
49. Stammberger U, Hamacher J, Hillinger S, Schmid RA. sCR1sLe(X) ameliorates ischemia/reperfusion injury in experimental lung transplantation. J Thorac Cardiovasc Surg 2000;120:1078-84.
50. Zacharowski K, Otto M, Hafner G, Marsh HC, Thiemermann C. Reduction of myocardial infarct size with sCR1sLe(X), an alternatively glycosylated form of human soluble complement receptor type 1 (SCR1), possessing sialyl Lewis x. Brit J Pharmacol 1999;128:945-52.
51. Kyriakides C, Wang Y, Austen WG, Favuzza J, Kobzik L, Moore FD, Hechtman HB. Moderation of skeletal muscle reperfusion injury by a sLe(X)-glycosylated complement inhibitory protein. Amer J Physiol Cell Physiol 2001;281:C224-C230
52. Kyriakides C, Wang Y, Austen WG, Favuzza J, Kobzik L, Moore FD, Hechtman HB. Sialyl Lewis(X) hybridized complement receptor type 1 moderates acid aspiration injury. Amer J Physiol Lung Cell M Ph 2001;281:L1494-L1499
53. Quigg RJ, Kozono Y, Berthiaume D, Lim A, Salant DJ, Weinfeld A, Griffin P, Kremmer E, Holers VM. Blockade of antibody-induced glomerulonephritis with Crry- Ig, a soluble murine complement inhibitor. J Immunol 1998;160:4553-60.
54. Rehrig S, Fleming SD, Anderson J, Guthridge JM, Rakstang J, McQueen CE, Holers VM, Tsokos GC, Shea-Donohue T. Complement inhibitor, complement receptor 1-related gene/protein y-Ig attenuates intestinal damage after the onset of mesenteric ischemia/reperfusion injury in mice. J Immunol 2001;167:5921-7.
55. Harris CL, Hughes CE, Williams AS, Goodfellow I, Evans DJ, Caterson B, Morgan BP. Generation of anti-complement 'prodrugs': cleavable reagents for specific delivery of complement regulators to disease sites. J Biol Chem 2003;278:36068-76.
56. McGrath Y, Wilkinson GWG, Spiller OB, Morgan BP. Development of adenovirus vectors encoding rat complement regulators for use in therapy in rodent models of inflammatory diseases. J Immunol 1999;163:6834-40.
57. Davoust N, Nataf S, Reiman R, Holers MV, Campbell IL, Barnum SR. Central nervous system-targeted expression of the complement inhibitor sCrry prevents experimental allergic encephalomyelitis. J Immunol 1999;163:6551-6.

58. Dreja H, Annenkov A, Chernajovsky Y. Soluble complement receptor 1 (CD35) delivered by retrovirally infected syngeneic cells or by naked DNA injection prevents the progression of collagen-induced arthritis. Arthritis Rheum 2000;43:1698-709.

59. Quigg RJ, He C, Lim A, Berthiaume D, Alexander JJ, Kraus D, Holers VM. Transgenic mice overexpressing the complement inhibitor Crry as a soluble protein are protected from antibody- induced glomerular injury. J Exp Med 1998;188:1321-31.

60. Matsushita M, Thiel S, Jensenius JC, Terai I, Fujita T. Proteolytic activities of two types of mannose-binding lectin- associated serine protease. J Immunol 2000;165:2637-42.

61. Jiang HX, Wagner E, Zhang HM, Frank MM. Complement 1 inhibitor is a regulator of the alternative complement pathway. J Exp Med 2001;194:1609-16.

62. de Zwaan C, Kleine AH, Diris JH, Glatz JF, Wellens HJ, Strengers PF, Tissing M, Hack CE, Dieijen-Visser MP, Hermens WT. Continuous 48-h C1-inhibitor treatment, following reperfusion therapy, in patients with acute myocardial infarction. Eur Heart J 2002;23:1670-7.

63. Caliezi C, Wuillemin WA, Zeerleder S, Redondo M, Eisele B, Hack CE. C1-esterase inhibitor: An anti-inflammatory agent and its potential use in the treatment of diseases other than hereditary angioedema. Pharmacol Rev 2000;52:91-112.

64. Kirschfink M, Mollnes TE. C1-inhibitor: an anti-inflammatory reagent with therapeutic potential. Expert Opin Pharmacother 2001;2:1073-84.

65. Horstick G. C1-esterase inhibitor in ischemia and reperfusion. Immunobiology 2002;205:552-62.

66. Sharma AK, Pangburn MK. Biologically active recombinant human complement factor H: Synthesis and secretion by the baculovirus system. Gene 1994;143:301-2.

67. Mikata S, Miyagawa S, Iwata K, Nagasawa S, Hatanaka M, Matsumoto M, Kamiike W, Matsuda H, Shirakura R, Seya T. Regulation of complement-mediated swine endothelial cell lysis by a surface-bound form of human C4b binding protein. Transplantation 1998;65:363-8.

68. Yoshitatsu M, Miyagawa S, Mikata S, Matsunami K, Yamada M, Murase A, Sawa Y, Ohtake S, Matsuda H, Shirakura R. Function of human factor H and I on xenosurface. Biochem Biophys Res Commun 1999;265:556-62.

69. Andersson J, Larsson R, Richter R, Ekdahl KN, Nilsson B. Binding of a model regulator of complement activation (RCA) to a biomaterial surface: surface-bound factor H inhibits complement activation. Biomaterials 2001;22:2435-43.

70. Weisman HF, Bartow T, Leppo MK, Marsh HC, Jr., Carson GR, Concino, M.F., Boyle MP, Roux KH, Weisfeldt ML, Fearon DT. Soluble human complement receptor type 1: in vivo inhibitor of complement suppressing post-ischemic myocardial inflammation and necrosis. Science 1990;249:146-51.

71. Shandelya SML, Kuppusamy P, Herskowitz A, Weisfeldt ML, Zweier JL. Soluble complement receptor type 1 inhibits the complement pathway and prevents contractile failure in the postischemic heart: Evidence that complement activation is required for neutrophil-mediated reperfusion injury. Circulation 1993;88:2812-26.

72. Smith EF, Griswold DE, Egan JW, Hillegass LM, Smith RAG, Hibbs MJ, Gagnon RC. Reduction of myocardial reperfusion injury with human soluble complement receptor type-1 (BRL-55730). Eur J Pharmacol 1993;236:477-81.

73. Homeister JW, Satoh PS, Kilgore KS, Lucchesi BR. Soluble complement receptor type-1 prevents human complement-mediated damage of the rabbit isolated heart. J Immunol 1993;150:1055-64.

74. Lazar HL, Bao YS, Gaudiani J, Rivers S, Marsh H. Total complement inhibition - An effective strategy to limit ischemic injury during coronary revascularization on cardiopulmonary bypass. Circulation 1999;100:1438-42.

75. Makrides SC, Nygren PA, Andrews B, Ford PJ, Evans KS, Hayman EG, Adari H, Levin J, Uhlen M, Toth CA. Extended in vivo half-life of human soluble complement receptor type 1 fused to a serum albumin-binding receptor. J Pharmacol Exp Ther 1996;277:534-42.

76. Kalli KR, Hsu PH, Bartow TJ, Ahearn JM, Matsumoto AK, Klickstein LB, Fearon DT. Mapping of the C3b-binding site of CR1 and construction of a (CR1)2-F(ab')2 chimeric complement inhibitor. J Exp Med 1991;174:1451-60.

77. Scesney SM, Makrides SC, Gosselin ML, Ford PJ, Andrews BM, Hayman EG, Marsh HC. A soluble deletion mutant of the human complement receptor type 1, which lacks the C4b binding site, is a selective inhibitor of the alternative complement pathway. Eur J Immunol 1996;26:1729-35.

78. Murohara T, Guo JP, Delyani JA, Lefer AM. Cardioprotective effects of selective inhibition of the two complement activation pathways in myocardial ischemia and reperfusion injury. Meth Find Exp Clin Pharmacol 1995;17:499-507.

79. Gralinski MR, Wiater BC, Assenmacher AN, Lucchesi BR. Selective inhibition of the alternative complement pathway by sCR1[desLHR-A] protects the rabbit isolated heart from human complement-mediated damage. Immunopharmacology 1996;34:79-88.

80. Lennon PF, Collard CD, Morrissey MA, Stahl GL. Complement-induced endothelial dysfunction in rabbits: Mechanisms, recovery, and gender differences. Amer J Physiol Heart Circ Phy 1996;39:H1924-H1932

81. Bao LH, Haas M, Boackle SA, Kraus DM, Cunningham PN, Park P, Alexander JJ, Anderson RK, Culhane K, Holers VM, Quigg RJ. Transgenic expression of a soluble complement inhibitor protects against renal disease and promotes survival in MRL/lpr mice. J Immunol 2002;168:3601-7.

82. Bao LH, Haas M, Kraus DM, Hack BK, Rakstang JK, Holers VM, Quigg RJ. Administration of a soluble recombinant complement C3 inhibitor protects against renal disease in MRL/lpr mice. J Amer Soc Nephrol 2003;14:670-9.

83. Holers VM, Girardi G, Mo L, Guthridge JM, Molina H, Pierangeli SS, Espinola R, Xiaowei LE, Mao DL, Vialpando CG, Salmon JE. Complement C3 activation is required for antiphospholipid antibody-induced fetal loss. J Exp Med 2002;195:211-20.

84. Hill J, Lindsay TF, Ortiz F, Yeh CG, Hechtman HB, Moore FD. Soluble complement receptor type-1 ameliorates the local and remote organ injury after intestinal ischemia-reperfusion in the rat. J Immunol 1992;149:1723-8.

85. Eror AT, Stojadinovic A, Starnes BW, Makrides SC, Tsokos GC, SheaDonohue T. Antiinflammatory effects of soluble complement receptor type 1 promote rapid recovery of ischemia/reperfusion injury in rat small intestine. Clin Immunol 1999;90:266-75.

86. Fruchterman TM, Spain DA, Wilson MA, Harris PD, Garrison RN. Complement inhibition prevents gut ischemia and endothelial cell dysfunction after hemorrhage/resuscitation. Surgery 1998;124:782-92.

87. Chavez Cartaya RE, Desola GP, Wright L, Jamieson NV, White DJG. Regulation of the complement cascade by soluble complement receptor type 1. Protective effect in experimental liver ischemia and reperfusion. Transplantation 1995;59:1047-52.

88. Pemberton M, Anderson G, Vetvicka V, Justus DE, Ross GD. Microvascular effects of complement blockade with soluble recombinant CR1 on ischemia/reperfusion injury of skeletal muscle. J Immunol 1993;150:5104-13.

89. Lindsay TF, Hill J, Ortiz F, Rudolph A, Valeri CR, Hechtman HB, Moore FD. Blockade of complement activation prevents local and pulmonary albumin leak after lower torso ischemia reperfusion. Ann Surg 1992;216:677-83.

90. Yeh CG, Marsh HC, Jr., Carson GR, Berman L, Concino MF, Scesney SM, Kuestner RE, Skibbens R, Donahue KA, Ip SH. Recombinant soluble human complement receptor

type 1 inhibits inflammation in the reversed passive arthus reaction in rats. J Immunol 1991;146:250-6.

91. Goodfellow RM, Williams AS, Levin JL, Williams BD, Morgan BP. Local therapy with soluble complement receptor 1 (sCR1) suppresses inflammation in rat mono-articular arthritis. Clin Exp Immunol 1997;110:45-52.

92. Goodfellow RM, Williams AS, Levin JL, Williams BD, Morgan BP. Soluble complement receptor one (SCR1) inhibits the development and progression of rat collagen-induced arthritis. Clin Exp Immunol 2000;119:210-6.

93. Mulligan MS, Yeh CG, Rudolph AR, Ward PA. Protective effects of soluble CR1 in complement-mediated and neutrophil-mediated tissue injury. J Immunol 1992;148:1479-85.

94. Lima MC, Prouvost-Danon A, Silva PM, Chagas MS, Calheiros AS, Cordeiro RS, Latine D, Bazin H, Ryan US, Martins MA. Studies on the mechanisms involved in antigen-evoked pleural inflammation in rats: contribution of IgE and complement. J Leukoc Biol 1997;61:286-92.

95. Szebeni J, Fontana JL, Wassef NM, Mongan PD, Morse DS, Dobbins DE, Stahl GL, Bunger R, Alving CR. Hemodynamic changes induced by liposomes and liposome-encapsulated hemoglobin in pigs - A model for pseudoallergic cardiopulmonary reactions to liposomes: Role of complement and inhibition by soluble CR1 and anti- C5a antibody. Circulation 1999;99:2302-9.

96. Rabinovici R, Yeh CG, Hillegass LM, Griswold DE, Dimartino MJ, Vernick J, Fong KLL, Feuerstein G. Role of complement in endotoxin/platelet-activating factor- induced lung injury. J Immunol 1992;149:1744-50.

97. Regal JF, Fraser DG, Toth CA. Role of the complement system in antigen-induced bronchoconstriction and changes in blood pressure in the guinea pig. J Pharmacol Exp Ther 1993;267:979-88.

98. Weiser MR, Pechet TTV, Williams JP, Ma MH, Frenette PS, Moore FD, Kobzik L, Hines RO, Wagner DD, Carroll MC, Hechtman HB. Experimental murine acid aspiration injury is mediated by neutrophils and the alternative complement pathway. J Appl Physiol 1997;83:1090-5.

99. Couser WG, Johnson RJ, Young BA, Yeh CG, Toth CA, Rudolph AR. The effects of soluble recombinant complement receptor 1 on complement-mediated experimental glomerulonephritis. J Amer Soc Nephrol 1995;5:1888-94.

100. Piddlesden SJ, Jiang SS, Levin JL, Vincent A, Morgan BP. Soluble complement receptor 1 (sCR1) protects against experimental autoimmune myasthenia gravis. J Neuroimmunol 1996;71:173-7.

101. Piddlesden SJ, Storch MK, Hibbs M, Freeman AM, Lassmann H, Morgan BP. Soluble recombinant complement receptor 1 inhibits inflammation and demyelination in antibody-mediated demyelinating experimental allergic encephalomyelitis. J Immunol 1994;152:5477-84.

102. Jung S, Toyka KV, Hartung HP. Soluble complement receptor type 1 inhibits experimental autoimmune neuritis in Lewis rats. Neurosci Lett 1995;200:167-70.

103. Kaczorowski SL, Schiding JK, Toth CA, Kochanek PM. Effect of soluble complement receptor-1 on neutrophil accumulation after traumatic brain injury in rats. J Cereb Blood Flow Metab 1995;15:860-4.

104. Pruitt SK, Baldwin WM, Marsh HCJ, Lin SS, Yeh CG, Bollinger RR. The effect of soluble complement receptor type 1 on hyperacute xenograft rejection. Transplantation 1991;52:868-73.

105. Xia W, Fearon DT, Moore FD, Schoen FJ, Ortiz F, Kirkman RL. Prolongation of guinea pig cardiac xenograft survival in rats by soluble human complement receptor type-1. Transplant Proc 1992;24:479-80.
106. Pruitt SK, Kirk AD, Bollinger RR, Marsh HC, Collins BH, Levin JL, Mault JR, Heinle JS, Ibrahim S, Rudolph AR, Baldwin WM, Sanfilippo F. The effect of soluble complement receptor type 1 on hyperacute rejection of porcine xenografts. Transplantation 1994;57:363-70.
107. Mikata S, Miyagawa S, Yoshitatsu M, Ikawa M, Okabe M, Matsuda H, Shirakura R. Prevention of hyperacute rejection by phosphatidylinositol- anchored mini-complement receptor type 1. Transpl Immunol 1998;6:107-10.
108. Pruitt SK, Bollinger RR. The effect of soluble complement receptor type 1 on hyperacute allograft rejection. J Surg Res 1991;50:350-5.
109. Pratt JR, Hibbs MJ, Laver AJ, Smith RAG, Sacks SH. Effects of complement inhibition with soluble complement receptor-1 on vascular injury and inflammation during renal allograft rejection in the rat. Am J Pathol 1996;149:2055-66.
110. Lehmann TG, Koeppel TA, Kirschfink M, Gebhard MM, Herfarth C, Otto G, Post S. Complement inhibition by soluble complement receptor type 1 improves microcirculation after rat liver transplantation. Transplantation 1998;66:717-22.
111. Pierre AF, Xavier AM, Liu MY, Cassivi SD, Lindsay TF, Marsh HC, Slutsky AS, Keshavjee SH. Effect of complement inhibition with soluble complement receptor 1 on pig allotransplant lung function. Transplantation 1998;66:723-32.
112. Gillinov AM, Devaleria PA, Winkelstein JA, Wilson I, Curtis WE, Shaw D, Yeh CG, Rudolph AR, Baumgartner WA, Herskowitz A, Cameron DE. Complement inhibition with soluble complement receptor type 1 in cardiopulmonary bypass. Ann Thorac Surg 1993;55:619-24.
113. Larsson R, Elgue G, Larsson A, Ekdahl KN, Nilsson UR, Nilsson B. Inhibition of complement activation by soluble recombinant CR1 under conditions resembling those in a cardiopulmonary circuit: reduced up-regulation of CD11b and complete abrogation of binding of PMNs to the biomaterial surface. Immunopharmacology 1997;38:119-27.
114. Rioux P. TP-10 (AVANT Immunotherapeutics). Curr Opin Investig Drugs 2001;2:364-71.
115. Zimmerman JL, Dellinger RP, Straube RC, Levin JL. Phase I trial of the recombinant soluble complement receptor 1 in acute lung injury and acute respiratory distress syndrome. Crit Care Med 2000;28:3149-54.
116. Moran P, Beasley H, Gorrell A, Martin E, Gribling P, Fuchs H, Gillett N, Burton LE, Caras IW. Human recombinant soluble decay accelerating factor inhibits complement activation in vitro and in vivo. J Immunol 1992;149:1736-43.
117. Christiansen D, Milland J, Thorley BR, Mckenzie IFC, Mottram PL, Purcell LJ, Loveland BE. Engineering of recombinant soluble CD46: An inhibitor of complement activation. Immunology 1996;87:348-54.
118. Christiansen D, Milland J, Thorley BR, Mckenzie IFC, Loveland BE. A functional analysis of recombinant soluble CD46 in vivo and a comparison with recombinant soluble forms of CD55 and CD35 in vitro. Eur J Immunol 1996;26:578-85.
119. Lanteri MB, Powell MS, Christiansen D, Li YQ, Hogarth PM, Sandrin MS, Mckenzie IFC, Loveland BE. Inhibition of hyperacute transplant rejection by soluble proteins with the functional domains of CD46 and Fc gamma RII. Transplantation 2000;69:1128-36.
120. Higgins PJ, Ko JL, Lobell R, Sardonini C, Alessi MK, Yeh CG. A soluble chimeric complement inhibitory protein that possesses both decay-accelerating and factor I cofactor activities. J Immunol 1997;158:2872-81.

121. Salerno CT, Kulick DM, Yeh CG, GuzmanPaz M, Higgins PJ, Benson BA, Park SJ, Shumway SJ, Bolman RM, Dalmasso AP. A soluble chimeric inhibitor of C3 and C5 convertases, complement activation blocker-2, prolongs graft survival in pig-to-rhesus monkey heart transplantation. Xenotransplantation 2002;9:125-34.
122. Kroshus TJ, Salerno CT, Yeh CG, Higgins PJ, Bolman RM, Dalmasso AP. A recombinant soluble chimeric complement inhibitor composed of human CD46 and CD55 reduces acute cardiac tissue injury in models of pig-to-human heart transplantation. Transplantation 2000;69:2282-9.
123. Sugita Y, Ito K, Shiozuka K, Suzuki H, Gushima H, Tomita M, Masuho Y. Recombinant soluble CD59 inhibits reactive haemolysis with complement. Immunology 1994;82:34-41.
124. Fodor WL, Rollins SA, Guilmette ER, Setter E, Squinto SP. A novel bifunctional chimeric complement inhibitor that regulates C3 convertase and formation of the membrane attack complex. J Immunol 1995;155:4135-8.
125. Quigg RJ, He C, Hack BK, Alexander JJ, Morgan BP. Production and functional analysis of rat CD59 and chimeric CD59-Crry as active soluble proteins in Pichia pastoris. Immunology 2000;99:46-53.
126. Jha P, Kotwal GJ. Vaccinia complement control protein: Multi-functional protein and a potential wonder drug. J Biosci 2003;28:265-71.
127. Marzari R, Sblattero D, Macor P, Fischetti F, Gennaro R, Marks JD, Bradbury A, Tedesco F. The cleavage site of C5 from man and animals as a common target for neutralizing human monoclonal antibodies: in vitro and in vivo studies. Eur J Immunol 2002;32:2773-82.
128. Jordan JE, Montalto MC, Stahl GL. Inhibition of mannose-binding lectin reduces postischemic myocardial reperfusion injury. Circulation 2001;104:1413-8.
129. Fiane AE, Videm V, Lingaas PS, Heggelungd L, Nielsen EW, Geiran OR, Fung M, Mollnes TE. Mechanism of complement activation and its role in the inflammatory response following thoraco-abdominal aortic aneurysm repair. Circulation 2003;108:849-56.
130. Takahashi K, Gordon J, Liu H, Sastry KN, Epstein JE, Motwani M, Laursen I, Thiel S, Jensenius JC, Carroll M, Ezekowitz RA. Lack of mannose-binding lectin-A enhances survival in a mouse model of acute septic peritonitis. Microbes Infect 2002;4:773-84.
131. Zhao H, Wakamiya N, Suzuki Y, Hamonko MT, Stahl GL. Identification of human mannose binding lectin (MBL) recognition sites for novel inhibitory antibodies. Hybrid Hybridomics 2002;21:25-36.
132. Collard CD, Vakeva A, Morrissey MA, Agah A, Rollins SA, Reenstra WR, Buras JA, Meri S, Stahl GL. Complement activation after oxidative stress - Role of the lectin complement pathway. Am J Pathol 2000;156:1549-56.
133. Lekowski R, Collard CD, Reenstra WR, Stahl GL. Ulex europaeus agglutinin II (UEA-II) is a novel, potent inhibitor of complement activation. Protein Sci 2001;10:277-84.
134. Stahl GL, Xu YY, Hao LM, Miller M, Buras JA, Fung M, Zhao H. Role for the alternative complement pathway in ischemia/reperfusion injury. Amer J Pathol 2003;162:449-55.
135. Tanhehco EJ, Kilgore KS, Liff DA, Murphy KL, Fung MS, Sun WN, Sun C, Lucchesi BR. The anti-factor D antibody, MAb 166-32, inhibits the alternative pathway of the human complement system. Transplant Proc 1999;31:2168-71.
136. Fung M, Loubser PG, Undar A, Mueller M, Sun C, Sun WN, Vaughn WK, Fraser CD, Jr. Inhibition of complement, neutrophil, and platelet activation by an anti-factor D monoclonal antibody in simulated cardiopulmonary bypass circuits. J Thorac Cardiovasc Surg 2001;122:113-22.

137. Undar A, Eichstaedt HC, Clubb FJ, Fung M, Lu MS, Bigley JE, Vaughn WK, Fraser CD. Novel anti-factor D monoclonal antibody inhibits complement and leukocyte activation in a baboon model of cardiopulmonary bypass. Ann Thorac Surg 2002;74:355-62.

138. Gupta-Bansal R, Parent JB, Brunden KR. Inhibition of complement alternative pathway function with antiproperdin monoclonal antibodies. Mol Immunol 2000;37:191-201.

139. HuberLang M, Younkin EM, Sarma JV, Riedemann N, McGuire SR, Lu KT, Kunkel R, Younger JG, Zetoune FS, Ward PA. Generation of C5a by phagocytic cells. Amer J Pathol 2002;161:1849-59.

140. Frei Y, Lambris JD, Stockinger B. Generation of a monoclonal antibody to mouse C5 application in an ELISA assay for detection of anti-C5 antibodies. Mol Cell Probes 1987;1:141-9.

141. Wang Y, Hu QL, Madri JA, Rollins SA, Chodera A, Matis LA. Amelioration of lupus-like autoimmune disease in NZB/WF1 mice after treatment with a blocking monoclonal antibody specific for complement component C5. Proc Natl Acad Sci USA 1996;93:8563-8.

142. Vakeva AP, Agah A, Rollins SA, Matis LA, Li L, Stahl GL. Myocardial infarction and apoptosis after myocardial ischemia and reperfusion: Role of the terminal complement components and inhibition by anti-C5 therapy. Circulation 1998;97:2259-67.

143. Wurzner R, Schulze M, Happe L, Franzke A, Bieber FA, Oppermann M, Gotze O. Inhibition of terminal complement complex formation and cell lysis by monoclonal antibodies. Complement Inflamm 1991;8:328-40.

144. Rinder CS, Rinder HM, Smith BR, Fitch JCK, Smith MJ, Tracey JB, Matis LA, Squinto SP, Rollins SA. Blockade of C5a and C5b-9 generation inhibits leukocyte and platelet activation during extracorporeal circulation. J Clin Invest 1995;96:1564-72.

145. Kroshus TJ, Rollins SA, Dalmasso AP, Elliott EA, Matis LA, Squinto SP, Bolman RM. Complement inhibition with an anti-C5 monoclonal antibody prevents acute cardiac tissue injury in an ex vivo model of pig- to-human xenotransplantation. Transplantation 1995;60:1194-202.

146. Thomas TC, Rollins SA, Rother RP, Giannoni MA, Hartman SL, Elliott EA, Nye SH, Matis LA, Squinto SP, Evans MJ. Inhibition of complement activity by humanized anti-C5 antibody and single-chain Fv. Mol Immunol 1996;33:1389-401.

147. Fitch JCK, Rollins S, Matis L, Alford B, Aranki S, Collard CD, Dewar M, Elefteriades J, Hines R, Kopf G, Kraker P, Li L, OHara R, Rinder C, Rinder H, Shaw R, Smith B, Stahl G, Shernan SK. Pharmacology and biological efficacy of a recombinant, humanized, single-chain antibody C5 complement inhibitor in patients undergoing coronary artery bypass graft surgery with cardiopulmonary bypass. Circulation 1999;100:2499-506.

148. Ames RS, Tornetta MA, Jones CS, Tsui P. Isolation of Neutralizing Anti-C5a monoclonal antibodies from a filamentous phage monovalent Fab display library. J Immunol 1994;152:4572-81.

149. Kola A, Baensch M, Bautsch W, Hennecke M, Klos A, Casaretto M, Kohl J. Epitope mapping of a C5a neutralizing mAb using a combined approach of phage display, synthetic peptides and site-directed mutagenesis. Immunotechnology 1996;2:115-26.

150. Amsterdam EA, Stahl GL, Pan HL, Rendig SV, Fletcher MP, Longhurst JC. Limitation of reperfusion injury by a monoclonal antibody to C5a during myocardial infarction in pigs. Amer J Physiol-Heart Circ Phy 1995;37:H448-H457

151. Tofukuji M, Stahl GL, Agah A, Metais C, Simons M, Sellke FW. Anti-C5a monoclonal antibody reduces cardiopulmonary bypass and cardioplegia-induced coronary endothelial dysfunction. J Thorac Cardiovasc Surg 1998;116:1060-8.

152. Wada K, Montalto MC, Stahl GL. Inhibition of complement C5 reduces local and remote organ injury after intestinal ischemia/reperfusion in the rat. Gastroenterology 2001;120:126-33.
153. Czermak BJ, Sarma V, Pierson CL, Warner RL, HuberLang M, Bless NM, Schmal H, Friedl HP, Ward PA. Protective effects of C5a blockade in sepsis. Nature Med 1999;5:788-92.
154. Huber-Lang MS, Sarma JV, McGuire SR, Lu KT, Guo RF, Padgaonkar VA, Younkin EM, Laudes IJ, Riedemann NC, Younger JG, Ward PA. Protective effects of anti-C5a peptide antibodies in experimental sepsis. FASEB J 2001;15:568-70.
155. Hopken U, Mohr M, Struber A, Montz H, Burchardi H, Gotze O, Oppermann M. Inhibition of interleukin-6 synthesis in an animal model of septic shock by anti-C5a monoclonal antibodies. Eur J Immunol 1996;26:1103-9.
156. Mohr M, Hopken U, Oppermann M, Mathes C, Goldmann K, Siever S, Gotze O, Burchardi H. Effects of anti-C5a monoclonal antibodies on oxygen use in a porcine model of severe sepsis. Eur J Clin Invest 1998;28:227-34.
157. Guo RF, HuberLang M, Wang X, Sarma V, Padgaonkar VA, Craig RA, Riedemann NC, McClintock SD, Hlaing T, Shi MM, Ward PA. Protective effects of anti-C5a in sepsis-induced thymocyte apoptosis. J Clin Invest 2000;106:1271-80.
158. Riedemann NC, Guo RF, Laudes IJ, Keller K, Sarma VJ, Padgaonkar V, Zetoune FS, Ward PA. C5a receptor and thymocyte apoptosis in sepsis. FASEB J 2002;16:U378-U392
159. Stevens JH, O Hanley P, Shapiro JM, Mihm FG, Satoh PS, Collins JA, Raffin TA. Effects of anti-C5a antibodies on the adult respiratory distress syndrome in septic primates. J Clin Invest 1986;77:1812-6.
160. Schmid E, Piccolo MTS, Friedl HP, Warner RL, Mulligan MS, Hugli TE, Till GO, Ward PA. Requirement for C5a in lung vascular injury following thermal trauma to rat skin. Shock 1997;8:119-24.
161. Laudes IJ, Chu JC, Sikranth S, HuberLang M, Guo RF, Riedemann N, Sarma JV, Schmaier AH, Ward PA. Anti-C5a ameliorates coagulation/fibrinolytic protein changes in a rat model of sepsis. Amer J Pathol 2002;160:1867-75.
162. Link C, Hawlisch H, Vilsendorf AMZ, Gyleruz S, Nagel E, Kohl J. Selection of phage-displayed anti-guinea pig C5 or C5a antibodies and their application in xenotransplantation. Mol Immunol 1999;36:1235-47.
163. Fung M, Lu M, Fure H, Sun W, Sun C, Shi NY, Du Y, Su J, Swanson X, Mollnes TE. Pre-neutralization of C5a-mediated effects by the monoclonal antibody 137-26 reacting with the C5a moiety of native C5 without preventing C5 cleavage. Clin Exp Immunol 2003;133:160-9.
164. Sprong T, Brandtzaeg P, Fung M, Paro A, Høyby EA, Michaelsen T, Aase A, van der Meer JW, van Deuren M, Mollnes TE. Inhibition of C5a-induced inflammation with preserved C5b-9-mediated bactericidal activity in a human whole blood model of meningococcal sepsis. Blood 2003; (in press; epublished July 24).
165. Rollins SA, Matis LA, Springhorn JP, Setter E, Wolff DW. Monoclonal antibodies directed against human C5 and C8 block complement-mediated damage of xenogeneic cells and organs. Transplantation 1995;60:1284-92.
166. Rinder CS, Rinder HM, Smith MJ, Tracey JB, Fitch J, Li L, Rollins SA, Smith BR. Selective blockade of membrane attack complex formation during simulated extracorporeal circulation inhibits platelet but not leukocyte activation. J Thorac Cardiovasc Surg 1999;118:460-6.
167. Lauvrak V, Brekke OH, Ihle O, Lindqvist BH. Identification and characterisation of C1q-binding phage displayed peptides. Biol Chem 1997;378:1509-19.

168. Roos A, Nauta AJ, Broers D, FaberKrol MC, Trouw LA, Drijfhout JW, Daha MR. Specific inhibition of the classical complement pathway by C1q-binding peptides. J Immunol 2001;167:7052-9.

169. Fryer JP, Leventhal JR, Pao W, Stadler C, Jones M, Walsh T, Zhong R, Zhang Z, Wang H, Goodman DJ, Kurek M, Dapice AJF, Blondin B, Ivancic D, Buckingham F, Kaufman D, Abecassis M, Stuart F, Anderson BE. Synthetic peptides which inhibit the interaction between C1q and immunoglobulin and prolong xenograft survival. Transplantation 2000;70:828-36.

170. Buerke M, Schwertz H, Seitz W, Meyer J, Darius H. Novel small molecule inhibitor of C1s exerts cardioprotective effects in ischemia-reperfusion injury in rabbits. J Immunol 2001;167:5375-80.

171. Szalai AJ, Digerness SB, Agrawal A, Kearney JF, Bucy RP, Niwas S, Kilpatrick JM, Babu YS, Volanakis JE. The Arthus reaction in rodents: Species-specific requirement of complement. J Immunol 2000;164:463-8.

172. Sahu A, Kay BK, Lambris JD. Inhibition of human complement by a C3-binding peptide isolated from a phage-displayed random peptide library. J Immunol 1996;157:884-91.

173. Morikis D, AssaMunt N, Sahu A, Lambris JD. Solution structure of Compstatin, a potent complement inhibitor. Protein Sci 1998;7:619-27.

174. Nilsson B, Larsson R, Hong J, Elgue G, Ekdahl KN, Sahu A, Lambris JD. Compstatin inhibits complement and cellular activation in whole blood in two models of extracorporeal circulation. Blood 1998;92:1661-7.

175. Fiane AE, Mollnes TE, Videm V, Hovig T, Hogasen K, Mellbye OJ, Spruce L, Moore WT, Sahu A, Lambris JD. Compstatin, a peptide inhibitor of C3, prolongs survival of ex vivo perfused pig xenografts. Xenotransplantation 1999;6:52-65.

176. Soulika AM, Khan MM, Hattori T, Bowen FW, Richardson BA, Hack CE, Sahu A, Edmunds LH, Jr., Lambris JD. Inhibition of heparin/protamine complex-induced complement activation by Compstatin in baboons. Clin Immunol 2000;96:212-21.

177. Ames RS, Lee D, Foley JJ, Jurewicz AJ, Tornetta MA, Bautsch W, Settmacher B, Klos A, Erhard KF, Cousins RD, Sulpizio AC, Hieble JP, McCafferty G, Ward KW, Adams JL, Bondinell WE, Underwood DC, Osborn RR, Badger AM, Sarau HM. Identification of a selective nonpeptide antagonist of the anaphylatoxin C3a receptor that demonstrates antiinflammatory activity in animal models. J Immunol 2001;166:6341-8.

178. Bautsch W, Hoymann HG, Zhang QW, MeierWiedenbach I, Raschke U, Ames RS, Sohns B, Flemme N, zuVilsendorf AM, Grove M, Klos A, Kohl J. Cutting edge: Guinea pigs with a natural C3a-receptor defect exhibit decreased bronchoconstriction in allergic airway disease: Evidence for an involvement of the C3a anaphylatoxin in the pathogenesis of asthma. J Immunol 2000;165:5401-5.

179. Drouin SM, Corry DB, Hollman TJ, Kildsgaard J, Wetsel RA. Absence of the complement anaphylatoxin C3a receptor suppresses Th2 effector functions in a murine model of pulmonary allergy. J Immunol 2002;169:5926-33.

180. Elsner J, Oppermann M, Czech W, Kapp A. C3a activates the respiratory burst in human polymorphonuclear neutrophilic leukocytes via pertussis toxin-sensitive G-proteins. Blood 1994;83:3324-31.

181. Kildsgaard J, Hollmann TJ, Matthews KW, Bian K, Murad F, Wetsel RA. Cutting edge: Targeted disruption of the C3a receptor gene demonstrates a novel protective anti-inflammatory role for C3a in endotoxin-shock. J Immunol 2000;165:5406-9.

182. Konteatis ZD, Siciliano SJ, Vanriper G, Molineaux CJ, Pandya S, Fischer P, Rosen H, Mumford RA, Springer MS. Development of C5a receptor antagonists - Differential loss of functional responses. J Immunol 1994;153:4200-5.

183. Finch AM, Wong AK, Paczkowski NJ, Wadi SK, Craik DJ, Fairlie DP, Taylor SM. Low-molecular-weight peptidic and cyclic antagonists of the receptor for the complement factor C5a. J Med Chem 1999;42:1965-74.

184. Arumugam TV, Shiels IA, Woodruff TM, Reid RC, Fairlie DP, Taylor SM. Protective effect of a new C5a receptor antagonist against ischemia-reperfusion injury in the rat small intestine. J Surg Res 2002;103:260-7.

185. Arumugam TV, Shiels IA, Strachan AJ, Abbenante G, Fairlie DP, Taylor SM. A small molecule C5a receptor antagonist protects kidneys from ischemia/reperfusion injury in rats. Kidney Int 2003;63:134-42.

186. Haynes DR, Harkin DG, Bignold LP, Hutchens MJ, Taylor SM, Fairlie DP. Inhibition of C5a-induced neutrophil chemotaxis and macrophage cytokine production in vitro by a new C5a receptor antagonist. Biochem Pharmacol 2000;60:729-33.

187. Short A, Wong AK, Finch AM, Haaima G, Shiels IA, Fairlie DP, Taylor SM. Effects of a new C5a receptor antagonist on C5a- and endotoxin-induced neutropenia in the rat. Brit J Pharmacol 1999;126:551-4.

188. Strachan AJ, Woodruff TM, Haaima G, Fairlie DP, Taylor SM. A new small molecule C5a receptor antagonist inhibits the reverse-passive arthus reaction and endotoxic shock in rats. J Immunol 2000;164:6560-5.

189. Strachan AJ, Shiels IA, Reid RC, Fairlie DP, Taylor SM. Inhibition of immune-complex mediated dermal inflammation in rats following either oral or topical administration of a small molecule C5a receptor antagonist. Brit J Pharmacol 2001;134:1778-86.

190. Woodruff TM, Strachan AJ, Dryburgh N, Shiels IA, Reid RC, Fairlie DP, Taylor SM. Antiarthritic activity of an orally active C5a receptor antagonist against antigen-induced monarticular arthritis in the rat. Arthritis Rheum 2002;46:2476-85.

191. Pellas TC, Boyar W, van Oostrum J, Wasvary J, Fryer LR, Pastor G, Sills M, Braunwalder A, Yarwood DR, Kramer R, Kimble E, Hadala J, Haston W, Moreira-Ludewig R, Uziel-Fusi S, Peters P, Bill K, Wennogle LP. Novel C5a receptor antagonists regulate neutrophil functions in vitro and in vivo. J Immunol 1998;160:5616-21.

192. Heller T, Hennecke M, Baumann U, Gessner JE, Vilsendorf AMZ, Baensch M, Boulay F, Kola A, Klos A, Bautsch W, Kohl J. Selection of a C5a receptor antagonist from phage libraries attenuating the inflammatory response in immune complex disease and ischemia reperfusion injury. J Immunol 1999;163:985-94.

193. Riley RD, Sato H, Zhao ZQ, Thourani VH, Jordan JE, Fernandez AX, Ma XL, Hite DR, Rigel DE, Pellas TC, Peppard J, Bill KA, Lappe RW, VintenJohansen J. Recombinant human complement C5A receptor antagonist reduces infarct size after surgical revascularization. J Thorac Cardiovasc Surg 2000;120:350-8.

194. deVries B, Kohl J, Leclercq WKG, Wolfs TGAM, VanBijnen AAJH, Heeringa P, Buurman WA. Complement factor C5a mediates renal ischemia-reperfusion injury independent from neutrophils. J Immunol 2003;170:3883-9.

195. Zhang X, Boyar W, Galakatos N, Gonnella NC. Solution structure of a unique C5a semi-synthetic antagonist: implications in receptor binding. Protein Sci 1997;6:65-72.

196. Baranyi L, Campbell W, Okada H. Antisense homology boxes in C5a receptor and C5a anaphylatoxin: a new method for identification of potentially active peptides. J Immunol 1996;157:4591-601.

197. Sumichika H, Sakata K, Sato N, Takeshita S, Ishibuchi S, Nakamura M, Kamahori T, Ehara S, Itoh K, Ohtsuka T, Ohbora T, Mishina T, Komatsu H, Naka Y. Identification of a potent and orally active non-peptide C5a receptor antagonist. J Biol Chem 2002;277:49403-7.

198. Biesecker G, Dihel L, Enney K, Bendele RA. Derivation of RNA aptamer inhibitors of human complement C5. Immunopharmacology 1999;42:219-30.
199. Hong K, Kinoshita T, Miyazaki W, Izawa T, Inoue K. An anticomplementary agent, K-76 monocarboxylic acid: its site and mechanism of inhibition of the complement activation cascade. J Immunol 1979;122:2418-23.
200. Miyagawa S, Shirakura R, Matsumiya G, Fukushima N, Nakata S, Matsuda H, Matsumoto M, Kitamura H, Seya T. Prolonging discordant xenograft survival with anticomplement reagents K76COOH and FUT175. Transplantation 1993;55:709-13.
201. Miyazawa H, Murase N, Demetris AJ, Matsumoto K, Nakamura K, Ye Q, Manez R, Todo S, Starzl TE. Hamster to rat kidney xenotransplantation - Effects of FK 506, cyclophosphamide, organ perfusion, and complement inhibition. Transplantation 1995;59:1183-8.
202. Kimura T, Andoh A, Fujiyama Y, Saotome T, Bamba T. A blockade of complement activation prevents rapid intestinal ischaemia-reperfusion injury by modulating mucosal mast cell degranulation in rats. Clin Exp Immunol 1998;111:484-90.
203. Kobayashi T, Neethling FA, Taniguchi S, Ye Y, Niekrasz M, Koren E, Hancock WW, Takagi H, Cooper DKC. Investigation of the anti-complement agents, FUT-175 and K76COOH, in discordant xenotransplantation. Xenotransplantation 1996;3:237-45.
204. Blum MG, Collins BJ, Chang AC, Zhang JP, Knaus SA, Pierson RN. Complement inhibition by FUT-175 and K76-COOH in a pig-to- human lung xenotransplant model. Xenotransplantation 1998;5:35-43.
205. Weiler JM, Edens RE, Linhardt RJ, Kapelanski DP. Heparin and modified heparin inhibit complement activation in vivo. J Immunol 1992;148:3210-5.
206. Fiorante P, Banz Y, Mohacsi PJ, Kappeler A, Wuillemin WA, Macchiarini P, Roos A, Daha MR, Schaffner T, Haeberli A, Mazmanian GM, Rieben R. Low molecular weight dextran sulfate prevents complement activation and delays hyperacute rejection in pig-to-human xenotransplantation models. Xenotransplantation 2001;8:24-35.
207. Olsson P, Sanchez J, Mollnes TE, Riesenfeld J. On the blood compatibility of end-point immobilized heparin. J Biomater Sci Polym Ed 2000;11:1261-73.

24

Activation and Inhibition of Complement by Immunoglobulins

Milan Basta
Neuronal Excitability Section, National Institute for Neurological Disorders and Stroke; National Institutes of Health, Bethesda, Maryland, U.S.A.

Abstract: Activation and augmentation of complement cascades are well-known functions of certain classes of immunoglobulins. On the other hand, pooled immunoglobulins in supraphysiologic concentrations have the ability to inhibit harmful biological effects of activated complement fragments by diverting them away from their targets to the fluid phase, where they may be subject to further inactivation. Scavenging appears to be mediated by immunoglobulin fragment-specific acceptor sites. Domains within constant region of F(ab)'2 seem responsible for anaphylatoxin binding and neutralization, while Fc fragments interact with C3b and C4b. The ability to attenuate complement fragment- induced immune damage cannot be correlated with any known phenotypic marker used today to categorize immunoglobulins and could serve as a basis for a new classification of immunoglobulins-strong versus weak inhibitors of complement fragment effects. The concept of dual effect of immunoglobulins on the complement system has implications for both novel physiologic functions of normal circulating immunoglobulins as well as clinical applications of high-dose intravenous immunoglobulin (IVIG).

Key words: immunoglobulins, complement cascades, anaphylatoxins, C3b/C4b, activation, scavenging, IVIG

1. INTRODUCTION

It has been a classic immunologic paradigm that specific immunoglobulins, following their binding to target antigens, trigger complement activation with subsequent cellular damage and initiation of the inflammatory reaction. In case of invasion by foreign microorganisms, such series of events is beneficial to the host, since it leads to the elimination of pathogens. However, the same sequence of events can be self-damaging if it is triggered under inappropriate circumstances, such as autoimmune reaction and/or over stimulation of the innate immunity by a pathogen. As it will be discussed in this chapter, immunoglobulins derived from the normal serum and modified for intravenous use in high doses (IVIG), have the ability to suppress and attenuate effects of activated complement fragments, including their pro-inflammatory capacity. Therefore, it appears that immunoglobulin molecules have ambivalent functions when it comes to their effects on the complement system and that the outcome (activation vs. inhibition) is determined by the immunoglobulin specificity.

2.   COMPLEMENT ACTIVATION BY IMMUNOGLOBULINS

Complement system can be activated through three distinct pathways and immunoglobulins have a role in initiation and or augmentation of each of these activation cascades.

Classical complement pathway is initiated when a conformational change in IgG and IgM molecules bound to their antigen activates the first complement component complex -C1q,r,s. This triggers a domino-like effect in which classical pathway complement components (present in serum as inactive pro-enzymes) get activated by the previous component in the system (1). Immunoglobulins of IgD, IgE and IgA isotypes do not have the capacity to activate complement through the classical pathway (2).

Among IgG subtypes, IgG1 and IgG3 are strong, IgG2 moderate activator of complement and IgG4 has no complement-activating properties at all (2). In general, IgG is not an efficient complement activator since C1 fixation requires two IgG molecules lying side-by-side in close proximity (so called "doublet"). The formation of a doublet occurs by chance; therefore, hundreds and thousands of IgG molecules have to be available in the process. On the other hand, a single IgM molecule, complexed with antigen on the cell surface, is sufficient to bind and activate C1; it was shown that as few as two IgM antibodies were sufficient to sensitize an erythrocyte (3).

Lectin pathway of complement activation is triggered when mannose–binding lectin (MBL) recognizes high-density arrays of terminal mannose residues on invading pathogens. Subsequent to MBL binding, MBL-associated serine proteases (MASP-1 and MASP-2) activate the classical pathway components 4 and 2 (4). MBL is structurally and functionally similar to C1q molecule of the classical pathway (1). Lectin pathway hemolysis was shown to be enhanced in-vitro by IgG, IgM and IgA molecules. Indicator sheep erythrocytes (E) coated with mannan (M) and sensitized with mannan-binding lectin (MBL), were exposed to anti-E hemolysin antibodies. This led to twofold enhancement of lectin pathway hemolysis when E-M-MBL was coated with IgM or IgA and fourfold when coated with IgG (5). In-vitro studies have demonstrated the ability of MBL to bind to polymeric IgA in a dose-dependent manner; this binding induced C4 and C3 cleavage upon addition of complement source (6). Certain patterns of IgG glycosilation (glycoforms) are associated with the lectin pathway of complement activation. There are two oligosaccharide chains in the Fc region of IgG molecules that have either 2 terminal galactose residues (G2 glycoform) one galactose and one N-acetylglucosamine (G1 glycoform) or 2 terminal N-acetylglucosamines (G0 glycoform). It is the last glycoform of IgG (G0), in which Fc carbohydrates terminate in N-acetylglucoasmine, that can activate complement via MBL (7). In rheumatoid arthritis, there is an increase of G0 glycoforms, thus enabling terminal N-acetylglucosamines to become exposed and accessible to MBL (7). Similarly, deglacosylated IgA1 ineracts with MBL and plays a pathogenic role in IgA nephropathy (8).

Alternative complement activation, unlike classical and lectin pathways, does not require specific recognition of foreign proteins. The alternative pathway bypasses early complement components of the classical cascade (C1, C4, and C2) in the process of C3 activation (1). Past that activation sequence, the activation follows the same chain of events as in the classical pathway (C5b-C9 and formation of the MAC complex). Immunoglobulins are not required for alternative complement activation, but are known to augment this cascade in different manners. Aggregated human monoclonal immunoglobulins of IgG, IgM, IgA and IgE classes are known to activate complement through the alternative pathway (2). IgG immunoglobulins in soluble immune complexes are good acceptors of C3b and form covalent complexes with these molecules (9). Such complexes are more efficient than C3b alone as precursors of the alternative pathway C3 convertase, causing prolonged amplification of the alternative pathway loop (10). Partial stability of these complexes is achieved by properdin that binds with increased avidity to such complexes (11). The C3 nephritic factor (C3NeF) is an autoantibody found in sera of patients with membranoproliferative hypocomplementemic glomerulonephritis and partial lipodystrophy. This is an antibody against the C3 convertase that forms a stable complex (C3bBbNeF) and leads into continuous activation and C3 consumption by the alternative pathway (2).

3.   INHIBITION OF COMPLEMENT BY IMMUNOGLOBULINS

Immunoglobulin molecules have no proven ability to inhibit complement activation; however, by scavenging activated and potentially harmful fragments of different complement components, exogenous immunolgobulins in high doses can exert attenuating effect in diseases and states in which these fragments play an important role in pathogenesis.

3.1   Scavenging of C3b/C4b

The theory of scavenging was first introduced by a series of experiments that showed that high doses of intravenous immunoglobulins can divert C3b and C4b away from target cells, thus preventing cell-surface assembly of the membrane attack complex and subsequent destruction (12). An in-vitro system was created in which corpusculate immune complexes (red cells sensitized with specific anti-erythrocyte antibodies) were used to both trigger complement activation and serve as targets for the uptake of C3b/C4b in whole serum. This uptake was effectively and in a dose-responsive manner inhibited by IVIG (13). Uptake inhibition was mediated by Fc fragments as shown in Table 1 and later mapped to a sequence within the CH3 domain of the IgG molecule (14).

Table *1*. Inhibition of C3/C4 uptake by IgG fragments and IgG purified from normal human sera.

Reagent	% Inhibition	
	C3b	C4b
F(ab)'$_2$	0	0
Fc	100	100
IVIG	25	20
IgG (1)*	97	93
IgG (2)	100	100
IgG (3)	95	95
IgG (4)	95	92
IgG (5)	91	88
IgG (6)	99	95
IgG (7)	88	87
IgG (8)	100	100

*The numbers in parenthesis indicate individual
healthy serum donors

C3b/C4b uptake inhibition was found to be an inherent ability of certain

IgG subsets unrelated to any known phenotypic categorization (Basta et al, unpublished data). Using monoclonal myeloma IgGs from all four subtypes with roughly equal distribution of kappa and lambda light chains, it was shown that the complement fragment uptake was inhibited by all subtypes within the same, 0%-100%, range of inhibition (Table 2).

Table 2. Inhibition of C3b/C4b uptake onto sensitized erythrocytes by individual myeloma proteins

Patient	Subclass	Light chain	% Inhibition C3b	C4b
1		λ	33	19
2		λ	50	35
3		κ	0	0
4		λ	50	10
5		κ	85	100
6	IgG1	κ	52	39
7		λ	90	78
8		κ	98	79
9		κ	35	30
10		κ	94	83
11		λ	30	0
12		κ	75	71
13		κ	5	0
14		κ	59	39
15	IgG2	λ	28	17
16		λ	0	0
17		κ	100	100
18		λ	100	100
19		κ	75	61
20		κ	73	39
21		κ	65	25
22	IgG3	κ	73	39
23		λ	70	23
24		λ	32	34
25		κ	0	0
26		λ	0	0
27		λ	47	19
28	IgG4	κ	0	0
29		κ	73	44
30		κ	67	36
31		κ	29	6

The magnitude of inhibition could not be correlated with IgG allotypes either, since monoclonal antibodies with the same allotypic marker exhibited both strong and weak inhibition of C3b/C4b deposition on target immune complexes (Table 3).

Interestingly, IgGs purified from healthy individuals showed high inhibition within a narrow range (87% to 100%) suggesting that efficient scavenging and functional predominance of high complement uptake suppressors in the normal imunoglobulin pool is important for homeostasis (Table 1). IgM and IgA molecules were shown to be, both on molar and weigh basis, much more efficient suppressors of C4 uptake than IgG (15).

Table 3. Inhibition of C3/C4 uptake by IgG allotypes

Ig Subclass	marker	% Inhibition	
		C3b	C4b
IgG1	z	94	85
	f	5	0
	f	75	71
	f	98	79
	f	10	5
IgG2	n+	100	78
	n-	100	95
	n+	29	10
IgG3	b	67	36
	b	93	74
	b	25	4
	b	87	75
	g	100	98
	g	32	34

Complement uptake was next quantitated in pre and post IVIG serum samples of patients suffering from diseases with varying degree of complement involvement in pathogenesis. In acute dermatomyositis (DM), Kawasaki disease and autoimmune hemolytic anemia (AIHA), pre-IVIG or baseline levels of C3b/C4b uptake (number of C3b/C4b molecules on target cells) were much higher than in patients with chronic DM and inclusion body myositis (IBM) (Table 4). Similarly, baseline uptake was significantly increased relative to disease controls and healthy individuals in sera of patients with Guillain-Barre syndrome and Myasthenia Gravis, neurological disorders with favourable response to IVIG (16). This finding suggests a rapid turnover of complement fragments as a consequence of continuous complement activation. In case of active DM and AIHA, the role of complement in the pathogenesis of endomyseal capillary damage (17) and C3 fragments on the surface of red cells (18), respectively, is well established, while the evidence of complement-mediated damage in

Kawasaki is still indirect (18). Baseline uptake data lend further support to the role of complement in pathogenesis of these diseases, especially since the beneficial effect of IVIG correlated with the high baseline complement uptake. IVIG therapy significantly reduced the number of C3b and C4b molecules on corpusculate immune complexes in active DM, Kawasaki disease and AIHA, but had no effect in chronic DM and IBM, both with a normal pre-IVIG uptake (Table 4).

Table 4. Complement uptake in pre and post IVIG serum samples from patients and disease controls

Disease	Pre-IVIG uptake*		Post-IVIG uptake		Post-IVIG inhibition
	Range	Mean	Range	Mean	%
Active DM (n=9)	2,032-61,646	12,190	1,646-9,707	2,350	70.6-93.4
Kawasaki (n=6)	13,919-21,358	19,120	9,053-18,242	12,120	13.4-57.6
AIHA (n=3)	25,071-69,812	54,123	18,196-53,860	32,263	21.7-51.5
Chronic DM (n=3)	1,418-2,220	1,986	1,466-2,223	1,896	0-2.3
IBM (n=5)	2,124-4,561	3,491	1,987-3,597	3,120	0-1.9

*Expressed as counts per minute, specific incorporation of radiolabeled anti-C3 antibodies into corpusculate immune complexes quantitated by gamma counter.

The above data suggest potential use of complement uptake assays in clinical practice to:
a) Detect complement activation and generation of fragments as a proof of the role of complement in pathogenesis, which in turn could influence the use of IVIG as the therapy of choice;
b) Monitor disease activity (high complement uptake in active DM, diminished or normal in chronic DM);
c) Determine response to IVIG therapy by demonstrating reduction of high baseline complement uptake and correlation between the half-life of IVIG, signs and symptoms of the disease and C3b/C4b uptake. In active DM, the initial post-IVIG decrease of C3 uptake (peaking at Day 2) is followed by a rebound towards pre-IVIG values three to four weeks later, correlating with the half-life of the infused immunoglobulins and gradual disappearance of the beneficial clinical effects of IVIG (19).

3.2 Accelerated Decay of C3b by IVIG

It was proposed that IVIG suppresses inflammation by inactivating C3b-containing complexes that cause further C3 activation via alternative pathway amplification loop (20). It is believed that C3b displaced away from immune targets by scavenging generates C3b-C3b-IgG (C3b2-IgG) complexes with fluid phase IgG (10). C3b has a variable affinity for native, non-aggregated IgG (21), a property that was confirmed by the results of the above complement uptake studies using myeloma immunoglobulins as C3b/C4b acceptors. Under those circumstances, some covalent C3b-IgG complex formation might occur and potentially lead to more complement activation via alternative C3 convertase. A proportion of exogenous immunoglobulins could then act by increasing the rate of C3b degradation by factors H and I to prevent more complement activation. The mechanism of such C3b decay acceleration remains yet to be elucidated.

3.3   F(ab)'₂-Mediated Neutralization of Anaphylatoxins

Biological activities of C3a and C5a anaphylatoxins, potent inducers and amplifiers of the inflammatory response, can be neutralized in the presence of F(ab)'₂ fragments (22). Anaphylatoxin acceptor sites reside within constant, non-antigen binding domains of these fragments (Figure 1).

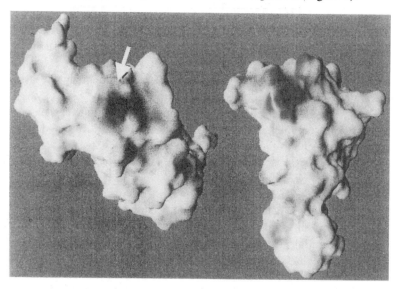

Figure 1. Molecular modeling of C3a/Fab binding sites. Tentative acceptor site within the constant region of Fab fragment (arrow) for an N-terminal domain of C3a (molecule to the right), based on the protonation state of both molecules and low-energy grid search as implemented in respective molecular modeling software programs.

Multiple in-vitro binding studies, animal models and molecular modeling have been employed to establish this hypothesis. Surface plasmon resonance (SPR) experiments have excluded contribution of specific anti C3a/C5a antibodies that might be present in commercial pools of intravenous immunoglobulins. SPR also determined that binding of C3a and C5a to immunoglobulin molecules was not affected by previous saturation of the binding sites with the specific antigen, implying the role of constant domains within Fab in mediating this binding. Physical association of C3a/C5a and F(ab)'$_2$ was documented by Western blotting as a shift in molecular weight of the complex. Immunoglobulin-anaphylatoxin interaction interfered with the ability of anaphylatoxins to engage their specific receptors, since C3a/C5a – induced calcium flux in human mast cells from the cell line HMC-1 and subsequent release of inflammatory mediators histamine and thromboxane were abrogated.

In-vivo evidence of anaphylatoxin neutralization by F(ab)'$_2$-containing immunoglobulin preparations was provided by showing decreased influx of inflammatory cells into bronchoalveolar compartments and lung tissue of mice subjected to asthma-like condition by ovalbumin (OVA) sensitization and OVA aerosol challenge. In a porcine model, injection of C5a induces severe cardiorespiratory distress that is lethal within minutes. Pre-treatment with F(ab)'$_2$-containing IVIG preparation prevents this reaction to occur even after administration of multiple lethal doses of C5a (Figure 2).

Addressing the issue of specificity of this anaphylatoxin-neutralizing effect by using appropriate control reagents in in-vitro and in-vivo experiments was of critical importance. It was shown that another abundant serum protein, albumin when used in equal amounts as IVIG, has no effect on biological activities of C3a and C5a, nor does the IVIG stabilizer or vehicle –glycine. Furthermore, IVIG preparations were assayed for specific anaphylatoxin inhibitors-carboxypeptidases N and R, that inactivate C3a and C5a by cleaving the penultimate arginine at the carboxyterminal part of these anaphyaltoxins. A sensitive colorimetric assay showed absence of these enzymes in IVIG preparations used, thus excluding the possibility that anaphylatoxin neutralization is due to simple inactivation (Table 5).

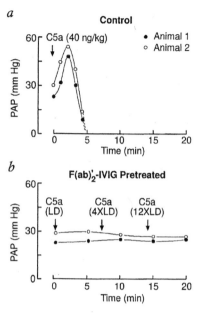

Figure 2. Inhibition of C5a-induced circulatory collapse in pigs Following the treatment of pigs (n=2) with 40 ng/kg of human recombinant C5a, pulmonary arterial pressure (PAP)was monitored (a). Pigs (n=2) were pretreated with 300mg/kg of F(ab)'2-containing IVIG prior to injection of the dose of C5a that was lethal for control animals and two additional adminsitrations of C5a given 7 minutes apart (b).

Table 5. Detection of carboxypeptidases in normal serum and immunoglobulin preparations

CP*	plasma	OD_{405}			
		$IVIG_{(1)**}$	$IVIG_{(2)}$	$F(ab)'_{2(1)}$	$F(ab)'_{2(2)}$
CPN	0.35±0.10	0	0	0	0
CPR	0.75±0.25	0	0	0	0

*carboxypeptidase;
** numbers in parenthesis indicate batches of IVIG and F(ab)'2 preparations;
F(ab)'2 stands for F(ab)'2 -containing preparation. Representative of three similar experiments

Therefore, neutralization of anaphylatoxins is an endogenous and specific effector function of immunoglobulin molecules not related to anti-anaphylatoxin antibodies or any other ingredient of IVIG preparations (contaminating molecules of IVIG preparations). Ig molecules seem to possess multiple binding sites for potentially harmful fragments of complement components. Acceptor sites for C3b/C4b (large fragments necessary for the completion of the classical complement cascade and cell lysis are situated within the Fc region of immunoglobulin molecule. On the other hand, constant region of F(ab)'$_2$ binds anaphylatoxins and renders them inactive.

4.   DISCUSSION

In summary, the concept that immunoglobulins may exert dual function when it comes to suppression or initiation of the inflammation via activated complement fragments is novel and fascinating. When a specific clone of plasma cells gets induced to secrete specific antibodies either against a pathogen or its own cells and tissues (under the circumstances of disturbed ability to differentiate between self and non-self), and leads to overstimulation of the innate immune system, the ensuing inflammatory reaction mediated by complement activation is suppressed by the remaining immunoglobulin clones that constitute the normal circulating immunoglobulin pool. The quenching of the self-destroying overstimulation of complement could be effected by this pool only up to the point of saturation. If the specific antibody continues to be secreted and create activated complement fragments, an infusion of exogenous Ig preparation in the form of IVIG then becomes necessary in clinical situations. This attenuation appears to be mediated by scavenging of activated complement fragments that can either directly damage host cells or initiate and augment the inflammatory reaction. In addition, covalent fluid phase complexes composed of diverted C3b and IgG molecule. that may lead to augmented C3 convertase assembly and alternative pathway activation, could be destabilized by the action of immunolgobulin molecules with high affinity for C3b. The ability to deviate complement fragments from their targets and receptors is not related to any known phenotypic categorization of immunoglobulin molecules (isotype, subclass, light chains or allotypes) and is clearly the unique property of a special subclass of immunoglobulins that crosses known immunoglobulin classification markers. The kinetics of complement fragment scavenging, as assayed by the in-vitro complement uptake system, may serve to determine complement involvement in pathogenesis, monitor the stage of the disease (active vs. chronic) and evaluate the effectiveness of the IVIG therapy. The importance of this concept reaches far beyond academic boundaries; it has immediate repercussions for novel clinical application of IVIG in numerous complement-mediated diseases and states with significant death and disability rate.

5. REFERENCES:

1. Volanakis, J.E.: Overview of the Complement System. In: The Human Complement System in Health and Disease 1st ed (Volanaksi, JE and Frank, M.M. editors) Marcel Dekker, Inc , New York-Basel-Hong Kong 1998, pp.9-32.
2. Frank, M.M., Fries, L.F.: Complement. In: Fundamental Immunology 2nd ed (Paul, WE, editor) Raven Press, New York 1989, pp. 686-687
3. Borsos, T., Rapp, HJ.: Complement fixation on cell surfaces by 19S and 7S antibodies. Science 1965; 150:505-507.
4. Wallis, R.: Structural and functional aspects of complement activation by mannose-binding protein. Immunobiology 2002; 205:433-445.
5. Suankratay, C., Zhang, Y., Jones, D., Lint, TF., Gewurtz, H.: Enhancement of lectin pathway haemolysis by immunoglobulins. Clin Exp Immunol 1999, 117:435-441.
6. Roos, A., Bouwman, L.H., van Gijlswijk-Janssen, D.J., Faber-Krol, M.C., Stahl, G.L., Daha, M.R.: Human IgA activates the complement system via the mannan-binding lectin pathway. J Immunol 2001; 167:2861-2868.
7. Malhotra, R., Wormald, M.R, Rudd, P.M., Fisher, P.B., Dwek, R.A, Sim, R.B.: Glycosylation changes of IgG associated with rheumatoid arthritis can activate complement via the mannose-binding protein. Nat Med 1995; 1:237-243.
8. Matei, L.: Plasma proteins glycosylation and its alteration in disease. Rom J Intern Med 1997; 35:3-11.
9. Gadd, K.J., Reid, K.B.M.: The binding of complement component C3 to antigen-antibody aggregates after activation of the alternative complement pathway in human serum. Biochem J 1981; 195:471-4...
10. Jelezarova, E., Lutz, HU.: Assembly and regulation of the complement amlification loop in blood: the role of C3b-C3b-IgG complexes. Mol Immunol 1999; 36:837-842.
11. Jelezarova E., Vogt, A., Lutz, HU.:Interaction of C3b(2)-IgG complexes with complement protein properdin, factor B and factor H: implications for amplification. Bichem J 2000; 349:217-223.
12. Basta, M. : Modulation of complement-mediated immune damage by intravenous immune globulin, Clin. Exp. Immunol 1996; 104:21-25.
13. Basta, M., Fries, L.F., Frank, M.M.: High doses of intravenous Ig inhibit in vitro uptake of C4 fragments onto sensitized erythrocytes. Blood 1989; 77:376-380.
14. Frank, M.M., Miletic, V.D, Jiang, H.: Immunoglobulin in the control of complement activation. Immunol Res 2000; 22:137-146.
15. Miletic, V.D, Hester, C.G, Frank, M.M.: Regulation of complement activity by immunoglobulin. I. Effect of immunoglobulin isotype on C4 uptake on antibody-sensitized sheep erythrocytes and solid phase immune complexes. J. Immunol 1996; 156:749-757.
16. Basta, M., Illa, I., Dalakas, M.C.: Increased in vitro uptake of the complement C3b in the serum of patients with Guillain-Barre syndrom, myasthenia gravis and dermatomyositis. J Neuroimmunol 1996; 71:227-229.
17. Kissel, J.T, Mendell, J.R., Rammohan, K.W.: Microvascular deposition of complement membrane attack complex in dermatomyositis. N Engl J Med 1986; 314:329-334.

18. Petz, L.D, Catlett, J.P., Lessin, L.S.: Hemolytic Anemias. In:Textbook of Internal Medicine 3rd ed (Kelley, W.N, editor) Lippincot-Raven, Philadelphia-New York 1997, pp. 1464-1467.
19. Basta, M., Dalakas, M.C.:High-dose intravenous immunoglobulin exerts its beneficial effect in patients with dermatomyosistis by blocking endomysial deposition of activated complement fragments. J Clin Invest 1994; 4:1729-1735.
20. Lutz, HU, Stammler, P., Jelezarova, E., Nater, M., Spath, P.J.: High doses of immunoglobulin G attenuate immune aggreagate-mediated complement activity by enhancing physiologic cleravage of C3b in C3bn-IgG complexes. Blood 1996; 88:184-193.
21. Lutz, H.U., Nater, M., Stammler, P.: Naturally occurring anti-band 3 antibodies have a unique affinity for C3. Immunology. 1993; 80:191-6.
22. Basta, M et al. F(ab)'2-mediated neutralization of C3a and C5a anaphylatoxins: a novel effector function of immunoglobulins. Nat Med 2003; 9:431-439

25

Engineering Control of Complement Inhibition at the Cell Surface

Richard A.G. Smith, Dirk Esser, Simon H. Ridley and Roberta Bradford
Adprotech Ltd., Chesterford Research Park, Saffron Walden, Essex, United Kingdom

Abstract: The role of complement regulation at the cell surface is reviewed and the desirability of being able to design exogenous therapeutic agents that function in this way is considered. An analysis of naturally occurring membrane proteins suggested that one particular type of membrane-localization mechanism (the myristoyl-electrostatic peptide switch) could be mimicked by minimization of the key molecular features involved and incorporation into relatively simple synthetic protein modification agents that could be attached to soluble proteins with retention of water solubility. This approach amounts to reconstruction of a membrane protein by substitution of the natural anchor by a more chemically tractable structure. It allows solution of a number of practical problems associated with production of recombinant membrane-interactive proteins and has permitted the development of one such protein (APT070, Mirococept) as a pharmaceutical agent. The membrane-binding properties of APT070 make it not only a potent regulator of complement activation but also permit it to be used in experimental and therapeutic situations where conventional soluble biopharmaceuticals are of limited use. Two such clinical applications of APT070 and the scope for application of other complement regulators such as CD59 in these reconstructed forms are also outlined.

Key Words: complement control, cell membrane, intrinsic action, therapy

1. INTRODUCTION: THE IMPORTANCE OF INTRINSIC ACTION

The complement system appears to have evolved primarily to provide protection for higher organisms against the acute threats posed by simpler organisms essentially all of which possess some form of cell membrane or genome-encapsulating structure. These threatening organisms include viruses, bacteria, fungi and yeasts and parasites both unicellular and more complex. In each case, the complement system provides one of the key components of "front-line" or innate immunity and permits immediate recognition of the potential invader as non-self without the requirement for a slow adaptive immune response. This is achieved by two main processes, the selective binding to arrayed non-mammalian carbohydrate structures that trigger the lectin pathway and the spontaneous unrestricted activation of the alternative pathway. In both cases, products are generated which label the invader as foreign (e.g. by attachment of C3b), achieve direct cytolysis (through formation of the membrane-attack or terminal complex [MAC]) or mediate indirect killing or removal of the labeled invader through recruitment and activation of macrophages, neutrophils and NK cells. This labeling and attack occurs at the outer membrane or capsule of the microorganism and the higher organism requires defenses to ensure that the highly amplifiable protease cascades of the complement pathways are not turned against itself. It is therefore not surprising that the restriction of complement activation to non-self surfaces is mediated by proteins which are intrinsic to the "self" cells of the higher organism. Intrinsically-acting complement regulators (IACRs) can be defined as negative regulators of complement activation which are either synthesised *in situ* or acquired externally so that they form a part of the cellular phenotype. It is also necessary to emphasis that IACRs must be localised on the outer membrane leaflet (or if located internally, be capable of rapid exteriorization upon perturbation of the self cell membrane). Furthermore, for maximum effectiveness IACRs need to be situated at locations on cell membranes or at cell-cell contact points which would be particularly vulnerable to unregulated attack by the complement system. The actual distribution of complement regulatory molecules such as CR1 on glomerular podocytes (1) and MCP on spermatozoa (2) suggests that such localization is of biological significance.

By being localized in the plane of the outer cell surface, IACRs acquire an advantage over fluid-phase extrinsically acting molecules which is highly relevant to therapeutic applications. The effective concentration of a membrane anchored protein within the space immediately above the membrane where convertases and MAC will form, is greatly increased and permits specific interactions of relatively low affinity in bulk solution to operate effectively at the membrane surface. There is a caveat which is that for such protein-protein interactions to be kinetically effective, the IACR must be mobile within the membrane bilayer phase (3) and/or must be capable of accessing the relevant binding site on (e.g.) C3b without having to detach from the membrane (which would have a serious thermodynamic cost). These considerations probably influence the choice of membrane anchoring mechanism (GPI versus transmembrane [TM] domains) and the size and structure of spacer regions between the membrane and the complement-regulatory domains in native IACRs (but see below). However, the limited published data on anchor-interchange in IACRs (4,5) suggests that as far as complement regulatory function is concerned, GPI and TM anchors are largely interchangeable.

The fact that nature employs soluble complement regulators, notably C1 esterase inhibitor, C4bp and Factor H, is of course partly due to the fact that complement activation can and does occur in the fluid phase but it may well also reflect steric contraints at the membrane surface. Intrinsic regulation at the C1r,s level, for example, would involve having to "reach up" from the membrane to the active sites of the enzymes above or around aggregated immunoglobulin and C1q. Some soluble regulators (notably Factor H) do act in a quasi-intrinsic fashion by binding non-covalently and relatively weakly to components of the outer cell membrane (such as heparans, ref 6). In one sense, this approach captures the best of both worlds and is an argument for using recombinant Factor H or C4bp therapeutically but it requires the maintenance of a high concentration of the relevant protein in plasma and hence is not a viable therapeutic option.

This chapter examines how novel types of IACRs can be designed and how they have been employed as therapeutics both experimentally and latterly in the clinic. The molecular approach employed is not restricted to the complement system and has much wider application.

2. MAKING INTRINSICALLY-ACTING PROTEINS

There are two main mechanisms for anchoring proteins to the membranes of eukaryotic cells. Firstly, additional sequences are added near the N- or C-termini of the polypeptide chain in which highly hydrophobic amino-acids predominate which fold into a helical structure in the presence of a lipid bilayer. One or more of these transmembrane (TM) helices then spans the membrane and anchors the hydrophilic extracellular or cytoplasmic domains in place. The thermodynamic driving force behind such stability derives from the increase in system entropy associated with the "expulsion" of water upon association of the hydrophobic components in the transmembrane helix. In the complement system, CR1 and MCP have single transmembrane helices whereas G-protein coupled receptors with important intracellular signalling functions such as C5aR and C3aR have 7-TM helices which are linked by extracellular or cytoplasmic peptide loops. The second major membrane-anchoring paradigm involves the glycosylphosphatidylinositol (GPI) anchor which is introduced postranslationally by a biosynthetic pathway triggered by a encoded processing signal at the C-terminus of the protein (7). The GPI anchor links a phosphorylethanolamine group to the protein C-terminus and this is followed by a glycan normally comprised of a trimannoside unit and glucosamine and terminated by an inositol phospholipid with generally two or three pendant fatty acyl groups. The latter provide the hydrophobic component for interaction with the lipid bilayer but it is probable that the glycan structure also provides additional features which contribute to the binding energy by interacting with other cellular components (for a review see 8). GPI anchors almost certainly have functions other than simple membrane anchoring and they have been implicated in protein sorting and apical localization (9).

In principle, it is straightforward to engineer TM sequences or GPI anchor signals into soluble proteins and express the products in heterologous hosts. However, bacteria do not have the GPI biosynthetic machinery and refolding of TM-containing proteins from inclusion bodies can be problematic. Retention of the membrane anchored product in the cell membranes of eukaryotic hosts results in the need to extract the protein with detergents and severely limits yields. Thus, although GPI anchored proteins have been prepared in experimental quantities by expression in baculovirus/insect cell systems (10) and in the slime mold *Dictyostelium* (11), neither process yields the gram/L level of production required for economic viability in a therapeutic agent. Even if workable levels of TM or GPI – anchored proteins can be generated, it is usually necessary to handle the products in the presence of detergents, which greatly complicates formulation and toxicological evaluation.

For all of these reasons, it became apparent that if IACRs were to become practical drugs, one approach would be to overexpress complement regulators in soluble forms and then attach a membrane anchor by an efficient post-translational step. Such anchors require the somewhat contradictory properties of good water solubility combined with high membrane affinity and a means of achieving this duality is the main subject of this chapter. An alternative approach to creating therapeutic IACRs is to fuse the complement regulators to other soluble proteins capable of functioning as high-affinity ligands for existing intrinsic membrane proteins. Examples of this targeting approach (such as CD59 – antibody fusions) are discussed elsewhere in this book (see chapter by T.Mollnes) and will not be analysed here. Such approaches generally suffer from the limitations imposed by the level of expression of the targeted membrane proteins and possible deleterious effects of fusion on their function.

3. MYRISTOYL-ELECTROSTATIC SWITCH PEPTIDES AND THE "METTAL" CONCEPT (PRODAPTIN™ TECHNOLOGY)

Certain intracellular proteins, exemplified by myristoylated alanine-rich C-kinase substrate (MARCKS), possess the ability to bind to the inner membrane leaflet of cells in which they are expressed (12). This binding is reversible and has been shown to be controlled by a kinase/phosphatase system which switches the net charge of a region of basic amino acids interspersed with serine (13). The other feature of this type of protein is the presence of a single myristoyl or palmitoyl group located at the C- or N-terminus and introduced by post-translation processing to give either amide bond linkage or linkage via a thiol ester (14). It was shown using deletion mutants (14,15) and with synthetic peptides (16) that the combination of a basic region and a hydrophobic group was critical for mediating binding to the inner membrane leaflet. The contributions to the overall membrane binding energy appeared to be additive and loss of the electrostatic interaction (of basic amino-acid side chains with acidic phospholipid headgroups) through a reduction in net local charge upon phosphorylation left the myristoyl group unable to mediate stable binding on its own. For the purposes of designing synthetic membrane localizing anchors that could be used to derive drug-like IACRs, the reversibility of this switch was not necessary and we realized (17,18) that the concept could be generalized as a molecular array in which a series of thermodynamically independent and additive weak interactions with the membrane were combined. This concept which was originally termed "membrane targeting through additive ligation" (METTAL) can be summarised as generating a series of reagents of the type:

$$(L_1)_n - (L_2)_m - - - (L_i)_x - R$$

Where L is a relatively low-affinity ligand for a one of a set of i contiguous molecular structures on the outer membrane surface and may be present in more than one copy (although n,m,x are not usually not more than 2). The array is terminated by a linker group R (usually a thiol) which permits covalent attachment of the soluble drug or protein. Examples of L include the fatty acyl groups and groups of lysine residues found in the myristoyl electrostatic switch but the range can be extended to other peptide ligands for membrane components such as intrinsic membrane proteins characteristic of particular cell types. The arrays can therefore be thought of as comprising the ligands for cognate membrane addresses or "molecular zip codes" (see below). It is worth noting that GPI anchors themselves can be viewed as belonging to this type of structural array (L_1 being the fatty acyl groups and L_2 the glycan units etc.).

A number of METTAL ligand arrays have been prepared at Adprotech and are known as Prodaptin peptides. One particular member of this set - APT542 - has been extensively applied to modification of proteins (18,19) and is characterised by a very hydrophilic peptide component containing a $(Lys)_6$ motif which more than balances out the hydrophobic contribution of the myristoyl group. Fig. 1 outlines the structure of the APT542 array and its role in the therapeutic agent Mirococept (APT070). This type of reagent is highly water soluble and meets the main requirements of a "GPI-anchor substitute" for localizing cargoes on negatively-charged phospholipid-containing membranes. Prodaptin reagents are made by modified solid-phase peptide synthesis and in most cases, linkage to the cargo is provided by a mixed activated disulfide function which reacts with free thiol groups introduced into proteins by site directed mutagenesis.

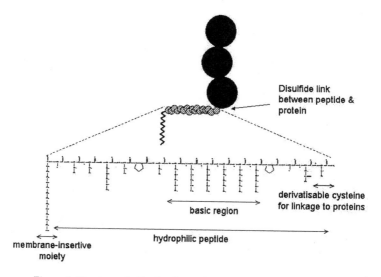

Figure 1. Structure of a Prodaptin peptide and its linkage to SCRs 1-3 of CR1

4.   TARGETING, TETHERING AND PAINTING

METTAL array reagents can be systematically varied using combinatorial chemistry to give a libraries of "tails" whose ability to discriminate between cells and organs *in vivo* can then be screened on an empirical basis. Currently, these libraries are quite diverse and such studies will not be described in detail here. However, it is fair to say that one feature that stands out as a property common to some tails is the co-localization of these materials with GPI anchored proteins in patterns reminiscent of lipid raft distribution (20). This observation may prove to be of considerable interest given the known concentration of receptors in lipid rafts (21). Preliminary studies *in vivo* have suggested that certain of these anchor reagents preferentially localize to certain organs (e.g. the kidney) and to certain tissues. However, the biodistribution patterns observed cannot be equated with the high-specificity targeting that can (sometimes) be achieved with monoclonal antibodies (for a discussion of different types of targeting, see e.g. ref 19). Rather, modification of proteins with these tails tends to retain the cargoes somewhat non-specifically to the vasculature (if administration is intravenous) and to cells in the immediate vicinity of the administration site if local delivery is employed. The function of the anchors is therefore probably better described as membrane tethering than membrane targeting. Duration of tethering varies with the route and site of administration and the nature of the tail but is typically hours to days. Internalization may also occur. Transfer of membrane-bound proteins between cells though direct cell-cell contact rather than dissociation and rebinding is termed "painting". The phenomenon has been well documented with GPI-anchored proteins but not with TM-anchored ones (22) and is thought to be particularly useful in transferring GPI anchored proteins to enucleate cells which do not synthesise them (23) – in other words, transferring IACRs via cell membranes. Further studies are needed to establish whether proteins modified with membrane-localizing tails do undergo painting.

5.   APT 070 (MIROCOCEPT): A NEW THERAPEUTIC COMPLEMENT REGULATOR

APT070 is derived from human CR1 (CD35) which has been extensively investigated in a soluble form (sCR1) as a fluid-phase therapeutic (24) as well as being the target of significant protein engineering efforts (25). Fig. 2 shows its derivation from the N-terminal three short consensus repeats (SCRs) of human CR1 expressed in *E.coli*. Some of the properties of this fragment and its conjugate with APT542 have been described previously

(18,19). SCRs (1-3) of CR1 corresponds to one of the three complement regulatory pharmacophores ("Site I") in CR1 ("Site II" being duplicated at SCRs (8-10) and (15-17) in the CR1 long homologous repeats B and C respectively (24,26). In our hands, SCRs(1-3) possesses significant decay accelerating activity and weak but detectable cofactor I activity against C3b and C4b (27 & unpublished) but these translate to a fluid-phase potency in anti-hemolytic assays which, in molar terms, is much lower (~2%) than that of the full-length soluble sCR1 (27). In view of the multiple complement regulatory sites in sCR1, this was not a surprising result. However, when terminated with an additional cysteine residue and linked to APT542 (see Fig. 1), the fragment becomes very much more potent in *cell-based* assays. For example the 50% inhibitory concentration for inhibition of classical pathway hemolysis in the standard sensitized sheep red blood cell (SRBC) assay decreases from around 20nM for SCRs(1-3) to 0.1 to 0.2 nM for APT070 (27 & unpublished) which is only slightly less potent than full-length sCR1 in the same assay. In fluid-phase complement activation assays, the potencies of APT070 and its unmodified precursor are essentially the same. Thus the membrane-anchoring process has the same effect as multimerisation of the C3b/C4b binding site in sCR1 that is consistent with the "increased effective concentration" mechanism noted in section 1. From a steric perspective however, the high potency of APT070 is remarkable because the location of the complement regulatory site has been brought so much closer to the membrane surface compared with native CR1 (see Fig. 2). Studies with human CD59 and rat CRRY both of which were expressed from bacteria and then tailed with APT542 with major increases in potency (28,29) suggest that convertase/MAC regulation (at least as measured by simple hemolytic assays) can be mediated by localising the relevant units close to the membrane surface and the relatively long "spacers" found in native CR1 and DAF may have other functions.

APT070 has been prepared for clinical evaluation in human disease and this process required development of a number of technologies which can be applied generally to therapeutic IACRs. Firstly, an efficient production process was needed for the precursor protein APT154. This was achieved by high-level expression under the control of the strong T7-RNA polymerase promoter in *E.coli* (30). Recombinant protein was deposited as inclusion bodies (IBs) at very high yields and the IBs then solubilized and refolded at high pH (27,30). Secondly, purification of refolded APT154 was followed by selective reduction of the *exo*-disulfide bond formed between the unpaired C-terminal cysteine and free cysteine from the refolding medium to give a form that could be reacted directly with the Prodaptin peptide APT542. Thirdly, the APT070 product could be prepared in a highly purified form by using purification methods such as hydrophobic interaction chromatography which exploit the fact that the added "tail" significantly alters local charge and hydrophobicity within the protein and acts as an "affinity tag" for purification purposes. APT070 has been formulated as a lyophilized product which real-time stability studies have shown to retain physical integrity and biological activity for more than two years under standard conditions. Overall, these processes have enabled the production of multi-gram batches of APT070 under conditions of current good manufacturing practice (cGMP) and they offer a good prospect that the agent (and similar IACRs) can be produced economically for the marketplace.

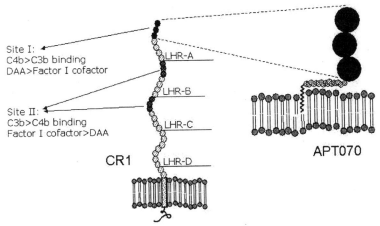

Figure 2. Derivation of APT070 from CR1 and location of Decay Accelerating Activity (DAA) and other functions in CR1

Given the unprecedented nature of APT070, it was a major concern that the safety and biodistribution parameters for such a product should be as well understood as possible before progression to human studies. Single and repeat-dose toxicokinetic studies demonstrated that clearance of APT070 given intravenously in rodents was rapid and biphasic with a terminal t½ around 1 hour and that peak concentrations (Cmax) and exposure (AUC) increased with dose in both rats and primates. APT070 was cleared slightly more slowly than unmodified APT154, an observation which is consistent with a relatively weak and reversible interaction of the tail with serum albumin which can also be demonstrated *in vitro*. Radiolabelled APT070 was distributed throughout the tissues with highest levels present in the kidneys where the agent was retained (in contrast to unmodified APT154 which was excreted in urine).

Formal toxicology studies have demonstrated that APT070 is a very well tolerated molecule when given acutely and subchronically according to standard protocols. As expected for a human protein in foreign species, APT070 was detectably immunogenic in rats but less so in primates and in neither species did the generation of antibodies produce overtly toxic effects or limit repeat dosing. No toxic effects attributable to extreme (or localized) complement inhibition have been observed.

The efficacy of APT070 as a complement regulator *in vivo* was first observed in a model of classical pathway-mediated acute shock induced in rats by intravenous administration of a polyclonal antibody directed against rat vascular tissue (R. Oldroyd et al., unpublished, see ref 31 for model). APT070 given prophylactically protected rats against the lethal effects of the antibody in a dose-responsive manner. Unmodified SCRs (1-3) showed some protective effect but this was much reduced. Subsequently, studies in a rat model of antigen-induced arthritis and rat isograft and allograft transplantation models indicated that APT070 was particularly suited to therapeutic situations where a local effect could be obtained through local administration (32,33). Again, in these models, the unmodified protein was without effect and these and other studies have demonstrated the ability of APT070 to be retained at the site of administration *in vivo*. The studies also form the basis for analogous proof-of-concept studies in human disease (see below). Further applications of APT070 are being explored as experience with this molecule in man has increased. These are generally focussed on acute treatment regimes (as in acute vascular leakage syndromes or cardiopulmonary by-pass) where some proof-of-concept has been provided using other agents and where the specific property of retention in particular tissues may be advantageous.

6.   HUMAN STUDIES

APT070 has been studied in a phase I, randomized, double blind, placebo-controlled, dose escalation study to evaluate safety, tolerability, pharmacokinetics and pharmacodynamics (PK/PD) in healthy male subjects. The objectives of the study were to evaluate the safety and tolerability of ascending, single, intravenous doses of APT070 and to assess the PK/PD characteristics in this study group. There were seven dose levels; from 2 to 100 mg APT070 with 6 subjects participating at each dose level - 4 subjects received active drug and 2 received placebo. The agent was well tolerated at these dose levels. PK analysis showed that the clearance rate decreased with increasing dose and this resulted in an increase in apparent half-life from about 70 mins at the 5 mg dose to around 230 min at 100 mg dose. Assay of active drug using the hemolytic CH50% test showed that only minor (<10%) depression of CH50% occurred at the lower doses (up to 10mg) and CH50% returned to pre-dose levels within 2h. At higher doses, up to ~40% reduction in CH50% was observed but the relationship between peak drug level and change in CH50% was markedly non-linear. In this protocol, CH50% is being reduced by drug carried over into the assay from the serum sample and this suggests that, in contrast to agents that are effectively depleting such as anti-C5 antibodies (34), APT070 has the potential to be used systemically at doses which do not completely disable the complement activation pathways. Only one subject (who received 100mg of APT070) showed any evidence of an antibody response and this was very weak.

A phase II study of the efficacy and safety of intra-articular, dose escalating injections of APT070 on the inflamed knee joint of patients with rheumatoid arthritis is also in progress. This is a multi-center, double blind, randomized, dose escalation study at three doses to be administered via intra-articular injection. 15 patients will be recruited to each dose group, randomized so that 12 patients receive APT070 and 3 patients receive placebo. Only patients receiving either no therapy or those stabilized on NSAID, DMARD and/or oral steroid therapy for at least 1 month are enrolled. The primary objective of this study is to determine whether APT070 has beneficial clinical effects as defined by the degree of improvement in pain at day 14. Secondary endpoints include time to relapse and the effects on APT070 on the changes in the complement system in synovial fluid. At the time of writing, the first cohort of this study has been completed and dose-escalation has been approved following a satisfactory safety profile in this cohort. The second cohort is near completion but this study is still blinded and no conclusions can be drawn about efficacy at this stage.

The third current study with APT070 is a multi-center, placebo controlled, double blind, single escalating dose, dose ranging, safety and efficacy study of the agent in the prevention of post transplantation renal graft dysfunction. The treatment arms are each planned to enrol 15 evaluable patients randomized (ratio 12:3) to APT070 or vehicle control. In this study APT070 is administered as a single dose as an *ex vivo* perfusion to the donor kidney prior to transplant of the organ into the recipient. The primary endpoint is safety in the context of the intensive and complex concomitant medication which transplant patients receive. Other than preliminary safety assessments (which appear to be satisfactory), no data is yet available from this study.

7.   OTHER IACRS

While APT070 is clearly the pathfinder molecule for this approach to therapeutic IACRs, it is not alone. In addition to the use of Prodaptin-modified rodent CRRY and CD59 for use in models of chronic disease (28,29), we have studied the modification of recombinant human DAF and human CD59 both derived by bacterial expression using the same approach of site-specific modification at the C-terminus. These materials are currently under evaluation. The hCD59 derivative makes use of a Prodaptin peptide distinct from APT542 which ensures a markedly altered biodistribution characterized by increased interaction with blood cells that is appropriate for protection of these cells against haemolytic complement challenge. Specifically, one such hCD59 derivative (APT3111) has been designed for replacement therapy in paroxysmal nocturnal hemoglobinuria. Its potency in reactive lysis and other assays is much greater than the precusor soluble hCD59. (S. Ridley et al., unpublished). Work on the bacterial expression of human DAF has yielded a biologically active form consisting of all four SCR domains with a C-terminal cysteine which has been crystallized and a full X-ray structure determined (35). hDAF(1-4)-cys has been modified with APT542 and been shown to bind to cells in a similar fashion to APT070. Like the CR1 fragment and CD59, this modified form of hDAF (APT2334) is much more active in anti-hemolytic assays than the unanchored hDAF(1-4)-cys (J. White et al., unpublished).

8.   CONCLUDING REMARKS

In principle it appears that any complement regulator or active fragment thereof can be modified using the Prodaptin technology and it is likely that the properties of increased potency and ability to be retained in tissues will be common to derivatives of all such proteins. The matching of complement regulator "cargo" and modification to proposed biological function in this way is not without challenges: firstly, the appropriate mechanism of complement regulation must be chosen, secondly the implications of intrinsic function at a disease site must be considered (along with the required duration of action) and thirdly, a means of delivering the material to that site must be found. We consider that the path taken by APT070 from original formulation of the METTAL concept through to the clinic opens a route to the rational design of complement regulatory therapeutics for a wide variety of diseases.

9. REFERENCES

1. Fearon DT. The human C3b receptor . Springer Semin Immunopathol. 1983; 6:159- 72
2. Simpson KL , Holmes CH. Differential expression of complement regulatory proteins decay-accelerating factor (CD55), membrane cofactor protein (CD46) and CD59 during human spermatogenesis. Immunology. 1994; 81: 452-61
3. Zhang F, Crise B, Su B, Hou Y, Rose JK, Bothwell A, Jacobson K. Lateral diffusion of membrane-spanning and glycosylphosphatidylinositol-linked proteins: toward establishing rules governing the lateral mobility of membrane proteins. J Cell Biol. 1991;115:75-84.
4. Lublin DM, Coyne KE. Phospholipid-anchored and transmembrane versions of either decay-accelerating factor or membrane cofactor protein show equal efficiency in protection from complement-mediated cell damage. J Exp Med. 1991;174: 35-44
5. Clissold PM, Ebling HJ, Lachmann PJ. Construction, expression and functional analysis of a glycolipid-linked form of CR1. Eur J Immunol. 1993;23: 2346-52
6. Spycher MO, Nydegger UE. Control of the immune complex-complement interaction by protein H of the alternative complement pathway and the natural inhibitor heparin. Eur J Immunol. 1984;14:276-9.
7. Low MG. Glycosyl-phosphatidylinositol: a versatile anchor for cell surface proteins. FASEB J. 1989;3:1600-8
8. Hwa KY. Glycosyl phosphatidylinositol-linked glycoconjugates: structure, biosynthesis and function. Adv Exp Med Biol. 2001;491:207-14.
9. Soole KL, Jepson MA, Hazlewood GP, Gilbert HJ, Hirst BH. Epithelial sorting of a glycosylphosphatidylinositol-anchored bacterial protein expressed in polarized renal MDCK and intestinal Caco-2 cells. J Cell Sci. 1995;108:369-77.
10. Davies A, Morgan BP. Expression of the glycosylphosphatidylinositol-linked complement-inhibiting protein CD59 antigen in insect cells using a baculovirus vector. Biochem J. 1993;295 :889-96
11. Ti ZC, Gooley AA, Slade MB, Bowers VM, Williams KL Purification of a membrane glycoprotein with an inositol-containing phospholipid anchor from Dictyostelium discoideum. J Biotechnol. 1990;16: 233-43
12. George DJ, Blackshear PJ. Membrane association of the myristoylated alanine-rich C kinase substrate (MARCKS) protein appears to involve myristate-dependent binding in the absence of a myristoyl protein receptor. J Biol Chem. 1992;267 24879-85
13. McLaughlin S, Aderem A. The myristoyl-electrostatic switch: a modulator of reversible protein-membrane interactions. Trends Biochem Sci. 1995;20: 272-6
14. . Hancock JF, Paterson H, Marshall CJ. A polybasic domain or palmitoylation is required in addition to the CAAX motif to localize p21ras to the plasma membrane. Cell. 1990; 63:133-9
15. Hancock JF, Cadwallader K, Paterson H, Marshall CJ. A CAAX or a CAAL motif and a second signal are sufficient for plasma membrane targeting of ras proteins. EMBO J. 1991;10:4033-9
16. Sigal CT, Zhou W, Buser CA, McLaughlin S, Resh MD. Amino-terminal basic residues of Src mediate membrane binding through electrostatic interaction with acidic phospholipids. Proc Natl Acad Sci U S A. 1994;91:12253-7.
17. Smith RA, Dodd I,Mossakowska DE. Conjugates of soluble peptidic compounds with membrane-binding agents. International Patent Publication 1998. No. WO 98/02454
18. Smith GP, Smith RA. Membrane-targeted complement inhibitors. Mol Immunol 2001; 38: 29-255

19. Smith RA. Targeting anticomplement agents. Biochem Soc Transactions. 2002; 30: 1037-1041.

20. Pralle A, Keller P, Florin EL, Simons K, Horber JK. Sphingolipid-cholesterol rafts diffuse as small entities in the plasma membrane of mammalian cells. J Cell Biol. 2000;148:997-1008.

21. Magee T, Pirinen N, Adler J, Pagakis SN, Parmryd I. Lipid rafts: cell surface platforms for T cell signaling. Biol Res. 2002;35:127-31

22. Medof ME, Nagarajan S, Tykocinski ML. Cell-surface engineering with GPI-anchored proteins. FASEB J. 1996 Apr;10(5):574-86

23. Liu T, Li R, Pan T, Liu D, Petersen RB, Wong BS, Gambetti P, Sy MS. Intercellular transfer of the cellular prion protein. J Biol Chem. 2002;277:47671-8

24. Weisman HF, Bartow T, Leppo MK, Marsh HC Jr, Carson GR, Concino MF, Boyle MP, Roux KH, Weisfeldt ML, Fearon DT. Soluble human complement receptor type 1: in vivo inhibitor of complement suppressing post-ischemic myocardial inflammation and necrosis. Science. 1990;249:146-51

25. Mossakowska DE, Smith RA. Complement receptors and their therapeutic applications. in: Recombinant Cell Surface Receptors: Focal Point for Therapeutic Intervention (ed. Browne MJ). 1996.R.G.Landes Company, Austin.

26. Krych M, Hauhart R, Atkinson JP. Structure-function analysis of the active sites of complement receptor type 1. J Biol Chem. 1998;273:8623-9.

27. Mossakowska D, Dodd I, Pindar W, Smith RA. Structure-activity relationships within the N-terminal short consensus repeats (SCR) of human CR1 (C3b/C4b receptor, CD35): SCR 3 plays a critical role in inhibition of the classical and alternative pathways of complement activation. Eur J Immunol. 1999;29:1955-65

28. Fraser DA, Harris CL, Williams AS, Mizuno M, Gallagher S, Smith RA, Morgan BP. Generation of a recombinant, membrane-targeted form of the complement regulator CD59: activity in vitro and in vivo. J Biol Chem. 2003;278:48921-7.

29. Fraser DA, Harris CL, Smith RA, Morgan BP. Bacterial expression and membrane targeting of the rat complement regulator Crry: a new model anticomplement therapeutic. Protein Sci. 2002;11:2512-21.

30. Dodd I, Mossakowska DE, Camilleri P, Haran M, Hensley P, Lawlor EJ, McBay DL, Pindar W, Smith RA. Overexpression in Escherichia coli, folding, purification, and characterization of the first three short consensus repeat modules of human complement receptor type 1. Protein Expr Purif. 1995;6:727-36.

31. de Carvalho IF, de Oliveira HL, Laus-Filho JA, Sarti W. Prevention of acute immunological lung lesion in rats by decomplementing treatment. Immunology. 1969;16:633-41

32. Linton SM, Williams AS, Dodd I, Smith R, Williams BD, Morgan BP.Therapeutic efficacy of a novel membrane-targeted complement regulator in antigen-induced arthritis in the rat. Arthritis Rheum. 2000;43:2590-7

33. Pratt JR, Jones ME, Dong J, Zhou W, Chowdhury P, Smith RA, Sacks SH. Nontransgenic hyperexpression of a complement regulator in donor kidney modulates transplant ischemia/reperfusion damage, acute rejection, and chronic nephropathy. Am J Pathol. 2003;163:1457-65.

34. Wang Y, Rollins SA, Madri JA, Matis LA. Anti-C5 monoclonal antibody therapy prevents collagen-induced arthritis and ameliorates established disease. Proc Natl Acad Sci U S A. 1995;92:8955-9.

35. Lukacik P, Roversi P, White J, Esser D, Smith GP, Billington J, Williams PA, Rudd PM, Wormald MR, Harvey DJ, Crispin MD, Radcliffe CM, Dwek RA, Evans DJ, Morgan BP,

Smith RA, Lea SM. Complement regulation at the molecular level: the structure of decay-accelerating factor.Proc Natl Acad Sci U S A. 2004;101:1279-84.

Index